HENRY OF HUNTINGDON
Anglicanus ortus

Henry, archdeacon of Huntingdon, England (*ca* 1088–*ca* 1154) has been admired for centuries as the author of the monumental *Historia Anglorum*. The recent discovery of the *Anglicanus ortus* opens a new window onto this important English author as well as onto the uses of poetry and the knowledge of medicine in medieval England. Written in Latin verse, the *Anglicanus ortus* describes the medicinal uses of 160 different herbs, spices and vegetables. Henry drew on centuries of learned medicine to compose this work, employing the medical knowledge of ancient authors like Pliny the Elder and Dioscorides and of medieval scholars like Walahfrid Strabo, Macer Floridus and Constantine the African. But this is no ordinary herbal: the work is staged first as a discussion between a master and a student walking around a garden, inspecting the plants in their separate beds, and then as an awkward performance by the same master before Apollo and a critical audience, seated in a theatre at the garden's centre. Beyond its didactic and performative aspects, the entire work is framed as a prayer to God's generative capacity and the rational order of nature. The search for that order is virtuous: as Henry himself says, 'Happy is he who can know the causes of things, especially whatever will be the cause of health.' This critical edition is based on the five extant manuscripts and includes a complete English translation on facing pages and a commentary on every poem. An extensive introduction traces the history and relation of the manuscripts, examines Henry's poetic skill and use of sources, and establishes the place of the *Anglicanus ortus* in a pivotal era in the history of medicine and natural philosophy.

BRITISH WRITERS OF THE MIDDLE AGES
AND THE EARLY MODERN PERIOD 3

Edited by

James P. Carley
York University
Pontifical Institute of Mediaeval Studies

Anne Hudson
University of Oxford

Richard Sharpe
University of Oxford

James Willoughby
University of Oxford

STUDIES AND TEXTS 180

HENRY OF HUNTINGDON

Anglicanus ortus

A Verse Herbal of the Twelfth Century

Edited and translated by

WINSTON BLACK

PIMS

PONTIFICAL INSTITUTE
OF MEDIAEVAL STUDIES

Bodleian Library
UNIVERSITY OF OXFORD

Acknowledgment

We gratefully acknowledge financial support from the Centre for Medieval Studies, University of Toronto in aid of the publication of this volume.

Library and Archives Canada Cataloguing in Publication

Henry, of Huntingdon, 1084?–1155
[Anglicanus ortus. English]
Anglicanus ortus : a verse herbal of the twelfth century / Henry of Huntingdon ; edited and translated by Winston Black.

(Studies and texts, ISSN 0082–5328 ; 180)
(British writers of the Middle Ages and the early modern period ; 3)
Includes bibliographical references and indexes.
Text in Latin with English translations on facing pages.
Co-published by: Bodleian Library.
ISBN 978–0–88844–180–5 (PIMS). – ISBN 978–1–85124–284–9 (Bodleian Library)

1. Herbs – Therapeutic use – Poetry – Early works to 1800. 2. Spices – Therapeutic use – Poetry – Early works to 1800. 3. Materia medica, Vegetable – Poetry – Early works to 1800. 4. Latin poetry, Medieval and modern – England – Translations into English. 5. Henry, of Huntingdon, 1084?–1155. Anglicanus ortus. English. 6. Medicine, Medieval – England. 7. Philosophy of nature – England – Early works to 1800. I. Black, Winston E., 1977– II. Bodleian Library III. Pontifical Institute of Mediaeval Studies IV. Title. V. Anglicanus ortus. English. VI. Series: Studies and texts (Pontifical Institute of Mediaeval Studies) ; 180 VII. Series: British writers of the Middle Ages and the early modern period ; 3

RS177.G7H45 2012 615.3'210942 C2011–905308–X

Published in North America by the Pontifical Institute of Mediaeval Studies, 59 Queen's Park Crescent East, Toronto, Ontario, Canada M5S 2C4 (www.pims.ca).

Published in Europe, including the United Kingdom, by The Bodleian Library, Broad Street, Oxford OX1 3GB (www.bodleianbookshop.co.uk).

For my father,

WALLACE BYRON BLACK (1918–1996),

who showed me the flowers and showed me the weeds.

W.E.B.
Knoxville, Tennessee
October 2011

Contents

Preface

My interest in Henry of Huntingdon predated the discovery of the *Anglicanus ortus* by several years. Both as an historian and as archdeacon of Huntingdon for nearly half a century, Henry played an important role in my doctoral research on the ecclesiastical government of Lincoln diocese. It is Henry's multi-faceted nature (discernible in few twelfth-century clerics) that has kept me coming back to him: he was at once clerical administrator, chronicler, courtier, husband and father, poet, botanist, gardener and gemmologist. I am hardly the first to follow Henry down one of his many paths of interest, and I hope many more will follow thanks to the publication of his verse herbal. I am grateful to many people for their assistance with this edition, but to none more than George Rigg, professor emeritus of the Centre for Medieval Studies, University of Toronto. In a show of generosity rare in academia, George offered me the opportunity in 2003 to make my first attempt at editing using Henry of Huntingdon's herbal, which he had recently discovered. A relatively small extracurricular assignment blossomed into a complete edition, fertilized by my discovery in 2005 of Henry's verse lapidary and staked up with more manuscripts of the herbal. All along, he has provided encouragement, insight and friendship. Thank you!

My discovery of three manuscript witnesses to the herbal is due in part to Frank Klaassen of the University of Saskatchewan, who hired me in 2003 to examine hundreds of manuscript catalogues in a search for medieval magical texts, as part of his project 'The Intellectual and Social History of Learned Magic 1300–1600,' funded by the Social Sciences and Humanities Research Council of Canada. In the process I was also able to familiarize myself with medical manuscript collections throughout the world, since herbs and spells often grew from the same bed in later medieval manuscripts. This project took on greater importance after I received encouragement from Diana Greenway; her edition of and excellent introduction to the *Historia Anglorum* are partly responsible for my fascination with Henry of Huntingdon and all things archidiaconal. Thanks are also due to Jonathan Black and Fred Unwalla of the Pontifical Institute of Mediaeval Studies, as well as to Fr James Farge, Bill Edwards and the late Caroline Suma of the Pontifical Institute of Mediaeval Studies Library. Jean Hoff and Megan Jones each provided keen eyes, cogent criticisms and kind words to improve my work. Michael Winterbottom helped vicariously through his conversations with George Rigg. Ruth Harvey, Fr Édouard Jeauneau, John Magee, James Carley, Richard Sharpe, Monica Green, Anne Van Arsdall, Florence Eliza Glaze, Grace Desa, Joseph Goering, Nicholas Everett, Jeannette Beer, Susan Crane, and Andrew Hicks all gave advice and encouragement. My mother, Jean Blashfield Black, offered the support only a mother can give, as well as the corrections only a professional editor can give. Most of all, I owe my thanks to my wife Dr Emily Reiner and to our own sprout Gabriel Alexander Black for their support, patience and love.

Introduction

The impulse to compose thousands of lines of verse on the medicinal attributes of plants both native and exotic is, perhaps, foreign to modern tastes. Indeed, the very notion of medical verse seems antithetical to the goals of both medicine and poetry as we now understand them. Yet this impulse was not uncommon in the Middle Ages, and in the ninth through thirteenth centuries there were many medical and botanical texts written in Latin verse, part of the larger genre of Latin didactic poetry.[1] The practice of putting technical information into verse served primarily as a mnemonic device: a poem is easier to recall than a prose treatise. This may be true of the verse herbal edited here, but as will become clear below, Henry of Huntingdon may have also composed his verses to entertain and for the sheer enjoyment of composition.

Henry of Huntingdon's verse herbal, which one scribe titled *Anglicanus ortus*, should be seen as one of the crowning achievements of medieval medical poetry and a key work in the spread north of the Alps of Salernitan medicine based on Greek and Arabic sources. The *Anglicanus ortus* is a large and ambitious work, treating (in its current form) 160 different medicinal herbs and spices in the context of 169 separate poems arranged into six books. This herbal is unique in the presentation of its information: names and attributes of plants are related by a narrator, at times arrogant or reluctant, to a student who occasionally poses or answers questions, against the background of an elaborate square garden and a theatre peopled with a demanding Greek god, an irate cook, a lecherous old man, and a flamboyant gem-wielding king.[2]

1 The didactic poem (*Lehrgedicht*) has been studied more thoroughly by German scholars than English. See Bernd Effe, *Dichtung und Lehre: Untersuchungen zur Typologie des antiken Lehrgedichts* (Munich 1977) for didactic Latin poetry of antiquity (pp. 194–204 for medical poetry) and Thomas Haye, *Das lateinische Lehrgedicht im Mittelalter. Analyse einer Gattung*, Mittellateinische Studien und Texte 22 (Leiden 1997) for medieval didactic poetry in Latin and the vernacular.

2 These characters are met in the prologues to Books 1 and 5, in poems 5.2.1–6, and in the interludes to Books 5 and 6 of the present work, as well as in poems 1 and 8 of Henry's lapidary *De gemmis preciosis*, published in Winston Black, 'Henry of Huntingdon's lapidary rediscovered and his *Anglicanus ortus* reassembled,' *Mediaeval Studies* 68 (2006), 43–87. See section 2.2 on 'Structure' below.

Henry's flair for verse, eagerness to include new sources of medical information, natural curiosity tempered with scepticism, and sense of humour all add shape and colour to the often drab field of medieval herbal medicine. Those already familiar with Henry of Huntingdon will find that the *Anglicanus ortus* adds a new facet to an already fascinating medieval author, and those familiar with the field of medieval medicine will find in Henry's herbal one of the most creative mixtures of old and new medical material from the start of a new era of rational medical theory.

Henry lived between the later eleventh and mid-twelfth centuries and thus wrote his herbal during a pivotal era in the history of medicine.[3] For the first time in centuries, formal medical theory, based in part on the writings of Galen and Aristotle, often through Arabic intermediaries, was being taught, first in southern Italy around Salerno and not long after in cathedral schools north of the Alps.[4] At the same time, older Latin medical works were being re-edited, carefully pruned, and rationally organized.[5] New translations and

3 The study of the 'renaissance médicale' (to borrow Danielle Jacquart's phrase) in both theory and practice during the long twelfth century has experienced a great deal of interest in the last quarter century, led especially by the studies of Jacquart, Monica Green, Faith Wallis, Michael McVaugh, Mark Jordan and Luis García-Ballester, to name just a few of the more prominent historians. Introductions to the topic include Danielle Jacquart, 'À l'aube de la renaissance médicale des XIe–XIIe siècles: L'*Isagoge Johannitii* et son traducteur,' *Bibliothèque de l'École des Chartes* 144 (1986), 209–40, and Mark D. Jordan, 'The construction of a philosophical medicine: Exegesis and argument in Salernitan teaching on the soul,' *Osiris*, 2nd series, 6 (1990), 42–61.

4 The foundational work on Salerno and the formal teaching of medicine practiced there is still Paul Oskar Kristeller, 'The school of Salerno: Its development and its contribution to the history of learning,' *Bulletin of the History of Medicine* 17 (1945), 138–94. The only accessible collection of Salernitan medical texts, while replete with inaccuracies, is Salvatore de Renzi's monumental *Collectio Salernitana*, 5 vols (Naples 1852–9; repr. Bologna 1967). Scholars have begun to reassess the utility of this collection and question the actual composition and distribution of the texts which de Renzi gathered, with perhaps too generous an embrace, for his collection. See *La* Collectio Salernitana *di Salvatore De Renzi*, ed. Danielle Jacquart and Agostino Paravicini Bagliani (Florence 2008), particularly the essay by Monica Green, 'Rethinking the manuscript basis of Salvatore de Renzi's *Collectio Salernitana*: The corpus of medical writings in the "long" twelfth century,' 15–60. On the early use of the Salernitan *Articella* collection at Chartres, see Jordan, 'The construction of a philosophical medicine.'

5 Most important in the eleventh century was the medical compilation of Gariopontus called the *Passionarius*, which has only recently begun to receive scholarly attention. See Florence Eliza Glaze, 'Gariopontus and the Salernitans: Textual traditions in the eleventh and twelfth centuries,' in *La* Collectio Salernitana *di Salvatore De Renzi*, ed. Jacquart and Paravicini Bagliani, 149–90. Glaze is currently working on an edition of the *Passionarius*. I thank Dr Glaze for sharing her work with me.

adaptations were made from Arabic and Greek medical texts, most notably by Constantine the African, a monk at Monte Cassino whose work Henry used. The process by which these new medical works, now collectively known as 'Salernitan,' were carried to northern Europe and England is still unclear, but within only a few decades of Constantine's death and Henry's birth (both perhaps in the 1080s) a wide variety of medical texts both new and old could be found in the libraries of northern religious houses and cathedrals.[6] In fact, English scholars seem to have been especially eager for the new Salernitan medical literature, so much so, in fact, that the question is not how did Salernitan texts reach England, but rather why did so many?[7]

The *Anglicanus ortus* is a product of these trends in academic medicine, both as a new reading (like the herbal of Macer Floridus) of older Latin texts and as a popularization of the newer Salernitan works. Yet the *Anglicanus ortus* should be understood not only in the light of medieval medicine, but also as part of the rebirth of classical verse for which the long twelfth century is justly famous.[8] Henry is a masterful poet, calling on the usual suspects (Virgil, Ovid, Horace, *etc.*), and casting himself as a new Martial by caustically remarking on his society and its medical customs in witty epigrams, or as a Statius reborn by bestowing an epic and heroic sweep on contemporary events or even on the curative properties of herbs. Like his older contemporaries (and also erstwhile archdeacons) Hildebert of Lavardin and Marbode of Rennes, Henry applied his poetic skill in several arenas: love lyrics, satire, moral verse, political commentary, epitaphs, and medical verse.[9] There is no doubt that Henry had a keen interest in medicine and the latest pharmacology, but unlike many medical authors, he was just as interested in practicing and presenting technical information with properly-scanned verse, the best classical allusions, and the cleverest turns of phrase. It is not as a *medicus* or *physicus* that Henry identifies himself, but as a *uates paupercule* (poem 5.2.6, line 4). Thus it is more a

6 Monica Green has supplied a table of twelfth-century manuscripts of Salernitan texts with Norman and English provenance in 'Rethinking the manuscript basis of Salvatore de Renzi's *Collectio Salernitana*,' 54–60.

7 On this phenomenon, see also Monica Green, 'Salerno on the Thames: The genesis of Anglo-Norman medical literature,' in *Language and Culture in Medieval Britain: The French of England, c.1100–c.1500*, ed. Jocelyn Wogan-Browne, with Carolyn Collette, Maryanne Kowaleski, Linne Mooney, Ad Putter, and David Trotter (Woodbridge 2009), 220–31. I am grateful to Dr Green for her personal correspondence on this issue, which she continues to pursue.

8 Janet Martin, 'Classicism and style in Latin literature,' in *Renaissance and Renewal in the Twelfth Century*, ed. Robert L. Benson and Giles Constable, with Carol D. Lanham (Cambridge, MA 1982; repr. Toronto 1991), 537–68.

9 Marbode's verse lapidary *De lapidibus* was the primary source for Henry's own verse lapidary *De gemmis preciosis*: see Black, 'Henry of Huntingdon's lapidary.'

self-deprecating poet and curious clerical administrator whom we will follow around the *Anglicanus ortus* than a rational physician of the new, Salernitan mode.

1. HENRY, ARCHDEACON OF HUNTINGDON[10]

1.1 *Biography*

Until recently, Henry of Huntingdon's only extant work was the *Historia Anglorum*, and thanks to it he has enjoyed centuries of well-deserved fame, not so much as a poet or archdeacon but as an historian. The *Historia Anglorum* was an influential work in Henry's own day, popular through the rest of the Middle Ages, and it remains a key witness to the social and political upheavals of Anglo-Norman England, particularly the 'Anarchy' of the 1140s. Many of the poems in the historical books of the *Historia Anglorum* are believed to have been written by Henry and show that he was a poet of no small skill,[11] but the discovery of the *Anglicanus ortus* now places Henry in the front ranks of Anglo-Latin poets. His now larger literary corpus shows the scope of erudition possessed by an ambitious medieval cleric educated in the liberal arts and philosophy before the rise of the universities.

Most of what we know about Henry must be gleaned from his *Historia Anglorum*, from a handful of charters he drafted or witnessed which still survive, and from a few passages in the *Anglicanus ortus*. He was born around the year 1088, possibly in the village of Little Stukeley outside of the town of Huntingdon, a cousin of the powerful Glanville family. He was therefore related to another archdeacon (of Lisieux), William de Glanville (died by 1113), and was likely an ancestor of Ranulf de Glanville (died by 1190), Henry II's chief justiciar. While descended from Norman nobility on his father's side, his mother was probably a native English woman and from her he learned to read English as well as French and Latin, a rare talent for a high-ranking Anglo-Norman cleric.

He was groomed from an early age for a career in the church: son of Nicholas, archdeacon of Huntingdon (an office with jurisdiction over the counties of Huntingdonshire, Cambridgeshire, and part of Hertfordshire), raised in the household of Robert Bloet, bishop of Lincoln (r. 1094–1123),

10 Most of the information provided here on Henry's life comes from the excellent introduction to Henry, Archdeacon of Huntingdon, *Historia Anglorum: The History of the English People*, ed. and trans. Diana Greenway (Oxford 1996), hereafter cited as *HA*.

11 A. G. Rigg describes what was known of Henry's poetry before the discovery of the *Anglicanus ortus* in 'Henry of Huntingdon's metrical experiments,' *Journal of Medieval Latin* 1 (1991), 60–72.

and educated in Laon with several other clerics who were destined to become archdeacons and bishops. While there he studied under the great exegete Anselm of Laon (d. 1117), as described in poem 1.12 on germander, where he perhaps crossed paths with Adelard of Bath (*ca* 1080–*ca* 1152).[12] It could have been in Laon that Henry was first introduced to natural philosophy in the form of native Latin works like the herbal of Macer Floridus or Greek and Arabic medical treatises translated or adapted by Constantine the African.

His father Nicholas died in 1110, soon after the lands of Cambridgeshire were removed from the archdeaconry for the creation of the new diocese of Ely, and Henry, aged about 22, succeeded his father as archdeacon over the now smaller archdeaconry of Huntingdon. For nearly half a century Henry was one of the eight archdeacons of the diocese of Lincoln, the largest in England and one of the largest in northern Europe. A member of the clerical elite, possessing a rich office with pastoral and legal responsibilities, he acted as an ecclesiastical judge on behalf of the bishop of Lincoln and had oversight of all the secular clergy within his archdeaconry (though the extensive lands of the abbey of St Albans were exempt from Henry's jurisdiction). Some of his charters survive; these show him monitoring clerical incomes and settling disputes over tithes and parish boundaries. He was also a teacher, running a song school in Huntingdon, which he was forced to give up to the canons of St Mary's of Huntingdon, who were able to claim a monopoly on education in the town.

He was apparently a happily married man and fathered at least one child,[13] though by the end of his life, clerical marriage and the direct inheritance of church offices would be seriously frowned upon, and eventually forbidden in canon law to clerics of his rank. He continued to hold the estate of Little Stukeley from Ramsey Abbey, which he passed on to his son Adam; it was kept in the family until 1231. This was probably his home, where his wife and son (and perhaps other children) lived, but he also held one or two other parcels of land. In the single reference to himself in the monumental *Historia Anglorum*, he gently mocks his wealth. With some allowance for poetic hyperbole, this passage is still a good indication of the quality of his manor: 'Your verses, bard Henry, are elegant, elegant your house, elegant your estate. Elegant your bedroom, elegant your orchards; look, your garden gleams with

12 Adelard mentions his time spent in Laon at the start of his *Quaestiones naturales* (Adelard of Bath, *Conversations with His Nephew*, ed. and trans. Charles Burnett [Cambridge 1998], 90–91), in which he gives a nuanced discussion of plants and their elemental qualities which may have influenced Henry's *Anglicanus ortus*.

13 See Nancy Partner, 'Henry of Huntingdon: Clerical celibacy and the writing of history,' *Church History* 42 (1973), 467–75, and *HA* xxvii–xxviii.

hundred-fold elegances'.[14] So he was a cleric of no small means, as befitting an archdeacon who was expected to travel frequently and entertain important guests.

Most archdeacons, in service to their bishops, were expected to have a significant level of literacy and some legal expertise. Henry's extensive education, both broad and deep, is obvious from his extant works. His son and grandson both bore the title *magister*, indicative of higher education (though not yet earning formal degrees), and his grandson was even named Aristotle, clearly a member of a family that appreciated learning. Henry's position often kept him at the side of the three bishops whom he served on journeys, at church councils, and at the cathedral in Lincoln. He even made a trip to Rome in 1139 with Theobald, archbishop of Canterbury, as a representative of Alexander 'the Magnificent', bishop of Lincoln from 1123 to 1148.[15] An archdeacon was also a canon of his cathedral, so Henry was expected to be present occasionally in chapter to sing his part of the Psalter (Psalm 77 in his case), bear witness to important charters, and participate in cathedral government.

Since bishops wielded not only ecclesiastical, but also political, authority, Henry was present at some state gatherings, often in the entourage of King Henry I (r. 1100–1135). He found himself in such company both as a high-ranking cleric and as an author of note. In poem 1.2 on basil Henry explains that he wrote a funeral oration for Queen Matilda, who died in 1118, which (if we can assume it was delivered at her funeral) is indicative of his high standing as a courtier and friend of the royal family from a relatively young age.[16] Henry grew old and at least locally famous in his office. Around 1154, a continuator of the *Liber Eliensis*, a witness for both Henry and his father's continuing importance in the new diocese of Ely, called Henry 'a most learned man of letters, venerable for his age and white hair'.[17] His last datable appearance comes in 1156, but he may have lived as late as 1164, in which year he was replaced by Nicholas de Sigillo as archdeacon of Huntingdon.[18]

14 *HA* 590–91. It is tempting to see the garden 'with hundred-fold elegances' as a veiled reference to the one hundred plants in Books 1–4 of the herbal, but it is probably mere coincidence.

15 Alexander was Henry's classmate in Laon and commissioned the *Historia Anglorum*.

16 The oration is found in *HA* 462–3.

17 'Unde quidam litterarum peritissimus senio atque canitie venerandus attestari perhibetur'. *Liber Eliensis*, ed. E. O. Blake, Camden Third Series 92 (London 1962), 125. This passage is in the second book of the *Liber Eliensis*, which the editor dates after 1154 (xlviii), so Henry would have been about sixty-six years old when this passage was written.

18 John Le Neve, *Fasti Ecclesiae Anglicanae, 1066–1300*, vol. 3: *Lincoln*, ed. Diana Greenway (London 1977), 26–30.

1.2 *Works*

Henry is believed to have penned numerous works, but until recently only the *Historia Anglorum* was known to survive. It is not necessary to review here the justifiably famous *Historia*, which has received accolades for centuries as a groundbreaking work of English history and, more recently, as a finely crafted piece of narrative, rhetoric, and propaganda.[19] Some of his other compositions, most of which remain lost, were youthful exercises in verse that he shared with his fellow archdeacon of Lincoln diocese, Walter of Leicester. Henry appended to one recension of his *Historia* a letter to Walter, titled *De contemptu mundi* ('On contempt for the world'), in which he outlines some of these works: 'In the joyful prime of our lives, I wrote for you a book of epigrammatic verse, and I also composed a poem on Love, which was worthy of your acceptance.' By the end of the letter we learn that Walter has died, and in his final funeral lament Henry addresses again the works he wrote for Walter: 'I, Henry, who bear garlands to you, first brought epigrams, next the contests of love, and then medicinal herbs.'[20]

The existence and scope of these works is confirmed by the sixteenth-century historian and bibliophile John Leland, who records that Henry wrote, apart from the *Historia Anglorum*, a variety of poems: eight books of epigrams, eight books on love, and eight books on herbs, spices, and gems (apparently united by a medical theme).[21] He may also have composed prose

19 Among the authors (apart from Greenway) who have studied the *HA* for its style, and not just for its historical content, see Nancy Partner, *Serious Entertainments: The Writing of History in Twelfth-Century England* (Chicago 1977), and Monika Otter, '*Prolixitas temporum*: Futurity in medieval history narratives,' in *Reading Medieval Culture: Essays in Honor of Robert W. Hanning*, ed. Robert Stein and Sandra Prior (Notre Dame, IN 2005), 45–67.

20 *HA* 618–19: 'Henricus tibi serta gerens, epigramata primum, / Prelia mox Veneris, gramina deinde tuli.'

21 'In epigrammatis et lusibus amatoriis aliquid memoria dignum praestitit. At non perinde se artificem probauit, secutus nescio quem recentiorem Macrum, in libro suo de herbis, cui subiecit et alios duos libellos, unum [[si recte memini]] de aromatibus, alterum de gemmis, in neutro assecutus gratiam quam ego optarem, illis tamen forsan temporibus, tanquam doctos et utileis multorum manibus assidue uersatos. . . . Sequitur index librorum qui ab illo scripti adhuc extant:

Epigrammaton libri octo
De amore libri octo
De herbis }
De aromatibus } libri octo,
De gemmis }

quibus et adiunxit compendiolum de ponderibus et mensuris.' John Leland, *De uiris illustribus / On Famous Men*, ed. and trans. James P. Carley, with the assistance of Caro-religious works, befitting a well-educated cleric, titled *De lege Domini* and *Super 'Beati immaculati'*.[22] Of his poetic works, the eight medical books and two books of epigrams survive. From a passage in the *De uiris illustribus*, we can see that Leland enjoyed Henry's epigrams and love poetry but had little time for the medical verse, for Henry 'did not prove himself a master to the same extent . . . in his book *On Herbs*.'[23] I would certainly disagree about Henry's lack of artistry in the herbal, but the loss of the books on love is a great one indeed. Perhaps Henry was ashamed of his youthful endeavours into frivolous topics and did not plan to share these poems with anyone but his close friend Walter of Leicester. Of the epigrams, only the last two books survive; he refers to the first six books as 'pleasant' (*iocunda . . . epigrammata*) and the final two as 'serious' (*seria*).[24] The serious nature of those books probably helped in their survival, for he republished them as books 11 and 12 of the *Historia Anglorum* as a moral, poetic epilogue.[25] The addition of the *Anglicanus ortus* to the *epigrammata seria* and occasional poems of the *Historia* confirms that Henry 'was much more than merely competent' as a Latin poet.[26] Were all of his lost works to survive, Henry would be considered first and foremost a poet (as he considered himself), who also wrote a history of the English.

2. THE *ANGLICANVS ORTVS*

Henry of Huntingdon's *Anglicanus ortus* is a verse compendium in eight books treating the medicinal properties and applications of herbs, spices, vegetables, gems, and stones, illustrated with classical allusions, Christian symbolism, and occasional historical or autobiographical digressions. This

line Brett, Studies and Texts 172, British Writers of the Middle Ages and the Early Modern Period 1 (Toronto and Oxford 2010), 334–6. He also quotes lines 11–14 from the Prologue to Book 1, which are discussed below in the commentary on that poem. Leland also recorded a manuscript of 'Henricus Huntindunensis de herbarum virtute carmine' at a hermitage called 'Coenobium S. Benedicti apud Fennicolas': *Joannis Lelandi antiquarii De rebus Britannicis collectanea*, ed. T. Hearne, 2nd ed., 6 vols (London 1770), 4. 29. See also Wolfgang Maaz, *Lateinische Epigrammatik im hohen Mittelalter. Literarhistorische Untersuchungen zur Martial-Rezeption* (Hildesheim 1992), 106–107, on this passage.

22 See *HA* cxii–cxvii for Greenway's discussion of the lost works.

23 John Leland, *De uiris illustribus*, trans. Carley, 335.

24 *HA* 804–805.

25 *HA* cxii–cxiv, 778–825. The second of the two books of *epigrammata seria* was also edited, with commentary, by Maaz, *Lateinische Epigrammatik im hohen Mittelalter*, 148–74.

26 *HA* cx.

compendium so described, however, has not been found in its entirety. Its existence as a work of poetry in eight books is attested only by John Leland's description discussed above, and the work has long been assumed to be lost.[27] Its structure, contents, and the identity of its author have been pieced together by a series of scholars over the last two decades. In 1987 John Harvey wrote about 'The square garden of Henry the poet,' based on the prose lists of herbs in a fourteenth-century medical miscellany in the British Library (Sloane 3468, hereafter *S*, fols. 32r–34v), but rejected the attribution of the herbal to Henry of Huntingdon.[28] A decade later Bernd Ruppel argued convincingly that the four books of poems in *S* (fols. 31r–105v) were indeed the work of the author of the *Historia Anglorum*.[29] This identification was confirmed by A. G. Rigg's discovery of six books *de herbis* in Prague, Knihovna metropolitní kapituly, M. VI 1359, fols. 1r–47v (hereafter *P*).[30] I subsequently discovered the lapidary *De gemmis preciosis* of books 7 and 8, which treat gems and stones, respectively, and endeavoured to reconstruct the eight books of the *Anglicanus ortus*. Books 7 and 8 are not included in this edition

27 That Henry intended the work to contain eight books is also supported by his statement in Book 12 of the *Historia Anglorum* (804–805, ed. and trans. Greenway): 'Since the number eight signifies lasting blessedness, it is only right that our works should be finished in that which we ourselves have finished.' ('Cum octonarius perpetuitatem beatitudinis significet, dignum est ut in eo opera nostra finiantur in quo et ipsi finiamur.')

28 John Harvey, 'The square garden of Henry the Poet,' *Garden History* 15 (1987), 1–11. This manuscript has been remarked on by several other historians as an interesting compilation of several herbals: Loren MacKinney, 'Medieval medical dictionaries and glossaries,' in *Medieval and Historiographical Essays in Honor of James Westfall Thompson*, ed. James Lea Cate and Eugene N. Anderson (Chicago 1938), 240–68, at 250 n24; Lynn Thorndike, *A History of Magic and Experimental Science*, 8 vols (New York 1923–58), 2. 438–9, 447–8; George R. Keiser, 'Reconstructing Robert Thornton's herbal' *Medium Ævum* 65 (1996), 35–53, at 52 n9.

29 Bernd Ruppel, 'Heinrichs von Huntingdon verschollenes Gedicht "De herbis",' *Mittellateinisches Jahrbuch* 32/2 (1997), 211; Ruppel, 'Ein verschollenes Gedicht des 12. Jahrhunderts: Heinrichs von Huntingdon "De herbis",' *Frühmittelalterliche Studien* 31 (1997), 197–213. The herbal in four books, as described by Ruppel, is also mentioned by Bernhard Schnell and William Crossgrove in Macer Floridus, *Der deutsche 'Macer.' Vulgatfassung mit einem Abdruck des lateinischen Macer Floridus 'De viribus herbarum'*, ed. B. Schnell with W. Crossgrove (Tübingen 2003), 33–4.

30 A. G. Rigg, 'Henry of Huntingdon's herbal,' *Mediaeval Studies* 65 (2003), 213–92; this also contains the prose lists in the Sloane manuscript used by Harvey in his 1987 article (Rigg, 'Henry of Huntingdon's herbal,' 288–92). See also Diana Greenway, 'Henry of Huntingdon as poet: The *De herbis* rediscovered,' *Medium Ævum* 74 (2005), 329–32.

of the *Anglicanus ortus*, as they do not survive in a good copy and have been printed elsewhere.[31]

2.1 *Authorship and Dating*

Several pieces of evidence point definitively to Henry of Huntingdon's authorship of these poems. Almost all of the poems shared by *P* and *S* are attributed to 'Henricus' or 'Henricus poeta' in their titles or in the margin and the author is addressed as 'Henrice' by the muse Erato in poem 2.10, line 41. In poem 1.5 on baldmoney the writer says that England made him into a poet (line 2, 'me reddidit Anglia uatem'). We are thus dealing with an English poet named Henry. This poet also tells us that he wrote funeral verses for Matilda, wife of King Henry I,[32] and the same king is addressed in Epilogue 2 to Book 4 (line 3), so our Henry was active between 1118 and 1135 (the deaths of Matilda and the king, respectively). He also says that Clio, muse of history, has crowned him with garlands (2 Prologue, lines 1–6), a statement in accord with Henry of Huntingdon's activity as an historian.

This poet describes his earlier works in the Prologues to Book 1, lines 1–2, and Book 5, lines 8–9, in a fashion almost identical to Henry's references to his earlier works in the *De contemptu mundi*:

> Henricus tibi serta gerens, epigramata primum,
> Prelia mox Veneris, gramina deinde tuli.
> (*HA* 618)

> Qui teneris ludens pueris epigramata scripsi,
> Quique canens iuueni seria scripta dedi,
> (1 Prologue, lines 1–2)

31 The poems on gems and stones are found in only one corrupt and incomplete manuscript, Oxford, Bodleian Library, MS Digby 69, fols. 192v–195r. I have edited its thirty-five lapidary poems in the journal *Mediaeval Studies* (Black, 'Henry of Huntingdon's lapidary'), where I argue that Henry wrote a total of forty poems in the lapidary which made up books 7 and 8 of the *Anglicanus ortus*. There are two other witnesses to the *Anglicanus ortus*: the oldest, Oxford, Bodleian Library, MS Digby 13, fols. 89v, 91r–92v, a twelfth-century prose redaction of fifty-one poems from books 1–4, has long been ascribed to Henry of Huntingdon; the fifteenth-century compilation of herbals in Cambridge, Trinity College, MS O. 9. 10 (James 1422), fols. 89r–108r, contains excerpts from poems in books 1–6. For a full description of the manuscripts see section 3, 'The Edition', below.

32 Poem 1.2, lines 4–5. As noted above, Henry of Huntingdon wrote an oration for the funeral of Queen Matilda (*HA* 462–3).

Cui, ludens Veneremque fugans et gramina plantans,
Ter nitui, . . .
(5 Prologue, lines 8–9)

Finally, verses in the prologue of Henry's *Historia Anglorum* are so similar to two passages in the herbal as to suggest either the same author or direct imitation:

Principium rerum, uegetatio, finis earum,
Hoc opus aspira, deduc finique precamur.
(*HA* 6)

Principium rerum, generacio, finis earum
hoc opus aspiret, deducat terminum, oro.
(Prose Prologue, 1–2)

Principium rerum, uegetacio, finis earum,
(5 Prologue, line 7)

All of this evidence, combined with many stylistic similarities between the herbal and the poetry in the *Historia Anglorum*, points decisively to Henry of Huntingdon's authorship of the *Anglicanus ortus*.

We do not know what Henry called his collection of medical poems. Leland described it as eight books covering three topics, 'De herbis, De aromatibus, De gemmis.'[33] Ruppel uses the name *De herbis* for the four-book herbal in *S* and Greenway uses the same name for the six-book herbal described by Rigg. But since Henry's lapidary poems (discovered after Ruppel and Greenway were writing) probably make up the two remaining books, that means Leland's *De aromatibus* is not a lost work but rather is Book 6 of the herbal already outlined by Rigg, which primarily treats exotic spices of the East. Therefore I think it is wise to read Leland's description not as a list of titles, but merely as an indication of what the work in eight books contains.

The only clue to the title found in the work itself is in the very last line of the herbal: 'Find the title of this work in the first entry of the first book.'[34] Herbals, like other medieval works, could be identified by their incipits (as in the twelfth-century pharmacological handbook *Circa instans*) or named after their first ingredients (like Henry Daniel's fourteenth-century work *Aaron*, discussed below). In the case of the present work, *Arthemisia* is the first herbal poem of the first book, and thus could be taken as a title, or perhaps *Mater*

33 See note 21 above.

34 6 Epilogue, line 6, 'In primo primi titulum deprendito libri.'

herbarum ('mother of herbs'), a common epithet for artemisia that is given in the first poem (on mugwort, a type of artemisia). Other possibilities are *Principium rerum*, from the opening couplet to the work's Prose Prologue, or *Flores*, a key word in the Prologue to Book 1 (line 14),[35] although the latter would be an unlikely title for a work which is dedicated not to flowers but to herbs and spices, and in which the differences between *flos*, *herba*, and *species* are usually made clear. The name *Anglicanus ortus* (*The English Garden*) is given by the scribe of *P*, the most complete manuscript, to the herbal in six books that he copied.[36] Henry probably never intended this title—it is a name that only someone outside England would give the work—but as it suggests both the provenance and subject of the work it seems a fitting one.

Henry composed the *Anglicanus ortus* in several stages, a fact apparent from the structure and organization of the books. Of the eight books on herbs, aromatics, and gems described by Leland, books 1–4, describing a hundred herbs, were written first and later seen as a single unit: in Epilogue 1 to Book 4, Henry refers to the 'hundred herbs' (*gramina centum*, line 1) and in the Book 5 Interlude, line 3, he makes another reference to the previous 'hundred.' These books were likely planned and written between 1118 and 1135. The former date is the death of Matilda, whose funeral is mentioned in poem 1.2, lines 4–5. The latter is the death of Henry I, addressed in the Epilogue 2 to Book 4, line 3. A narrower date range may be suggested in the Prologue to Book 2, where Henry says that Clio, goddess of history, has already bestowed garlands on him. Rigg has taken this to mean that Henry had already written his *Historia Anglorum*, which appeared in its first form in 1129.[37] If that is true, then we can significantly narrow the date range of books 1–4 to 1129x1135. As Diana Greenway has stressed, however, Henry had a tendency to revise his works.[38] It is possible, even likely, that Henry wrote the several prologues and epilogues after he wrote many of the individual herbal poems, as he crafted an ever more elaborate structure for the entire work. Therefore, the reference in Epilogue 2 to Book 4 to King Henry returning from wars in Normandy only provides a *terminus post quem* of 1124 for that particular poem and not for the entire work.[39]

The final four books were clearly written later. In Book 6 he treats the one hundred herbs of Books 1–4 as a distinct work, referring the reader to 'that

35 Suggested by Rigg, 'Henry of Huntingdon's herbal,' 288.

36 Following the two epilogues after Book 4, the scribe of *P* added 'Sequitur quintus liber Anglicani orti' (fol. 32r). The verso of the flyleaf reads 'Macer orti anglici' as does the title of an index of herbs compiled by the scribe of *P* at the top of fol. 48r.

37 Rigg, 'Henry of Huntingdon's herbal,' 262; *HA* lxvi–lxvii.

38 Greenway, 'Henry of Huntingdon as poet,' 330–31.

39 See the commentary on Book 4, Epilogue 2, for more on this reference.

book which contains one hundred herbs' (6.1.12, 38, 'ille liber qui centum continet herbas'). Books 5 and 6 were designed to continue the herbal, adding more herbs, vegetables, and eastern spices, while Books 7 and 8 treat gems and stones. These later books could have been written any time from the mid-1130s to the mid-1150s. Greenway (writing before the lapidary was discovered) suggested that Books 5 and 6 were written in the 1140s or even the early 1150s.[40] This is likely, and those dates probably also hold true for Books 7 and 8.

The pattern of the work's survival in the manuscripts also confirms the separate composition of the first and final four books. The alphabetical herbal in *S* and the prose redaction in Oxford, Bodleian Library, MS Digby 13 (hereafter *O*) are both based on books 1–4. *P* contains the complete herbal of books 1–6 and Cambridge, Trinity College, MS O. 9. 10 (hereafter *T*) has excerpts from all of books 1–6. Finally, Oxford, Bodleian Library, MS Digby 69 (hereafter *D*) contains herbal poems only from books 5 and 6 as well as the only witness of the lapidary poems that probably made up books 7 and 8.[41] It is difficult to tell without further manuscript evidence if Henry wrote and published books 5–8 together or if 5–6 and 7–8 were written and appeared separately. Even if the last four books were originally published together, they were eventually separated by readers or scribes who desired only an herbal or only a lapidary. This convoluted manuscript history is indicative not only of Henry's patterns of writing and publication but possibly also of readers' changing interests in and demands of an herbal text.

2.2 *Structure*

As the previous discussion of dating suggests, one of the most distinctive qualities of the *Anglicanus ortus* is its organizational structure, that is, the intentional relationship between books and groups of poems.[42] Henry carefully planned the number and relation of the books as well as the placement of many poems within each book, a major improvement over his primary source and model, the later eleventh-century *De viribus herbarum* of Macer Floridus. Macer's *De viribus* (hereafter 'Macer') treats 77 herbs with no separate books and in no order apart from grouping the exotic spices in the last twelve

40 Greenway, 'Henry of Huntingdon as poet,' 331.

41 I have entertained a more complex theory of production in Black, 'Henry of Huntingdon's lapidary,' 53–4, but until firmer evidence appears we cannot speak certainly about the order in which Henry wrote and published the several versions of the herbal and lapidary.

42 First outlined by Rigg, 'Henry of Huntingdon's herbal,' 217–18, and expanded upon in Black, 'Henry of Huntingdon's lapidary,' 53–7.

poems.[43] Henry's herbal contains six books describing 160 herbs, vegetables, and spices, totalling 3386 lines. He also wrote a prose prologue (found only in *S*), which seems unfinished or poorly transcribed (see the commentary on the prose prologue below at pp. 342–3). With two exceptions, each poem is dedicated to a single plant or medicinal ingredient, an arrangement also used by Macer and by Walahfrid Strabo in his ninth-century poem *Hortulus*.[44] The first four books make a cohesive unit, each containing a prologue and twenty-five herbal poems (if we treat the one poem on hyacinth and narcissus as a double entry, 4.1–2), covering a total of a hundred herbs, followed by two epilogues which also serve as an introduction to the books that follow.

Books 5 and 6 are of different lengths and display a more elaborate, partially duodecimal organization: each has a prologue and is separated into two unequal parts by an interlude (so the numbering of poems given below changes from two digits, *e.g.* 4.12, to three, *e.g.* 5.2.5). Book 5 contains eighteen poems divided into two sections of twelve and six, while Book 6 contains forty poems divided into two sections of twelve and twenty-eight. This gives us a total of 169 separate poems and 158 ingredients discussed in the six books of the herbal. The concluding poem, however, states that 160 herbs and eastern spices are found in the garden (6 Epilogue, lines 1–2). The missing two items of *materia medica* can be found in Epilogue 1 to Book 4 (vine, lines 3–8, and squirting cucumber, lines 9–12).[45]

Henry seems to have planned a comprehensive medical work covering two hundred different items of *materia medica*, divided evenly between a hundred items in books 1–4 (less the two in Epilogue 1 to Book 4) and another hundred in 5–8, if we include the two in the epilogue and assume that the lapidary which comprised the final two books contained forty stones and gems. Since we have no complete manuscript of the work and since the one manuscript of the poems on gems and stones is apparently incomplete and not in its intended sequence, this structure remains conjectural.

43 The relationship between poems nos. 66–77 in the *De viribus herbarum* to the rest of the herbal is discussed by William C. Crossgrove, 'Zur Datierung des "Macer Floridus"', in *Licht der Natur. Medizin in Fachliteratur und Dichtung. Festschrift für Gundolf Keil zum 60. Geburtstag*, ed. Josef Domes, Bernhard D. Haage and Werner E. Gerabek (Göppingen, 1994), 55–63. He argues they are a later addition, possibly by a second author.

44 Poem 4.1–2 treats hyacinth and narcissus, while Epilogue 1 to Book 4 includes vine and squirting cucumber. Poem 6.2.25 treats the mineral *nitrum* (soda), though it appears Henry did not know what it was. See notes 70 and 73 below for more on Macer and Strabo.

45 It is not clear if the two plants described in Epilogue 1 to Book 4 were composed with the first redaction of the herbal, or if they were added to bring the total to 160.

The guiding metaphor for the structure of Henry's herbal is a square garden, and it was this arrangement that first caught the attention of John Harvey in 1987. Henry describes the garden in his Prose Prologue:

> Therefore I set forth the example of a sumptuous garden. Since it is square, let there be a lake in the middle, in which you can see fish swim. In the middle of the lake there is a seat, a kind of theatre, fending off Phoebus's rays with interwoven vines.[46]

The garden is also described as square at the end of the herb lists in *S* (fol. 34r): 'Henrici Poete centum herbarum. De xxv herbis que sunt in boriali parte orti sui quadranguli' ('[List] of the one hundred herbs of Henry the Poet. The twenty-five herbs which are in the northern part of his square garden').[47] Even though the compiler or scribe of *S* had taken the poems out of their original books and placed them in alphabetical order, he was aware of the structure of the original herbal: four books of twenty-five herbs each, represented by a garden of four beds placed according to the cardinal directions. Once the reader is introduced to the garden, he is escorted around it, like a student by his master, beginning in the north quadrant. Henry, as narrator and teacher, explains each plant and occasionally points out its place in a bed. He is especially keen to introduce the twenty-first plant in each of books 1–4, perhaps because he liked to alliterate on *uiginti uisis* (having seen twenty), which he does in each case.[48] Henry ends Book 1 by stating, 'An end is given here to the northern side.'[49] From this point we move in a circle around the garden to the eastern or western bed (he is not specific on the direction, but, for the sake of convenience, we shall assume the movement was clockwise), then to the southern side, where he begins Book 3: 'Dittany takes up the standard on the emerald cloister's southern side.'[50] A diagram of the garden and the narrator's path is reconstructed in Illustration 1.[51]

We return to the theatre, first seen in the Prose Prologue, in Epilogue 1 to Book 4, lines 1–3:

46 Prose Prologue, lines 47–50, 'Exemplum ergo delicati proponimus orti. Qui cum quadratus sit, in medio eius lacus sit, in quo pisces natare uideas. In medio uero laci sedes est quasi theatrum, palmitibus conductis Phebo resistens.'

47 Rigg, 'Henry of Huntingdon's herbal,' 288–9.

48 The first lines of poems 1.21, 2.21, 3.21, and 4.21.

49 Poem 1.25, lines 21–22, 'Lateri finis boreali / Hic datur.'

50 Poem 3.1, lines 1–2, 'In uiridi claustro uexillum tollit ab austro / Diptanum.'

51 This diagram first appeared in Black, 'Henry of Huntingdon's lapidary,' 52.

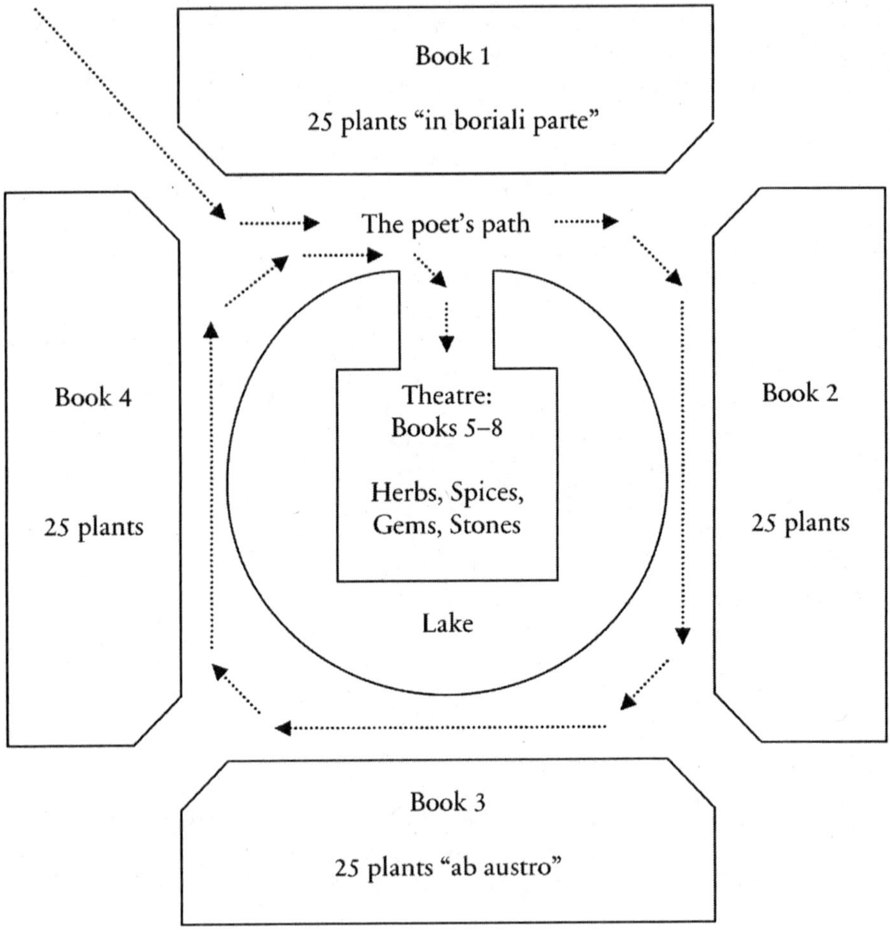

Illustration 1: The Square Garden

> If the one hundred herbs do not already bore the viewer,
> now seek out the theatre, though small, which you'll admire
> in the middle of the garden.[52]

Although Henry may have originally intended the theatre only as decoration for his garden, it now becomes the focus and stage for the rest of the work. It

52 'Tedia ni tulerint cernenti gramina centum, / Iam theatrum pete, sed modicum, medio quod in orto / Suspicies.'

is in the theatre that Henry the Narrator plans to declaim on more herbs, spices, gems, and stones in the second half of the *Anglicanus ortus*. He makes these plans explicit in the Prologue to Book 5 in the form of a prayer to the creator of all plants (*plasmator eorum*, 5 Prologue, line 2) imitating the opening of the Prose Prologue:

> ... the beginning of things, their growth, and their end, You,
> for whom I strove three times, playing with, and fleeing Venus,
> and planting herbs, and for a fourth I've woven a squared book,
> in which I recite three times four of the common herbs,
> as many spices, and as many gems and stones ...
>
> (5 Prologue, lines 7–11)[53]

The square garden of books 1–4, then, is to be reflected in the 'squared book' (*quadratum . . . libellum*) composed of books 5–8: in the former set of four books the narrator guides the reader through four beds of twenty-five plants each and in the latter set of four he intends to describe four groups (herbs, spices, gems, stones) of twelve ingredients each, but now in the calm of a shaded portico. Apollo appears in the theatre and shows his approval of Henry's plan by decorating him with the subjects of his speech:

> He [Apollo] bound my temples thrice with flowering garlands:
> 'So it may be more pleasing now,' he said, 'I'll insert gems in these,
> and I'll intersperse the gems with precious stones:
> how much splendour, and what great power, lies in these!
> Your right hand, bearing beautiful garlands for a sceptre,
> will hold godlike herbs, which the people have and do not understand.
> And that they may be more pleasing, I shall add aromas of the East:
> Such garlands I provide my servants and such sceptres too.'
>
> (5 Prologue, lines 14–21)[54]

53 Principium rerum, uegetacio, finis earum,
Cui, ludens Veneremque fugans et gramina plantans,
Ter nitui, quarto quadratum texo libellum,
In quo uulgares recito ter quatuor herbas,
Tot species, totidem gemmas totidemque lapillos ...

54 Hic michi florigeris ter cinxit tympora sertis:
'Nunc magis ut deceat, hiis gemmas insero,' dixit,
'Gemmas preclaris interpellabo lapillis:
Quantus splendor inest predictis, tanta potestas.
Serta decora gerens, pro sceptro dextra tenebit
Diuinas, quas uulgus habet nec iudicat, herbas.
Que magis ut placeant, Orientis aromata iungam:
Talia serta meis et talia sceptra ministro.'

This scene is intentionally ridiculous, for we will find that Henry is not quite up to Apollo's task, and it sets the stage for some of the herbal's most surprising and humorous aspects, the repeated device of an interruption from the audience. After describing twelve herbs (poems 5.1.1–12), Henry indulges in a round of arrogant self-congratulation—'I'll be read through the entire world, I'll have an eternal name!'[55]—only to be interrupted by a character simply called 'a certain cook' (5 Interlude, line 7). The Cook, probably meant to represent Henry's favourite poet Martial,[56] heaps scorn on Henry, whom he repeatedly addresses as 'Envy' (*liuor*),[57] and takes over the rest of the book (5.2.1–6) in order to speak about the medical attributes of common kitchen vegetables.[58]

After a grudging reconciliation with the Cook, Henry takes up his task again, now relating twelve spices (6.1.1–12), the 'aromas of the East' mentioned by Apollo. Another interruption (Interlude to Book 6) follows in which Henry is scolded, this time more gently, by an old man. It is not clear who he is supposed to be: perhaps Apollo in disguise or Constantine the African, the eleventh-century translator of Greek and Arabic medical texts whose *Liber graduum* ('Book of Degrees') Henry used for much of Book 6 and his lapidary.[59] The second part of this book (6.2.1–28) is apparently given in the voice of the Old Man (although there is no dialogue as there was in Book 5 between Henry and the Cook), who ends Interlude 6:

55 5 Interlude, line 6, 'Orbe legar toto nomenque perenne tenebo!'

56 Wolfgang Maaz details Henry's devotion to Martial in *Lateinische Epigrammatik im hohen Mittelalter*, 103–74.

57 Henry had similarly personified *liuor* in his epigram 'De statu suo' (*HA* 792–4, lines 13–16).

58 This section, dedicated to vegetables rather than medical herbs, may owe something to the late antique letter of Anthimus on the qualities of foods, particularly vegetables, found in several manuscripts of the ninth to twelfth centuries: *Anthimi De observatione ciborum ad Theodoricum regem Francorum epistula*, ed. and trans. Eduard Liechtenhan, Corpus medicorum Latinorum 8. 1 (Berlin 1963). I have found no clear correlation between the two works, however, and the structure is more likely a product of Henry's literary imagination.

59 Rigg, 'Henry of Huntingdon's herbal,' 286; Black, 'Henry of Huntingdon's lapidary,' 56. On the history and circulation of the *Liber graduum* see Faith Wallis, 'The ghost in the *Articella*: A twelfth-century commentary on the Constantinian *Liber Graduum*,' in *Herbs and Healers from the Ancient Mediterranean through the Medieval West: Essays in Honor of John M. Riddle*, ed. Anne Van Arsdall and Timothy Graham (Aldershot, forthcoming).

I will add what the Arab once taught,
and what the Chinese and Indian, travelling among them.
(6 Interlude, lines 12–13)[60]

The herbal concludes with a short verse epilogue, discussed above, in which the 160 medicinal items of books 1–6 are treated as the subject of a coherent work:

The flowering garden, enclosing one hundred and sixty
eastern spices and herbs that love the earth, is done.
(6 Epilogue, lines 1–2)[61]

2.3 *Relations between Poems*

The previous section addressed the structure of the herbal as a whole, that is, in the relationship between the books. Within each book Henry also developed an internal structure by indicating the place of poems within their book or bed (first, sixth, twenty-first, and so on) and the similarities and differences between groups of herbs. Unlike Macer's *De viribus herbarum* in which each of the poems stands on its own with little or no connection to the others, most of Henry's poems are understood best in the specific order of the edition below, providing a narrative for the teacher and student in the square garden, and an established *ductus* for the reader to follow. In many poems, Henry indicates the relationship of the herb to the previous one, and he often groups two or more poems together on the basis of the herbs' appearance, curative properties (*e.g.* diuretic), Galenic qualities (*e.g.* all hot in the fourth degree), or religious association (*e.g.* the Virgin Mary's violet, rose, and lily). In some cases, he simply indicates that his audience should follow him to the next plant in the garden: basil is said to

60 'Quod Arabs quondam, quod Serus et Yndus / Inter eos peregrinantes, docuere reponam.'

For more on the possibility that the Old Man or the *Arabs* is supposed to be Constantine, see Black, '"I will add what the Arab once taught": Constantine the African in Northern European medical verse,' in *Herbs and Healers*, ed. Van Arsdall and Graham.

61 'Floriger eoas species, herbas philogeas / Centum sex decies claudens concluditur ortus.' The structure of the lapidary in books 7–8 is not entirely clear but in one of the surviving poems, Henry is interrupted by Evax, mythical king and expert on gems. It is likely that Henry continued the pattern of twelve poems followed by an interruption and further poems; see Black, 'Henry of Huntingdon's lapidary,' 59–60. A complete copy of the lapidary or of the entire *Anglicanus ortus* is needed to verify this theory.

be *post matrem* (poem 1.2, line 1), since it follows artemisia, called *herbarum matrem* (poem 1.1, line 1). In many poems, he describes the numerical placement of the plant within its bed, most notably the twenty-first poem in books 1–4, each of which begins 'Viginti uisis' ('Having seen twenty'). Table 1 lists every instance in which poems are described by their placement or linked to one another by some named similarity or difference.

2.4 *Sources*

Henry, as a writer, has been aptly described as a 'weaver.'[62] Little of his known work—be it history, herbal, or lapidary—can be considered entirely original; rather, he wove allusions, paraphrases, and direct quotes from numerous sources into a fabric that is uniquely his own. He even makes this weaving explicit in the Prologue to Book 5, where he describes his plan for the book ('I've woven a squared book, in which I recite three times four of the common herbs') and in the opening of his letter *De contemptu mundi* ('I also composed [*contexui*] a poem on Love').[63] He is hardly ashamed of this extensive borrowing. This manner of 'weaving' is common to many medieval authors; indeed, it was an accepted method of composition to borrow extensively from numerous authorities.

As should also be expected of a well-educated medieval cleric, Henry liberally seasoned his herbal with classical quotations and allusions. The classical authors used in this work are virtually identical to those employed in his *Historia Anglorum*: Virgil, Horace, Ovid, Lucan, Juvenal, Statius, and Martial are employed most often.[64] As is common in medieval works, it is difficult to tell whether an allusion is intentional or if Henry knew some classical authors so well that their language was merely part of his 'writer's toolbox.' In some cases, however, Henry is explicit about his source: he names Ovid (1.10, 7; 6.1.9, 23) and Virgil (1.6, 3; 2.17, 16; 3.1, 5; 4.1–2, 35) several times. Henry expects his reader to be familiar with their works, pointing to passages relevant to his herbal: 'What did tuneful Ovid sing, while plucking wings from Love? "Gather eye-sharpening Rues."'[65] Other poems, like 4.1–2 on hyacinth

62 *HA* lxxxv. Greenway estimates that 'For about 75% of the *History*, Henry was entirely dependent on the work of other writers.'

63 5 Prologue, lines 9–10, 'quadratum texo libellum, / In quo uulgares recito ter quatuor herbas . . . '; *HA* 584–5, 'Carmen etiam in amorem acceptabile contexui' (Greenway translates *contexui* as 'composed' but it also means 'wove together').

64 Quotations from most of these authors could be found in the copy of Priscian kept at Lincoln cathedral; see *HA* xxxiv–xxxvi.

65 Poem 1.10, lines 7–8: 'Naso suaue canens, dum pennas demit Amori, / Quid cecinit? "Sumas acuentes lumina rutas".'

The quotation is taken from Ovid's *Remedia amoris*, line 801.

Table 1: Indicators of Internal Structure

Poem(s) and line(s)	Herb(s)	Indicating phrase or relation	Refers to poem
1.1, 1–2	*Arthemisia*	*primo limite . . . pretulimus orto*	
1.2, 1	*Ozyma*	*post matrem*	1.1
1.3, 2–10	*Crocus*	*Crocus* claims to be superior to *ozyma*	1.2
1.10, 1	*Ruta*	*decimo . . . agello*	
1.11, 1	*Ysopum*	*undenum*	
1.14–15	*Buglossa, Sanicla*	Both used to heal wounds	
1.16–17	*Costus, Anglica costus*	Same name	
1.18, 1	*Beta maior*	*Ordine que sequitur*	
1.19, 1	*Beta minor*	*Betam beta minor . . . sequitur*	1.18
1.21, 1	*Petroselinum*	*Viginti uisis*	1.1–20
1.21, 3–10	*Petroselinum*	Compared to *apium*	1.20
1.22, 1	*Solsequium*	*cernitur ordine certo*	
1.25, 1	*Mirtus*	*Vltima iam partis . . . borealis*	
2.1, 2	*Mandragora*	*Iure locanda prius*	
2.2–4	*Elleborum album, Elleborum nigrum, Azimum*	All three herbs aid mental health	
2.3, 1	*Elleborum nigrum*	*Elleborum subit elleboro, nigro subit album* (White and Black Hellebore together)	2.2
2.6, 1	*Carui*	*Stat carui sexto . . . lecto*	

Table 1: Indicators of Internal Structure (*Continued*)

Poem(s) and line(s)	Herb(s)	Indicating phrase or relation	Refers to poem
2.9–11	*Viola, Rosa, Lilium*	Emblems of the Virgin Mary	
2.11, 1	*Lilium*	Compared to *rosa*	2.10
2.12, 1	*Celidonia*	*spacio . . . duodeno*	
2.16–17	*Pulegium, Serpillum*	Both are hot and dry in the third degree (2.17, 2)	
2.21, 1	*Viola hyemalis*	*Viginti . . . uisis*	2.1–20
2.22, 1	*Basilisca*	*Proximus extollit locus*	
2.25, 1	*Ligusticum*	*Finis in aduentum*	
3.2–3	*Feniculum, Anetum*	Nearly identical plants	
3.5, 1–2	*Nimphea*	*Quinta libro detur . . . datur quinto . . . lecto*	
3.8–9	*Yris, Yreos*	Two kinds of iris	
3.10, 1	*Menta*	Hot and dry like *yris*	3.8
3.13–14	*Raphanus, Radix*	Two kinds of radish	
3.16–17	*Altea, Sinula*	Two kinds of mallow	
3.18, 1	*Piretrum*	*Sinula si nulla* (pun on previous plant's name)	3.17
3.21, 1	*Sclarega*	*Viginti uisis*	3.1–20
3.21–22	*Sclarega, Sclarega maior*	Two kinds of clary	
4.3, 1	*Sinapis*	*Tercia stat sinapis*	
4.4, 1	*Eruca*	*Erucam synapi similem*	4.3

4.5, 1	*Lactuca*	Hot *eruca* compared to cold *lactuca*	4.4
4.6–10	*Satureia, Nasturcium, Ameos, Psillium, Coriandrum*	Three very hot herbs followed by two very cold	
4.7, 1	*Nasturcium*	*Septima stant . . . nasturcia*	
4.11–12	*Lupinum, Fenugrecum*	Effective against wine, use of military metaphors	
4.13, 1	*Papauer*	*Miconius stat tredecimus*	
4.19–20	*Meu, Ciperus*	Diuretics	
4.21, 1	*Valeriana*	*Viginti uisis*	4.1–20
4.25, 1	*Savina*	*Vltima procedit*	
5 Interlude		*herbas . . . duodenas*	5.1.1–12
5.2.1–6	*Cepa, Porrum, Caulis, Atriplex, Petrosilinum, Allium*	Culinary vegetables	
6.1.1, 4	*Piper*	*Principio*	
6.1.2, 3	*Mirra*	*Post piper*	6.1.1
6.1.5–6	*Cynnama, Cassia*	Nearly identical spices	
6.2.4–5	*Storax, Mastix*	Gums or resins	
6.2.16, 1	*Squilla*	*Squilla gradu quo thus manet*	6.2.15
6.2.17, 2	*Siler*	*Stat quo squilla gradu*	6.2.16
6.2.18–19	*Dragagantus, Diagridium*	Famous antidote ingredients	

and narcissus, are filled with classical allusions; Ovid was the obvious source for tales about youths transformed into flowers and Henry could not resist the urge to join two such flowers into one impressive poem.[66] Likewise, Henry explains in poem 3.1 that poets can provide useful medical information, such as when Virgil described how Aeneas healed an arrow wound with dittany.

While Henry might be indebted to classical authors for much of his style, he is dependent on a number of herbalists and medical authors for the content of most of the poems in the *Anglicanus ortus*. He stresses at the end of his prose prologue that all of his information is taken from 'authorities'.[67] In Epilogue 2 to Book 4, lines 7–21, he proudly lists his alleged sources:

> But lest you think that we have brought here falsehoods,
> if you wish to learn their authors, I have written
> what was sung by Phoebus, Phoebus's son, by Olympius the author,
> by Themison, by Apollodorus, by the Sisters,
> or what was sung by eminent Hippocrates, divinely sick,
> by Prodymus, Chrysippus too, and by the mighty Pliny,
> what Justus mentions, what Galen has foretold,
> and what Xenocrates, whom philosophy adorns,
> what Cato, Pythagoras, and Palladius asserted,
> what Stephen, what Mellitius of the honeyed mouth,
> and Asclepius, father of medicine, a splendid author,
> what Dioscorides, what Philo, what Menemachus,
> what polished Macer, and Macer's follower Strabo,
> what Oribasius orders, matching the known to the unknown,
> or what others teach . . . .[68]

66 See Rigg, 'Henry of Huntingdon's herbal', 273–4, for more on this poem's sources.

67 'Sciatis autem utique hic apposita ex auctoritatibus sumpta', lines 51–2.

68 At ne uana putes nos hic commenta tulisse,
Autores si uis istorum noscere, scripsi
Quod Phebus Pheboque satus, quod Olympius autor,
Quod Themeson, quod Apollodorus cecinere, Sorores,
Siue quod excellens Ypocras, diuinitus eger,
Quod Prodymus, quod Crisipus, et quod Plinius ingens,
Quod memorat Iustus, quod diuinat Galienus,
Et quod Xenocrates quem philosophia uenustat,
Quod Catho, Pittagoras, Palladius asseruere,
Quod Stephanus, quod melliti Mellicius oris,
Asclepiusque, pater medicine, splendidus autor,
Quod Dyascorides, quod Philo, quod Menetamus,
Quod Macer nitidus, Macrique pedissequa Stabus,
Nota quod ignotis iubet Oribasius equans
Siue alii . . . .

While this catalogue suggests that Henry drew laboriously on an entire library of medical authors, he never read, and probably never even had access to, most of their writings. The names come, along with his botanical information, from just a few sources, most of which prove to be much later than these Greek and Roman philosophers.

Diana Greenway was correct in postulating that Henry's herbal would be dependent on Macer Floridus's *De viribus herbarum*.[69] The majority of poems in books 1–5 and the first half of Book 6 are based on poems by Macer. Henry used almost every poem from Macer's herbal, and he imitates the division of Macer's herbal between herbs and spices (though that division is the only structure given to the *De viribus herbarum*). All of Macer's poems on spices (nos. 66–77) are used in Henry's Book 6 on spices, apart from no. 67, 'Pyrethrum,' used for Henry's poem 3.18, and no. 74, 'Costus,' which Henry did not use. Henry acknowledges his debt to Macer and Walahfrid Strabo (whom he calls *Stabus*), in whose 'famous footsteps' (*clara* ... *uestigia*, poem 1.9, line 4) he says he is proud to be walking. Henry even teases his liberal borrowing from these herbalists through the voice of the Cook in poem 5.2.6 on garlic: 'And what is Macer to you? You mock it all, then you steal, and aping another, you boast it as your own!'[70] Of the 157 herbal poems in books 1–6 (*i.e.* not including the prologues, epilogues, and interludes), seventy-five are adapta-

69 *HA* cxiv–cxv; *Macer Floridus De viribus herbarum*, ed. Ludwig Choulant (Leipzig 1832), reprinted in facsimile with German translation, *Höhepunkte der Klostermedizin. Der 'Macer Floridus' und das Herbarium des Vitus Auslasser,* trans. Johannes Gottfried Mayer and Konrad Goehl (Holzminden 2001). It is generally accepted that Macer was not the classical poet Aemilius Macer, but rather is the pseudonym of Odo Magdunensis (Odo of Meung), a cleric in the Loire region writing in the late eleventh century. The identification of 'Macer' with Odo of Meung was made by Cyrill Resak in his dissertation *Odo Magdunensis, der Verfasser des 'Macer Floridus' und der deutsche Leipziger Macer Text* (Leipzig 1917). The epithet 'Floridus' seems to have been added by twelfth-century scribes. See Bruce P. Flood, Jr, 'Macer Floridus: A medieval herbalism,' PhD diss. (University of Colorado, 1968); Flood, 'The medieval herbal tradition of "Macer Floridus",' *Pharmacy in History* 18 (1976), 62–6; and Flood, 'Pliny and the medieval "Macer" medical text,' *Journal of the History of Medicine and Allied Sciences* 32 (1977), 395–402. William Crossgrove, in 'Zur Datierung des "Macer Floridus",' has tentatively suggested a new chronology of production for *De viribus herbarum*: poems 1–49 and 51–65 were composed perhaps any time after the death of Walahfrid Strabo but before the publication of Constantine the African's medical works ca. 1070–85, and poems 50 and 66–77, along with some additions to the older entries, depend on Constantine's work and are therefore at least late eleventh century in date. This would, of course, deny authorship of most of the work to Odo of Meung.

70 Poem 5.2.6, lines 30–31: 'Multa cauillans / Furaris iactasque tuum imitans alienum!'

tions of Macer's poems.[71] Henry's treatment of Macer ranges from direct copying in a few instances (1.9, 21 and 5.1.8, 4) or mere rewordings, to complete and creative overhauls (*e.g.*, 1.9, 12–22 and 3.11, 3–9).

After exhausting Macer's herbal, Henry drew primarily from Walahfrid Strabo's *Hortulus*, the herbal of Pseudo-Apuleius (also known as Apuleius Barbarus or Apuleius Platonicus), and one or more works of Constantine the African.[72] Five poems (1.6, 1.16, 2.18, 3.7, 3.21) are based primarily on Strabo's *Hortulus*, and some poems which are primarily dependent on Macer also contain lines derived from the *Hortulus*.[73] The small number of poems which Henry borrowed directly from Walahfrid Strabo's *Hortulus* is outweighed by the overall influence of the *Hortulus* on the *Anglicanus ortus*. Much of Henry's tone, style, and rhetoric in the herbal seem to be in conscious imitation of the *Hortulus*, in which a personable narrator guides an unnamed guest around his garden. Strabo's narrator likewise interjects witty and devotional comments into a primarily medical discussion of his plants. Given the obvious impact the *Hortulus* had on Henry, it is curious that he would borrow so little from it. Perhaps he was dissatisfied with the limited amount of medical information, while nonetheless impressed by its style.

Another five poems (1.18, 1.22, 2.1, 2.20, 3.12) are based on passages in the late Antique herbal of Pseudo-Apuleius. Henry never mentions Apuleius by name; he may have found this herbal without attribution or under another author's name, such as Galen or Dioscorides, to whom many medieval medical works were pseudonymously ascribed. Book 6 is dedicated to 'eastern spices,'[74] and introduces a new source, Constantine the African's *Liber graduum* (also called *De gradibus*). Poems in the first section (6.1.1–12) come

71 Henry may have been using an extended, perhaps distinctly English, redaction of Macer, since several of Henry's lines (2.19, 8 and 2.23, 21–25) are based on lines that Ludwig Choulant rejected from his edition of *De viribus herbarum* (Choulant used manuscripts from only Dresden, Leipzig, and Wolfenbüttel).

72 Walahfrid Strabo, *Hortulus*, ed. Cataldo Roccaro (Palermo 1979); Pseudo-Apuleius is published in *Antonii Musae De herba vettonica liber, Pseudoapulei Herbarius, Anonymi De taxone liber, Sexti Placiti Liber medicinae ex animalibus*, ed. Ernst Howald and Henry E. Sigerist (Leipzig 1927), 15–225, 287–98 (entries from this edition will be cited both by the number given by the editors and by the page number of the edition); Constantine's *Liber graduum* is found in some manuscripts as part of the *Practica* section of his adaptation of the *Pantegni* of 'Alī ibn al-'Abbās al-Maǧūsī, first printed in the works of Isaac Israeli, *Opera omnia Ysaac* (Lyons 1515), 2. 78r–86r. It also circulated as an independent work, with small changes, and was printed as a separate work in *Constantini Africani . . . Opera* (Basel 1536–9), 2. 342–87. I have used the later edition unless otherwise indicated.

73 Poems 2.7, 2.10, 2.16, 2.23, 2.25, 3.8, 3.10, and 3.18.

74 *Eoas species* is used at 6.1.1, line 1, and repeated in the Epilogue to Book 6, line 1.

from Macer and Constantine, but nearly every poem in the second section (6.2.1–28) is drawn from the *Liber graduum*. We can only conjecture how and when Henry obtained a copy of this work. The *Liber graduum* was part of Constantine's medical encyclopaedia *Pantegni* but also circulated independently. It seems likely that Henry obtained a copy of this work after he wrote books 1–4, since there is no definite sign of Constantine's influence in the first half of the *Anglicanus ortus* outside of what he could have learned from Macer's herbal. The two poems in books 1–4 (3.20, 4.7) that appear to have information from Constantinian works may have been augmented by Henry himself or a scribe at a later date, or his copy of Macer could already have been modified with Salernitan material.

The remaining poems are more difficult to trace. It appears that Henry used several other works, or possessed a medical florilegium containing some or all of the following works: Pliny's *Natural History* (perhaps 1.22, 4.12, 4.14, 4.15; see discussion below in section 2.5.5) or an abbreviation of it like Robert Cricklade's *Defloratio Plinii*;[75] Latin translations of works by the Byzantine physicians Alexander of Tralles and Oribasius;[76] and one of the two Latin versions of Dioscorides' *De materia medica*, most likely the eleventh-century

75 Pliny the Elder, *Natural History*, ed. and trans. H. Rackham, W. H. S. Jones, and D. E. Eichholz, 10 vols, Loeb Classical Library (Cambridge, MA 1938–63); *Roberti Crikeladensis Defloratio Naturalis historiae Plinii Secundi*, ed. Bodo Näf (Berlin 2002). While Robert's work is dedicated to the new king Henry II (1154), it may have been finished earlier. See L. D. Reynolds's comments on the manuscript tradition of Pliny in *Texts and Transmission: A Survey of the Latin Classics*, ed. L. D. Reynolds (Oxford 1983), 307–16. Although only a few poems have passages which seem to be dependent on Pliny or one of his redactors, it is tempting to think that Henry and Robert, who became prior of St Frideswide's, Oxford, in 1141, may have crossed paths and even shared manuscripts.

76 Gerhard Baader, 'Early medieval Latin adaptations of Byzantine medicine in Western Europe,' *Dumbarton Oaks Papers* 38, Symposium on Byzantine Medicine (1984), 251–9, at 252. See also Alain Touwaide, 'Oreibasios,' in *Der neue Pauly*, ed. Hubert Cancik and Helmuth Schneider (Stuttgart 1996–2003), 9. 15–16. The original Greek works of Oribasius, with French translation of select parts, with two early medieval Latin translations of the *Synopsis* and *Euporistes*, are published in *Oeuvres d'Oribase*, ed. U. C. Bussemaker and C. Daremberg, 6 vols (Paris 1851–76), at 5. 799–927 (*Synopsis* 1–3, ed. A. Molinier), 6. 2–402 (*Synopsis* 4–9, ed. A. Molinier), and 6. 403–626 (*Euporistes*, ed. A. Molinier). The Latin Oribasius exists in 'old' and 'new' recensions, discussed by Henning Mørland, *Die lateinischen Oribasiusübersetzungen*, Symbolae Osloenses, Supplement 5 (Oslo 1932). The first part was edited in *Oribasius Latinus (Erster Teil)*, by H. Mørland, Symbolae Osloenses, Supplement 10 (Oslo 1940). M. L. Cameron includes the Latin Oribasius among the medical works available in Anglo-Saxon England: 'The sources of medical knowledge in Anglo-Saxon England,' *Anglo-Saxon England* 11 (1983), 135–55, at 138–9.

alphabetical version attributed to Constantine the African.[77] The Latin alphabetical redaction of Dioscorides was sometimes bound with the Latin Oribasius in British manuscripts, and Henry may have worked from such a compilation.[78] One manuscript, now partially lost, that would have given us a very good idea of the sort of compilation Henry might have used is London, British Library, MS Cotton Galba E. IV.[79] The manuscript, of English provenance and once owned by the Elizabethan magician Dr John Dee, is a collection of medical works from the last quarter of the twelfth century which once contained twenty-six titles, but now retains only nine after mutilation. Dr Dee's own manuscript catalogue informs us that among the missing works were Constantine's *Liber de herbis* (apparently a different work than his *Liber graduum*), Dioscorides' *De virtutibus herbarum*, Oribasius's *De virtutibus herbarum*, Macer's *Versus de virtutibus herbarum*, and Constantine's *Liber graduum*. Clearly Henry was not the only twelfth-century cleric interested in compiling these medical works. While the sources of most of Henry's poems can be traced, this still leaves a significant number of poems which seem to be original for the most part[80] or for which I have not yet found a source.[81]

Another possible source is the medical poem of Quintus Serenus (often appearing with the cognomen Sammonicus) who wrote his *Liber medicinalis* in the third or fourth century.[82] The *Liber medicinalis* survives in at least fourteen copies, mostly of the ninth and tenth centuries.[83] While Serenus's work

77 On these versions see John Riddle, 'Dioscorides,' *Catalogus translationum et commentariorum: Mediaeval and Renaissance Latin Translations and Commentaries* 4 (1980), 1–143, at 20–27. The alphabetical Dioscorides is printed in Dioscorides, *De materia medica* (Colle 1478), reprinted in Lyons in 1512. This early printed version, however, contains the glosses and additions of Pietro d'Abano, made *ca* 1300, found only in Paris, Bibliothèque nationale de France, MS Lat. 6820, fols. 1–72. I have also used for reference the unglossed version in Cambridge, Jesus College, MS Q. D. 2 (44), fols. 17–145.

78 For two examples, see Richard Sharpe, 'List of identifications' (version of 10/09/08) under 'Dioscorides' and 'Oribasius,' part of the British Medieval Library Catalogues project available online at <http://www.history.ox.ac.uk/sharpe/index.htm>.

79 Described in Marius, *On the Elements*, ed. and trans. Richard C. Dales (Berkeley 1976), 7–10.

80 Poems 1.2, 1.3, 1.8, 1.23, 2.13, 2.21, 3.1, 4.1–2, 4.17, and 4.24.

81 Poems 1.4, 1.5, 1.15–17, 1.19, 1.21, 1.25, 2.4, 2.6, 2.8, 2.15, 2.19, 2.22, 2.24, 3.4, 3.5, 3.9, 3.13, 3.14, 3.22, 4.8, 4.9, 4.11, 4.15, 4.19, 4.21, 4 Epilogue 1, 5.1.9, 5.1.12, 5.2.5, 6.1.10, 6.2.19, and 6.2.26. I am assuming that overtly medicinal or botanical passages are not original to Henry's observation but were taken from another author.

82 Quintus Serenus, *Liber medicinalis*, ed. and trans. R. Pépin (Paris 1950). Pépin dates the work between the end of the second century and the first decade of the fourth (*Liber medicinalis*, x). For a more recent discussion of its date, see D. R. Langslow, *Medical Latin in the Roman Empire* (Oxford 2000), 64.

83 Quintus Serenus, xlviii.

is therapeutic, organized by disease rather than by herb, it does share some similarities with the *Anglicanus ortus*. Most obviously, it is composed of numerous short poems, all in hexameters. There are also some distinctive features and words shared by Henry and Serenus that do not occur in Strabo or Macer. Both works are dedicated to *Phebe*, Apollo Phoebus, as the founder of medicine (Henry, Prologue to Book 1, line 11; Serenus, line 1). At a purely grammatical level, both Serenus and Henry prefer to make orders in the future imperative, a form not employed in other Latin herbals: for example, *curato*, *misceto*, *tractato* (Serenus, lines 81, 150, 249) and *assumito*, *addito*, *sumito* (Henry, poem 1.3, lines 14 and 21; poem 1.22, line 17). Both prefer to use the epithets *cum Baccho* and *Lyeo* instead of Macer's pedestrian *cum vino* (to name a few instances, Serenus, 150, 197, 225, 1072, and Henry, 1.9, 32; 1.24, 14; 2.11, 30; 2.25, 6; 3.23, 6). The most convincing similarity is the shared ingredient of goat's milk. Henry includes it only in his poem on clary: 'Huius enim succus niuee cum lacte capelle . . .' (3.22, 3). Serenus employs this ingredient in many recipes, usually with the same phrase, 'cum,' 'vel,' or 'de lacte capellae' (lines 197, 229, 312, 565, 872, 1076). These similarities suggest that Henry had access to a copy of Serenus's herbal, but perhaps because it was not organized by plant, Henry did not actively imitate it.

2.5 *Treatment of Sources and Compositional Methods*

Henry's treatment of his material ranges from the delightful to the banal, from inspired explorations of nature's virtues to mere paraphrases of Macer. In the former category, herbs speak for themselves in the first person (strawberries, 2.15; elecampane, 3.15). In some poems he demonstrates his love of classical culture: he makes fanciful comparisons of herbs to ancient myths (periwinkle, 1.23; dittany, 3.1; fennel, 3.2; hyacinth and narcissus, 4.1–2), converses with the muse Erato (rose, 2.10), personifies herbs as bellicose warriors (lupin and fenugreek, 4.11 and 4.12), and transforms the difficult identification of an herb into a Horatian legal battle (feverfew, 3.4). Only a few poems are explicitly Christian; he recalls flowers blooming at Christmas (winter violet, 2.21), describes the three emblematic flowers of the Virgin (sweet violet, 2.9), and explores the mysteries of the virgin birth and the paradox of Holy Father-as-Son (St Mary's seal, 4.24). A few earthly women are introduced to the poems, such as when he tenderly recalls the late Queen Matilda and her

Table 2: Medical Sources of the *Anglicanus ortus*

I have provided Table 2 as a convenient reference to the main sources which Henry used for his medical information. I do not supply here literary sources (Ovid, Virgil, *etc.*), which can be found in the commentaries on the individual poems below. In the cases where I am relatively certain that Henry's poem or a significant portion of it is entirely original, I have noted it as such. I have placed a question mark next to those poems for which I believe Henry had an outside source which I have not yet discovered. Passages from Macer are recorded with their poem and line numbers as found in Choulant's edition, those from Strabo according to their line numbers in the edition of Roccaro, and those from Pliny according to book and paragraph in Rackham's Loeb edition of the *Natural History* (see notes 70, 73, 76). Passages from Constantine the African are given according to pages in *Constantini Africani . . . Opera* (Basel 1536–9). Unless otherwise indicated, references to Constantine come from his *Liber graduum* in vol. 2 of the *Opera*.

***Anglicanus ortus*, poem numbers and titles**		**Main medical sources (with title and lines if relevant)**
1	Prologue	Original
1.1	'Arthemisia'	Macer no. 1, 'Artemisia,' 1–30
1.2	'Ozyma'	Original
1.3	'Crocus'	Original
1.4	'Laureola'	?
1.5	'Baldemonia'	?
1.6	'Ambrosia'	Strabo, 'De Ambrosia,' 369–74
1.7	'Origanum'	Macer no. 38, 'Origanum,' 1285–324
1.8	'Lauandula'	Original
1.9	'Saluia'	Macer no. 24, 'Salvia,' 870–81
1.10	'Ruta'	Macer no. 7, 'Ruta,' 267–331
1.11	'Ysopum'	Macer no. 45, 'Ysopum,' 1503–31
1.12	'Camedreos'	Macer no. 59, 'Chamaedrys,' 1903–17
1.13	'Camomilla'	Macer no. 14, 'Chamomilla,' 549–91
1.14	'Buglossa'	Macer no. 34, 'Buglossa,' 1127–38
1.15	'Sanicla'	?
1.16	'Costus'	?
1.17	'Anglica costus'	?
1.18	'Beta maior'	Pseudo-Apuleius no. 36, 'Herba Personacia'
1.19	'Beta minor'	?
1.20	'Apium'	Macer no. 8, 'Apium,' 332–65
1.21	'Petroselinum' [no. 1]	?
1.22	'Solsequium'	Pseudo-Apuleius no. 49, 'Herba Heliotropia' Pliny 22. 57–61
1.23	'Paruenca'	Original
1.24	'Strucion'	Macer no. 26, 'Ostrutium,' 907–27

Anglicanus ortus, poem numbers and titles		Main medical sources (with title and lines if relevant)
1.25	'Mirtus'	?
2	Prologue	Original
2.1	'Mandragora'	Pseudo-Apuleius no. 131, 'Effectus herbae mandragorae'
2.2	'Elleborum album'	Macer no. 56, 'Elleborus albus,' 1774–1832
2.3	'Elleborum nigrum'	Macer no. 57, 'Elleborus niger,' 1833–58
2.4	'Azimum'	?
2.5	'Pastinaca'	Macer no. 37, 'Pastinaca,' 1264–84
2.6	'Carui'	?
2.7	'Dragantea'	Macer no. 54, 'Colubrina,' 1728–65
2.8	'Saxifraga'	?
2.9	'Viola'	Macer no. 40, 'Violae,' 1342–94
2.10	'Rosa'	Macer no. 21, 'Rosa,' 776–807 Strabo, 'De Rosa,' 400–401 (of 392–428)
2.11	'Lilium'	Macer no. 22, 'Lilium,' 808–42
2.12	'Celidonia'	Macer no. 52, 'Chelidonia,' 1690–1708
2.13	'Pigmentum'	Original
2.14	'Vetonica'	Macer no. 11, 'Betonica,' 429–91
2.15	'Fraga'	?
2.16	'Pulegium'	Macer no. 16, 'Pulegium,' 626–77
2.17	'Serpillum'	Macer no. 39, 'Serpillum,' 1325–41
2.18	'Pipera'	Strabo, 'De Agrimonia,' 359–68
2.19	'Benedicta'	?
2.20	'Conferba'	Pseudo-Apuleius no. 59, 'Herba Confirma'
2.21	'Viola hyemalis'	Original
2.22	'Basilisca'	?
2.23	'Abrotanus'	Macer no. 2, 'Abrotanum,' 31–51
2.24	'Taneticum'	?
2.25	'Ligusticum'	Macer no. 25, 'Ligusticum,' 882–906 Strabo, 'De Lybistico,' 229–35
3	Prologue	Original
3.1	'Diptannus'	Original
3.2	'Feniculum'	Macer no. 17, 'Feniculum,' 678–710
3.3	'Anetum'	Macer no. 10, 'Anethum,' 395–428
3.4	'Febrifuga'	?
3.5	'Nimphea'	?
3.6	'Asarum'	Macer no. 46, 'Asarum,' 1532–68
3.7	'Macedonia'	Strabo, 'De Cerfolio,' 235–47
3.8	'Yris'	Macer no. 43, 'Iris,' 1456–88 Strabo, 'De Gladiola,' 217–28
3.9	'Yreos'	?
3.10	'Menta'	Macer no. 47, 'Mentha,' 1569–84 Strabo, 'De Menta,' 284–99

Anglicanus ortus, poem numbers and titles		Main medical sources (with title and lines if relevant)
3.11	'Absinthium'	Macer no. 3, 'Absinthium,' 52–114
3.12	'Balsama'	Pseudo-Apuleius no. 106, 'Herba Sisimbrium'
3.13	'Raphanus'	?
3.14	'Radix'	?
3.15	'Enula'	Macer no. 44, 'Enula,' 1489–1502
3.16	'Altea'	Macer no. 9, 'Althaea,' 366–94
3.17	'Sinula'	Macer no. 62, 'Malva,' 1962–92
3.18	'Piretrum'	Macer no. 67, 'Pyrethrum,' 2086–2108
3.19	'Centaurea'	Macer no. 53, 'Centaurea,' 1709–27
3.20	'Marrubium'	Macer no. 42, 'Marrubium,' 1437–55 Constantine, *Opera* (Basel 1536), 1. 205
3.21	'Sclarega'	Strabo, 'De Sclarega,' 275–83
3.22	'Sclarega maior'	?
3.23	Nepta'	Macer no. 15, 'Nepeta,' 592–625 Pseudo-Oribasius 1. 129, 'Antidotum Diacalamentum'
3.24	'Portulaca'	Macer no. 19, 'Portulaca,' 748–64
3.25	'Semperuiua'	Macer no. 18, 'Acidula,' 711–42
4	Prologue	Original
4.1–2	'Iacinctus et Narcissus'	Original
4.3	'Sinapis'	Macer no. 35, 'Sinapi,' 1139–1200
4.4	'Eruca'	Macer no. 31, 'Eruca,' 1016–36
4.5	'Lactuca'	Macer no. 20, 'Lactuca,' 765–75
4.6	'Satureia'	Macer no. 23, 'Satureia,' 843–69
4.7	'Nasturcium'	Constantine, 'Nasturtium,' 384 Macer no. 30, 'Nasturtium,' 988–1015
4.8	'Ameos'	?
4.9	'Psillium'	?
4.10	'Coriandrum'	Macer no. 29, 'Coriandrum,' 957–87
4.11	'Lupinum'	?
4.12	'Fenugrecum'	? (Pliny 24. 184–8)
4.13	'Papaver'	Macer no. 32, 'Papaver,' 1037–86
4.14	'Git'	? (Pliny 19. 167–68; 27. 121)
4.15	'Gazara'	? (Pliny 27. 113–17)
4.16	'Pionia'	Macer no. 49, 'Paeonia,' 1605–40
4.17	'Aquileia'	Original
4.18	'Verbena'	Macer no. 58, 'Verbena,' 1859–1902
4.19	'Meu'	?
4.20	'Ciperus'	Macer no. 48, 'Cyperus,' 1585–1604
4.21	'Valeriana'	?
4.22	'Boragum'	Macer no. 50, 'Barrocus,' 1641–63
4.23	'Aristologia'	Macer no. 41, 'Aristolochia,' 1395–1436
4.24	'Palma Christi'	Original
4.25	'Savina'	Macer no. 12, 'Sabina,' 492–506

Anglicanus ortus, poem numbers and titles		Main medical sources (with title and lines if relevant)
4	Epilogue 1	?
4	Epilogue 2	Original
5	Prologue	Original
5.1.1	'Plantago'	Macer no. 5, 'Plantago,' 196–266
5.1.2	'Urtica'	Macer no. 4, 'Urtica,' 115–60
5.1.3	'Iusquiamum'	Macer no. 61, 'Iusquiamus,' 1933–61
5.1.4	'Cerifolium'	Macer no. 27, 'Cerefolium,' 928–46
5.1.5	'Lapaphum'	Macer no. 63, 'Paratella,' 1993–2014
5.1.6	'Senecion'	Macer no. 51, 'Senecion,' 1664–89
5.1.7	'Maurella'	Macer no. 60, 'Maurella,' 1918–32
5.1.8	'Ysatis'	Macer no. 55, 'Gaisdo,' 1766–73
5.1.9	'Cynoglossa'	?
5.1.10	'Lolium'	Macer no. 64, 'Lolium,' 2015–28
5.1.11	'Cicuta'	Macer no. 65, 'Cicuta,' 2029–55
5.1.12	'Lappa'	?
5	Interlude	Original
5.2.1	'Cepa'	Macer no. 33, 'Cepa,' 1087–1126
5.2.2	'Porrum'	Macer no. 13, 'Porrum,' 507–48
5.2.3	'Caulis'	Macer no. 36, 'Caulis,' 1201–63
5.2.4	'Atriplex'	Macer no. 28, 'Atriplex,' 947–56
5.2.5	'Petrosilinum' [no. 2]	?
5.2.6	'Allium'	Macer no. 5, 'Allium,' 161–95
6	Prologue	Original
6.1.1	'Piper'	Macer no. 66, 'Piper,' 2056–85 Macer no. 68, 'Gingiber,' 2109–10
6.1.2	'Mirra'	Constantine, 'Myrrha,' 359
6.1.3	'Spicanardus'	Macer no. 75, 'Spica,' 2182–2203
6.1.4	'Garrofilum'	Macer no. 72, 'Gariofilus,' 2141–6
6.1.5	'Cynnama'	Macer no. 73, 'Cinnama,' 2147–64
6.1.6	'Cassia'	Constantine, 'Cassia fistula,' 346–7 Constantine, 'Cassia lignea,' 369
6.1.7	'Galanga'	Macer no. 70, 'Galanga,' 2125–30
6.1.8	'Zeduar'	Macer no. 71, 'Zedoar,' 2131–40
6.1.9	'Ciminum'	Macer no. 69, 'Cyminum,' 2111–24
6.1.10	'Ceroton'	?
6.1.11	'Liquiricia'	Constantine, 'Liquiritia,' 347
6.1.12	'Aloe'	Macer no. 77, 'Aloë,' 2233–69
6	Interlude	Original
6.2.1	'Balsamum'	Constantine, 'Balsamus,' 356–7
6.2.2	'Agaricum'	Constantine, 'Agaricus,' 346
6.2.3	'Amomum'	Constantine, 'Amomum,' 376
6.2.4	'Storax'	Constantine, 'Styrax,' 351
6.2.5	'Mastix'	Constantine, 'De Mastice,' 354

Anglicanus ortus, poem numbers and titles		Main medical sources (with title and lines if relevant)
6.2.6	'Anisum'	Constantine, 'Anisum,' 376
6.2.7	'Genciana'	Constantine, 'Gentiana,' 367
6.2 8	'Euforbium'	Constantine, 'Euphorbium,' 381
6.2.9	'Folium'	Constantine, 'Lolium' [= 'De folio'], 361
6.2.10	'Cardamomum'	Constantine, 'Cardamomum,' 347
6.2.11	'Reu'	Constantine, 'Rheum,' 354
6.2.12	'Epitimum'	Constantine, 'Thymum' [*sic*], 368
6.2.13	'Sagapinum'	Constantine, 'Sagapinum,' 373
6.2.14	'Squinantum'	Constantine, 'Squinantum,' 372
6.2.15	'Thus'	Macer no. 76, 'Thus,' 2204–32
6.2.16	'Squilla'	Constantine, 'Scilla,' 362
6.2.17	'Siler'	Constantine, 'Seseleon,' 364
6.2.18	'Dragagantus'	Constantine, 'Dragagantum,' 360–1
6.2.19	'Diagridium'	?
6.2.20	'Amoniacum'	Constantine, 'Amoniacum,' 375
6.2.21	'Bdellium'	Constantine, 'Bdellium,' 359
6.2.22	'Acorus'	Constantine, 'Acorus,' 355
6.2.23	'Camphora'	Constantine, 'Camphora,' 370
6.2.24	'Nux muscata'	Constantine, 'Nux muscata,' 355
6.2.25	'Nitrum'	Constantine, 'Nitrum,' 384
6.2.26	'Thimus'	?
6.2.27	'Anacardus'	Constantine, 'Anacardi,' 382
6.2.28	'Calamus aromaticus'	Constantine, 'Calamus aromaticus,' 357
6	Epilogue	Original

herb garden (basil, 1.2), or discusses love and the conquest of beautiful maidens (periwinkle, 1.23; columbine, 4.17). In the least modified poems, though, Henry has merely rearranged Macer's words, or has at most provided synonyms for medical terms (*e.g.* oregano, 1.7, and chamomile, 1.13). Some poems are not based on earlier sources and seem drawn from Henry's daily sensory experience: in lavender (1.8), he describes how its pleasing odour protects clothing and books; in the first of two poems on parsley (1.21) he gives delicious recipes for spiced goat and pork; in the poem on meadowsweet (2.13) he provides a recipe for spiced mead; and he describes spicing his wine with germander (1.12) during his student days in Laon.

In some poems Henry shows his originality on the didactic, rather than literary, side. In the very first herbal poem (1.1) Henry glosses Macer's technical vocabulary in the manner of a teacher speaking to a student: after mentioning *opium* he asks of his student or reader, 'What do they call *opium*? "The drink that takes your sense away."'[84] He employs the same tool—one not found in Macer—to explain the possibly unfamiliar medical terms *menstrua*, *steras*, and *hicterici* (poem 1.1, lines 15, 20, 23). This technique is used particularly with feminine medical terms (his expected audience would be solely male clerics or regulars), as in a lengthy explanation of *secundae*, afterbirth, at 3.8, 24–9, in the poem on iris. In a pair of poems, he takes to task the methods of ancient herbalists. Why do the philosophers, he asks in his poem on herb bennet ('Benedicta,' 2.19), name plants according to their shape (*e.g. auricula leporina* = hare's ear) when the common folk wisely name them after their virtues (*benedicta* = herb bennet, *i.e.* 'the blessed herb')? Likewise, the many powers which comfrey (2.20) shares with other herbs provide Henry with a platform to speak on variations of the four humours and on God's reasons for placing useful herbs all around the world.

Since Henry definitely used the works of four different medical authors and possibly those of several others in his herbal, he had to treat each of his sources differently if he was to adapt them into his own style of verse. Naturally, more obvious changes were involved in adapting Constantine's and Pseudo-Apuleius's prose works into verse than in adapting the verse works of Strabo and Macer. Nonetheless, in the case of each author used, Henry took different steps in making the information provided his own. In the following sections I review several cases that illustrate Henry's compositional method by comparing Henry's source and his final product.

2.5.1 *Macer Floridus*

The *De viribus herbarum* of Macer Floridus is Henry's most important source, providing material for about half of the poems in Books 1–5 of the *Anglicanus ortus*. Since Henry used 76 of Macer's 77 poems, only a few examples must suffice to demonstrate Henry's methods of composition when using Macer. Of all of Henry's sources, Macer's poems are the least changed and, for the most part, the longer the poem is in Macer the less Henry has changed it. Henry preserves most of Macer's recipes and ingredients without significant changes, usually rearranging the material and providing synonyms, as can be seen in the following selections:

84 Poem 1.1, line 25: 'Quid dicunt opium? "Que tollit pocio sensum."'

Macer no. 52, 'Chelidonia,' 1699–1703
Florentis succus cum melle coquatur in aere
Igne levi, spumam donec proiecerit omnem
Et quasi crassitiem mellis decoctio sumat;
Utilius nullum dicunt oculis medicamen,
Quos caligo nocet, si sint hoc saepe perunct.

Henry 2.12, 'Celidonia,' 6–9
... Succum florentis in ere
Iunctum melle coquas dum spumam perdat et inde
Crassiciem quamdam mellis decoccio sumat.
Vtilius nichil est oculis caligine pressis.

Macer no. 46, 'Asarum,' 1535–40
Provocat urinam, potataque menstrua purgat,
Hocque modo iecoris medicatur sumpta dolori,
Hydropicosque iuvat, sciasim fugat hausta frequenter,
Et vulvae morbis decoctio subvenit eius.
Dicitur ictericum potata repellere morbum,
Elleborique modo vomitu praecordia purgat ...

Henry 3.6, 'Asarum,' 5–9
Prouocat urinam stipatam flecmate grosso,
Yctericos sed et ydropicos, sciasim quoque sanat.
Pota eciam iecori fit certa medela dolenti;
Menstrua pota uocat, uuluas decoccio sanat,
Et uomitu uelud elleborum precordia purgat.

Macer no. 50, 'Barrocus,' 1641–6
Herbam, quam Graeci dixerunt Mellisophyllon,
Barrocum nostri dicunt vulgariter; illa
Prae cunctis apidbus gratissima dicitur herbis.
Nec gaudere magis ullius flore videntur;
Contritis foliis apium si vasa perungas,
Non fugient ...

Henry 4.22, 'Boragum,' 1–4
Boragum nostri quam 'mellisoffilos' Achiui
Dicunt. Hec apibus cunctis est gracior herbis,
Cui si lac iungas et earum uasa perungas
Non fugient: remanere solent per eam fugientes.

Macer no. 71, 'Thus,' 2227–30
Vim memorem cerebri proprio confortat odore,
Origano iunctum si quis commasticet ipsum,
Humores nocuos capitis per sputa repellit,
Allevat ista gravem capitis purgatio linguam.

Henry 6.2.15, 'Thus,' 2–4
Vim cerebri memorem confortat odore beato.
Origano iunctum qui masticat hoc capitales
Humores per sputa iacit; sic lingua leuatur.

In all of the preceding examples, Henry has condensed the information in Macer into fewer lines while still preserving the necessary details. In other cases, Henry repeats the essential information from Macer but in a more expanded, poetic fashion, such as when he describes the qualities of oregano in four lines where Macer used two:

Macer no. 38, 'Origanum,' 1285–6
Origani vires calidae siccaeque leguntur,
Tertius huic in utroque gradus conceditur esse.

Henry 1.7, 'Origanum,' 1–4
Origani uis exigui feruere probatur;
Origani calor eximii siccare putatur.
Tercius in sicca uirtute gradus datur illi,
Tercius in calida, quociens petit hanc medicina.

Henry has doubled each of Macer's lines by using anaphora (*Origani . . . Origani*, *Tercius in . . . Tercius in*), added descriptive adjectives to the herb (*exigui . . . eximii*), and personified *medicina* in line 4. Such changes are common to many of Henry's poems.

The most typical change Henry makes to Macer's poems, after the initial paraphrasing, is to add a new introduction or conclusion with more details about the herb or in which he places the herb in a wider philosophical, religious, or mythical context. In poem 1.11, 'Ysopum' (hyssop), before a paraphrase of Macer's 'Ysopum,' 1503–31, Henry describes Solomon's praise of hyssop and gives a biblical justification for hyssop's virtues (lines 1–9).[85] In poem 3.2, 'Feniculum,' he compares fennel's great size to the Giants of classical mythology (lines 1–7) before closely adapting Macer's 'Feniculum,' 678–710. In a longer example, in poem 3.3, 'Anetum' (dill), Henry prefaces a paraphrase of Macer's 'Anethum,' 395–428, with a 22-line cosmological exploration of why fennel (in the previous poem, 3.2) and dill look so similar yet effect different cures. Henry's poem 3.17, 'Sinula' (based on Macer's 'Malva,' 1962–92) has a new introduction of seven lines in which he connects the twisting manner in which curled mallow grows to its ability to remove corruption from a patient.

Some poems are a pastiche of sources with Macer providing the core information. For example, in Henry's poem 1.9, 'Salvia' (sage), only lines 12–22 are based on Macer ('Salvia,' 870–81). Lines 1–11 are original, in which he praises sage and the wisdom of Strabo and Macer, both of whom also praised it, and lines 26–35 give a recipe for an antidote featuring sage (the source of which I have not found). In a similar fashion, the middle of Henry's poem 1.12, 'Camedreos' (germander), is based on Macer's 'Chamaedrys,' lines 1903–17, but with an introduction (lines 4–7) describing how Henry and fellow students in Laon mixed the herb into their wine, and a conclusion (lines 19–23) giving the antidote *dyacamedreos* which features germander (not given in Macer). Such a recipe for an antidote featuring the subject herb has

85 All biblical quotations in Latin come from the Vulgate. English quotations are from the New International Version.

been added by Henry in several instances after a paraphrase of one of Macer's poems, as in 3.20, 'Marrubium' (horehound; based primarily on Macer's 'Marrubium,' 1437–55), with a ten-line description of the antidote *dyaprassion* (apparently from Constantine), or 3.23, 'Nepta' (catnip; Macer's 'Nepeta,' 592–625), with the added antidote (lines 26–33) *dyacalamentis* (from Pseudo-Oribasius).

In a few cases, Henry has used Macer's material as the basis for an entirely new poem, and he does this most effectively by creating a dialogue. In some cases, the herb itself speaks, in some Henry adds a voice, and in others authorities from the past or pagan deities speak (as will be seen below in Henry's 'Rosa'). For his poem 3.15, 'Enula' (elecampane), Henry turns Macer's straightforward didactic poem into a conversation between the plant and him:

Macer no. 44, 'Enula,' 1489–93, 1499–1502

Enula, quam Graecus Elnam vocat Eleniumque
Dicitur a medicis, est forma cognita cunctis.
Humida vis eius et fervida dicitur esse,
Humor habere gradum primum, fervorque secundum . . .
. . . Eius radicum pulvis cum melle voratus
Tussim compescit, orthopnoicisque medetur;
Cum succo rutae si sumitur eius,
Affirmant ruptis quod prosit potio talis.

Henry 3.15, 'Enula,' 1–7

'Enula, que tibi uis, quam uulgus nominat elnam?'
'Vis michi feruescens et uis michi contigit humens;
Primo prima gradu uiget atque secunda secundo.'
'Enula, quanta potes, nisi nulla potes, manifesta.'
'Puluis radicum prodest cum melle mearum
Inflatis aut ortomicis, tussique et anhelis,
Et meus et rute succus ruptis medicatur.

Henry begins his poem the same way as Macer, but has apostrophized *Enula*. The medical information is the same, but *Enula* relates it in the first person as an answer to Henry's questions.

One of the most dramatic adaptations of Macer is poem 2.10, 'Rosa,' in which the phrase *flos florum*, used by both Macer and Strabo, is the focus of a conference between the muse Erato, Henry, Macer, and Strabo. Below is a comparison of portions of Henry's poem with portions of Macer's and Strabo's poems on the rose:

Macer no. 21, 'Rosa,' 776–88

Dici flos florum nobis Rosa iure videtur,
Quod specie cunctos praecedat odoreque flores.
Non tamen haec specie tantum nec odore iuvare

Henry 2.10, 'Rosa,' 12–18, 32–40

Sic Dea. Sic Macer: 'Florum flos esse uidetur,
Quod forma pariter precedat odoreque flores.'
'Dic et, Stabe, precor. Sic non grauis irruat ymber,

Nos valet, at variis non adiuvat illa medelis,
Eius sicca gradu vis est et frigida primo.
Compescit sacrum, si trita apponitur, ignem,
Sic quoque, si stomachus calet aut praecordia, sedat;
Fluxum matricis cum vino stringit et alvi,
Illius succum collyria plurima quaerunt,
Et siccae pulvis morbis bene subvenit oris,
Infrictus per se tantum cum melleve mixtus.
Omnes fervores superaddita trita coërcet
Ipsa recens, vel si mulsae commixta bibatur.

Strabo, 'De Rosa', 396–401
Haec, quia non Tyrio Germania tinguitur ostro,
lata nec ardenti se Gallia murice iactat,
lutea purpurei reparat crementa quotannis
ubertim floris, tantum qui protinus omnes
herbarum uicisse comas uirtute et odore
dicitur, ut merito florum flos esse feratur.

Non fera girouaget pegaseos incola fontis,
Dum per amena tui lustras uestigia Macri.'
Sic Dea. Sic Stabus: 'Sic ui, sic uincit odore
Flores, ut merito florum flos esse feratur.' . . .
' . . Flos rosule marcet, uis nullo tempore marcet:
Puluis habet quod flos habuit—uigor equus utrique.
Huius opes et opus colliria multa requirunt;
Infrictus puluis langoribus obuiat oris.
Si caleat stomachus, caleant si uiscera, prosit.
Fluxum matricis, fluxum conterminat alui;
Vt reliquos ignes, sacros exterminat ignes.
Omnis trita recens feruores destruit omnes;
Mitigat ipsa recens si mulse mixta bibatur.'

This poem presents a rare case of Henry quoting his sources (Macer in lines 12–13 and Strabo in 17–18), although in both cases Henry has paraphrased part of the source lines (Macer 776–7 and Strabo 400–401, respectively). Comparison shows that while Henry's medical information comes from Macer's relatively dry report, his highly artificial tone is clearly indebted to Strabo. But where Strabo turns his poem to religious themes, addressing the Virgin and her similarity to the lily and the rose, Henry almost mockingly populates his poem with as many classical pagan figures and locations as possible: Erato, Tempe, Pegasus, Parnassus, Pindus, Aganippe, Etna (see the commentary to poem 2.10 below for more on these examples). In the end, however, Henry uses all of the medical information in Macer's poem, and in those lines he returns to his usual, less creative paraphrasing, *e.g.* Henry's lines 35–8 are very close to Macer's 781–5; Henry simply changes the order of remedies and provides some synonyms.

As should be clear from the preceding comparisons, there are a wide variety of ways in which Henry adapted material from Macer's herbal. This list is not exhaustive and in the commentaries on the poems below I indicate other ways in which Henry has condensed, expanded or otherwise modified Macer's poems.

2.5.2 *Walahfrid Strabo*

Henry's adaptation of Walahfrid Strabo's *Hortulus* is curious and markedly different from his adaptation of Macer. As noted above, even though much of Henry's style is similar to Strabo's, only five of Henry's poems are based primarily on poems in the *Hortulus*, and only two of those treat the same plants as their main sources (1.6, 'Ambrosia,' and 3.21, 'Sclarega'). The other three poems which are based on lines from the *Hortulus* treat different plants than their sources: Henry's poem 1.16 ('Costus') takes material from Strabo's 'De Sclarega' (lines 275–83), 2.18 ('Pipera') from Strabo's 'De Agrimonia' (lines 359–68), and 3.7 ('Macedonia') from Strabo's 'De Cerfolio' (lines 235–47). Henry's adaptation of Strabo's 'De Sclarega,' on clary sage, shows his ability to take a small amount of information in his source and stretch it into a much longer work—in this case, two separate poems. Below is Strabo's poem next to the two of Henry's it inspired:

Strabo, 'De Sclarega,' 275–83

Hic umbrosa nouos inter sclarega uirores,
stipite preualido assurgens, ramosque comasque
altius extollit. Quae quamuis rarius ulli
quaesita auxilio, medicorum paene putetur
effugisse manus, dulci tamen indita caldae
et vires et odorati fermenta saporis
prestat; eam iuxta hortensis non extima costi
silua latet, stomachique moras uentremque salubri
prouocat auxilio radicis munere coctae.

Henry 3.21, 'Sclarega'

Viginti uisis uiridis sclarega uidetur!
A medicis dulci calde conferre putatur
Et uires et odorati fermenta saporis.
Dat rauco sclarega sonum clarissima clarum
Sed nec pulmoni nec uisceribus fit inepta.
Hec et multa potest que uel tacuere scientes
Vel non nouerunt (nec cuncta sciunt sapientes).

Henry 1.16, 'Costus'

Ortensis costi sedes prefulget in orto,
Est etenim costum species a nomine cuius
Herba trahit nomen, quasi non deceat speciosam
Nomine signari nisi preclare speciei.
Si numeras herbas redolentes hanc numerabis;
Si numeras medicis acceptas hanc numerabis,
Huius enim radix fuerit si cocta parumper
Aut oleo uel aqua (si munus desit oliue)
Prouocat auxilio stomachum uentremque salubri.
Et quia sunt multi qui nolunt credere multis
Ambiguaque fide tarde raris quoque credunt,
Ne finxisse putent, uerbum non amplius addam.

Comparison shows that Henry adapted or directly copied every part of Strabo's poem, but added much more to each of his two new poems and gave each a new focus. Strabo's main interest in clary sage was its shape and, while he does mention its heating virtue and flavour, he does not specify the cures it could effect. Henry, in his poem on the same herb, has borrowed the description of the plant's *dulci calde* and simply copied outright Strabo's line 280, but has added three specific cures, not bothering at all to describe the plant's appearance. Strabo is not named, and his material is now referred to unnamed *medicis*. The final two lines of Henry's 'Sclarega' make much more sense when read in light of Henry's source: he seems to be criticizing Strabo (as one of the *scientes* or *sapientes*), who shows that he 'does not know everything' (*nec cuncta sciunt*) by not providing specific remedies in his poem.

The final three lines of Strabo's 'De Sclarega' mention a new plant, cost; Henry used these lines for part of a poem dedicated entirely to this plant. Lines 1, 7, and 9 of Henry's 'Costus' clearly come from Strabo's 'De Sclarega,' but the rest of Henry's poem is original. In lines 2–4 he explores why a herb and a spice have the nearly identical names *costus* and *costum*, and in lines 5–6 he adds a poetic flourish announcing the herb's pleasant odour and medicinal qualities, which in turn leads to the medical information borrowed from Strabo. Henry, though, in line 8 adds a detail to the remedy, specifying that cost can be cooked in oil or water, when Strabo simply said the root should be cooked. In the final three lines of the poem on cost Henry as usual adds a remark about belief and authority, just as he does at the end of his poem 3.21 on clary sage. Henry's composition of these two poems indicates certain patterns in how he used the *Hortulus*: he admired Strabo's poetic skill but found him lacking in medical information. While Henry adds medical details and commentary on medical authorities, he usually simplifies the verse itself. Strabo tended to employ the more tortuous classical literary devices, such as enjambment, synchysis and hyperbaton, which Henry rarely employs in the herbal.

2.5.3 *Pseudo-Apuleius*

The herbal of Pseudo-Apuleius provided Henry with much of the medical information he was looking for without any of the graceful style of a Strabo. Henry thus adds little technical information to the five poems based directly on Pseudo-Apuleius, but had to exercise his poetic muscles to put that information into verse. Henry clearly enjoyed providing synonyms for each plant, usually at the start of a poem, and Pseudo-Apuleius was one of the best sources for those synonyms. For example, Pseudo-Apuleius gives the many names of 'Herba Personacia' (no. 36, pp. 81–2) after its cures: 'A Graecis dicitur prosopis, alii Bachhion, alii elefantosis, alii elefas, Itali personacia, alii bardana, alii manifolium, Galli betilolen, Daci riborasta.' Henry greatly simplifies this list in his poem 1.18, 'Beta maior,' but places the synonyms at the start of the poem (lines 1–4) and makes the plant's multiple names one of its key features:

> Ordine que sequitur hec 'personatia' Rome,
> 'Prosopes' a Grecis, a uulgo 'beta' uocatur.
> Nec mirum si, tam Grecis quam nota Latinis,
> Splendeat et presit cum multis sepeque prosit.

After this the poem is a relatively straightforward versification of the seven remedies given by Pseudo-Apuleius, but as he is wont to do, Henry adds a comment at the end of the poem (lines 15–17) about his medical authorities and whether he believes them:

> Sed quid ego? Cum certa lego, non hec nego, sed cum
> Talia conspicio, non funditus assero laudans
> Talia sumere, sumpta probare, probata tenere.

Nor should we be surprised that in these wholly original lines Henry shows off his poetic skill, employing a curious triple rhyme in line 15 which does not rhyme with the caesura, which is in turn echoed by the three-stage rhetorical climax in the final line.

In a similar fashion, Henry based most of his poem 2.1, 'Mandragora,' on Pseudo-Apuleius no. 131 (pp. 222–5), 'Effectus herbae mandragorae,' but added an introduction (lines 1–10) in which he explains in detail the similarities between a mandrake root and the human body, a fact which Pseudo-Apuleius does not mention, most likely assuming his readers know it already. Henry heightens the almost magical sympathy between man and root by borrowing liberally from Ovid's *Metamorphoses* in these lines (see the commentary to poem 2.1 below). But when Henry comes to the famous description of how to gather the mandrake without being killed by its deadly scream, he condenses Pseudo-Apuleius's twenty-two lines of prose to a mere six lines of verse (lines 12–17) and casts doubt (as he often does) on the truth of the story (*non hoc tamen assero firme*, line 12). The rest of Pseudo-Apuleius's passage is a list of remedies which Henry apparently found more rational and acceptable, for he closely paraphrases them in verse for the rest of the poem (lines 18–36).

In three other poems (1.22, 2.20, 3.12) Henry uses Pseudo-Apuleius to add medical information to passages not of a strictly medical nature. In the example below, Henry understood (probably incorrectly) Pseudo-Apuleius's *sisimbrium* (horsemint) to be a synonym for the famous *balsama*, or balsam:

Pseudo-Apuleius no. 106 (p. 189), 'Herba Sisimbrium'

1. Ad uesicae dolorem et stranguiriam. Herbam sisimbrium contritum excepto suco scripulos II, febricitanti ex aqua calida, non febricitanti ex uino potui dabis, remediabis mire.

Henry 3.12, 'Balsama'

Balsama scribantur multo lustrata decore;
Balsama scribantur grato dilecta sapore;
Balsama scribantur que precellant et odore.
Hoc et 'terralis' solet atque 'sisimbria' dici.
Hinc faciet succum procurator febrientum,
Cuius aqua scrupulos calida geminos det anhelis;
Quod si uesice dolor aut stranguria subsit,
Cum uino succum dabis et morbos releuabis.

Not surprisingly, Henry praises the odour and flavour of *balsama* with anaphoric repetition in lines 1–3, and uses those marvellous qualities as an explanation (*Hinc*, line 5) for the medicinal remedies in lines 5–8 which he learned from Pseudo-Apuleius. In a similar fashion, Henry's poem 1.22, 'Solsequium' (calendula), is primarily about the flower's miraculous ability to follow the sun and only lines 16–21 relate its medicinal qualities as learned from Pseudo-Apuleius no. 49 (pp. 99–100), 'Herba Heliotropia,' while much of Henry's poem 2.20, 'Conferba' (comfrey), is a general discussion of humoural medicine and herbal remedies and only lines 17–24 paraphrase the remedies in Pseudo-Apuleius no. 59 (pp. 112–13), 'Herba Confirma.' In these cases we can see that Henry valued the medical information provided by Pseudo-Apuleius but had to change the stilted Late Antique Latin dramatically so that the material fit into his more artful literary production.

2.5.4 *Constantine the African*

Twenty-eight of Henry's poems (perhaps twenty-nine: poem 6.2.26 is in question), all found in Book 6, are based on entries from Constantine the African's *Liber graduum*.[86] Most of these poems are relatively short (shorter than most poems based on Macer) and present little information beyond what is in the *Liber graduum*. Usually Henry summarizes the spice's medicinal virtues, rearranging the order of Constantine's material, yet still providing most of his remedies in a condensed fashion. Where Henry does add material, he adds his usual praises of the plant's virtues, apostrophizes it, or refers its medicinal qualities to God or *Natura*. For example, in poem 6.2.3, 'Amomum' (bastard cardamom), Henry versifies a brief entry in the *Liber graduum*, but devotes

86 A more detailed discussion of how Henry, Macer, and other authors versified Constantine's *Liber graduum* is found in Black, '"I will add what the Arab once taught": Constantine the African in Northern European medical verse'.

four lines of new material to introducing the spice as 'gift of God', costly and famous for both its odour and its virtues:

Constantine, 'Amomum', 376	**Henry 6.2.3, 'Amomum'**
Amomum calidum et siccum in tertio gradu. Muliere in eius apozemate sedente, dolor uuluae placabitur. Pessarium illud operatur, et menstrua prouocat. Apozema potatum, optimum est epilepticis, nephreticis et podagricis.	Dulce Dei donum, mirabile fraglat amomum Quod quam famosum tam crediderim preciosum. Hoc igitur famam preciumque meretur odore; Si non esset odor, reniteret utrimque uigore, Nam uicium dire solet extirpare podagre Eius si fuerit tantum decoccio pota, Sic et nefreticis et sic prodest epilensi. Subdita si uulue mulieris forte sedentis Hec decoccio sit, uulue dolor adnichilatur. Hec et multa potest, que longum multa referre. Tercius huic gradus est in ui sicca calidaque.

We can see here a typical example of how Henry adapted material from Constantine, using it as the core of his poem, while adding new information and a religious context. There is no indication in Constantine's entry that *amomum* has a pleasing odor; he no doubt expected his readers to know this and so there was no need to state the fact. For Henry, its marvellous odour is central to his depiction of the spice, so he begins the poem with lines praising that aspect, which are made all the more dramatic by the internal and end rhymes. Constantine almost always states a herb's Galenic degrees at the start of an entry, as he does in this case, but Henry has moved that detail to the end of his poem. Moreover, Henry expands Constantine's brief statement that 'Apozema potatum, optimum est . . . podagricis' into all of lines 4–7 of his poem, and he has replaced both instances of *apozema* with the more common word *decoccio*, which has the added benefit of scanning in hexameter verse. It is not clear why Henry omitted Constantine's emmenagogue, but since he never uses the word *pessarium* (frequently used by Constantine), perhaps he simply omitted a statement he did not understand.

In a similar case, most of Henry's poem 6.2.1 (lines 5–31), 'Balsamum' (balm of Gilead), is a paraphrase of Constantine's 'Balsamus' (356–7), but with the following lines as introduction:

> Sunt summi precii prestancia balsama mire,
> Sunt et opis summe medicancia balsama mire.
> Hec Natura parens summo dotauit honore,
> Omnis et hec mundus summo dignatur odore.

Constantine, writing a practical pharmacological manual, probably intended for a learned physician, does not indulge in elaborate hyperbole or invocations of supernatural beings. Henry, however, is writing poetry and the famous spice balsam gives him the opportunity to attribute its marvellous odour and medicinal virtue to the power of 'Mother Nature' (*Natura parens*).

One of the poems based on Constantine (6.1.6, 'Cassia') is unique in that Henry composed it from two different entries. This poem shows how thoroughly Henry could, when inclined, rework prose sources into a poem. Constantine devoted separate entries to *cassia fistula* (fruit) and *cassia lignea* (bark). Henry recognized that these two ingredients belonged to the same plant and condensed their attributes into a single poem dedicated to the entire plant (I have italicized those lines based on Constantine's 'Cassia fistula'):

Constantine, 'Cassia fistula,' 346–7

Cassia fistula mediocris est inter calidum et frigidum. Vnde Galenus: medicina temperata aequali compositioni uel complexioni similis neque in calidum, neque in frigidum et humidum et siccum potest iudicari. Proprie choleram rubeam purgat, acumen sanguinis extinguit, et apostema ex eo genitum dissoluit. Gargarizata apostemata gulae et faucium curat, praecipue si misceatur cum succo stringni.

Constantine, 'Cassia lignea,' 369

Cassia lignea calida et sicca in tertio gradu. Stomachum, epar, uulnera, et omnia principalia membra confortat, oppilationem aperit, et grossos humores et uentositatem dissoluit, urinam et menstrua prouocat. Muliere in eius apozemate sedente, mox uulua confortatur. Suffumigata ex ea, dolor uuluae placatur, et eius oppilatio aperitur. Si uero cum medicina laxatiua misceatur, ad eijciendos grossos humores, iuuat. Cum melle temperata et super dura et humida apostemata imposita ea dissoluit et curat. Cleopatra cinnamomum alithinum pro cassia lignea, et cassiam ligneam pro cinnamomo posuit. Dioscorides duplum pondus cinnamomo pro uno cassiae poni iussit.

Henry 6.1.6, 'Cassia'

Cassia non eadem que cassia fistula confert,
Cassia namque gradu feruet siccatque secundo
Sed Galienus ait quod cassia fistula prestet
Inter utrosque gradus. Calidam nec iudicat ipsam,
Nec frigescentem, nec humentem, neque siccam—
Tanta temperie dedit hanc Natura uigere.
Cassia sumpta iecur confortat, * * * * sterasque
Cunctaque primatum retinencia corpore membra
At rubeam coleram bene cassia fistula purgat.
Cassia confortat ualide muliebria membra
Eius si tepido sint apozimate fota;
Sanguinis extinguit uim cassia fistula diram.
Cassia uentosas dissoluit rite querelas;
Soluit apostema sic cassia fistula durum
Quod cruor ipse creat, nec quicquid soluit ut ipsa.
Cassia purificans grossis humoribus obstat;
Rumpit apostema bene cassia fistula bucce.
Cassia si ueniat, fugit opilacio uulue;
Gargarizetur si cassia fistula curat
Eque gingiuas, fauces uuasque tumentes
Et melius stringni succus si iungitur illi.
Vix igitur uideas quenam precellit earum
Viribus excelsis eque uires utriusque.
Cinnama Cleopatra, si desit cassia, ponit
At Dyascoride aliter nam cinnama duplat;
Cinnama si desint eadem, te, cassia, ponit.
Elige quem pocius (nam summus uterque) sequaris.

Henry could have versified Constantine's two entries merely in the order they were written, but he has instead thoroughly blended the two, alternating between *cassia fistula* and *cassia* (for *cassia lignea*) in order to compare their respective qualities and effects: *cassia fistula* in lines 3–6, 9, 12, 14–15, 17, and 19–21, and *cassia lignea* in lines 2, 7–8, 10–11, 13, 16, and 18. The poem is thus more effectively didactic than Constantine's entries, as it presents the reader with multiple ingredients taken from a single tree. By means of this series of comparisons, Henry can outline for the practicing physician or apothecary important conclusions that could be missed by reading Constantine's two entries separately: the *lignea* and *fistula* effect different cures, *cassia fistula* is remarkable and very useful for its overall balance of qualities (*temperies*), yet both are excellent for their numerous virtues. By providing these alternating comparisons of the parts of cassia, Henry's poem serves in many ways as a gloss or commentary on its source.

2.5.5 *Pliny the Elder*

An unresolved question concerning Henry's sources is whether or not he used Pliny the Elder's *Natural History*. Four poems (1.22, 4.12, 4.14, 4.15) contain passages which are more similar to the *Natural History* than to any other source I have found, but none of them are so close as to prove definitively that it was indeed the source. Because there is still doubt about this issue, it is useful to present here all the passages in question so that another may be able to make a definite connection:

Pliny 22. 57 Heliotropi miraculum saepius diximus cum sole se circumagentis etiam nubilo die, tantus sideris amor est. Noctu velut desiderio contrahit caeruleum florem.	**Henry 1.22, 'Solsequium,' 1–4** Herbe florentis que cernitur ordine certo 'Solsequia' est nomen nobis, elitropia Grecis. Aureus huic flos est quem tanto nutrit amore Vt uix cogat eum uel yemps inuisa perire.
Pliny 24. 184 Vis eius siccare, mollire, dissolvere. Sucus decocti feminarum pluribus malis subvenit, sive duritia sive tumor sive contractio sit vulvae, foventur, insidunt. Infusum quoque prodest. **Pliny 24. 186** Farinam feni cum hordeo aut lini semine decoctam aqua mulsa contra vulvae cruciatus obiecit idem inposuit imo ventri.	**Henry 4.12, 'Fenugrecum'** Insilit in cetum, mollire studens, fenugrecum; Duricias mollit collecturasque resoluit; Si tamen alteam, maluam quoque iunxeris illi, Quas bene sola domat melius sociata domabit. Semen item lini cum polline iungitur illi: Non encathisma restabit ad hoc cataplasma. Cum fenugreco caulem tundas et aceto: Molliet artheticos gratum cataplasma dolores Et poterit seuam saltem lenire podagram.

Pliny 24. 187

Si vero cum malva decoquatur postea addito mulso, potus ante cetera vulvis interaneisque laudatur, quippe cum vapor quoque decocti plurimum prosit

Pliny 19, 167–68

Git pistrinis, anesum et anetum culinis et medicis nascuntur . . . hoc [*i.e.* papaver] et panis rustici crustae inspergitur, adfuso ovo inhaerens, ubi inferiorem crustam apium gitque Cereali sapore condiunt.

Pliny 27. 121

Semen [*i.e.* pelecinos] in siliquis fert corniculorum modo aduncis ternis quaternisve, quale git novimus, amarum, stomacho utile. Additur in antidota.

Henry 4.14, 'Git'

Git cornute, tuos depromit Musa triumphos!
Quatuor aduersis in celum cornibus audes
Tendere, collectis in summam uiribus arcem,
In qua grana locas mirum latura saporem.
Hic in pane sapor panem longe meliorat
Et causa effectum preciosa parat preciosum.

Pliny 27. 113, 116

Qui plura genera polygoni faciunt hanc marem intelligi volunt appellarique a multitudine seminis aut densitate fruticis. . . . Quartum genus silvestre appellatur, paene arboris modo frutex . . .

Henry 4.15, 'Gazara,' 1–3

Gazara uero quid est, namque herba putatur et arbor?
Arbor namque potest herbas imitata uocari
Consimilisque potest herba arboribus reputari.

Comparison of the four passages by Henry with the relevant passages by Pliny shows that some similarities are in description alone: both Pliny and Henry remark how one variety of *polygonum* or *gazara* (both probably names for a knotgrass) could be mistaken for a tree, and both note that *git* is added to breads. Some similarities are in both description and vocabulary, as in the case of the great love felt between the sun and both Pliny's *heliotropum* (*tantus . . . amor*) and Henry's *elitropia* (*tanto . . . amore*), or when both describe git's seed as resembling four horns ('corniculorum modo aduncis ternis quaternisve' at Pliny 27. 121; 'Git cornute . . . / Quatuor aduersis in . . . cornibus' at Henry 4.14, 1–2). All of these cases of shared description could be attributed to coincidence, if we assume Henry knew the plants in question and made the same observations as Pliny. However, coincidence cannot explain the numerous parallels between Henry's and Pliny's descriptions of fenugreek. According to Henry, fenugreek 'duricias mollit collecturasque resoluit' (line 2), while Pliny's language is almost the same: 'mollire, dissolvere . . . duritia.' Pliny calls for *malva* (mallow) to be added to fenugreek in order to treat similar conditions of the womb, and Henry does as well (line 3). Finally, both authors call for fenugreek to be mixed with linseed, although they seem to be for different cures (*vulvae cruciatus* in Pliny, *encathisma* in Henry; see the commentary on poem 4.12, line 6). In conclusion, there is no single phrase in Henry's poems which stands out as obviously dependent on Pliny, but the similarities noted above are too close to ignore.

2.6 *Metre, Rhyme and Rhetoric*

Henry wrote the *Anglicanus ortus* as much as an exercise in verse as a medical manual. A. G. Rigg, before his initial discovery of the herbal, had already marked Henry as a 'versatile and imaginative poet.'[87] Henry's poetic style, dependent primarily on dactylic hexameters, occasionally as leonines with internal and end rhymes, was typical of the late eleventh and twelfth centuries. He has much in common with nearly contemporary poets like Reginald of Canterbury (died after 1109) or those in northern France such as Hildebert of Lavardin (1056–1133), Baudri of Bourgueil (Baldricus of Dol, 1046–1130), Marbode of Rennes (1035–1123), and Macer Floridus (later eleventh century), Henry's main source.[88] Henry's verse lapidary is primarily an imitation of Marbode's own verse lapidary,[89] while Henry's master at Lincoln cathedral was one Albinus,[90] recruited from the cathedral of Angers in the Loire region, from whom he would have learned grammar, poetics, and rhetoric as they were practiced in northern France in the late eleventh century. The poetry of this circle is known for its humanism and for the combination of classical themes and metres with contemporary poetic devices like alliteration and disyllabic rhymes.[91]

Henry used unrhymed dactylic hexameters for all poems on herbal ingredients. Only in the prologues does he use other metres, showing off his metrical talents:[92]

87 A. G. Rigg, *A History of Anglo-Latin Literature, 1066–1422* (Cambridge 1992), 40.

88 On Reginald, see Rigg, *A History of Anglo-Latin Literature*, 24–30; Michael Lapidge, 'Some Latin poems as evidence for the reign of Athelstan,' *Anglo-Saxon England* 9 (1981), 61–98, at 67–9; and *HA* cxi–cxii. On the influence of Hildebert, Baudri, and Marbode in England, see Rigg, *A History of Anglo-Latin Literature*, 63–4. A still-useful survey of these eleventh-century poets can be found in F. J. E. Raby, *A History of Secular Latin Poetry in the Middle Ages*, 2 vols (Oxford 1934; repr. Oxford 1997), 1. 307–55.

89 Black, 'Henry of Huntingdon's lapidary,' 64–5.

90 *HA* xv.

91 This discussion of metre is indebted to Rigg's Appendix on Anglo-Latin metre in *A History of Anglo-Latin Literature*, 313–29, which is illustrated with examples of Henry's verse in the *Historia Anglorum*.

92 Henry's talent for a variety of classical and modern metres, as displayed in the *Historia Anglorum*, is explored by Rigg in 'Henry of Huntingdon's metrical experiments.'

Prose Prologue, opening couplet	Elegiac couplet
1 Prologue	Elegiac couplets
2 Prologue	Rhymed couplets in imitation of Boethius, *De cons. phil.* 1 met. 2
3 Prologue	Sapphics
4 Prologue	Adonics
5 Prologue	Dactylic hexameters
6 Prologue	Elegiac couplets

Alliteration is one of his favourite devices, and is evident in his very first poem in the *Historia Anglorum* ('O Adonai,' in *HA* 6–9). In the *Anglicanus ortus* alliteration is often used in the first line of a poem to start it off with a flourish: 'laudata lauandula lecto' (1.8, 1), 'Viginti uisis uiridis sclarega uidetur!' (3.21, 1), 'Gratificat gratos galanga' (6.1.7, 1), 'Cum calamus sit aromaticus uirtute coruscus' (6.2.28, 1). In poem 4.21 on valerian, Henry takes every opportunity to alliterate and pun *ualeriana* with forms of *ualere* (lines 4, 5, 12), compounded by another *uiginti uisis* since it is the twenty-first poem of the book. Elision is uncommon, but there are a few examples, such as 'Preterea innumeris perhibent occurrere morbis' (1.9, 23), or, in an extreme case, 'Arthetica, in manibus ciragra, in pedibusque podagra' (1.10, 38), where he seems to be showing off how many words he can fit into one hexameter line.

Anaphora and parallel structure are not uncommon and are used to reiterate important points or an impressive turn of phrase. In poem 1.16, lines 5–6 begin and end in the same manner:

Si numeras herbas redolentes hanc numerabis;
Si numeras medicis acceptas hanc numerabis . . .

Elsewhere, all of lines 17–24 of poem 3.18 begin with 'Hoc iuuat'; lines 15–17 of poem 5.1.9 begin with 'Hec oculos ualide'; and in poem 4.23, lines 11–16 and 17–20 begin with 'Hec in aqua' and 'Cum uino,' respectively. In Epilogue 1 to Book 4, three lines (10–12) on the caper spurge begin with 'Lactea lacteridis' ('milky Caper Spurge'). Alliteration and repetition might grow monotonous to modern ears, but they show an artistry and attention to detail that Macer Floridus lacked in his verse herbal.

Henry occasionally uses rhyme, often in the first line of a poem, but sometimes wherever the mood strikes him or the words allow. Leonine hexameters—rhyming between the caesura and end—are common throughout: 'Hoc eciam dentes curabis sepe dolentes' (1.11, 28), 'Cum locio splenem purgare simulque lienem' (1.13, 29), or 'Destruit ad plenum uictor quodcumque uenenum' (1.22, 21). Only rarely do leonines appear in pairs:

Hinc non maiestas, non est minuenda potestas,
Nec minuendus honor dum claram reddere conor.

(1.10, 5–6)

Some rhymes highlight the importance (or discomfort) of a cure, such as the following example, used twice: 'Et reddet sanum si tantum subditur anum' (3.17, 18), 'Illius et sanum reddet subiecta per anum' (3.19, 7). A favourite rhyme seems to have been *figmenta—pigmenta*, also used twice (2.15, 9, and 4.24, 9–10). Elsewhere he employed repetition of a final syllable (not exactly rhyme) throughout a couplet, as in this case with seven words ending in *-is*:

Nobis herba nimis multis accepta medelis,
Emplastris, solet antidotis dari preciosis . . .

(5.1.3, 26–7)

Less common are lines such as the following with *caudati* end rhymes:

Hac etenim ueniente fugit, uenit hac fugiente.
Hec estate uiret, bruma uiret ille rigente . . .

(1.3, 6–7)

Huc illucque means, remeans quoque, sinula salue,
Nulli certa loco, species clarissima malue!

(3.17, 1–2)

There is one example of an impressive *cruciferi*, where the caesura of one line rhymes with the end of the other, and *vice versa*:

Dum radians Phebus rapidi tenet ora Leonis,
Sicque quater denis debet feruere diebus.

(1.7, 40–1)

Henry also combines end rhymes with more experimental metrical forms, such as *trinini salientes* ('jumping threesomes') where there are two caesurae in each line and both rhyme, or lines without caesurae that consist of three units (hence, *tripertitus*), the first of which are dactyls (*dactylici tripertiti*) or dactyls followed by spondees (*hexametri tripertiti*). In the first case, a pair of *trinini salientes* rhymes at each caesura and each end:

Vim piperis, uim gingiberis similes perhibemus
Vnde tuam, piper, atque suam uim consociemus

(6.1.1, 11–12)

In this second case, he combines two three-unit lines without caesurae with an internal rhyme in the first two units of each; in the first line the two rhyming units are dactyls, in the second a spondee and a dactyl:

> Preterea, munitus ea, medicamine grato
> Empicos et pleureticos cum melle iuuato.
>
> (1.17, 9–10)

He also mixed forms. For example, he ends a normal end-rhymed pair with a *dactylicus tripertitus*:

> At ciperi solus puluis melliue coherens
> Vlcera sordida, uulnera putrida purgat inherens.
>
> (4.20, 16–17)

In poem 2.18, *Pipera*, he wraps two *hexametri tripertiti* around a normal hexameter:

> Flos niueus, flos exiguus, flos undique densus,
> Cuius si uires queras paucis tibi subdam:
> Vulnera mundat, mundaque sanat, sana colorat.
>
> (2.18, 6–8)

The first line is particularly masterful in that the second and third *flos* each end a spondee but begin a new phrase, pulling the reader forward in an aggressive manner at odds with the topic of delicate white flowers.

Henry similarly wraps special lines around a normal hexameter in poem 1.18, where he wants to emphasize his rational thinking. He begins with a triple rhyme which leads to a rhetorical and grammatical climax supported by *dactylici tripertiti*:

> Sed quid ego? Cum certa lego, non hec nego, sed cum
> Talia conspicio, non funditus assero laudans
> Talia sumere, sumpta probare, probata tenere.
>
> (1.18, 15–17)

An extreme example of his experimentation can be found in poem 3.1 on dittany, where he combines a *dactylicus tripertitus* with *trinini salientes*:

> Hec simul omnibus una sequentibus eminet herba,
> Vnde prehit sceptrumque uehit splendore superba.
>
> (3.1, 3–4)

The combination of one line without caesura followed by another with two creates one of the cleverest couplets in the entire work, as the line seems to march jerkily along with dittany, sceptre held aloft. Henry was not afraid to use any topic at hand to exercise his poetic skills.

2.7 *Henry of Huntingdon and Twelfth-Century Medicine*

The *Anglicanus ortus* belongs to the tradition of herbals called 'simples,' in which each entry or poem treats the attributes of only one herb or spice, which is administered alone or as the featured ingredient in a compound. This model was perfected by Dioscorides in his *De materia medica*, which was widely imitated in both the Greek and Latin herbal traditions. The classical Latin work with the greatest influence on medieval herbalism was Pliny the Elder's *Natural History*, in which Pliny recorded the virtues of hundreds of separate plants, especially in Books 24–7. The works of Dioscorides and Pliny would form the backbone of early medieval herbal literature, and no significant changes would occur in European herbal medicine until the translation of new works from Arabic in the eleventh and twelfth centuries which changed European medicine in terms of content, introducing a wide range of Middle Eastern and Asian *materia medica* to the older Mediterranean tradition, and in terms of method, reintroducing and popularizing Hippocratic and Galenic medical theory.

In Henry's herbal, like most others, *herba* refers broadly to any ingredient used in *materia medica*, including spices, trees, fruits, gums, aromatics, animal parts, and even stones and gems. As is the case with most medieval herbals, the reader is assumed to be familiar with the herbs, and therefore the poems cannot be used easily for botanical identification or the practical collection of herbs. The appearance and shape of the plants are rarely described except in relation to the name (such as *cynoglossa*, hound's-tongue, poem 5.1.9, lines 1–5) or in cases where it might easily be confused with another plant (pleasant *camomilla* and stinking *amaruscus*, 1.13, 5–9).

Most poems follow a common pattern:

1) an introduction to the herb, its varieties and synonyms (Latin, Greek, or *uulgus*, *i.e.* Norman French);
2) a comparison to other herbs, often the one immediately preceding it;
3) an explanation of its qualities (hot or cold and dry or wet) and their respective strengths (first through fourth degree) according to Galenic pharmacotherapy;[93]

93 On the medical system of four qualities in four degrees, best known through Galen, see Erich Schöner, *Das Viererschema in der antiken Humoralpathologie*, Sudhoffs Archiv, Beiheft 4 (Wiesbaden 1964), and Georg Harig, *Bestimmung der Intensität im medizinischen system Galens: ein Beitrag zur theoretischen Pharmakologie, Nosologie und Therapie in der galenischen Medizin* (Berlin 1974).

4) and, finally, the longest section, a description of the therapeutic uses of the herb, often separated into simple remedies for individual parts of the body followed by those for the whole body. Many of the poems provide remedies following the *a capite ad calcem* pattern typical of ancient and medieval medical receipts. Occasionally complex recipes, called 'antidotes' by Henry and other herbalists, which feature the main ingredient at hand are included at the end of the poem.[94]

Many herbals, like those of Dioscorides and Pseudo-Apuleius, also include descriptions of a plant's habitat and appearance. Henry rarely gives this sort of information.

As a work of botany or medicine, the *Anglicanus ortus* is highly derivative and contains little original material. It is as a work of creative literature, representative of changing views of nature in the twelfth century, however, that the *Anglicanus ortus* deserves to be known. During Henry's lifetime and the following generation, a flurry of works which could be called creative natural philosophy appeared: Adelard of Bath's *Quaestiones naturales*, Bernardus Silvestris's *Cosmographia*, Alan of Lille's *De planctu Naturae*, and the sequences of Hildegard of Bingen, to name a few.[95] All of these works share a new view of nature as an intelligible system of universal laws which is indelibly a part of God, yet can work independently of Him. It is common for these authors to personify *Natura* as a goddess or a daughter of God. Henry's poem can be seen as a forerunner of this philosophical and literary movement, though not yet a full member. He is more interested in showing his classical learning than any familiarity with contemporary philosophy, which nonetheless did exercise some influence on his understanding of medicine.

His literary influences appear dramatically as characters: Apollo, god of doctors, prepares wreaths for Henry, who humorously portrays himself as the inept poet laureate of herbal medicine, and the poet Martial appears as an irate Cook, scolding Henry for ignoring the kitchen vegetables.[96] God and

94 For a concise history of the medieval medical recipe, see the introduction to Tony Hunt, *Popular Medicine in Thirteenth-Century England* (Cambridge 1990), 1–16.

95 The *Quaestiones naturales* are printed in Adelard of Bath, *Conversations with His Nephew*, 81–227; Bernardus Silvestris, *The* Cosmographia *of Bernardus Silvestris*, trans. Winthrop Wetherbee (New York 1973); Alan of Lille, *The Plaint of Nature*, trans. with commentary by James J. Sheridan, Mediaeval Sources in Translation 26 (Toronto 1980). For a discussion of nature in Hildegard's sequences, see Peter Dronke, *Poetic Individuality in the Middle Ages. New Departures in Poetry, 1000–1150*, 2nd ed. (London 1986), 159–60. Key studies of the concept of *natura* in the twelfth century are Peter Dronke, 'Bernard Silvestris, Natura, and personification,' *Journal of the Warburg and Courtauld Institutes* 43 (1980), 16–31, and George D. Economou, *The Goddess Natura in Medieval Literature* (Cambridge, MA 1972; repr. with a new introduction, Notre Dame, IN 2002).

96 On the cognomen *Cocus* for Martial see Maaz, *Lateinische Epigrammatik im hohen Mittelalter*, 262–7.

the Virgin Mary also make brief appearances, but fleetingly, as if they do not really belong in a work of natural philosophy. The new emphasis on nature—seen in Henry's familiarity with newer scientific works such as William of Conches's *Philosophia Mundi* and the translations of Constantine the African—is present, however, and most apparent in the frequent appearance of Nature herself, personified. Unlike Apollo and the Cook, she does not speak, but it is she who endows plants with medicinal properties, dictates the arrangement of the garden, balances the qualities of plants and through that balance helps heal an imbalance of humours in our bodies.

For the most part, the curative properties of herbs are not questioned or examined in any detail; it is assumed that Nature, that aspect of God that governs the ordered, physical universe, has given every plant a specific function and it is up to the philosopher to discover it. In only a few poems does Henry venture into more difficult terrain, tentatively approaching questions of theoretical medicine or even cosmology. In poem 2.20 on comfrey he tries to settle doubts about 'why He who granted every good would give the same power to so many herbs.'[97] He answers this doubt with a brief exposition of Galenic medicine, explaining the four humours and four qualities which govern every body and every plant. In his poem on dill (3.3), Henry uses the similar appearance of dill and fennel as a path to loftier themes, discussing the relationship of *hyle*, or primal matter, and the elements. While reminiscent of Claudian's passage on the elements in *De raptu Proserpinae* and Boethius's Platonic hymn 'O qui perpetua,'[98] it also shows that Henry was familiar with recent developments in natural philosophy. Natural bodies are composed not of elements, he explains, but of *elementata* (the 'elementing' or 'elementated'), indivisible particles of matter upon which the elemental properties have been impressed. We cannot see the actual elements, but rather the products of their conjunctions and conflicts, the 'elementated' matter of the sublunar realm, which are composed of the immaterial qualities hot, cold, wet, and dry, which cannot exist in the sensible world apart from matter. This word *elementatum* made its first appearance before 1129, in William of Conches's *Philosophia Mundi*.[99]

Henry's tone is often lighthearted, as if this tour around his garden were only an amusing diversion, but a serious goal underlies much of the work: explaining the causes and principles of nature as most clearly indicated by the effects of medicinal herbs on the human body. Henry shows some affinity with the new generation of natural philosophers, who were intent on reaching God not by the rejection of the world, but by understanding it in all its

97 Poem 2.20, lines 1–2: 'Qui dedit omne bonum cur graminibus tot eandem / Vim dederit quidam dubitant.'

98 Claudian, *De raptu Proserpinae* 1. 246–68 (*Claudii Claudiani Carmina*, ed. John Barrie Hall [Leipzig 1985], 300–301); Boethius, *De cons. phil.* 3 met. 9.

99 See the commentary to poem 3.3 for a fuller discussion of this fascinating passage.

complexities. It may have been while studying under Anselm at the cathedral school of Laon that he gained an appreciation for rational inquiry into God's universe, and read *quaestiones naturales*, like those of Seneca and Adelard of Bath, questions about the natural world posed for the sake of constructing a coherent picture of a rational creation.[100] Since much of the new twelfth-century learning came through medical works being translated into Latin, it is not surprising that a student like Henry would have turned to *physica*, or medicine, as a suitable path toward understanding nature.[101] Jerome Bylebyl has traced the development of the term *physica* in antiquity and the Middle Ages, showing that it is precisely in the later eleventh and early twelfth centuries—the period of Henry's education—that in philosophical texts *physica* comes to mean medicine rather than natural philosophy or cosmology.[102]

We can clearly see in the Prologue to Book 4 that Henry is part of this intellectual movement:

> So also in writings
> two things
> are rightly thought
> to surpass all equally:
> healing Physic
> and saving Ethics. . . .
> . . . the saviours are
> Physic for the flesh,
> Ethics for the mind—
> the former if care is not kept
> of the flesh, the latter
> if care is not kept of the mind.[103]

100 On the history and development of the literature of *quaestiones*, see Brian Lawn, *The Salernitan Questions. An Introduction to the History of Medieval and Renaissance Problem Literature* (Oxford 1963).

101 *Cf.* Richard McKeon, 'Medicine and philosophy in the eleventh and twelfth centuries: The problem of elements,' *The Thomist* 24 (1961), 211–56; Mark D. Jordan, 'The construction of a philosophical medicine: Exegesis and argument in Salernitan teaching on the soul,' *Osiris*, 2nd series, 6 (1990), 42–61.

102 Jerome J. Bylebyl, 'The medical meaning of *physica*,' *Osiris*, 2nd series, 6 (1990), 16–41.

103 4 Prologue, lines 7–12, 31–36:
Sic quoque scriptis
Bina preesse
Iure putantur
Omnibus eque
Phisica sanans,
Ethica saluans. . . .
. . . Phisica carnis,

By Physic (*phisica*) he means medicine, and medicine is the best foundation for building a comprehensive philosophy of nature. We can see this emphasized in the Prologue to Book 6, where Henry puts a twist on the famous line from Virgil's *Georgics* (2. 490):

> Happy is he who can know the causes of things,
> especially whatever will be the cause of health.[104]

Henry would have agreed with his contemporary William of Conches, who expressed outrage at his fellow clerics who rejected this search for natural causes as somehow irreligious.[105] Henry, filled with this same investigative spirit, boldly states in that same poem:

> I properly judge them insane who were able to learn
> the articles of health but did not wish to learn.[106]

To Henry of Huntingdon and like-minded students of nature, the search for causes in no way detracted from the glory of God, and leaving an illness simply in God's hands when medicinal herbs grow nearby is suicide, not devotion.

2.8 *The Herbal's Legacy*

Henry of Huntingdon's *Anglicanus ortus* enjoyed a small degree of popularity for the rest of the Middle Ages, but it could never match the *De viribus herbarum* of Macer Floridus in terms of distribution, copying, and translation.

Ethica mentis,
Saluificatrix,
Que nisi carnis,
Hec nisi mentis
Cura tenetur.

104 6 Prologue, lines 1–2: 'Felix qui potuit rerum congnoscere causas, / Precipue quicquid causa salutis erit.'

105 Marie-Dominique Chenu, 'Nature and man: The Renaissance of the twelfth century,' in M.-D. Chenu, *Nature, Man, and Society in the Twelfth Century. Essays on New Theological Perspectives in the Latin West*, ed. and trans. Jerome Taylor and Lester K. Little (Toronto 1997), 1–48, at 9.

106 6 Prologue, lines 5–6: 'Arbitror insanos proprie monimenta salutis / Qui didicisse queunt nec didicisse uolunt.'

All the manuscripts of the *Anglicanus ortus* but one are English and even the fifteenth-century manuscript found in Prague (*P*, described below, 60–61) may owe its existence to a Bohemian scholar who accompanied Anne of Bohemia to England at the time of her marriage to Richard II in 1382, and carried the text from England back to his homeland after Richard's death. This is evidently the case with manuscripts of John Wycliffe's works.[107] Two of the manuscripts (*D* and *T*, described below, 61–2 and 63) indicate that Henry's work was used to supplement Macer's herbal. In both of those manuscripts, small portions of the *Anglicanus ortus* are found appended to or integrated with copies of Macer.

Like many works of natural philosophy, the *Anglicanus ortus* was translated into the vernacular in the later Middle Ages. Portions of it were translated into prose in two English herbal collections of the fourteenth century: a Middle English 'Macer' found in eight manuscripts,[108] and an herbal known as *Aaron* (after its first entry), by the Dominican physician Henry Daniel, which is found in two manuscripts.[109] The Middle English 'Macer' (cited in the apparatus as EMA, *i.e.* 'English Macer Additions') is primarily a prose translation of Macer Floridus. When the translator ran out of Macer, he turned to a book which he explicitly describes as not being by Macer: after the passages based on Macer the translator writes, 'Now folowiþ a fewe herbes of whiche Macer tretyþ nat of, atte leste þey ben nat founden in þe cours of Macer book,' and in the table of contents found at the end of the work, 'Lo here be þe names of þe herbes þe whiche be nat founde in þe book of Macer.'[110] This book was Henry of Huntingdon's herbal. The translator pro-

107 See, for example, Alfred Thomas, *Anne's Bohemia: Czech Literature and Society, 1310–1420*, with a foreword by David Wallace (Minneapolis, MN 1998).

108 These are described and edited by Gösta Frisk in *A Middle English Translation of Macer Floridus De viribus herbarum* (Uppsala 1949). Several other manuscripts of the Middle English Macer have since been found. See David Moreno Olalla, '*The fautys to amende*: On the interpretation of the *explicit* of Sloane 5, ff. 13–57, and related matters,' *English Studies* 88 (2007), 119–42, at 121 n17.

109 The two manuscripts of the *Aaron* (London, British Library, MS Arundel 42 and MS Additional 27329) are very different from one another and may represent two distinct versions of the work. Dr E. Ruth Harvey of Toronto is currently preparing an edition. I am grateful to her for sharing her transcriptions of the *Aaron* with Rigg and me, and for extracting references to 'Henry the Englishman.' See also John H. Harvey, 'Henry Daniel: A scientific gardener of the fourteenth century,' *Garden History* 15 (1987), 81–93; and George R. Keiser, 'Through a fourteenth-century gardener's eyes: Henry Daniel's herbal,' *Chaucer Review* 31 (1996), 58–75.

110 *A Middle English Translation of Macer Floridus De viribus herbarum*, ed. Frisk, 189, 201. Frisk was not able to identify the source of these passages.

vides prose versions of twenty-seven[111] of Henry's poems, usually highly abbreviated, giving little more than Henry's cures. Since the translations are taken from books 1–4 and 6 of the *Anglicanus ortus*, the translator may have had a complete version of the work in eight books (and ignored the lapidary) or a six-book version like that found in *P*.

Henry Daniel likewise used entries from both Macer's and Henry's herbals, among the works of many other herbalists. Daniel quotes directly from eighteen[112] of Henry's poems and took information from all of books 1 through 6.[113] Daniel cites Henry by name at several points as 'Henricus Anglicus,' 'Henricus Englisch,' 'Henri,' and 'Henr. Englisch, leche and noble poete.' Henry Daniel knew Macer's and Henry's herbals very well, and compared the information each provided on the same plant, using one to supplement the other. When necessary, I have employed the translations of both EMA and Henry Daniel for help in my own translation and in understanding the most corrupt or difficult passages of the Latin original.

In the end, Henry's herbal was not a source for new medical knowledge and would never supersede the medical works of Macer Floridus and Constantine the African. Judging by the greater popularity of Macer's herbal over Henry's, most medieval physicians who could read such works were looking for simple and accessible guides, easily recalled, to a manageable number of the better-known herbs and spices. Henry's herbal was too monumental, complex, and even entertaining to serve as a practical handbook. It is unlikely

111 The plants are described in the following order (EMA, 189–200) and are given with the name and location of Henry's original poem: Sanicle ('Sanicla,' 1.15), Pympernolle ('Pipera,' 2.18), Baldemoyne ('Baldemonia,' 1.5), Beta ('Beta minor,' 1.19), Rodewort ('Solsequium,' 1.22), Tansey ('Taneticum,' 2.24), Laureole ('Laureola,' 1.4), Liquorice ('Liquiricia,' 6.1.11), Notemuge ('Nux muscata,' 6.2.24), Mirtus ('Mirtus,' 1.25), Saffron ('Crocus,' 1.3), Carui ('Carui,' 2.6), Saxifrage ('Saxifraga,' 2.8), Benet ('Benedicta,' 2.19), Ditayne ('Diptannus,' 3.1), Fetherfoy ('Febrifuga,' 3.4), Bawme ('Balsama,' 3.12), Millemorbia ('Nimphea,' 3.5), Nepe ('Raphanus,' 3.13), Radissh ('Radix,' 3.14), Sclarye ('Sclarega,' 3.21), Femygrek ('Fenugrecum,' 4.12), Git ('Git,' 4.14), Azara ('Gazara,' 4.15), Valerian ('Valeriana,' 4.21), Lupinus ('Lupinum,' 4.11), Ambrosiana ('Ambrosia,' 1.6).

112 This list includes only Henry Daniel's most extensive citations from the *Anglicanus ortus*: 'Cicuta' (5.1.11), 'Beta maior' (1.18), 'Plantago' (5.1.1), 'Viola' (2.9), 'Gazara' (4.15), 'Garrofilum' (6.1.4), and 'Palma Christi' (4.24) are used in BL Additional 27329; 'Nepta' (3.23), 'Nux muscata' (6.2.24), 'Crocus' (1.3), 'Cassia' (6.1.6), 'Centaurea' (3.19), 'Solsequium' (1.22), 'Cynoglossa' (5.9), 'Saxifraga' (1.22), 'Saluia' (1.9), and 'Fenugrecum' (4.12) are used in BL Arundel 42; and 'Anglica costus' (1.17) is used in both. A complete study of Henry Daniel's use of the *Anglicanus ortus* must await the publication of the *Aaron*.

113 See Rigg, 'Henry of Huntingdon's herbal,' 224 and n25, for more on the relations between Henry Daniel and Henry of Huntingdon.

that this would have bothered him; he clearly enjoyed composing verses on a wide range of topics and sharing them with his close companions, like Walter of Leicester, before moving on to another topic that fascinated him.

3. THE EDITION

Portions of the *Anglicanus ortus* survive in five manuscripts, which I describe here with the sigla used in this edition and their respective shelfmarks:

S = London, British Library, MS Sloane 3468, fols. 31r–105v (*s.* 14)

This manuscript contains a medical collection of the fourteenth century, most likely of English provenance. After a copy of another popular medical poem, the *Regimen sanitatis Salernitanum* (fols. 6r–27r), and an excerpt of Bernard de Gordon's *Lilium Medicine* (fols 27r–31r)[114] comes an alphabetical compilation of three separate herbals: Macer Floridus, prose selections from the herbal of Pseudo-Apuleius (attributed to 'Grosthede,' *i.e.* Bishop Robert Grosseteste of Lincoln), and the first four books of *Anglicanus ortus* (less 1.3, 2.22, 2.24, 4.24, 4.25, and 4 Epilogues 1–2).[115] The entries have been taken out of their original order and arranged alphabetically.[116] The Latin names of the plant and the author (*Macer, Henricus, Grosthede*) are recorded, sometimes incorrectly, both above and beside each entry in a different hand. *S* is the only witness to the prose prologue and the prologue to Book 1 of the *Anglicanus ortus*. Among the verse prologues, which are gathered together in *S* (fols. 32r–34r), are four prose lists of herbs (printed in Rigg, 288–92) that conform for the most part to the original order of herbs in books 1–4 as found in *P*. These lists provide evidence that the compiler of *S* was aware of the original arrangement of the *Anglicanus ortus*, but felt the entries were more useful in an alphabetical format. The manuscript also contains various prose and verse passages on weights and measures, indicating that the collection was intended, and likely used, for practical application by a physician or apothecary.

114 Luke Demaitre, *Doctor Bernard de Gordon: Professor and Practitioner* (Toronto 1980), 193.

115 A similar compilation, made of Macer's and Henry's herbals with additions from several other sources, is found in another English manuscript of the early fifteenth century (*T*, discussed below).

116 The contents of this manuscript and their arrangement were first noted by Valentin Rose, 'Ptolemaeus und die Schule von Toledo,' *Hermes* 8 (1874), 327–49, at 330–31 n3. The manuscript, arrangement, and authors are discussed more fully by Haye, *Das lateinische Lehrgedicht*, 325–6.

P = Prague, Knihovna metropolitní kapituly, MS M. VI. 1359, fols. 1r–47v (*ao.* 1443)[117]

The only manuscript produced outside England is also the most complete. A medical manuscript of 103 leaves, *P* contains books 1–6 of *Anglicanus ortus* as its primary text, preserving the organization and order intended by Henry. Hans Walther records this manuscript under the incipit of poem 1.1, 'Arthemisia,' which helped Rigg identify the work.[118] The herbal is followed on fols. 48r–49v by a table of contents alphabetized by first letter, in at least two hands, with various interlinear and marginal notes in Czech. The entire work was foliated, apparently by the original scribe, in Arabic numerals and these are indicated after each plant name in the table of contents. The verso of the flyleaf identifies the work as 'Macer orti anglici' ('Macer of the English Garden'), as does a note at the top of fol. 48r, which suggests that any herbal could be called a 'Macer.'[119] The Latin and Czech names of the plants are given in the margins and nearly every poem has several marginal notations in Latin indicating the various cures given.

The scribe was one Martinus de Tissnow, who also went by the name Wenceslaus de Crumpnaw. He completed the first part of the manuscript in 1443 in the Bohemian city of Humpolec, now in the Czech Republic: 'Explicit hoc opus finitum per manus Martini de Tissnow scriptum in Humpolecz anno domini 1443° feria quinta ante festum Nicolai' (fol. 47v). The manuscript contains three other works: Constantine the African's *Liber graduum*, here called 'Tractatus Constantini de medicinis simplicibus secundum ordinem alphabeti' (fols. 50r–75v), and the 'Tractatus de Pestilentia' (fols. 76r–87v) and 'Tractatus de Pulsibus' (fols. 88r–102v) of Bernard de Gordon.[120] These are followed by medical notes and more lines from the *Regimen sanitatis Salernitanum* in several hands (fols. 102v–103v). There is no colophon for the *Liber graduum*, but the scribe names himself at the end of both of Bernard

117 Briefly described in Adolf Patera and Antonín Podlaha, *Soupis rukopisu Knihovny Metropolitní kapitoly pražské*, 2 vols (Prague 1910–22), 2. 252–63.

118 Hans Walther, *Initia carminum ac versuum Medii Aevi posterioris Latinorum. Alphabetisches Verzeichnis der Versanfänge mittellateinischer Dichtungen*, 2nd ed. (Göttingen 1969), no. 7710; Rigg, 'Henry of Huntingdon's herbal,' 214. The collection was studied, however, nearly two centuries ago by Kaspar Sternberg, *Abhandlung über die Pflanzenkunde in Böhmen*, 2 vols (Prague 1817–18), who was most interested in the Bohemian scribe. Sternberg prints the final poem, the Epilogue to Book 6, in full as well as lines 1–2 of poem 1. 5, *Baldemonia*, to show that the author was English (*Abhandlung*, 64–5).

119 The Middle English herbal of John Lelamour in London, British Library, Sloane 5 is likewise called a 'Macer.'

120 See Demaitre, *Doctor Bernard de Gordon: Professor and Practitioner.*

de Gordon's treatises, which he says he finished in 1444 before heading to Padua to study canon law.[121] A later hand added, 'Qui promotus est in doctorem anno 1449 et obbit anno D<omi>ni 1460 in die s. Lucie ex vixit XXXV annos' (fol. 102v). If the dates and ages are correct, Martin/Wenceslaus was remarkably only eighteen years old when he began the manuscript. He is recorded in three other manuscripts now in Prague, and in one colophon he is named as a *doctor decretorum* and dean of Prague.[122] The scribe, marginalia, and orthography all indicate that the manuscript has not wandered far from its original site of production in the vicinity of Prague.

D = Oxford, Bodleian Library, MS Digby 69, fols. 192r–192v (*s.* $13^{ex}/14^{in}$)

This manuscript of 222 folios contains an extensive collection of recipes, charms, notes, and medical treatises. Tony Hunt outlines thirty separate items from this collection in 'The collection of medical receipts in MS Oxford, Bodleian Library Digby 69', in *Popular Medicine in Thirteenth-Century England* (Cambridge 1990), 311–24. Henry's herbal poems are found only on fol. 192. This short herbal is a collection of sixteen poems containing portions of poems in Henry's books 5 and 6, namely 5.1.1 (lines 57–64), 5.1.2 (lines 22–5, 27–30, 36–7), 5.1.9 (all), 5.1.12 (all), 5.2.2 (lines 12–14), 5.2.3 (lines 12–13, 31–40, 45–54), 5.2.5 (lines 14–16), 5.2.6 (lines 1–2, 5–6, 22–5, 30–31, 33–7), 6.2.16 (lines 5–6), 6.2.18 (all), 6.2.20 (all), 6.2.21 (lines 1–4), 6.2.23 (all), 6.2.24 (all), 6.2.25 (all), and 6.2.26 (all). A note at the top of fol. 192r indicates that the scribe gathered these poems as a supplement to the copy of Macer on fols. 66–80 of *D*: 'de naturis istarum et aliarum herbarum <quae> non sunt in Mac<ro>' ('on the natures of these and other herbs <which> are not in Macer'). The first poem begins in the middle of Henry's poem on plantain ('Plantago', 5.1.1). The scribe has cut lines from most of the poems, but this witness does provide three lines not found in *P* (5.1.9, 15 and 17; 5.1.12, 3), the only other exemplar for books 5 and 6. There is nothing to indicate that

121 'Finivit Venceslaus quondam Martini de Crumpnaw anno D<omi>ni MoCCCCXLIIII. Eodem anno in crastino s. Bartholomei exivit de Crumpnaw ad studium Paduam, habens annos etatis sue XVI in translacione s. Venceslai' (*P* fol. 87v). 'Finitus per Venceslaum Martini de Crumpnaw anno D<omi>ni 1444 ante festum Assumpcionis. Eodem anno ivit ad studium Paduam in jure canonico, sequenti die post Bartolomei. Qui continuans in studio per I annum et VIII menses rediit in Crumpnaw, promotus in baccalarium, habens annos etatis sue XVIII' (*P* fol. 102v). The explicits are recorded (with some errors) by the Bénédictins du Bouveret, *Colophons de manuscrits occidentaux des origines au XVIe siècle*, 6 vols, Spicilegii Friburgensis Subsidia 2–7 (Fribourg 1965–1982), no. 13308.

122 Bénédictins du Bouveret, *Colophons de manuscrits occidentaux*, nos 18680–82.

these are new additions by the scribe, so I have assumed they are original to Henry and were missed or unavailable to the scribe of *P*.

After the herbal poems are thirty-five poems (fols. 192v–195r) treating the medicinal and magical attributes of gems and stones. This is the sole known witness to Henry's *De gemmis preciosis*, which I have published in *Mediaeval Studies* 68 (2006), where I argue that these poems made up most of books 7–8 of his *Anglicanus ortus*. The lapidary is followed by astrological, magical, and medical notes in Latin (fols. 195r–196r) and an Anglo-Norman geography of Asia and Africa (fols. 196r–201r). An edition of the last work is planned by Dr Brent Pitts of Meredith College.[123] The manuscript begins with a collection of recipes primarily in Latin, but an English charm on fol. 6v is discussed by T. M. Smallwood, 'The transmission of charms in English, Medieval and Modern,' *Charms and Charming in Europe*, ed. Jonathan Roper (Basingstoke 2004), 11–31, at 24.

O = Oxford, Bodleian Library, MS Digby 13, fols. 89v, 91r–92v (*s.* 12)

The oldest witness to Henry's medical writings is a prose redaction called 'Exceptiones [*sic*] de libro Henrici' in the manuscript, appended to a copy of Macer's herbal. This witness has long been identified correctly, though no one has acknowledged its importance; the catalogue *Codices Digbeiani* gives its title and states that it is 'from the book of herbs compiled by Henry of Huntingdon, as Leland and others write.'[124] The 'Digby Excerptor,' as I call him in the commentary, abbreviated fifty-one of the herbal poems, drawn only from books 1–4 of the *Anglicanus ortus*. This selection suggests an affinity with manuscript *S*, which also contains only books 1–4. Though the excerpts are written as prose, fifty-three lines of poetry have been preserved mostly intact within the abbreviated entries. I have printed the entire 'Exceptiones' in the Appendix below and included the relevant passage from the 'Exceptiones' in the *apparatus criticus* of each corresponding poem. Also of interest in this manuscript is a collection of nine herbal poems by another author found between the two sections of 'Exceptiones' on fols. 90r–91r. The poems treat

123 Personal correspondence, 11 December 2008.

124 '"Excerptiones de libro Henrici" de herbis variis. f. 91. Ex libro Herbarum compilato, ut Lelandus aliique scribunt, per Henricum de Huntingdon.' William D. Macray, *Catalogi codicum manuscriptorum Bibliothecae Bodleianae, pars nona: codices a viro clarissimo Kenelm Digby, Eq. Aur., anno 1634 donatos, complectens: adiecto indice nominum et rerum* (Oxford 1883), 10. In the annotated reprint of Macray's catalogue the editors say that it is 'Not by Henry of Huntingdon' (R. W. Hunt and A. G. Watson, *Bodleian Library Quarto Catalogues*, vol. 9: *Digby Manuscripts*, part 2: *Notes on Macray's Descriptions of the Manuscripts* [Oxford 1999], 11).

the herbs *titimallum*, *rafanus*, *pentaphilon*, *diptannum*, *pimpinella*, *rosmarinum*, *consolida*, *luvestica* and *millefolium*. All but the poem on rosemary (*rosmarinum*) are also found in *T*, described below.

T = Cambridge, Trinity College, MS O. 9. 10 (James no. 1422), fols. 89r–108r (*s.* 15)

This manuscript, like *S*, contains a compilation of several herbals. The compilation is part of an extensive medical-astrological miscellany of 144 folios. The manuscript is filled throughout with drawings, notes, signatures, and pen tests of one William Feelde, writing during the reign of Elizabeth I (he produced several unflattering portraits of the queen in the margins). John B. Friedman used astrological material in this manuscript for 'Alice of Bath's astral destiny: A re-appraisal,' *Chaucer Review* 35 (2000), 166–81.[125]

The 'Trinity Compiler,' as I call him, gathered or composed ninety poems on herbs with information from Macer Floridus, Henry of Huntingdon, Pseudo-Apuleius, Constantine the African, and other sources not yet identified (perhaps *Circa instans* and the *Antidotarium Nicolai*, among others). Every poem treats an herb except the last, on the signs of death: 'Signa naturalia cuiuscumque morientis.' Fifty-one of the poems are based on Macer, often just copies of the poems with a few lines added or removed. Twenty poems include excerpts from Henry's poems and these are drawn from books 1–4 and 6 of the *Anglicanus ortus*. Two poems are combined from the work of both Macer and Henry. The eighteen others are by an unknown herbalist who is worth identifying, as eight of these poems also appear in manuscript *O* (fols. 90r–91r) with the 'Exceptiones de libro Henrici' described above. The explicit of *T* (fol. 108r) identifies the work as 'Macer herbarum versificatus,' yet another indication that any herbal in the later Middle Ages could be called a 'Macer.'

Since the Trinity Compiler often extensively rewrites his sources and is a poor Latinist, *T* is not a useful witness to the *Anglicanus ortus*, but I do record important variant readings for the twenty-one relevant poems. The poems and lines used by the Compiler are as follows: 1.2 (lines 2–3, 12, 14), 1.3 (lines 14–22), 1.6 (lines 8–9), 1.21 (lines 1–4, 21–31), 1.22 (lines 9–14, 16–18, 21), 1.25 (lines 2–3, 13–14, 16), 2.1 (lines 4–5, 11, 19–31, 35–36), 2.6 (lines 2–3, 9–10), 2.15 (lines 2, 5), 2.18 (lines 1–2, 5–8), 2.24 (lines 1–4), 3.4 (lines 1–11), 3.12 (all, lines 1–8), 3.24 (line 4), 4.1–2 (lines 25–28), 4.9 (lines 8–12), 4.12 (lines 2–9), 4.15 (all, lines 1–9), 4.21 (lines 2–11), 4.24 (lines 1–3, 8), 6.2.10 (lines 7–9, 12).

125 The manuscript also contains a 'doggerel' version of John of Burgundy's fourteenth-century work *De Epidemia*. See Lister M. Matheson, '*Médecin sans frontières?* The European dissemination of John of Burgundy's plague treatise,' *ANQ* 18/3 (2005), 17–28, at n16.

* * * * *

The purpose of this edition is to provide a reconstruction of the complete herbal portion of the *Anglicanus ortus* (books 1–6) in its final form of perhaps *ca.* 1150. This version is extant in no manuscript, although *P* is closest to what I believe Henry intended. I have collated *D*, *P*, *S*, and *T* (where relevant), those exemplars which are still in verse; only two of these, *P* and *S*, reproduce the contents of complete books and only *P* gives entire books in the original order. Readings from the 'Exceptiones' found in *O* are given only when the verse manuscripts are deficient. In most cases the scribe of *O* has changed the phrasing too drastically for his prose redaction to be useful for this edition. There are few cases of shared error which would point to a clear relationship among the manuscripts, so I have not ventured to create a stemma. Neither of the key witnesses, *P* or *S*, is consistently dependable for reconstructing the text. *P* preserves many lines that were unavailable to or missed by the scribe of *S*; the reverse is rare. The scribe of *S*, moreover, seems to have been unduly influenced by his transcription of Macer's poems alongside Henry's. Since he was copying both simultaneously, words and entire lines from Macer have slipped into Henry's poems. The introduction of lines from Macer into Henry's work may also have been a problem for earlier scribes, as Macer's work was known far more widely. The entire Macer tradition needs to be investigated more thoroughly to determine which versions of Macer existed in early twelfth-century England, and which one Henry may have used. Several lines (*e.g.* 2.23, 21–3) indicate that both Henry and his Middle English translator had on hand versions of Macer different from Choulant's edition.

A. G. Rigg edited in 2003 the whole or part of twenty-six of Henry's poems and the Prose Prologue using *P* and *S*, the two manuscripts known to him at the time.[126] For this edition I have preserved the arrangement of books and poems determined by Rigg, emending his edition of those poems where necessary from *D*, *O*, and *T*. He has continued to provide helpful suggestions, as has Michael Winterbottom, both of whose emendations (from private conversation and correspondence) are noted in the *apparatus criticus*. I have retained the numbering system introduced by Rigg, but have replaced his Roman numerals with Arabic numerals. For each poem, I have given its location in manuscripts *D*, *P*, *S*, or *T* (where applicable), the titles given in the manuscripts, if any, a transcription of the prose 'Exceptiones' in *O* when it exists. Below the facing translation I provide a brief statement of the poem's main source, if known, and an *apparatus fontium*. For poems in books 1–4, I have also noted when a poem does not appear in manuscript *P* or *S*. More extensive commentary on each poem can be found after the edition.

126 Rigg, 'Henry of Huntingdon's herbal,' 247–88.

I also provide a title for each poem from the primary name or names in Latin. Usually there is clear agreement between the manuscripts about the name, varying only slightly in orthography, but sometimes completely different names are given, such as known variants (*Semperuiua* in *P* and *De Barba Iouis* in *S* for 3.25, or *Melissa* in *P* with *De Borago* in *S* for 4.22), significantly different spellings (*bethonica* [*P*] or *uetonica* [*S*] in 2.14), or simply wrong entries (*De Febrifugo* [*S*] for *Nimphea* in 3.5). In some cases I use the name or spelling given at the start of the poem if it makes more sense than the titles (such as masculine *Abrotanus* in poem 2.23 rather than neuter *Abrotanum* at the head of *P*, fol. 15v).

In terms of spelling, each manuscript varies greatly from the others in the difficult orthography of exotic plants and diseases. I have generally followed spellings in *S*, the older of the two key manuscripts, and based on those spellings in books 1–4, I have emended, as necessary, errors and alternate spellings in books 5 and 6 (which *S* does not reproduce) to make the orthography consistent. In some cases I have had to resort to spelling employed in the editions of Macer Floridus or Constantine when all of Henry's exemplars have proven corrupt. The scribe of *P* used a large W in place of both U and U-U. I have silently changed these instances to U when *P* is the only exemplar. I have retained the letter Y, used often by *P*, only in a few instances, such as words of Greek origin, or where both *P* and *S* consistently use it (as in *yris*, *ozyma*, *cynoglossa*).

4. TRANSLATION AND IDENTIFICATION OF PLANTS AND DISEASES

I have provided a line-by-line translation of the herbal in which I have endeavoured to keep it readable enough for anyone interested in the history of herbal medicine and accurate enough to be used as a gloss by the student of medieval Latin. In only a few cases where the difficult Latin syntax is not easily reproducible in English do the lines of the edition and translation not match. Wherever possible I have translated into blank iambic verse; it is difficult to reproduce quantitative verse in English (as witnessed by several painful attempts in the sixteenth and seventeenth centuries or Samuel Taylor Coleridge's amusing notes in hexameters to Dorothy and William Wordsworth). While the iambs into which English can naturally fall give a different feeling from the dactylic hexameter, they still preserve, I hope, some of the pulse felt by readers of the Latin. Henry occasionally abandons his classical styling and indulges in rhymes or alliteration; I have also rhymed or used alliteration in a few such cases, but only when it does not force the English too far from an accurate translation.

One of the most difficult issues for the translator of a Latin technical work is identifying and translating the many terms taken directly from other languages (usually Greek) with no equivalent in modern English or, what is more problematic, terms which still exist but with a different meaning. Jerry Stannard outlined the process an editor of a medieval medical text (in his case, a glossary) must go through for identifying plants: '[W]hen one encounters a strange or unfamiliar Latinized plant name, glossed with an equally unknown Anglo-Norman or Middle English synonym, one must first identify both the original name, probably Greek, *and* the Mediterranean plant which it denoted.'[127] In the case of words supposedly from Greek or in the language of the 'people' (*i.e.* Norman French), I have kept the term used by Henry (or changed the spelling slightly to match his source more closely), since these words may well have been as foreign to readers in the twelfth century as in the twenty-first century; they would have been read at the time as belonging to another language and culture. As a further complication numerous names are given to the same plant in both medieval Latin and modern English. Wherever possible, I have translated what seems to be the most common Latin name of the herb into the most common English name, leaving all other names given in Latin. Wherever it seemed reasonable, I have translated those names described as *latine* or *romane* into English, but kept those described as *grece* as Henry wrote them.

We also find terms for medical conditions derived from the Greek, such as *ortopnoicus* (1.24, 9), *ciliacus* (1.25, 16) and *emoptoicus* (5.1.1, 22) which in some cases I have given simply in modernized spelling ('orthopneic,' 'coeliac,' 'haemoptic').[128] It should be understood that these terms (especially *ciliacus*) do not necessarily refer to the modern conditions bearing the same names (*e.g.* coeliac disease). Finally, there is the difficulty of translating puns and etymologies based on a Latin word or phrase, many of which can be traced back to the *Etymologiae* of Isidore of Seville. In most cases, the pun or etymology is not reproducible in a readable translation and I have resorted to an explanation in the commentary.

I am not a professional botanist nor is this volume intended to be a medical or botanical reference work. For each poem, I have given the standard English and botanical Latin (usually Linnaean) name or names of the plant I think most closely approximates what Henry is describing. My primary guide in plant identification has been Maud Grieve's *A Modern Herbal*,[129] which is

127 Jerry Stannard, 'A fifteenth-century botanical glossary,' *Isis* 55 (1964), 353–67, at 355.

128 D. R. Langslow has created an excellent glossary of such Greek medical terms as found in classical Latin texts in his *Medical Latin in the Roman Empire*, 474–512.

129 Maud Grieve, *A Modern Herbal. The Medicinal, Culinary, Cosmetic and Economic Properties, Cultivation and Folklore of Herbs, Grasses, Fungi, Shrubs and Trees with All Their Modern Scientific Uses*, 2 vols (New York 1931; repr. Middlesex 1980).

distinctly unmodern and British in its selection and treatment of plants, and therefore well suited for the task of identifying Henry's herbs.

The medieval understanding of what constituted a uniquely identifiable plant is different from our own, now usually influenced by modern scientific taxonomy and accessible nature guides. Where Henry distinguishes between *species* (in the medieval philosophical, rather than taxonomical, sense), he uses different criteria than we would. In poem 2.5 the parsnip, skirret, and wild carrot, each of which now belong to a different genus, are for Henry the three species of *pastinaca* because they all have long roots which are good 'for food' (*pastu*). Conversely, in poems 3.3 on *anetum* (dill) and 6.1.10 on *ceroton* (perhaps carob), he employs a sense of *species* that sounds distinctly modern, though is probably indicative rather of the nascent Latin Aristotelianism of the twelfth century than of any sort of modern scientific differentiation: '... you'll see genus transform into species, species into lower classes, and then pass right back again'; 'Carob is a genus distinguished into species ...'.[130] Wherever Henry has named and described a plant, sometimes the identification is obvious and definite, and has been so for many centuries, as in the difference between types of artemisia: mugwort (1.1), southernwood (2.23) and wormwood (3.11). Sometimes we might see several or many species within a genus or family: modern science has identified, or even engineered, many different kinds of rose or lily (2.10 and 2.11), not to mention numerous kinds of mint (3.10) and houseleek (3.25). Some plants might not even exist at all, like the *yreos* (3.9), a plant apparently invented from a misunderstanding of the Greek genitive of *iris*.

It must be added, of course, that no treatment or remedy described in the *Anglicanus ortus* should be tried. Henry's poems reflect the medical theories and practices of another age with a far different understanding of plants, disease, our bodies, and their respective places in God's universe.

130 Poem 3.3, lines 14–15: 'Et genus in speciem, species in subteriora / Pertransire uides et retransire.' Poem 6.1.10, line 1: 'Est ceroton genus in species diuersificatum ...'.

Sigla and Editorial Conventions

D	Oxford, Bodleian Library, MS Digby 69, fols. 192r–192v
O	Oxford, Bodleian Library, MS Digby 13, fols. 91r–92v
P	Prague, Knihovna metropolitní kapituly, MS M. VI 1359, fols. 1r–47v
S	London, British Library, MS Sloane 3468, fols. 31r–105v
T	Cambridge, Trinity College, MS O. 9. 10, fols. 89r–108r

add.	addidit
corr.	correxit
exp.	expunxit
in mg.	in margine
om.	omisit
Rigg	Emendations made by A. G. Rigg in 'Henry of Huntingdon's herbal' or in private communication
s.l.	supra lineam
transp.	transposuit
Winterbottom	Suggestions made by Michael Winterbottom in a letter to A. G. Rigg, 17 May 2004

< >	Editorial addition
[ ]	Editorial deletion
{ }	Folio number (in Appendix)
†	Problem in text
* * * *	Illegible text

Abbreviations

Agnus Castus	*Agnus Castus. A Middle English Herbal Reconstructed from Various Manuscripts*, ed. Gösta Brodin (Uppsala 1950)
Alphita	*Alphita, a Medico-Botanical Glossary*, ed. J. L. G. Mowat, Anecdota Oxoniensia. Mediaeval and Modern Series, vol. 1, part 2 (Oxford 1887)
André	Jacques André, *Les noms de plantes dans la Rome antique* (Paris 1985)
Antidotarium Nicolai	*Eene Middelnederlandsche Vertaling van het Antidotarium Nicolaï (Ms. 15624–15641, Kon. Bibl. te Brussel)*, ed. W. S. van den Berg (Leiden 1917) [Includes a transcription of the Latin *editio princeps*, Venice 1471]
Black	Winston Black, 'Henry of Huntingdon's lapidary rediscovered and his *Anglicanus ortus* reassembled,' *Mediaeval Studies* 68 (2006), 43–87
Boethius, *De cons. phil.*	Boethius, *De consolatione philosophiae*, in *The Theological Tractates; The Consolation of Philosophy*, ed. and trans. H. F. Stewart and E. K. Rand, Loeb Classical Library (Cambridge, MA 1962)
Circa instans	*Liber de simplici medicina dictus circa instans*, in Johannes Serapion, *Practica Jo[hannis] Serapionis dicta Breviarium* (Venice 1497), fols. 186r–211v
Constantine	Constantine the African, *Liber graduum*, in *Constantini Africani . . . Opera* (Basel 1536–9), 2. 342–87, and in *Opera omnia Ysaac* (Lyons 1515), 2. 78r–86r [Cited by page number of the Basel edition unless otherwise noted]
CSEL	Corpus scriptorum ecclesiasticorum latinorum (Vienna 1866–)
Daniel Additional	Henry Daniel, *Aaron*. London, British Library, MS Additional 27329, fols. 4–236
Daniel Arundel	Henry Daniel, *Aaron*. London, British Library, MS Arundel 42, fols. 3–92

Digby Excerptor	*O*
Dioscorides	*Pedanii Dioscuridis Anazarbei, De materia medica libri quinque*, ed. Max Wellmann, 3 vols (Berlin 1906–14; repr. Berlin 1958)
DMLBS	*Dictionary of Medieval Latin from British Sources*, ed. R. E. Latham, D. R. Howlett, *et al.*, 13 fascicles (London 1975–)
EMA (= English Macer Additions)	*A Middle English Translation of Macer Floridus De viribus herbarum*, ed. Gösta Frisk (Uppsala 1949)
Grieve	Maud Grieve, *A Modern Herbal*. 2 vols. (New York 1931; repr. Middlesex 1980)
HA	Henry, Archdeacon of Huntingdon, *Historia Anglorum*, ed. and trans. Diana Greenway (Oxford 1996)
Hunt	Tony Hunt, *Plant Names of Medieval England* (Cambridge 1989)
Isidore, *Etym.*	Isidore of Seville, *Etymologiarum sive originum libri XX*, ed. W. M. Lindsay (Oxford 1911)
Latin Alphabetical Dioscorides	*Index librorum in presenti volumine contentorum Dyoscoridis exactissimi indagatoris fidelissimique scriptoris virtutum simplicium medicinarum liber CCCCCCCXVII continens capitula: cum nonnullis additionibus Petri Paduanensis in margine libri notatis. Eiusdem Dyoscoridis de naturis et virtutibus aquarum tractatus unus* (Lyons 1512) [Unglossed version in Cambridge, Jesus College, MS Q. D. 2 (44), fols. 17–145. References are to the glossed version unless otherwise noted]
Latin Dioscorides	'Der Longobardische Dioskorides des Marcellus Virgilius,' ed. Konrad Hofmann and T. M. Auracher, in *Romanische Forschungen* 1 (1882), 49–105, continued by Hermann Stadler, 'Dioscorides Longobardus,' *Romanische Forschungen* 10 (1897), 181–247, 369–446; 11 (1899), 1–121; 13 (1901), 161–243; with indices in 14 (1903), 601–36 [References are to volume and page]
Laud Herbal	*The Laud Herbal Glossary*, ed. J. Richard Stracke (Amsterdam, 1974)
Macer	*Macer Floridus De viribus herbarum*, ed. Ludwig Choulant (Leipzig 1832); repr. in *Höhepunkte der Klostermedizin. Der 'Macer Floridus' und das Herbarium des Vitus Auslasser*, trans. Johannes Gottfried Mayer and Konrad Goehl (Leipzig 2001)

Martial, *Ep.*	Martial, *Epigrams*, ed. and trans. D. R. Shackleton Bailey, 3 vols, Loeb Classical Library (Cambridge, MA 1993)
Oribasius	*Euporistes* 2, ed. A. Molinier (Paris 1876), in *Oeuvres d'Oribase*, ed. U. C. Bussemaker and C. Daremberg, 6 vols (Paris 1851–76), at 6. 424–626
Ovid, *Met.*	Ovid, *Metamorphoses*, trans. Frank Justus Miller, 2 vols, Loeb Classical Library (Cambridge, MA 1951)
PL	Patrologiae cursus completus: Series Latina, ed. J.-P. Migne, 221 vols (Paris 1844–64)
Pliny	Pliny the Elder, *Natural History*, ed. and trans. H. Rackham, W. H. S. Jones, and D. E. Eichholz, 10 vols, Loeb Classical Library (Cambridge, MA 1938–63) [Cited by book and paragraph number]
Pseudo-Apuleius	*Antonii Musae De herba vettonica liber, Pseudoapulei Herbarius, Anonymi De taxone liber, Sexti Placiti Liber medicinae ex animalibus*, ed. Ernst Howald and Henry E. Sigerist (Leipzig 1927) [Cited by number and by page of Howald and Sigerist's edition]
Pseudo-Oribasius	*Oribasii Medici de Simplicibus Libri Quinque*, Book 4, in *Physica S. Hildegardis* (Strasbourg 1533), 122–233
Quintus Serenus	Quintus Serenus, *Liber Medicinalis*, ed. and trans. R. Pépin (Paris 1950)
Rigg	A. G. Rigg, 'Henry of Huntingdon's herbal,' *Mediaeval Studies* 65 (2003), 213–92
RMLWL	R. E. Latham, *Revised Medieval Latin Word-List from British and Irish Sources* (1965; repr. with supplement, London 1980)
Rufinus	*The Herbal of Rufinus*, ed. Lynn Thorndike with Francis S. Benjamin, Jr (Chicago 1946)
Strabo	Walahfrid Strabo, *Hortulus*, ed. Cataldo Roccaro (Palermo 1979)
Trinity Compiler	*T*

HENRY OF HUNTINGDON

Anglicanus ortus
The English Garden

<PROLOGVS>

Principium rerum, generacio, finis earum
hoc opus aspiret, deducat terminum, oro.

Quod et religiosis et secularibus, licet diuersissimis, aptum, tamen proposui unum, † et est * * * * multis in quibus differunt † nec inutile est. Ad rem pertinet apponere religiosis, namque tria sunt effectiua: oracio, operacio, datum. Vtuntur hiis peruersi, sed aliter: religiosi ut thesaurizant, peruersi ut fallant. Quod ut elucescat, uespera diurnos actus cuiusque discuciat hoc modo. Discussio iusti secum: 'Septies hodie laudem dixi Domino. Post hoc opus optimum in Domino feci; ex hinc de datis a Deo partem suis reddidi; modo suus utilis cum laudibus tamen eiusdem nocturna silencia peto.' Item discussio alterius: 'Oraui mane summo ut prosperarer, et factum est. Aurum et argentum coaceruaui michi, et, quod carius est, possessionem nemoribus riuisque coruscam, quam in eternam hereditatem posteris meis ad laudem et honorem nominis mei dedi. Huius ergo diei gaudia in splendoribus uini et epularum recolamus.'

Loquar igitur prius ad primum: 'Hodie, frater, astutissime negociatus es. Singula namque uerba que in laudem Domini dixisti, in sempiterno reposita sunt thesauro. Minima illarum non deficiet in eternum. Operacio quoque diurna quam ad bonos usus direxisti, celesti reposita est armario. Minima pars subsistet in secula; quod autem de iuste adquisitis Domino errogasti, multiplici fenore accumulatum reseruatur. Minimus quadrans aureum tibi confert talentum nunquam defecturum. Hec omnia reperies in die necessitatis, que huic mundo est insensibilis.'

Ad alium quoque loquar: 'Dum aurum et argentum possessionemque tibi hodie lucratus es, circa nichilum et inane occupatus es: mallem te dormisse. Transiit actus, transiet gaudium, transiet memoria. Vbi est quod egisti? Nichil agis, nichil inuenies in die necessitatis, in die miserie et calamitatis! O fatue, iuueni tibi thesaurizasti que candidissima tibi uidebantur, etatis autem tempore tesaurum accepturus, quid inuenies?'

<PROLOGVS> *S* 31r–32r [no title] | [not in *P*] *First edited by Rigg, 248–51.*

24 reperies] *Rigg*, reperiens *S* 30 que] *Rigg*, quia *S* 31 uidebantur] *Rigg*, uidebatur *S* 32 inuenies] *Rigg*, inueniens *S*

Prose Prologue

May Generation, the beginning of things and their end,
inspire this work, and bring it to a close, I pray.

I have set forth a single work suitable for both the religious and the secular, although they are very different, † and [. . .] in which they differ, † nor is it without use. It is fitting to place it before the religious, for there are three effective things: prayer, service, giving. The wicked use these things, but in a different way: the religious in order to gather up treasure, the wicked in order to deceive. In order to clarify this, let [each one] plead in the evening for his acts during the day in this manner: The argument of the just man with himself: 'Seven times today I have praised the Lord. After this I did a great work in the Lord. After this, out of those things given by God I gave a part to his people. Now, as His useful servant, I seek the silence of the night, yet with praises to Him.' Likewise, the argument of the other: 'In the early morning I prayed that I might prosper, and it was done. I have heaped up gold and silver for myself, and, what is more precious, a property glittering with groves and streams, which I have given in perpetual inheritance to my heirs for the praise and honour of my name. Therefore let us recall the joys of this day in the splendours of wine and feasting.'

I shall speak first to the first one: 'Today, brother, you have conducted business very shrewdly. Each word that you have spoken in praise of the Lord has been laid up in an eternal treasury. The least of these praises will never fail. The daily service which you have directed to good uses has also been placed in a heavenly storehouse. The least part will survive through the ages; that which you have paid out to the Lord from your just acquisitions is kept and heaped up with interest many times over. The least farthing bestows on you a talent of gold that will never fail. All these things you will find on the day of need, which cannot be perceived by this world.'

I will also speak to the other: 'While you gained gold, silver, and a property for yourself today, you have been occupied with nothing and to no purpose; I would rather you had slept. The act is done, the joy will pass, the memory will fade. Where is that which you have done? You are doing nothing; you will find nothing on the day of need, on the day of misery and disaster! O fool, you have treasured up for yourself as a young man those things which seemed fairest to you, but in the time of old age what will you find when you are about to receive your treasure?'

Beatus igitur sapiens in uiis suis, maledictus fatuus in cecitate sua! Licet tamen horum tam diuersa sint opera, idem tamen aliquando boni bene, mali male, faciunt. Sicut in eius orti cultu quem iustus ad hoc componit, ut frigida cibis emendorum loco prosint. † Inepta ut frigidum morbis asserit. † Presto medicamina. Multis enim hec uulgaria magis profuerunt quam antidota sumptuosa. Si autem et in hiis bonus delectetur, nonne consuetudinis naturalis est ut bonum bona delectent? Malus autem, cui omnia cooperantur in malum, dum malos ad usus uel ingluuiei uel uoluptatis ortum componit, circa nil occupatur, ut assolet.

Iam uero, quia et religiosis et secularibus scribimus, cum hucusque religiose dixerimus, secularibus suo modo dicamus. Quem non delectet tam uarius color herbarum, tam uarius odor florum, tam uarius medendi usus, tam uarius saporum lusus? Quem non delectet uarietas earum dum pullulant, dum excrescunt, dum concipiunt, dum germinant, dum parturiunt? Exemplum ergo delicati proponimus orti. Qui cum quadratus sit, in medio eius lacus sit, in quo pisces natare uideas. In medio uero laci sedes est quasi theatrum, palmitibus conductis Phebo resistens. Ortum tamen si sani tam pulcrum neglexeritis, infirmi utile non negligetis. Sciatis autem utique hic apposita ex auctoritatibus sumpta.

34 sint *corr. e* sunt *S* 35 orti *corr. ex* ortu *S* 36 cibis *corr. e* cibus *S* prosint] *Rigg*, prosunt *S* 37 asserit *corr. ex* asseris *S* 47 delicati] *Rigg*, dilecati *S* 51 negligetis] *Rigg*, negligis *S* auctoritatibus *corr. ex* auctoritateibus *S*

Blessed therefore is the man wise in his ways, cursed the fool in his blindness! Although their works are so different, nevertheless sometimes the good do the same thing well and the bad do it badly, just as in the cultivation of his garden, which the just man arranges for this purpose: so that cold things may be good as foods in place of things that must be bought. † He asserts they are useless for diseases . . . † I bring forth medicines. For these common medications were more useful to many than expensive antidotes. But if the good man also delights in these, is it not the custom of nature that good things should delight the good man? The wicked man, however, for whom all things work together for evil, when he arranges a garden for the wicked purposes of greed or pleasure, is busying himself with nothing, as usual.

But now, because I am writing for both the religious and the secular and since I have spoken till now in a religious manner, let me now speak to seculars in their own manner. Who is not delighted by such a varied colour of herbs, such a varied smell of flowers, such a varied application of healing, such a varied play of flavours? Who is not delighted by their variety when they sprout, grow, conceive, produce buds, and bear fruit? Therefore I set forth the example of a sumptuous garden. Since it is square, let there be a lake in the middle, in which you can see fish swim. In the middle of the lake there is a seat, a kind of theatre, fending off Phoebus's rays with interwoven vines. If you should neglect so fair a garden when you are well, you will not neglect a useful one when you are sick. I want you to know that what is set out here is taken in every instance from authorities.

1 <PROLOGVS LIBRI PRIMI>

Qui teneris ludens pueris epigramata scripsi,
  Quique canens iuueni seria scripta dedi,
Primo docens, postremo iuuans, nunc maius utrisque
  Construo quod senibus subsidietur opus.
Iure puer pueris, iuuenis iuueni, documenta
  Cum dederim, senibus dem documenta senex—
Nec senibus solum, <tamen> hoc specialius illis
  (Est etenim morbus ipsa senecta) fero.
Rite senes, casu iuuenes puerique teruntur;
  Ergo puer, iuuenis me seniorque legant!
Vatum magne parens, herbarum, Phebe, repertor,
  Vosque quibus resonant Tempe iocosa dee,
Si michi serta prius edera florente parastis,
  Ecce meos flores—serta parate—fero.

1.1 ARTHEMISIA

Herbarum matrem, quam primo limite ponit
Nature racio digne, pretulimus orto.
Tres species Diascorides pronunciat huius:
Hec monolos, hec eptapolos est, illa tagantis.
Hanc prius Arthemim (quam dicimus esse Dianam)
Inuenisse ferunt, hinc arthemisia greco
Nomine nomen habet, que cum sit magna decore,
Effectu maior, natura maxima mater,
Quatuor ergo modis deducere menstrua fertur;

1 <PROLOGVS LIBRI PRIMI> *S* 32r: [no title] | *Leland* (lines 11–14 in *De uiris illustribus*, ed. Carley, p. 336) | [not in *P*] *First edited in full by Rigg*, 251–2.

2 quique] *Rigg*, qui *S* seria] *scripsi*, serta *S* 4 senibus] *scripsi*, seminibus *S* : satis *Rigg* 7 tamen] *add. Rigg*, *om. S* 9 teruntur] *Rigg*, *tri*untur *S* 10 ergo] *Rigg*, hoc *S* 12 Tempe] *Leland et Rigg*, tempora *S* 13 parastis] *Leland et Rigg*, paractis *S* 14 parate] *Leland et Rigg*, parare *S*

1.1 ARTHEMISIA *P* 1r–1v: Arthemisia | *S* 43r–43v: De Artemesia. Henricus

1 quam] te *P* 2 pretulimus] *scripsi*, preferrimus *PS* 3 Dyaschorides *P* pronuncciat *P* 4 hec . . . hec] hoc . . . hoc *S* mollodos *S* epthaphilos *S* tagangtis *S* 5 dicimus] diuina *P* Dianam] diam *S* 6 artemesia *S* 7 magno *S* 8 effectu] *scripsi*, effectum *S* : est tam *P*

1 Prologue of the First Book

I, who once wrote playful epigrams for boys of tender age,
who gave to youths some songs of sombre note,
at first a teacher, then a guide, now construct a work
better than those two to be of help to older men.
I rightly gave instructions as a boy to boys, a youth to youths,
now old, I give this treatise for older men to use—
I write not only for the aged, yet especially for them
(indeed, old age itself is also a disease).
The old wear down, as is right, but boys and youths by mischance,
therefore let boy and youth and elder read my work!
O Phoebus, mighty father of poets and discoverer of herbs,
and goddesses, whose echo merry Tempe rings,
if you first made wreaths for me of flowering ivy,
look here: I bring my blooms for you. Prepare the wreaths!

1.1 Mugwort, *Artemisia vulgaris* L.

We bring up to the garden's front the mother of all herbs,
whom the law of Nature rightly places in the frontmost row.
Wise Dioscorides announces three varieties:
Monolos first, and next *Eptapolos*, and that one is *Tagantis*.
They say that Artemis—whom we do call Diana—
discovered it, hence it is known by the Grecian name
of Artemisia, and since she's great in beauty,
and greater in effect, the greatest mother by her nature,
therefore she's said to bring out menses in four ways;

1 <PROLOGVS LIBRI PRIMI> / **Prologue of the First Book** *Original*
1 *Cf.* Boethius, *De cons. phil.* 1 met. 1 11 *Cf.* Ovid, *Remedia amoris*, 76

1.1 ARTHEMISIA / **Mugwort** *Macer, 'Artemisia', 1–30*
2 *Cf.* Cicero, *De officiis* 3.23

Matribus auxilio digne succurrit amico:
Siue terendo diu uino coniuncta bibatur,
Siue sit ipsius decoccio sumpta frequenter,
Siue fouere uelis morbum matricis eadem,
Siue uirens eadem uentri de nocte ligetur.
Scis quid menstrua sint? 'Mulieris mense redundans
Vnoquoque cruor, Phebeque noua superundans,
Qui si non aliquo fluat ut solet impediente
Excurratue nimis morbus generatur utrimque.'
Emollire steras solet artemisia duras.
Quid dixere steras? 'Os matricis stera grece
Dicitur; hoc morbo fit dura tumensque grauante.'
Adiuuat hictericos cum uino sumpta frequenter.
Quid sunt hicterici? 'Qui galuiciem paciuntur.'
Hec opio pressis cum uino subuenit hausta.
Quid dicunt opium? 'Que tollit pocio sensum.'
Plinius hanc adipi strumis apponere iunctam
Precipit aut ipsam uino potare solutam.
Vrinamque mouere docet lapidemque fugare
Et si contritam uino coniunxeris herbam
Hiis fieri morbis uinum medicabile dixit.
Affirmant quidam, quisquis potauerit ipsam,
(Non affirmo tamen) quod nec nocuum medicamen
Huic noceat, nec cum nocuo medicamine carmen.
Hec affirmo tamen, quod gratus sit sapor illi
Cum uino iuncte, gratoque probetur odore,
Quod bibitum pectus reparat, precordia curat.

10 matribus . . . amico *om. P* 11 uino diu *S* 13 morbos *P* 15 scis quid] sis quis *S* muliere *S* 16 Phebeque] febeque *S* 17 inpediaente *P* 18 excurrat ne *S* 19 seras *S* arthemysia *P* 21 hoc] hec *P* tumescensque *S* 23 icterici *S* caluiciem *P* 24 hec] hoc *S* 26 adypi *P* 27 aut] an *P* 28 lapidesque *S* 29 coniuncteris *S* 30 uinum] unum *P* 31 illam *S* 33 cum] est *P* 34 hec] *scripsi*, hoc *PS* affirmat *S* 35 probatur *S*

it rightly succours mothers with assistance as a friend.
By grinding long and mixed with wine it should be drunk,
or if a decoction of it is frequently imbibed,
or if you wish to foment a sickness of the womb with it,
or if it is tied, when green, to the belly in the evening.
Do you know what *menses* are? 'A woman's blood which flows
in every month, and flows again each time Phoebe shines anew,
and if it doesn't flow as it should (blocked by some impediment),
or if it runs too fast, disease will come in either case.'
Artemisia is apt to make hardened *steras* soft.
What do they say that *steras* are? '"Mouth of womb" is *stera*
to the Greeks. By this burdensome disease it hardens and it swells.'
The jaundiced are made well by Artemisia taken frequently in wine.
Who are the 'jaundiced'? 'Those who suffer yellowness.'
When drunk with wine, this helps those slowed down by opium.
What do they call *opium*? 'The drink that takes your sense away.'
Apply this, so Pliny orders, mixed with lard on sores
from scrofula, or drink it dissolved in wine.
He teaches that it moves the urine and forces out the stone
and if you mix this herb, well ground, with wine
he claimed this wine is curative for these diseases.
So some affirm (though I do not!) that neither a harmful
medicine, nor magic spell provided with that wicked cure,
will injure whosoever drinks this herbal wine.
Yet I affirm these things: that when the herb is steeped in wine
its flavour is agreeable, as proven by the pleasing smell,
and when imbibed repairs the chest and cures the diaphragm.

26 Pliny 26. 24

1.2 OZYMA

Ozyma post matrem preelecta sequi meruerunt;
Hec rutam foliis, hec thus imitantur odore,
Saluia, te flore sed te, celidonia, lacte.
Anglorum Matillis honor, decus et dolor orbis,
Cuius funereum mea dant epigramata carmen,
Solam delicias inter ponebat habendas,
Olle tellurem, telluri semina mandans.
Sic cum uere nouo mire frondesceret, illa
Nocte frequens thalamo, de luce locabat in orto,
Nocte gelu uitans et crescere luce ministrans,
Nocte suam redolens et luce uidens basileam,
Nam basilea solet uel basilicon uocitari.
Eius si uires queras nec sint tibi tanti
Tantus splendor, odor, uires dissoluere uiri
Letiferi pote uires possunt basilee.

1.3 CROCVS

Ecce crocus redolens liuoris carpitur igne!
Basilicon foliis et flore crocus superextat;
Ambo decore pares, neuter superatur odore,
Et conferre comas et concertare parati.
Se tamen iste fere sociare cauet basilee,

1.2 OZYMA *P* 1v: Ozyma | S^1 45v: De Basilica. Henricus | S^2 75r–75v: De Ozoma. Henricus | *T* 96v–97r: Gariofilatum (*sic*) *First edited by Rigg, 252–3, from P and S.*

Exceptiones (*O* 91r): Ozima uel basilea uel basilico est herba foliis rute similis, thuri odore, saluie flore, celidonie lacte. Contra letiferam potionem hausta ualet.

1 ozima *S* 2 hec . . . hec] hoc . . . hoc S^1S^2 imitantur] jimitatur (?) *T* 3 saluia] sic alma S^1S^2 set S^2 4 Matilon *P* honor] et *add. P* 5 carmen] carnem S^1 6 habendas] habundans S^1 : habundas S^2 8 mirum *P* 9 locabit S^2 10 uitens S^2 13 eius] cuius S^1S^2 sint] sunt S^1S^2 15 letiferi pote] letili potes S^1

1.3 CROCVS *P* 1v–2r: Crocus | [not in *S*] | *T* 96v: Galbo

Exceptiones (*O* 91r): Crocus messe surgit, uere cedit i<bi> hoc basilee contraria. Huius flores lacti muliebri commisce: qua mixta, diu seruata, oculos patientes superunge et multum proderit. Item contra letiferam potionem sicut basilea ualet. Item admisce ei thus et nigellam et hoc in mulsa coque et sciasim superponendo curabit. Picture etiam apta est ut medicine.

3 neuter *corr ex.* ne ter *P et add.* neuter *s.l.*

1.2 Basil, *Ocymum basilium* L.

And Basil, very choice, deserves to follow her Mother;
she imitates Rue in leaves, but Frankincense in odour,
and Sage, she mimics you in bloom, and Celandine, in juice.
Matilda, honour of the English, the world's glory and its grief,
whose funeral song is in my book of epigrams,
placed it alone among delights worth keeping,
when she put soil into a pot and seeds into that soil.
So when in early spring the leaves—a marvel—grew, she kept
it often in her room at night, in the garden during day,
to shun the cold of night and help it grow with light,
in darkness smelling, and in daylight seeing, her *basilea*,
(for most times it is called *basilea*, or *basilicon*).
But if you inquire about its strength, still unimpressed
with such great splendour and such scent, the power of Basil,
when in a drink, can dissipate the power of deadly poison.

1.3 Saffron Crocus, *Crocus sativus* L.

Look here: the fragrant Crocus is seized with envy's fire!
First Basil wins the day with leaves, then Crocus with his bloom;
in beauty both are matched and neither is surpassed in scent—
they both are set to join their blades and come to blows!
Yet Crocus is wary even to associate with Basil,

1.2 OZYMA / **Basil** *Original*
4–5 *Cf.* Martial, *Ep.* 11. 13. 5

1.3 CROCVS / **Saffron Crocus** *Original*

Hac etenim ueniente fugit, uenit hac fugiente.
Hec estate uiret, bruma uiret ille rigente,
Hec cum pulchra dies, hic cum nequit herba uirere.
Vere crocus cedit, procedunt ozyma uere;
Messe crocus surgit, procumbunt ozyma messe.
Hic igitur uires iactat crocus auxiliares:
'Me Natura parens non solum pellere morbos
Constituit. Cum multa queam non multa reponam?
Qui langues oculos flores assumito nostros,
Lac muliebre simul, nec cum lacti muliebri
Iungi dedignor; que cum simul associata
Et seruata diu fuerint, oculos superunge;
Sic oculos sanus uideas, uitesque uenena,
Nec tibi fiat opus misere leso basilee
Amplius! Admisce mecum thus atque nigellam,
Admixtos mulsa coquito, sic addito coxe
Quam uexat sciasis; sciasis uexabitur eque.
Pictori tamen an medico specialior exto?
Par que sum medico sum pictori specialis,
Nam res picture meliorem nulla colorem
Conferet excepta (quis enim nescit?) basilea.'

1.4 LAVREOLA

Lauri laureolas non dedignantur amenas,
Ex re nomen habent quia lauri laureolarum:
Corticibus cortex certare nitorque nitori
Et folium foliis et honor uideatur honori.
Hanc dedit eternum uiridi gaudere iuuenta

8 hic] hoc *P*   14 languens *T*   flores assumito nostros] illius sumito flores *T*   17 oculis superadde *T*   18 oculis *T*   20 admissa *T*   mecum] illi *T*   21 addita cere *T*   22 quam] *scripsi*, quem *P* : que *T*   sciasis²] scyasis *P*

1.4 LAVREOLA   *P* 2r: Laureola | *S* 65v: De Laureola. Henricus

Exceptiones (*O* 91r): Laureola est herba sic dicta quia lauro est similis, tamen in multis, tamen quia semper uiret. Cuius semen Persius coconidion dixit. Hinc optima fit potio que intima purgans per inferiora, et lenis est et non periculosa.

1 lauri] laurea *S*   dedignetur *S*   2 qui *P*   laureolari *P*   3 nitori] uitori *S*   5 iumenta *S*

for when she comes he flees and he returns when she departs.
She grows in summer, he is green with winter's chill,
so she in lovely days, and he when grass forgets to grow.
Come spring the Crocus will retreat and Basil will advance;
in harvest time watch Crocus rise and Basil fall.
And here the Crocus launches his auxiliary troops:
'Mother Nature brought me up to do more than fight
disease. Since I can do so much, why don't I tell it all?
You who suffer in your eyes, take up our blooms
with mother's milk (nor do I show disdain to mix
with mother's milk); and once the two are mixed
and preserved a while, anoint the eyes:
with eyes now clean, you shall see, and poisons you'll avoid,
nor should you ask when you're injured for wretched Basil
anymore! Mix Frankincense with me and Cockle too,
then cook this mixture in some mead, apply it to the hip
which sciatica disturbs, and sciatica will be equally disturbed.
Yet am I considered dearer to the physician or the painter?
As special as I am for art, I'm the same for physic, too,
for nothing grants a better colour to a painted work
except—But who is there who does not know?—*basilea.*'

1.4 Laureole (= Spurge Laurel), *Daphne cnidium* L.

It is not for laurels to disdain the pleasant Laureoles,
for laurel is a species of the genus Laureole:
so bark with bark and sheen with sheen apparently contend,
and leaf will vie with leaves, one honour fighting honour.
The begetter of Nature granted that Laureole

7 Pliny 21. 34; *cf.* Lucan, *De bello civili* 1. 17 20–22 Macer 2025–6

1.4 LAVREOLA / **Laureole** *Source unknown*
2 *Cf.* Ovid, *Amores* 1. 8. 3; Marbode of Rennes, *De lapidibus*, 420

Nature genitor, nec uritur ergo calore,
Frigore nec squalet. Animosi Persius oris
Semen predicte dixit cocognidon herbe—
Hoc testantur idem medici simul atque poete.
  Hinc fieri fertur preciose pocio laudis,
Intima que purgans pellit per subteriora,
Si quid obest stomacho, pulmoni uisceribusque.
Si grauis efficiat ne prosit pocio morbus—
Namque nihil medicina docet quod semper ubique
Omnibus eueniat—nunquam tamen ista nocebit,
Cum multe multis uel summi causa doloris
Sint uel supreme festinans clausula mortis.

1.5 BALDEMONIA

Compatriota tibi dat, baldemonia, laudes:
Anglia te speciem, me reddidit Anglia uatem,
Tam renitens herbis quam non obscura poetis.
Te quamuis ude soleant nutrire paludes,
Vis quibus humectans et frigida noscitur esse,
Vis tibi desiccans et feruida dicitur esse.
  Hanc multi speciem gaudent gestare salubrem,
Vt si forte dolor turbauerit intima cordis
Aut subito pectus moueat stomachumque lacescat,
Cor sanet, pectus releuet, stomachum refocillet,
Quod solo conferre solet non irrita morsu.

6 nec] non *S*   7 nec] que *S*   8 coconidio *S*   9 hoc] hec *S*   10 ferunt *S*   14 nil *S*   15 tamen] sed *P*   17 uel] *add.* sint *S*   suppreme *S*

1.5 BALDEMONIA   *P* 2r: Baldemonia | *S* 45v–46r: De Baldemonia. Henricus *Edited by Rigg*, 253–4.

Exceptiones (*O* 89v): Baldemonia est species sicce et frigide nature. Hec comesta cordis, pectoris, stomachi dolores curat. Cor sanat, pectus releuat, stomachum refocillat.

(*O* 91r): Baldemonia feruida et sicca licet in palude oriatur que frigida est et humida. Cor sanat a dolore quolibet, pectus releuat, stomacum confortat. Solo morsu facit quod gingiber gariofilum piretrum cinnama, nam quod agunt empte facit hec inuenta palude, quodque datur pretiis, dat baldemonia gratis.

4 ude] reicere (?) *S*   9 moueat stomachumque lacescat] relue (!) stomachum refocillet *S*   10 releuet stomachum refocillet] moueat stomachum ne lacescat *S*

rejoice forever in greenest youth, so never
is it burned by heat, nor is it rimed by frost.
Persius, with lively tongue, called its seed *cocognidon*—
doctors likewise, with the poets, give witness to this too.
From this is said to come a drink of precious praise,
which purges all the insides and drives through to lower parts,
if anything is blocking the intestines, stomach, lungs.
If a sickness is so heavy that this potion does no good—
for physic teaches that nothing is of benefit
to everybody, everywhere—yet this will never harm,
although for many patients cures are the cause
of greatest pain, even hastening the final close of death.

1.5 Baldmoney (also Spignel), *Meum athamanticum* Jacq.

Your countryman, Baldmoney, sings your praises,
for England made you a spice, and me into a poet,
England, as splendid in herbs as she is not unknown for bards.
And although damp fens—which are known to have
a cold and humid strength—are wont to nourish you,
they say a hot and drying power belongs to you.
Many rejoice to carry this health-bringing spice,
for if perchance a pain disturbs the hollows of the heart
or suddenly provokes the stomach and moves the chest,
this heals the heart, revives the stomach and relieves the chest,
which it can grant (and not in vain) with a single bite.

7 *Cf.* Ovid, *Amores*, 1. 15. 19   8 *Cf.* Pliny 27. 70   11 *Cf.* Dioscorides 4. 146

1.5 BALDEMONIA / **Baldmoney** *Source unknown*
4 *Cf.* Ovid, *Met.* 1. 418

Gingiber hiis parue sunt et gariofila cure,
Nec piretrum precii constat nec cinnama magni,
Nam quod agunt empte, facit hec inuenta palude,
Quodque datur preciis, dat baldemonia gratis.

1.6 AMBROSIA

Ambrosiam licet ordinibus discernere pulcris,
Cuius ab antiquis celeberrima mencio constat,
Cuius nec Maro siluit laudes nec Homerus,
Cuius in excelsis diis est sapor unicus ipsis.
Hec tamen illane sit quam Pyerides coluere
Laudibus inmodicis dubitant qui credere nolunt.
Huic tamen insignem medicorum dogmata laudem
Contribuunt: tantum quod demat pota cruoris
Corporibus quantum potus in corpora † uergit. †

12 gingiber hiis] gingiberis *S* et *om. S* gariophila *P* 13 cinama *S* 14 nam quod] namque *S* hec *om. S*

1.6 AMBROSIA *P* 2v: Ambrosia | *S* 38r: De Ambrosia. Henricus poeta | *T* 90v–91r: Ambrosia

Exceptiones (*O* 89v): Ambrosia herba que tantum cruoris potata tollit, quantum de ipsa bibitur.

(*O* 91r): Ambrosia pulcris ordinibus discernitur. Tantum demit cruoris quantum inde potatur.

2 cuius] eius *P* celeberima *S* 3 cuius] eius *P* nec . . . nec] non . . . nec *S* 4 cuius] eius *P* diis *om. P* est] et *P* 5 illane sit] illa nescit *S* 6 nolunt] uolunt *S* 7 huic tamen] ast huic *P* 8 demat] donat *P* : deuiat *T* 9 quantus *S* uergit] uirginis *S* : uerbis *T*

Cloves and Ginger are petty cures compared to this,
and neither Cinnamon nor Pellitory have much worth at all,
for what these, purchased, perform, this fen-born herb can do,
and what is offered for a price, Baldmoney gives for free.

1.6 Ragweed, *Ambrosia artemisiifolia* L.

One may now distinguish Ambrosia in her beautiful rows,
whose naming by the ancients continues with great fame,
whose praises Maro did not keep silent, nor Homer too,
for its flavour is unique among the gods on high.
Yet some (those who do not wish to believe) are in doubt that it
is Ragweed that Pierus's daughters cultivate with boundless praise.
Still, the doctrines of physicians grant great praise to this,
because when drunk it presses as much blood
out of bodies as the drink poured into bodies.

1.6 AMBROSIA / **Ragweed** *Strabo, 'De Ambrosia', 369–74*
1 Strabo, 'De Agrimonia', 361 9 *Cf.* Ovid, *Ex Ponto* 1. 9. 52

1.7 ORIGANVM

Origani uis exigui feruere probatur;
Origani calor eximii siccare putatur.
Tercius in sicca uirtute gradus datur illi,
Tercius in calida, quociens petit hanc medicina.
Origani succus iunctus cum lacte dolorem
Auribus extirpat si diffundatur in aures.
Naribus inuisum capiti prodire cruorem,
Infusus nari, coget si iungitur yri.
Ore diu tentus plagis medicabitur oris,
Dente diu tritus denti medicabitur egro.
Fauces et tumidas siccando comprimit uuas.
Origani puluis tussim cum melle repellit,
Cum calida morsus stomachi (loquor agnita) lenit,
Vrine prodest et lumbricis nocet haustum,
Omnibus hec tandem ualet interioribus herba.
Crure superpositus cum farris polline succus
Sepe fugat sciasim; si non fugat at premit illam.
Quid quibus in membris det habes; quid corpore toto
Donet habe: fugat ydropisim siccatque tumorem.
Cum mulsa bibitum (fuerit si pondere sumptum
Oxifali) coleram coget deponere nigram.
Deducit bibitum, deducit menstrua tritum,

1.7 ORIGANVM *P* 2v–3r: Origanum | *S* 74v–75r: De Origano. Henricus

Exceptiones (*O* 91r): Origanum calidum et siccum in tertio gradu. Lacti coniunctum et in aures infusum dolorem extirpat. Naribus infusum cruorem prodire coget si iungitur iri. Ore diu tentum plagis medicabitur oris, dente diu tritum denti medicabitur egro. Fauces et tumidas siccando comprimit uuas. Puluis eius cum melle tussim pellit. Cum calida morsus stomachi lenit, urine prodest, lumbricos pellit. Omnibus interioribus ualet potata. Cum farris polline coxe appositum sciasim fugat uel opprimit. Fugat ydropisim et tumorem. Cum mulsa pondere oxifabi sumptum coleram nigram purgat. Deducit menstrua bibitum uel tritum uel coctum suffumigatum. Albo cum uino dat ne digestio tardet. Pruritus, acoras, maculas, elixatura eius delet. Si carice iuncta bibatur, sudorem eicit. Luxatis uel contusis superaddita membris lana repleta prius oleo iunctis et aceto, succis eius. Decoctio ipsius in uino frequenti potu mortiferos morsus fugat. Cum mulsa potatur aconita. De succo eius et cepis et rossiriaco confectio talis ad solem in ere ponitur Phebo ente in Leone. Sic .xiiii. diebus feruere. Exinde subdita lecto non patitur nocuum accedere.

2 eximius *P* 3 tercius . . . illi] *om. P* 4 quocies *P* 6 exstrirpat *S* 7 inuisum] infusam *S* 8 cogit *P* 9 plagas *P* 11 tumidas] mundas *S* comprimet *S* 12 tussim puluis *S* 13 liquor *S* 17 ipsam *S* 18 dat *P* 19 donet habe] donec habere *S* necatque *P* 20 multa bibit *S*

1.7 Oregano, *Origanum heracleoticum* L.

The power of diminutive Oregano is shown to heat,
and by this heat remarkable Oregano is known to dry.
The third degree in virtue dry is granted unto it,
and third in virtue hot, whenever medicine seeks it out.
The juice of Oregano, when mixed with milk, eradicates
an aural pain if it is poured into the ears.
If mixed with Iris and placed inside a nostril,
it will force hated blood of the head flowing out the nose.
Held long inside the mouth, it heals oral wounds,
or ground up with the teeth awhile it heals an ailing tooth.
It subdues a swollen throat or uvula with drying power.
The powder of Oregano with honey drives away a cough,
with hot water softens stomach gripes (I know of what I speak),
when drunk, it's good for urine and will harm your stomach worms,
and in the end, this herb is good for everything inside.
The juice with flour, when placed atop the shin, often drives out
sciatica, or checks it if it does not drive it out.
  You have its gifts for separate parts, now take what it bestows
to the entire body: it drives off dropsy and dries out swelling.
When drunk with mead, it forces melancholy to recede
if one should take it at the measure of a vinegar-cup.
It brings out menstrual courses if drunk, or when ground

1.7 ORIGANVM / **Oregano** *Macer, 'Origanum', 1285–1324*

Si mulier trita uel cocta se fouet herba.
Albo cum uino dat ne digestio tardet;
Hictericis ualet in lauacris decoccio talis.
  Quid ferat interius dixi; nunc dicere restat
Quid ferat exterius fiamque uel ordine gratus.
Hoc in quo coquitur si sepius amne lauentur
Pruritus, acoras, maculas et talia delet.
Origani succo si carica iuncta bibatur
Poris sudorem producit: cognita testor.
Luxatis uel contusis superaddita membris
Lana repleta prius oleo iunctis et aceto,
Origani succis, eque iuuat hec, iuuat illa.
Ipsius fugat in uino decoccio sumpta
Mortiferos morsus, fuerit si pota frequenter;
Potum cum mulsa premit infrendens aconitum.
Iungitur hic succus cepis et rosiriaco;
Ponitur ad solem confeccio talis in ere,
Dum radians Phebus rapidi tenet ora Leonis,
Sicque quater denis debet feruere diebus.
Dempta sub hoc Phebo fuerit si subdita lecto,
Non animal nocuum poterit contingere lectum
(Vt perhibent quibus expertum est uel fingere gratum).

1.8 LAVANDVLA

Fulget odorifero laudata lauandula lecto.
Hanc peplis regina suis, hanc ponere gaudet
Clericus in libris; hanc qui studio preciosas
Conseruat uestes inponit uestibus ipsis.
Hinc peplum, libri, uestes redolent ut ab ipsis

23 si mulier] similiter *P*   fouet] probat *P*   25 lauacro *P*   26 quid . . . gratus] quid ferat interius fiamque uel ordine gratus *S*   28 hoc] hic *P*   31 proris *P*   congnita *P*   32 luxatis] elixatis *S*   35 ipsius . . . sumpta] *om. P*   37 multa *P*   aconita *P*   40 radians] feris *add. et. exp. P*   44 peribent *P*   gratum] est *add. S*

1.8 LAVANDVLA   *P* 3r: Lauendula | *S* 65r: De Lauandula. Henricus

Exceptiones (*O* 91r): Lauandula, herba odorifera unde et libris et uestibus imponi aptissima.

1 falget *P*   2 peplis] prelis *S*   gaude *S*   4 conseruat] hostes *add. P et exp.*   uestibus] istis *add. S*   5 peplum] *scripsi*, pepla *P* : preli *S*   libri] codices *S*

if the woman applies the herb ground down and cooked.
It guarantees digestion never slows, if taken with white wine;
such a decoction placed in baths is good for those with jaundice.
  Its properties inside I gave, and now it's left to say
what it grants outside, and may I be pleasing in this way.
If you often wash in water in which this herb is cooked,
it destroys itching, ulcers, blemishes and all such things.
And if a fig is mixed with Oregano juice and drunk
it produces sweat from pores: I stand witness to the facts.
Wool, first soaked in oil mixed with vinegar and Oregano juice,
and applied to bruised or dislocated limbs,
can help the former just as well as it can help the latter.
A decoction of Oregano taken in your wine,
if it's drunk frequently, drives off death-bringing bites;
when drunk with mead it presses out the gnashing aconites.
The juice is mixed with Onions and with powdered sumac;
such a potion should be placed in open air, beneath the sun,
when radiant Phoebus holds the mouth of rapid Leo,
and in such a way it ought to heat for forty days.
Removed from under Phoebus, if placed beneath a bed,
no harmful beast can dare to touch the bed—or so relate
those to whom it's proven, or to whom it's pleasing to pretend!

1.8 English Lavender, *Lavandula vera* D.C.

Lavender, well-praised, is shining in her scented bed.
A queen rejoices to place this inside her royal robes,
a cleric inside his books; one who would keep with care
his precious garments enfolds this in his clothes.
Robes and books and clothing are so redolent of it, that if

40 *Cf.* Martial, *Ep.* 1. 2. 1; Martial, *Ep.* 6. 93. 3; Ovid, *Met.* 2. 81

1.8 LAVANDVLA / **English Lavender** *Original*

Ipsam si demas, absens uideatur adesse.
Hec dotes tantas tanto contraxit odore
Vt si mater ei uires Natura dedisset
In medicamentis nichil equum tradere quisquam
Posse uidetur. Vix ergo superba medetur.

1.9 SALVIA

Si constat mundi precio preciosior omni
Firma salus, quis lilifagum queat appreciari
Cuius firma salus donum—prestacio—letum?
Primam, clara sequens Macri uestigia Stabus
Primam, clarificans extollit carmine Macer,
Macer cui uiridem dedit orti cura coronam,
Huius enim uires—est uatum signifer ille—
Nosceret egregie (quid enim non nouerat ille?).
Edidit insignem cum fama perpete uersum:
'Cur moriatur homo cum saluia crescat in orto?'
   Quos tamen hec morbos specialius arguat audi:
Cum mulsa potata solet iecur exhilarare,
Cum uino tussim ueterem laterisque dolorem
Curat, sed tepido tepidum coniungito succum.
Vulneribus nimio que manant sanguine tritam
Consocies, perhibent cursum remanere cruoris.
Hoc eciam crines dicunt nigrescere succo
Si fuerint uncti cura sub sole frequenti.
Hec tibi certa scias, quod si certissima poscas:

7 contraxit] constructa *S*   9 nil *S*   quisquam] cuiquam *S*   10 posse uidetur] possem tradetur   uix] nil *S*

1.9 SALVIA *P* 3r–3v: Lilifagus | *S* 91r–91v: De Saluia. Henricus

Exceptiones (*O* 91r–91v): Saluia saluberrima trita cum lilifago, uetonica, tanetico, feniculo, cerfolio, marrubio, absinthio, centaurea, plantagine, lappa. Hec omnia amplo uase loca, uino pleno. Hinc bibe cotidie ciffulum in mane. Hec medicina .X. herbarum dicitur contra quodlibet morbum.

1 constat] omni *add. et exp. P*   2 salus *om. S*   3 cuius . . . letum] *om. P*   prestacio] *scripsi*, predacio *S*   4 primam] primea *S*   5 primam] primea *S*   7 est] cum *P*   8 noceret *S*   9 perprete *S*   10 cur moriatur] infirmatur *S*   12 yecur *P*   16 consociant *P*   cursum] curam *S*   remouere *P*   18 cura] iura *S*   fruenti *S*   19 certas *S*   quod si] nunquam *P*

you take away the herb, when absent it still seems present there.
It has drawn together such great gifts with so great an odour
that if Mother Nature had endowed it with some powers
in medicine, it seems no one could supply
its equal. Therefore haughty, she can scarcely heal.

1.9 Sage, *Salvia officinalis* L.

If health assured is valued as more precious
than any price in the world, who could put a price
on Sage, whose happy gift (its guarantee) is health assured?
Famous Macer extolled it as first, celebrating it in song,
and Strabo called it first, walking in Macer's famous steps,
that Macer, to whom Gardening gave a verdant crown,
for its powers (he is the poets' standard bearer!)
he would know full well, for what did he not know?
He published this great verse of unending fame:
'Why would a man die when Sage grows in his garden?'
  Yet hear what maladies Sage censures especially well:
when drunk with mead the liver it refreshes,
with wine it cures a nagging cough or aching in the side
—but mix its juice, when warm, with the wine, when warm.
Should you apply it ground to wounds which seep
with excess blood, they say the flow of blood is stayed.
They also say that hair is blackened with its juice
if anointed with repeated care beneath the sun.
Know these things as certain, but if you demand very certain things:

1.9 SALVIA / **Sage** *Macer, 'Salvia', 870–81*
10 *Regimen sanitatis salernitanum*, in *Collectio Saleritana* (ed. de Renzi) 5. 31, 1102

Menstrua fert, mouet urinam, depellit abortum,
Pruritus uulue curat uirgeque uirilis,
Si foueantur eo coquitur quo saluia uino.
Preterea innumeris perhibent occurrere morbis
Hanc, laudare tamen plus docta nequit medicina
Quam laudare solet, certans garrire, coquina.
  Vis rem perfectam, uis claram, uis memorandam
Noscere perpetue que sit tibi causa salutis?
Lilifagum lege, uetonicam lege taneticumque,
Feniculum lege, cerfolium lege marubiumque,
Absinthii, centhauree, plantaginis adde
Gramina, cum lappa tere. Iuncta simul bene trita
Amplo uase loca; uas Bachi munere comple.
Hinc cifulum bibe cotidie sed mane supremo;
Sic quosuis morbos, sic quasuis effuge pestes.
Herbarum solet ista decem medicina uocari.

1.10 RVTA

Ruta decens decimo ramos extendit agello,
Ruta decens semper, ramos uiridissima semper.
Vim desiccantem, uim fertur habere calentem.
Forte gradum queres? Gradus illis tercius heret–
Hinc non maiestas, non est minuenda potestas,
Nec minuendus honor dum claram reddere conor.
  Naso suaue canens, dum pennas demit Amori,
Quid cecinit? 'Sumas acuentes lumina rutas.'
Ergo quid melius uel quid specialius implet,
Lumina nunc acuens, nunc te, Cytharea, retundens?
Nil horum melius, neutrum specialius eque.
  Tercia succedit probitas quam sepe probaui:

20 repellit *S*   aborsum *P*   22 qua *S*   24 medicinis *P*   27 noscere] nosse *P*   28 taneticumque] *scripsi* (*cf.* tanetico, *O 91r*) : tanetumque *PS*   29 ferniculum *S*   30 centauree *S*   33 suppremo *S*

1.10 RVTA   *P* 3v–4v: Rutha | *S* 89v–90v: De Ruta. Henricus   *First edited by Ruppel,* 207–208, *from only S. ll. 1–2 transp. P*

4 illi *P*   heret] hec est *S*   5 hinc] hoc *P*   9 ergo] hoc *S*   10 te *om. P*   citharea retundit *S*   11 nil . . . eque] *om. S*

it brings out menses, moves the urine, and expels a foetus,
it cures an itching of the vulva and of the manly rod,
if they are washed in wine in which the Sage was cooked.
They relate, moreover, this cures diseases without number,
yet learned Medicine knows not how to praise it more
than Kitchen, garrulous and quarrelsome, is apt to praise.
  Do you want to know a perfect thing, a famous thing,
a memorable thing that is a source of lasting health?
Take Sage, take Betony, and take Tansy too,
take Fennel, Chervil, and pick Horehound too,
add the seeds of Wormwood, Centaury, and Plantain;
thus grind with Dock. Place these things, ground well together,
in a spacious vase, and fill the vase with Bacchus's gift.
Drink a spoonful of it daily, but only at the height of morning,
and thus chase away any disease, thus drive out any plague.
This recipe is often called the 'Ten-Herb Medicine.'

1.10 Rue, *Ruta graveolens* L.

Rue fittingly extends its branches in the tenth plot,
Rue, always proper, ever greenest in its branches.
It is said to have a drying power and a heating power.
Do you ask, perchance, the grade? The third degree belongs to these—
from it neither majesty nor strength should be diminished,
nor is honour to be diminished while I strive to make it famous.
  What did tuneful Ovid sing, while plucking wings
from Love? 'Gather eye-sharpening Rues.'
Therefore what satisfies better, what more specifically,
now sharpening eyes, now deflecting you, Cytherean Venus?
No other can serve better, nor any quite as specifically.
  A third proof comes next, which I have often tested:

1.10 RVTA / **Rue** *Macer, 'Ruta,' 267–331*
1 *Cf.* Ovid, *Amores* 3. 1. 9 7–8 Ovid, *Remedia amoris* 801–802

Tres sumo ramos, sumptos macero, maceratos
Febris in accessu dono donandoque curo.
  Illi quarta datur preciose gloria laudis:
Pota uenena potest uel cruda comesta fugare.
Hoc mustela docet, que si serpentibus atris
Confligat, prius hanc comedit; mox prelia uincit.
Rex Mitridates Ponti, uitare uenena
Dum uellet, foliis uiginti rute solebat
Cum pauco sale, cum caricis geminaque iuglanti
Ieiunus uesci, postquam securus edebat.
  Quatuor hee prime sunt uires ordine rute.
Nunc reliquas tractare libet, temptare licebit:
In corio maligranati comprime succum
Rute, mox tepefac aurique infunde dolenti.
Huius item succum nimio que sanguine manant
Naribus infundas; cessabit currere sanguis.
Ruta rapit stomachi morbos si sepe bibatur,
Tussim compescit, tardancia menstrua purgat
Expellitque moram partus—certissima dico.
Hanc in aqua coquito, post iungas acre lyeum:
Sic procurrentis compescit tormina uentris.
Pulmones sanat sic sumptum, pectora purgat,
Curat pleureticos (in costis hii paciuntur),
Sic eciam fugat artheticam sciasimque. Quid hec sunt?
'Morbus enim coxe sciasis, cubitisque uocatur
Arthetica, in manibus ciragra, in pedibusque podagra.'
Si coquis hanc oleo, lumbricos pota repellit.
Quid sunt lumbrici? 'Vermes longi stomachales.'
Matricem iuuat hec intestinumque morantem
Vnguen clisterio si diffundatur in illis.
Huic quoque si iungas uinum iuuat hanc, iuuat illum.
Cum lauri foliis hanc coniungas bene tritis:

13 sumo] *scripsi*, summo *S* : summe *P*   sumpto *S*   macce macceratos *P*   14 accensu *S*   16 commesta *S*   18 commedit *P*   19 mytridates *P*   poti *S*   uenena *bis S*   20 uiginti] XX *P*   rete *S*   21 cum . . . iuglanti] *om. S*   iuglanti] *scripsi*, uiglanti *P*   22 postquam] post quos *S*   24 tractare] uelit *add. et exp. P*   25 maligranati] mali grauati *P*   26 infude *P*   27 mandant *P*   29 rapi *S*   30 compellit *S*   32 aquam *S*   iungas] aqua *add. et exp. P*   acre lyeum] accelienum *S*   33 procurrentis] *scripsi*, procurantis *P* : procurentis *S*   compescis *S*   34 pulmonem *P*   35 plureticos *S*   36 artericam *S*   quid hec sunt] uocatur *S*   38 aterica *S*   40 sunt] sit *P*   41 matriciem *S*   42 unguen] *scripsi*, unguem *PS*   43 hunc *P*

I pick three branches, I boil them when picked, once boiled
I give them at the onset of a fever, and I cure with such a gift.
  A fourth glory of precious praise is given to it:
when drunk or eaten green it is able to drive out poisons.
The weasel teaches this who, if he does battle
with serpents dark, eats this first; soon it wins its battles.
When the King of Pontus, Mithridates, wished
to avoid poisons he liked to eat twenty leaves of Rue
with a little salt, with figs and two walnuts,
all on an empty stomach; afterwards he ate secure.
  These are the first four powers of Rue, in order.
Now I am free to discuss the rest, if allowed to try:
press juice of Rue juice in a pomegranate skin,
next heat it a little and pour it into an aching ear.
Likewise pour its juice into noses which flow
with too much blood; the blood will cease to flow.
Rue destroys stomach diseases if often imbibed,
checks a cough, purges delayed menstrual courses,
and expels the afterbirth—I speak most certain things.
Cook this in water and afterwards add vinegar:
thus it restrains the pains of a runny stomach.
Taken thus it cleans the lungs, purges the chest,
cures the pleuritic (those who are suffering in the ribs),
so also it drives out arthritis and sciatica. What are they?
'The disease of the hip is called *sciatica*; in the elbows
it is called *arthritis*, in the hands *ciragra*, in the feet *podagra*.'
If you cook this with oil and drink it repels *lumbrici*.
What are *lumbrici*? 'Long worms found in the stomach.'
This helps the womb and a sluggish intestine if
an ointment of it is injected into them with a clyster.
If you blend wine with this, it helps the former, helps the latter.
Add this to well-ground laurel leaves;

19–22 *Cf.* Quintus Serenus 1061–8

Appositis testes potes hiis curare tumentes.
Necnon cum caricis in uino concoque rutam,
Sic ualet ydropicis si nocte quidem superaddas.
  Vnguentum rute scribam: miscere iuuabit
Ceruse necnon oleo te, ruta, rosato.
Scis cerusa quid est? 'Conbustum sic uoco plumbum.'
Hoc unguen mire laudis sacrum fugat ignem,
Conterit et dertam que dicitur 'herpeta' grece.
Hoc 'acoras' delet—capitis sic ulcera Grecus
Que pingui fluitant humore solet uocitare.
Naribus inpositum fugat ozinas. Hee quoque quid sunt?
'Vlcera que fetent in naribus abdita curuis.'
  'Paganon' in greca uocitatur ruta loquela;
Antidotum sic conficitur diapaganon inde:
Quantum de ruta sola, piper atque ciminum
Et nitrum iungunt; hec ut iungant, prius assant.
Mox assata terunt contritaque melle resoluunt.
Hoc iecur et renes, latus et pectus bene curat.
Roborat hoc stomachum quo prompte digerat escas,
Hoc bilem lenit, uentrem sine tormine mollit.
Hoc, si ruta ualet (immo, quoniam ualet), hoc est:
† Cetera non minime tibi sit res maxima cure. †

1.11 YSOPVM

Nunc licet undenum Salomonis gloria primum
Dat scriptis ysopum. Cunctas huic sublocat herbas,
Sublocat arboreos cetus et te quoque, cedrus.
Quod si non etas delesset opus preciosum,

45 curare] iuuare *P* 46 in] et *P* conquoque *S* 47 idropicis *P* quidem] quaque *P* 48 unguentum] ungium *S* 49 rosato] sosato *S* 51 unguem *S* 52 dentam *P* herpeta] hec peta *S* 53 hoc] hec *P* 54 quod *S* 55 inpositum] infusum *P* ozinas] orinas *P* hee] hec *P* quoque] quo *S* 56 fetent] fecerit *S* addita *P* 57 pagamon *P* grea *S* 58 conficiunt *S* 58 dyapagamon *P* 59 cuminum *S* 61 terunt] tremunt *S* 62 iecur et renes latus] latus et renes yecur *P* curat *corr. e* curant *P* 63 quo prompte] quod forte *P* digerat] *scripsi*, dirigat *P* : degerat *S* 64 bilen *S* 65 hoc . . . hoc] hec . . . hec *P* immo quoniam ualet] ymmo ualet quam ualet *P* : immo ualet o ualet *Rigg* est] et *P*

1.11 YSOPVM *P* 4v–5r: Isopus | *S* 105r–105v: De Ysopo. Henricus
1 nunc] nos *S* 2 huic] hoc *P* subleuat *S*

apply these and you can cure swollen testicles.
You can also cook Rue with figs in wine; thus it is good
for those with dropsy if you apply it every night.
I will describe an ointment made of Rue: it will help to mix
you, Rue, with oil-of-Rose and *cerusa*. Do you know
what *cerusa* is? 'This is the name I give burnt lead.'
This ointment of marvellous praise drives out Holy Fire,
and it clears those scabs which are called *herpes* in Greek.
This destroys *achores*—a Greek is thus apt to name
the ulcers of the head which flow with a fatty humour.
Placed in the nose it ejects *ozinas*—and what are they?
'Polyps which fester hidden within curved noses.'
Rue is called *paganon* in the Greek language;
so from it the antidote *diapaganon* is made:
they mix the same amount of Rue alone, then Pepper,
Cumin and Soda; so that they blend, they roast them first.
Next, they grind them, roasted, and mix them ground with honey.
This cures the liver and kidneys well, the sides and the chest.
It strengthens the stomach so that it promptly digests foods,
it softens bile and soothes the belly without pain.
This, if the Rue is good (or rather, since it is good), is this:
† no other may be the greatest matter for your smallest cure. †

1.11 Hyssop, *Hyssopus officinalis* L.

The glory of Solomon gives Hyssop (although it is eleventh
here) the first place in his writings. He placed all other herbs below,
and placed below it the arboreal crowd and, Cedar, even you.
If time had not destroyed this precious work,

1.11 YSOPVM / **Hyssop** *Macer, 'Ysopum', 1503–31*
1–9 1 Kgs. 4: 33

Non hunc non alios opus esset scribere libros.
Nunc ysopi tractetur honor. Rex atque propheta,
Versificus tam carminibus quam tempore primus,
Solius meminit: gramen uenerabile, salue,
Salue, graminei decus et iactancia cetus!
  Hic cum multa queat specialiter interiorum
Dicitur antidotum. Calet et siccat: gradus illi
Tercius extat in hiis. Decoccio graminis huius
Sicut sicca simul ficus cum melle coquatur;
Adiuuat omnimodas pulmonum sumpta querelas,
Sumpta potest aqua tussimque ptysimque fugare
In pectus capitis que distillacio fecit.
Lumbricos perimit, reicit potata catharrum,
Hausta prius raucum reddit clarissima clarum.
Hec quoque si puluis melli datur omnia curat,
Tensaque cum uino sumptum precordia laxat,
Et fugit absque mora ledens tumor interiora.
Oximel huic iunctum stipatum prouocat aluum;
Forcius hunc solues istis si cardama iunges.
Ipsum cum nitro cum ficu contere sicca:
Hoc iuuat ydropicos et splen tumidum cataplasma.
Elixum apponas: liuores limpidat omnes.
Accendas ysopum: fumo sonitus perit auris.
Hoc eciam dentes curabis sepe dolentes
In quo decoquitur si confoueantur aceto.
Siccum siue uirens ysopum si sepe bibatur,
Hinc calor eximius (ni fallat fama) paratur.

1.12 CAMEDREOS

Grece 'camedreos' et 'germandreia' latine
Diceris, herba uirens semper, breuis, acris, odora,
Sicca calensque: gradus tibi tercius est in utroque.

6 yzopi *P* 9 certus *S* 10 hic] hoc *S* inferiorum *S* 14 pulmonium *P* 15 ptysimque] *scripsi*, sitimque *P* : tysimque *S* 18 raucum] ranem *S* 22 iunctum] uictum *P* 24 ficcu *S* 25 cathaplasma *P* 26 elyxim *P* 27 parit *S* 28 eciam] in *S* curabit *P* 29 conficiantur *S* 30 succum *S* 31 calor] *scripsi*, color *PS* nisi *S* paratur] paciatur *S*

1.12 CAMEDREOS *P* 5r: Camedreos | *S* 48v–49r: Cametreos. Henricus *Lines 1–7 were first edited by Rigg, 254–5.*

1 cametreos *S* gamandrea *P* 2 semper *om. S*

there would be no need to write this nor other books.
Let Hyssop's honour now be treated! That king and prophet,
a poet first in both his poetry and his time,
mentioned it alone: Hail, venerable herb,
hail, glory and boasting of this grassy gathering!
Since it is good especially for many problems of the inner parts,
it is called an 'antidote'. It heats and dries,
and has the third degree in these. A decoction of its seed
should be cooked like a dry fig in honey:
it helps out every sort of lung complaint when taken
and drunk with water it drives away consumption and the cough
which a dripping in the head has made inside the chest.
When drunk it kills stomach worms and drives out a catarrh;
when this most famous herb is first imbibed it makes a sore throat clear.
If powdered Hyssop is added to honey it cures all these things as well,
and taken with wine it loosens a tightened diaphragm;
even a harmful tumour found inside flees without delay.
Honey-vinegar mixed with Hyssop loosens constipation,
and if you add some Cress, you will loosen it even more.
Grind this herb with Soda and dried figs:
as a plaster this assists the dropsical and a swollen spleen.
Apply it boiled: it clears up all your bruises.
Burn Hyssop and a ringing of the ears vanishes with the smoke.
With this you will also cure teeth which often hurt
if they are rubbed with vinegar in which this herb was cooked.
If Hyssop, dry or green, is often taken in a drink,
a mighty heat is produced from this (if rumour does not lie).

1.12 Wall Germander, *Teucrium chamaedrys* L.

Germander, you're called *germandreia* in Latin and *camedreos*
in Greek, an herb ever green, low-lying, bitter, aromatic,
both dry and hot: your degree is third in each.

7 Henry of Huntingdon, *HA* 12. 1, 29 (pp. 806–807); 1 Chr. 16: 7–36

1.12 CAMEDREOS / **Germander** *Macer, 'Chamaedrys', 1903–17*

Bis genito sociare deo te Gallia sueuit,
Nam te Lauduni—dum mellea flumina poto
Fontibus Anselmi manancia—sepe solebam,
Sepe solebatis Bacho superaddere, ciues.
Si mixta poteris aqua depellis abortum,
Conquassata iuuas. Si mixta bibaris aceto
Ydropicis sic succurris, sic menstrua purgas,
Sic splen desiccas, sic seuis morsibus obstas,
Omnibus hiis eciam trita et superaddita prodes.
Te cum melle terunt et tritam melle reponunt,
Vulnus ut immundum purges licet inueteratum,
Et cum melle tuo superungunt lumina succo
Hecque sibi dempta reddunt caligine clara.
Te tritam miscent oleo corpusque perungunt
Vt sic frigdorem pellas reuocesque calorem.
Antidotum dyacamedreos sic inde paratur:
Camedreos binas et bracteos accipe denas
Ast unam piperis, edere mirreque. Sed ista
Tandem conficies, dragmam iunges ydromellis.
Hec sciasi—mire nequaquam—proficit eque.

1.13 CAMOMILLA

'Anthemis' grece que dicitur hanc 'camomilla'
Romani dicunt. Hec magni nominis esse
Fertur apud Grecos quod et Esclapius docet ipse.
Scribitur hec feruere gradu siccareque primo,
Sic herbe similis quam dicit plebs amaruscum
Vt si conspicias amaruscum cum camomilla,
Hic camomilla tibi uideatur et hec amaruscus,

4 genite *P* seuit *S* 5 te *om. P* Lauduni *S*] Laudumi *P* : laudaui *Rigg* pote *P* 6 Ancelmi *S* 7 soledabis *S* Bacco *P* 8 aborsum *P* 9 cum quassata uinas *S* 10 ydropisis *S* 11 splende siccas *S* 12 prodest *P* 13 terunt] terre *S* reponunt] repellunt *P* 15 superungant *S* 17 trita *P* 18 frigorem *P* *ll. 19–23 om. S* 23 mire nequaquam] *scripsi*, mirre nec quidquam *P*

1.13 CAMOMILLA *P* 5r–5v: Camomila | *S* 48r–48v: De Camomilla. Henricus
1 antemis *P* que] qua *S* 2 hec] hoc *S* 3 aput *P* et *om. P* 4 feruere] seruire *S* 5 similis] simul *S* dicit] docet *S* amaroseum *S* 6 si] sic *S* amaroseum *S* 7 hic] hec *P* amaroseus *S*

France was wont to blend you with the Twice-Born god,
for while I was drinking the honeyed rivers
flowing from the fonts of Anselm, I was often apt
(and you, citizens of Laon, were often apt) to mix you so.
  If you are drunk, when mixed with water, you expel a foetus,
and you heal bruises. If mixed with vinegar and drunk,
you thus assist the dropsical and purge the menstrual courses,
thus you dry the spleen and counteract savage bites,
and when ground and applied you're good for all these things.
They grind you with honey and apply you ground with honey
to purge an unclean wound, albeit very old.
They anoint the eyes with honey and your juice,
and render them clear after the cloudiness is removed.
They mix you ground with oil and anoint a body
so you thus force out the cold and recall the warmth.
  The antidote *dyacamedreos* is prepared from it like this:
take two parts of Germander and ten parts Juniper,
but one each of Pepper, ivy, and Myrrh. And finally
mix all these things together and add a dram of honey-water.
This is just as good for sciatica, a thing by no means surprising.

1.13 Chamomile, *Chamaemelum nobile* (L.) All.

The Romans call this herb Chamomile which is called
anthemis in Greek. It is said to be of great fame among
the Greeks, which Aesculapius himself makes known.
This herb is described as heating and drying in the first degree,
so similar to the herb which the crowd call *amaruscus*
that if you should see *amaruscus* with Chamomile,
the former would seem Chamomile to you, the latter *amaruscus*.

4 Ovid, *Met.* 3.317 6 Jerome, *Ep.* 49.13 (ed. Hilberg and Kamptner); Pseudo-Virgil, *Culex* 78 (ed. Fairclough)

1.13 CAMOMILLA / **Chamomile** *Macer, 'Chamomilla', 549–91*

Quorum si temptes ut discernantur odores
Non magis a tenebris lucem distare uidebis!
Hec thuri similis, fetentibus ille cicutis,
Suauibus hec uiolis, squalentibus hic colubrinis.
  Hanc si quis sumat cum uino tormina sedat,
Inflatum reprimit stomachum cum melle iugata,
Sicque rapit squamas uultu decoccio sumpta.
Prodest hictericis mire iecorisque querelis.
Morsibus hec obstat cum uino pondere dragme.
Vrine ualet et lapidi decoccio, purgat
Menstrua, cum uino potata depellit abortum.
Si medicus commasticet hanc et postea ponat
Egilopas curat, sed et ulcera sordida purgat.
Si coquis hanc oleo sanas ypocondria feda;
Hoc unguen febrem pellit sed frigora lenit.
Quod si forte caput febris feruore grauatum
Vlcera que Grecus uocat 'exantumata' prodat,
Deficient illa uirtute tua, camomilla.
Plinius hanc dicit, si quadraginta diebus
Et bis quaque die sumatur pondere dragme
Cum uini ciatis albi clarique duobus,
Cum locio splenem purgare simulque lienem.
  Tres illi species auctores esse fatentur:
Floribus hee clarent, nam cum flos aureus illis
Omnibus in medio sit circumcingitur ille
Vel niueis uel purpureis foliisue nigellis.
Nigris et niueis sunt purpurei meliores.
Nec sine nomine sunt: 'leucantemon' datur albis
Et nigris 'crisantemon.' Est purpureorum
'Anthemys' proprie nomen quod et est generale.

10 hec] hoc *S*   simul fetentes *S*   ille] *scripsi*, illa *PS*   11 hec] hoc *S* : *om. P*   uiollis *S*   hic] hec *S*   13 iugata] *scripsi*, iugatum *PS*   15 mirre *P*   18 depellit] repellit *S*   19 si] sic *S*   21 oleo] febrem pellit uel frigora leuit *add. et exp. S*   ipocondria *S*   22 unguem *S*   23 febres *S*   24 uocat] uatat *S*   exantumiata *S*   26 dicit *om. S*   28 ciatis] sciathis *S*   29 purgat *P*   30 autores *P*   31 ille *P*   35 leucatemon *S*   36 et] at *S*   37 antemis *S*   et est] *scripsi*, est et *P* : est *S*

But if you try to distinguish their odours
you'll see that day does not differ more from night!
Chamomile is similar to Incense, *amaruscus* to stinking Hemlock,
the former to sweetest Violets, the latter to filthy Dragon Arums.
If you take this with wine it settles stomach cramps,
when mixed with honey it prevents a bloated stomach,
and used in a decoction it removes scales from the face.
It marvellously benefits the jaundiced and liver complaints.
Taken at a dram's weight with wine it works against bites.
A decoction is good for urine and the stone, it purges
menstrual courses, and drunk with wine it expels a foetus.
If a doctor chews and afterwards applies this,
it heals tumours of the eye, and also purges filthy ulcers.
If you cook this in oil you clean a fouled abdomen;
this ointment dispels a fever, but also soothes a cold.
But if perchance a head, burdened by a fever's fire,
produces ulcers which the Greeks call *exanthemata*,
they will disappear by your virtue, O Chamomile!
Pliny says that if this is taken for forty days,
twice on every day, and at the weight of a dram,
with two spoonfuls of clear, white wine,
it purges both the spleen and liver through the urine.
The authorities say there are three varieties:
they are distinguished by their flowers, for although the flower
is golden in the middle for all of them, it is surrounded
by petals of either white or red or nearly black.
The red are better than the purple or the white,
nor are they without a name: *Leucanthemum* is given
to the white, and to the purple *Chrysanthemum*. *Anthemis*
is proper to the reds, but the name is also general.

1.14 BVGLOSSA

'Lingua bouis' Rome, 'buglossa' uocatur Athenis.
Vulneribus mire ius huius proficit herbe,
Vt si non aliud quid haberet, nominis esset
(Et merito) magni, meritis nunc maxima multis.
Mixtus aque succus tepide si sumitur herbe
Quos stabilis uexat sciasis mire ualet egris.
Pulmonum nocuos humores pota repellit,
Quod si cardiacum colere dat copia nigre,
Adnichilabit eum. Fuerit si pota frequenter
Sic coleram purgat rubeam, feruore perustam.
Illam si maceres et uino des maceratam
Sicque bibas, memorem cerebri uim seruat et auget.
Plinius affirmat hoc, quod decoccio reddat
Letos conuiuas hac si conuiuia spargas.

1.15 SANICLA

Huic merito sanicla subest, quod uulnera sanat.
Vulnera quod sanet merito sanicla uocatur.
Hec in sanando uirtutis uulnera tante
Dicitur ut, stomacho nunquam dignata morari,
Perforet, exundans stomachi penetralia, carnes,
Ossa simul, uulnusque petens in uulnere prodat.
Talem conspicies qualem potauerat eger
Dum proprius uigor huic superato corpore restat.
At si transierit caput inclemencia ferri

1.14 BVGLOSSA *P* 4v–6r: Buglossa | *S* 67v–68r: De Lingua bouis. Henricus

2 ulneribus *S* ius] *scripsi*, uis *PS* 3 non] nil *P* aliud quid] aliquid quid *S* 5 tepidus *P* 10 perustum *P* 12 uim] inde *S* 13 hoc] *scripsi*, hec *PS* 13 quod] que *S* 14 conuiuia] conuiua *S*

1.15 SANICLA *P* 6r: Sanicula | *S* 92v–93r: De Sanicla. Henricus

Exceptiones (*O* 91v): Sanicla dicitur quod uulnera sanet. Hec omnia penetrans per plagam exit qualiter bibitur. At <c>apite sauciato cauenda est ne uulnera querendo pelliculam cerebri perforet et cerebrum turbando sauciatum interficiat.

1 huic] fuit *S* sanet *P* 3 uulnere *S* 4 dignatur *P* 5 exundas *S* stomacum *S* 6 patens *P* perdat *S* 7 conspiciens *S* 8 proprius uigor huic] color huic prius *S* 9 inclemencia] in dementa *S*

1.14 Ox-Tongue (Bugloss), *Anchusa arvensis* L.

The Ox-Tongue of Rome in Athens is called *buglossa*.
The juice of this herb is marvellously good for wounds,
so that if it had nothing else, it still would have a great
reputation (and worthily), now the greatest for its many merits.
If the juice of the herb is taken, mixed with tepid water,
it's very good for patients whom persistent sciatica bothers.
When drunk, it repels painful humours of the lungs,
but if an abundance of black bile creates heartburn,
this will destroy it. If it should be drunk frequently
it thus purges red bile, burning it up with heat.
If you boil it, give it boiled with wine, and drink it thus:
it preserves and amplifies the brain's power of memory.
Pliny affirms that a decoction renders partygoers
happy if you should sprinkle the banquet hall with this.

1.15 Wood Sanicle, *Sanicula europaea* L.

Sanicle rightly is found next to this because it heals wounds.
Since it sanitizes wounds, it is properly called Sanicle.
It is said to be of such great power in healing wounds
that it never deigns to remain inside the stomach,
but, overflowing the stomach's inner parts, it pierces the flesh,
and seeking bones and wounds alike, it comes out in the wound.
You will see there exactly what the patient had imbibed,
provided its native vigour remains, once the body is overcome.
But if the cruelty of a sword should cut through a skull,

1.14 BVGLOSSA / **Ox-Tongue** *Macer, 'Buglossa', 1127–38*
13 *Cf.* Pseudo-Dioscorides, *De herbis femininis* cap. 2, 'Buglossos' (ed. Kästner, 591)

1.15 SANICLA / **Wood Sanicle** *Source unknown*

Hanc moneo caueas, nec enim, dum uulnera querens
In caput ascendit, cerebro cerebrique fideli
Pellicule seruatrici fortissima parcet
Nullaque cura sibi, cerebrum si turbet et eius
Pelliculam rumpat, qua rupta rumpitur eger.

1.16 COSTVS

Ortensis costi sedes prefulget in orto,
Est etenim costum species a nomine cuius
Herba trahit nomen, quasi non deceat speciosam
Nomine signari nisi preclare speciei.
Si numeras herbas redolentes hanc numerabis;
Si numeras medicis acceptas hanc numerabis,
Huius enim radix fuerit si cocta parumper
Aut oleo uel aqua (si munus desit oliue)
Prouocat auxilio stomachum uentremque salubri.
Et quia sunt multi qui nolunt credere multis
Ambiguaque fide tarde raris quoque credunt,
Ne finxisse putent, uerbum non amplius addam.

11 ascendens *P*   13 eius] amens *S*

1.16 COSTVS *P* 6r: Costus | *S* 54r: De Costo. Henricus

Exceptiones (*O* 91v): Costus herba hortensis nomen habens a costo quod species est quia speciosa est et bene redolens, escis preelecta. Eius radix oleo uel aqua cocta stomacum et uentrem constipatum salubriter soluit.

1 hortensis . . . horto *S*   3 protrahit *P*   4 signare *S*   5 numeres *S*   6 si . . . numerabis] *om. S*

I advise you to beware of this, for, while it seeks out wounds
and ascends into the head, it's very strong and will not spare
the brain and the brain's faithful, protective skin.
There is no cure for this, if it disturbs the brain and tears apart
its little skin, for once that's cut, the patient is cut short.

1.16 Cost (Costus Root), *Costus speciosus* J. König

The seat of Garden Cost is outstanding in the garden,
for *costum* is the spice from which the herb
receives its name, as if it did not suit a lovely herb
to be named after anything but a famous spice.
If you collect sweet-smelling herbs, you will gather this,
if you collect the doctors' favourites, you will gather this,
for if its root is cooked a little while with oil
(or with water, if the olive's gift is lacking),
it rouses the esophagus and stomach with wholesome aid.
And because many do not wish to believe many things,
or believe things rarely with a thin and tardy faith—
lest they think me a liar—I will add no more.

12 *Cf.* William of Conches, *De philosophia mundi* 4. 24 (PL 172: 95)

1.16 COSTVS / **Cost** *Source unknown*
1, 7–9 *Cf.* Strabo 281–3 12 *Cf.* Ovid, *Fasti* 6. 3–4; Horace, *Satires* 1. 1, 121

1.17 ANGLICA COSTVS

Herba subit costo que dicitur 'Anglica costus,'
Anglica nam costus a Gallis fertur; ab Anglis
Hanc quasi despiciant, Scotorum dicitur herba.
Non despecta tamen, non uilis debet haberi,
Que condimentis et odoribus est aliena,
Cum medicinali tociens sit munere plena.
Namque solet, si purpureo sit iuncta lyeo,
Pectoris ardores, cordis sedare dolores.
Preterea, munitus ea, medicamine grato
Empicos et pleureticos cum melle iuuato.

1.18 BETA MAIOR

Ordine que sequitur hec 'personatia' Rome,
'Prosopes' a Grecis, a uulgo 'beta' uocatur.
Nec mirum si, tam Grecis quam nota Latinis,
Splendeat et presit cum multis sepeque prosit.
Cum uino ueteri si personatia detur
Morsus anguinos, morsus sanat colubrinos.
Trita diu radix, sed cum sale, menstrua purgat.

1.17 ANGLICA COSTVS *P* 6r: Costus Anglica | *S* 38v: De Anglica costus. Macer (*sic*) *Edited by Rigg, 255.*

Exceptiones (*O* 91v): Est alia que dicitur costus Anglica que a Gallis despectiue Scottorum dicitur herba. Condimentis tamen et odoribus grata. Purpureo uino mixta pectoris ardores, cordis dolores sedat. Empicis et pleureticis cum melle prodest.

1 herba] uerba *S* que] qui *S* 3 schotorum *P* 5 que condimentis] super condumentis *S* 6 tocies *P* sit *om. S* 7 iuncta] mixta *S* lieo *P* 9 pretereas *P* munitus] inimicus *S* 11 plureticos *S* iuuato] iuuaret *P*

1.18 BETA MAIOR *P* 6v: Betha | *S* 46v: De Beta maiore. Henricus

Exceptiones (*O* 91v): Personatia est herba que a grecis persopes, a uulgo beta uocatur. Cum uino ueteri morsus anguinos et colubrinos sanat. Radix diu trita cum sale menstrua purgat; radix eius cum spina siccis nata locis equali pondere commixta morsum canis rabidi curat. Preterea sumpto ciatho bete et duobus ciathis mellis, uetus ulcus sanatur.

1 hec] herba *P* personancia *S* 2 persopes *S* a] autem *S* beta] *scripsi*, betha *P* : beata *S* 4 sepe prositque *P* 5 ueteri uino *S* personancia *S* 6 anguineos *P* 7 trida *S*

1.17 English Cost/Costmary, *Tanacetum balsamita* L.

There follows Cost an herb called English Cost.
It's labelled by the French as English Cost, but by the English
it is called the 'Herb of Scots' as if a thing despised.
But that herb should not be deemed despicable or vile
which is unsuitable for seasonings or perfumes,
since it is so often filled with the gifts of medicine.
For it is accustomed, if added to purple wine,
to settle burnings of the chest and pains within the heart.
Moreover, guarded by this herb, aid those with abscesses
and pleurisy by this pleasing medicine with honey.

1.18 Burdock, *Arctium lappa* L.

The herb which follows in succession is called *personatia*
in Rome, *prosopes* by Greeks, and Burdock by the crowd.
No wonder if it, as famous to Latins as to Greeks,
is distinguished and powerful since it's often good for many things.
If Burdock is given with old wine
it cures snake bites and serpent stings.
The root, when ground awhile with salt, purges menses.

1.17 ANGLICA COSTVS / **English Cost** *Source unknown*

1.18 BETA MAIOR / **Burdock** *Pseudo-Apuleius no. 36, 'Herba Personacia' (pp. 81–2)*

Que siccis innata locis est accipe spinam,
Prosopes equali radicem pondere pone;
Sic rabidi morsum canis euades superatum.
Preterea ciatum bete, ciatos quoque mellis
Sume duos, sumptisque uetus sanabitur ulcus.
Hiis foliis cinctum sanari febricitantem
Affirmant quidam, uetiti non credere quicquam.
Sed quid ego? Cum certa lego, non hec nego, sed cum
Talia conspicio, non funditus assero laudans
Talia sumere, sumpta probare, probata tenere.

1.19 BETA MINOR

Betam beta minor lecto sequitur tamen equo:
Beta minor foliis, minor effigie, minor actu.
Si dolor aut uulnus capitis turbauerit arcem
Hanc medici celerem perhibent conferre salutem.
Hanc igitur medicaminibus cunctis sapientes
Que capiti prosunt, simul et theodoricon addunt.
Quid theodoricon est? 'Preciosum sic Galienus
Nominat antidotum contra capitis nocumentum.'

8 que] quod *S* 9 prosopes] per sopes *S* pone] preme *P* 10 rapidi *S* 11 bethe *P* 12 summe *P* 13 cinocum *P* febricitatem *S* 15 quid] quem *S* cum] dum *S* 17 summere *P* tenete *S*

1.19 BETA MINOR *P* 6v [no title] | *S* 46v: De Beta minore. Henricus

Exceptiones (*O* 91v): Est alia beta minor foliis, effigie, uiribus, si tamen dolor aut uulnus capud turbauerit, cito subuenit. Vnde et omnibus capitis medicaminibus simul et Theodoricon additur. Theodoricon est precisoum antidotum contra capitis passionem.

1 betam] betham *P* beta] *scripsi*, betha *P* : beata *S* sequitur tamen equo] sequetur equino (?) *P* 2 beta . . . actu] *om. P* 3 archam *P* 5 medicantibus *S* 6 que] quod *S* 7 preciosis *S*

Take the thorn which is found in arid places
and add an equal weight of Burdock root;
thus you will overcome and escape the bite of a rabid dog.
Moreover, take a teaspoon of Burdock and two of honey;
after these are taken a lingering ulcer will be healed.
Some, opposed to disbelieve anything, affirm
that a feverish person bound with these leaves is healed.
But what of me? When I read established facts, I don't deny them,
but when I see such things, not praising out of hand, I state
that you take such things, prove once taken, and keep once proven.

1.19 Lesser Burdock, *Arctium minus* Bernh.

Lesser Burdock follows Burdock yet in an equal bed:
lesser in leaves, lesser in shape, and lesser in effect.
If a pain or wound disturbs the top of your head,
the doctors claim this grants a speedy remedy.
Hence wise men add this herb to every medicine,
including *theodoricon*, which helps the head.
And what is *theodoricon*? 'In such a way did Galen
name the antidote of value for an injury to the head.'

15–17 *Cf.* Henry of Huntingdon, *HA* 9. 1 (p. 622)

1.19 BETA MINOR / **Lesser Burdock** *Source unknown*

1.20 APIVM

Sic apium—quod apex uictoris ferre solebat
Dum ueterum clari fierent de more triumphi—
Herba triumphalis nullique secunda medelis
Ingenti fastu procedit; gramina spectant
Alcius extantem celoque inpune minantem.
Hanc prius Althydes cum cuncta simul superasset
Presumpsit galea subter lucente coronam.
Hanc alii studuere sibi uel morte suprema
Querere quam Greci 'selinon' dixere periti
Et calide sicceque simul uirtutis habetur;
Tercius huic in utroque gradus sanxitur ab istis.
Delet feruorem stomachi sedatque tumorem
Potum sicque poris manifeste pellit apertis
Si stomachus uentum generauit forte nociuum.
Compescit uomitum, compescit tormina uentris
Si sibi commixtum limphe iungatur acetum.
Vrinas potata ciet tam cruda comesta
Quam si contritum semen sit forcius haustum
Sed magis hoc radicis aget decoccio sumpta.
Splen eciam tumidum iuuat ydropisimque, iecurque
Feniculi succus si detur ei sociatus.
Herba uenenatos perimit fortissima morsus,
Quod si uel semen uel apozima sumitur eius
Preualet hocque modo tussis sedatur anhela.
Vnaquaque die si discindat febris egrum,
Cum limpha dabis huic apium: linquet febris egrum.
Si fuerit trita cum succo candida mica
Sanabit tumidum noctu superaddita lumen,
Hocque modo mammis prodesse tumentibus aiunt.
Preterea succus farris cum polline iunctus
Oui cum lacrimo purgabit uulnus et ulcus.

1.20 APIVM *P* 6v–7r: Apium | *S* 40v–41r: De Apio. Henricus
1 sic] hic *S* 2 ueterum] *scripsi* (*cf.* Macer 333), ueterem *P* : uetere *S* morte *P* 4 iungenti *S* fastu] in estu *P* 6 prior *S* alcades *S* 7 lucente] supprema *add. et exp. S* choronam *P* 8 studere *S* 9 querere] quod rere *S* pariti *S* 10 habetur] *scripsi*, haberi *PS* 11 sanccitur *P* istis] idem *S* 13 potum sicque poris] pota sic et paris *S* 14 generaret *P* 19 hoc] hec *P* 21 sociatur *S* 23 apozyma *P* 24 hocque] hoc *S* anhela sedatur *P* 25 discindat] *scripisi*, discendat *S* : discentat *P* eger *S* 26 liquet *S* eger *S* 29 timentibus *S* ayunt *P* 30 farris] sarris *S* 31 oui] diu *S* lacrima *P*

1.20 Celery (Smallage), *Apium graveolens* L.

And thus Celery—which the victor's helmet used to bear,
according to ancient custom, when great victories were won—
a triumphal herb, second to none for cures,
steps forward in great pride: the herbs see it standing high
above them and projecting toward the sky, unchallenged.
Hercules first wore this as a crown, under a glittering helm,
when he had overcome all things at one time.
Others have endeavoured, even at death's door,
to seek this for themselves, which learned Greeks called *selinon*;
it is thought to be in virtue both hot and dry—
they established that it is the third degree in each.
When drunk, it stops a burning in the stomach and reduces
swelling, and thus it clearly forces harmful wind
out from the open pores if the stomach by chance created it.
It suppresses vomiting and curbs the stomach pains
if vinegar mixed in water is blended with it.
It expels urine when drunk, consumed either raw
or better yet if the ground seed is drunk,
but a decoction of the root when taken does this more.
It also helps a swollen spleen, dropsy and the liver
if the juice of Fennel is mixed with it and given.
This most powerful herb counteracts poisoned bites,
but if its seed or a salve made out of it is used,
it is even stronger and in this manner a hacking cough is settled.
If a fever tears at the patient every single day,
give Celery to him with water: the fever will leave the patient.
If white bread crumbs are ground with Celery juice
they will clean a swollen eye if applied at night,
and in this manner they say it's good for swollen breasts.
Moreover, Celery juice mixed with wheaten flour,
and with an egg white, will purge a wound or ulcer.

1.20 APIVM / Celery *Macer, 'Apium',* 332–65
5 *Cf.* Silius, *Punica* 4. 2   7 Exod. 25: 27

Si tamen emplastrum superaddas sepius istud,
Feda superpositam lentigo diffugit herbam.
Hac color opacis amissus redditur egris
Si comedant crudam ieiuni sepius herbam.

1.21 PETROSELINVM

Viginti uisis patet—aspice—petroselinum;
Hoc Danai dicunt, fama testante, 'triannem.'
Est apio similis foliis, uirtute, colore;
Distat et inde parum foliis, uirtute, colore.
Conuenit huic foliis, quoniam sunt equa figuris;
Dissidet et foliis, quia non sunt equa staturis.
Conuenit huic uirtute, ualens ea que ualet illa;
Dissidet et uirtute quod hac sit forcior illa.
Est color hiis similis, quod et ista uirescat et illa;
Dissimilis color est, quod paulo magis uiret illa.
At proprium Natura suo dat petrosilino,
Vnde et nomen habet, quod petram pota repulset.
Hec solet antidotis, nec sepius ulla, reponi.
  Transierim de more cocos, nisi clamet Apollo:
'Accersi, Talia, cocos, medicique recedant!'
Nec spernit cocus ille cocos epigramata scribens,
Quem dum forte sequor, nomen uatis adipiscor.

32 emplaustrum *S*   istud] illud *S*   33 diffugit] umbram *add. et. exp. P*   34 color *corr. e* calor *S*   opacis] obectis *Ṣ*   ammissus *P*   35 crudam] uiridem *P*

1.21 PETROSELINVM   *P* 7r–7v: Petroselinum | *S* 78v–79r: De Petrosillino. Henricus | *T* 102v: Petrosilinus *First edited by Rigg, 256–8, from P and S.*

Exceptiones (*O* 91v): Petroselinum greci triannem uocant. Hec apio similis est foliis, uirtute, colore, non tamen adeo fortis nec adeo uiridis. Sic dicitur quod petram pota repellat. Antidotis adhibetur. Hec est optima arietinis carnibus, sociata puleio, nasturcio, uel potius illi que ius danna uulgo dicitur. Addito costo, modico pipere, hec arietino iure conficiantur et erit sapor optimus. Ad porcinam uero carnem aliter: petroselinum, lilifagum, satirea, nasturcium (si desit ius danna). Conterantur his succis; adde piper et cuminum. Sic porcina tibi caro frigida iocundissime comedatur.

1 petrosillum *S*   2 hec *S*   danay *P*   5 quoniam . . . figuris] quia hec sunt equa figuris *post corr. P*   *ll. 6–7 transp. et corr. P*   6 non] nec *S*   7 que] qua *Rigg*   8 quod] qui *S*   *ll. 9–10 transp. S*   13 hec . . . reponi] *om. S*   14 cocos] coquo *S*   15 cocos] coquo *S*   16 cocus ille] *Rigg*, ille cocus *P* : coquis ille *S*   cocos] coquos *S*   epigmata *P*   17 dum *S*] cum *P* : si *Rigg*   uates *S*

Yet if you often apply that plaster over it,
an ugly freckle flees the herb applied on top.
This herb returns to pale patients the colour they have lost
if, on an empty stomach, they often eat the uncooked herb.

1.21 Parsley (no. 1), *Petroselinum crispum* (Mill.) Nyman

Now that we've seen twenty, look here, Parsley appears!
The Greeks call it *triannis*, so rumour relates.
It's similar to Celery in leaves, virtue and colour,
and it differs from it a little in leaves, virtue, and colour.
It agrees with it in leaves, since they are of the same shape;
and it differs in leaves, because they are of a different size.
It agrees with it in virtue, capable of what that one can do;
and it differs in virtue because that one is stronger than this.
Their colour is similar, because this and that are green;
their colour is dissimilar, for that is a little greener.
But Nature gives to her Parsley a power of its own,
whence it has its name: when drunk it drives out the stone.
This is apt to be placed in antidotes—no other more often.
  I would, of course, have passed over the cooks, but Apollo cries out:
'Thalia, fetch the cooks and order the doctors to depart!'
Nor did that cook who wrote in epigrams spurn the cooks,
and perhaps as long as I follow him, I'll earn the name of poet.

1.21 PETROSELINVM / **Parsley** *Source unknown*
3 *Cf.* Rabanus Maurus, *De rerum naturis* 19.9 15 *Cf.* Martial, *Ep.* 7.17.4; Strabo 324–5

Hec arietinis est optima carnibus herba,
Optima porcinis. Si queras quomodo, dicam.
Primo tibi primas signabo, secundo secundas.
Accipe puleium, nasturcia, petrosilinum;
Que tamen herba solet uulgo 'ius danna' uocari
Si presens fuerit, hanc, non nasturcia, sumes.
Hiis addes costum modicumque piper sociabis;
Hec arietino misceri iure licebit.
Non arietinis sapor hoc erit apcior ullus
Carnibus, ut perhibent super artibus hiis studiosi.
Accipe lilifagum, satureiam, petrosilinum
Et nasturcia, uos nisi sit 'ius danna' propinqua.
Hiis succis perfunde simul piper atque ciminum.
Sic porcina tibi caro frigida si comedatur,
Non sapor hoc alius iocundior efficiatur.

1.22 SOLSEQVIVM

Herbe florentis que cernitur ordine certo
'Solsequia' est nomen nobis, elitropia Grecis.
Aureus huic flos est quem tanto nutrit amore
Vt uix cogat eum uel yemps inuisa perire.
Hec aperit florem, nam diligit ille calorem,
Meridie; noctu, nam uitat frigida, claudit.
Vergit et ad solem preclarum mane cacumen,
Vergit ad occasum cum Phebus tendit ad imum.

18 hec arietinis] hoc anetum *S* 21 nasturcium *P* petrosillinum *S* 22 que] quod *S* tamen . . . uocari] solet herbarum wlgo sic danna summes *P* danna] dampna *T* 23 non] et *P* 25 hec arietino] hoc arriemio *S* 26 arietinis *om. Ŝ* 28 satureia *P* petrosillinum *S* 29 et . . . propinqua *om. P* 30 cuminum *S* 32 efficiatur] associatur *S*

1.22 SOLSEQVIVM *P* 7v: Solsequium | *S* 57v: [no title] | *T* 104v: Solsequium

Exceptiones (*O* 91v): Solsequia grece elitropia dicitur, cui est flos aureus. Vix bruma superabilis sed qui et meridie aperitur nocte clauditur. Cacumen eius ad solem tam orientem quam occidentem uergitur. Hic quacumque die uidebitur uidentem febris acuta non inuadet et quicumque predictam febrem patitur folium dimidiumque folii suma[n]t, bis genito sumptam macerent, potent maceratam. Hoc in principio prodesse dicunt si luxus cuiquam contingat solesequii folia potata succurrent. Puluis eius uel herbe succus in uino bibitus omne uenenum destruit.

2 helytropia *P* 4 yems *P* perire] parumper *P* 5 hec] hoc *S* 6 frigora *S* 7 preclare *S* 8 ymum *P*

This is the best herb for mutton, the best for pork.
If you ask the method, I will tell you. I'll indicate for you
the first meats in the first place, the second in the second.
  Take Pennyroyal, Cress, and Parsley;
yet if that herb which the crowd is apt to call *ius danna*
should be present, use it and not the Cress.
Add Cost to these and mix in a bit of Pepper;
you can now mix these with the mutton drippings.
There will be no other flavour better suited to mutton,
or so they relate who are devoted to these arts.
  Take Basil and Savory and Parsley
and Cress, unless *ius danna* is near to you.
Mix together Pepper and Cumin with these juices.
In such a way, if you are eating cold pork,
no other flavour would be made more pleasing than this.

1.22 Calendula (Pot Marigold), *Calendula officinalis* L.

The name of the flowering herb that is seen in proper succession
is Calendula to us and *heliotropia* to the Greeks.
Golden is its flower which it nourishes with such love
that even hated winter can scarcely make it die.
This herb opens its flower at midday because it loves the heat,
and closes it at night because it shuns the cold.
It turns its shining head toward the sun in the morning,
and turns it to the west when Phoebus moves to the depths.

1.22 SOLSEQVIVM / **Calendula** *Pseudo-Apuleius no. 49, 'Herba Heliotropia' (pp. 99–100)*
1–8 *Cf.* Aldhelm, 'Eliotropus' (*The Riddles of Aldhelm*, ed. Pitman, 28) 3 *Cf.* Ovid, *Met.* 1. 496 7 *Cf.* Ovid, *Met.* 4. 270

Vis igitur flori mirabilis esse putatur
Vt quacumque die florem perspexeris almum
Non te preripiet que febris acuta uocatur
At uulgus gystam non indigne uocat illam.
Qui tamen hoc morbo, non hac uisa, rapiuntur
Mox sibi dimidium folii, folium quoque sumant,
Bis genito sumptam macerent, potent maceratam.
Hoc in principio quidam prodesse fatentur
Si luxus cuiquam contingat: sumito tundens
Solsequii folia; succurrent protinus illa.
Quod si plura petis, puluis mollissimus eius
Aut herbe succus uino iunctus bibitusque,
Destruit ad plenum uictor quodcumque uenenum.

1.23 PARVENCA

Hoc nemus umbrosum uiridis paruenca decorat,
Corpore parua quidem, sed uiribus insuperata,
Et quoniam matrem scelus est odisse, perornat,
Vestit, amat terram semperque incumbit amanti.
Sunt que lasciuo transcendant aera motu,
Matreque despecta longe longeque recedant.
Hec petit hanc, fugit hec. Non sic Peneia Daphne
Phebeos tactus fugiebat aquasque petebat

11 proripiat *S* 12 at] aut *S* gestam *S* illam] istam *T* 13 hoc] hec *P* rapiuntur] moriuntur *T* 14 folii folium *transp. T* sumant] sumunt *S* : summant *P* 15 bis genito] *scripsi*, bis geniti *P* : *om. S* sumptum *P* potent maceratam *om. P* 16 quidam] ipsam *P* : quosdam *T* 17 cuiquam] cuidam *T* sumito tundens *om. P* 19 puluer *S* mollissimus] melli *P* eius *om. P* 21 uictor] uincens *T*

1.23 PARVENCA *P* 7v–8r: Pervinca | *S* 77v–78r: De Paruenca. Henricus *First edited by Rigg, 258–60.*

Exceptiones (*O* 89v): <P>aruinca est herba immo dicta quod alias uincat. Hec uincit guttam.

(*O* 91v): Paruenca humilis et parua matrem tegit, ornat. Aerem fugiens terre incumbit, unde et pro mutuo habet quolibet tempore flores in mediis etiam niuibus, purpureis uiolis uix cedentes. Tactu dicitur puellas allicere. Victoriola etiam uocatur quia guttam uincit; cesas in uulnere carnes uincire fertur.

4 amanti] amare *S* 5 lasciua *P* 6 recedunt *P* 7 petit] perit *S* hec²] hanc *P* non . . . Daphne] preemeses non sic *P* Peneia] *supplet Rigg*, preemeses *P* : ponera *S* 8 phebeos] feboos *S* tactus] currus *P* *ll. 9–10 om. S*

The strength of the flower is therefore considered wonderful,
so that on whatever day you see this propitious bloom,
the fever, which is called an 'ague' but the common people
not unworthily call 'gout', will not carry you off too soon.
Yet those who do not see it and are seized by this disease
should soon pick a leaf and a half for themselves,
boil it mixed with the Twice-Born God, and drink it, boiled thus.
Some report that this is beneficial from the start
if someone suffers a dislocation: pick and grind
the leaves of Calendula and they will help immediately.
But if you seek more, the finest powder of the herb
or its juice, blended with wine and drunk,
victorious, destroys completely any venom.

1.23 Periwinkle, *Vinca minor* L.

Green Periwinkle decorates this shady grove,
small indeed in body, but in powers unsurpassable,
and since it is a crime to hate one's mother, she adorns,
clothes, and loves and ever lies upon the loving earth.
There are things which climb the air with lusty leap,
despise their mother and recede far and farther away.
She seeks her, flees the air. Not so did Peneus's daughter,
Daphne, running fast, flee Phoebus's touch and seek

1.23 PARVENCA / **Periwinkle** *Original*
1 *Cf.* Ovid, *Met.* 7.75 7–10 *Cf.* Ovid, *Met.* 1.452–567, 5.379–424

Currendo patrias; non sic Proserpina Ditis
Amplexus fugiens matrem peritura petebat,
Vt paruenca pudens terram petit, aera linquit.
  Vnde et mater ei tantos congessit honores,
Vt quocunque uelit florescat tempore. Cernas
In niuibus mediis paruence sidera parue,
Purpureis uiolis uix supponenda colore,
Vnde et mira potest. Quod possit mira, probarunt
Multi qui teneras hanc incantando puellas
Et tangendo sibi subdunt certamine leni.
Inuite cupiunt quod amant odisse puelle,
Nolentesque uolunt uenerem, noluntque uolentes.
Quid uobis opus est nolentes nolle, puelle?
Quid uobis opus est odisse, precor, quod amatis?
Dum uenerem paruenca mouet, parete mouenti!
† Quod si ultro uultis dabit ultro quaeque uelitis.
Ergo quibus dabitis? Hilares date linthea uentis!
Et bene quod uultis perfecte laudo—uelitis,
Ne sit et ipsa grauis frustra restando uoluptas. †
  Hactenus hec. Victoriolam uictoria namque
Hoc dedit inuicte nomen, tam uincere guttam
Quam uincire, ferunt, cesas in uulnere carnes.
Et ne longa tibi generem fastidia longis,
Hoc quicunque legis, nil amplius hinc tibi sumes!

1.24 STRVCION

Strucion 'ostricium' plebs, turbans nomina, dixit.
Siccat et accendit. Succus cum melle iugatus
Extrahit humores capitis si nare trahatur,

11 pudens *om. S* liquit *S* 12 mater] matet *S* 13 tempore] *add.* curas *et. canc. P* 14 sidera] *add.* mag *et. canc. P* 15 uiolis] *scripsi* (*cf. O 91v*), niueis *P* : mollis *S* : miniis *Rigg* 16 mira . . . mira] mirra . . . mirra *P* 20 noluntque uolentes] uoluntque nolentes *S* 21 quid . . . puelle *om. P* nolle] *Rigg*, nobis *S* 22 opus . . . precor] odisse precor opus *P* 23 paruenca] paruum que *P* parere *S* 24 ultro uultis] multum multis *S* ultro quaeque] *Winterbottom*, utroque *P* : ultro *S* *ll. 25–26 om. S* 28 uictoriolam *corr. ex* uictaoriolam *S* 29 hoc] hec *P* inuicte] in mente *S* 30 uincire ferunt] uincere fere *S* 32 leges *S* nichil *P* summes *P*

1.24 STRVCION *P* 8r–8v: Strucion | *S* 97r: De Struction. Henricus
1 struction *S*

her native waters; not so did Persephone, about to die,
flee the Plutonian embrace and seek her mother,
as modest Periwinkle seeks the earth and flees the air.
  Therefore her mother granted such great honours to her,
that she flowers at whatever time she wishes. You may see
Periwinkles like little stars in the midst of snow,
hardly to be subject to the purple Violets in colour,
and for this reason it can do great things. That it can do such things,
many have proven, who, by enchanting and touching her,
subdue tender maidens for themselves in the gentle battle.
Unwilling girls desire what they love to hate,
the unwilling long for sex, and the willing no longer want.
Girls, what need do you have to be unwilling and not to wish?
What good is it, I ask, for you to hate what you do love?
When Periwinkle kindles lust, give heed to the mover!
† But if you desire freely, it will give freely what you desire.
So to whom will you give? Happily give sails to the winds!
And I wholly praise what you properly desire—may you desire,
lest pleasure herself be a burden as you resist in vain. †
  Enough of this. Since victory bestows the name
victoriola on this, unconquered, they say it both
can conquer gout and bind up flesh cut in a wound.
And lest I make long boredom for you with lengthy words,
whoever reads this, you'll take no more away from here!

1.24 Masterwort, *Peucedanum ostruthium* L.

The people, corrupting names, called *strucion ostricium*.
It dries and heats. The juice, when mixed with honey,
draws out humours of the head if taken up the nose,

1.24 STRVCION / **Masterwort** *Macer, 'Ostrutium',* 907–27

Per se quin eciam puluis si nare trahatur
Sternutamentum uelut elleboro replicatur.
Cum uino iecoris morbo radix medicatur
Quem 'sclirosim' Greci durum dixere tumorem.
Hocque modo prodest tussi splenisque tumori,
Ac ortopnoicis, languor quibus ipse iacere
Abstulit atque dedit—nolintue uelintue—sedere.
Sic eciam lapides uesice frangere dicunt,
Menstrua sic lociumque mouet, uel subdita tantum
Matrici talique modo depellit abortum.
Preterea ualet hictericis uel mixta lyeo
Vel si nare trahas cum succo lac muliebre.
Succus cum uino si iungitur atque polenta
Percurare feras testatur Phisica lepras,
At si consocies succum cum polline quem dant
Ordea sicque addas emplastri more dolori
(Si credas medicis) curatur pustula queuis.
Dotibus ex tantis hanc Angli 'pontificalem'
(Vt digne dicant) herbam cognomine dicunt.

1.25 MIRTVS

Vltima iam partis mirtus retinet borealis,
Mirtus tam pulcre Veneri quam laurea Phebo
Grata, sedens lecto terre (quod aquas amet) equo.
Nam lectos genibus reliquos uideas licet equos
(Ne, si discernas uel odores cominus herbas,

4 per . . . trahatur *om. S* 5 uelud *P* 7 quem . . . tumorem *om. S* sclirosim] *supplet Macer 911*, sclirosi *P* : *om. S* 9 ac ortopnoicis] atrotopnoicis *S* tacere *P* 12 lociumque] locium *S* 14 uelet yctericis *S* 16 iungi *S* 18 conficias *P* succus *S* 22 digno *S*

1.25 MIRTVS *P* 8v: Mirtus | *S* 71r–71v: De Mirto. Henricus | *T* 100r: Mirtus *First edited by Rigg, 260–61, from P and S.*

Exceptiones (*O* 91v): Mirtus in palude oritur calida tamen et uenerem mouens. Hec licet amara grata tamen, nam eius decoctio cum tisana et succo plantaginis ad terciam partem decocta dissentericos et ciliacos curat. Si poma quercus his apponantur, tormina omnia sedantur, si uicturus sit eger.

1 retinet] reciit *S* borialis *S* 2 pulcra *T* 3 terre . . . equo] *scripsi*, terre quod aquas amat equo *Rigg* : tene quas aut quas amas equo *P* : quod aquas amet equos *S et add.* terre *in mg.* : terre quod aquos amet equo *T* 4 nam . . . equos *om. S* uideas] *Rigg*, uideat *P*

but even if the powder by itself is taken up the nose,
sneezing is forced out as if by Hellebore.
The root with wine cures the liver disease
whose hard tumour the Greeks called *sclerosis*.
And in this manner it is good for a cough, a tumour of the spleen,
and for the orthopneic, from whom weariness itself stole lying down
and made them sit—whether they would or not!
Thus they also say it breaks up bladder stones,
thus it moves menstrual courses and urine, or if taken alone
into the womb, in such a manner it expels a foetus.
Moreover, it is helpful for the jaundiced either mixed with wine
or if you take up your nose mother's milk mixed with its juice.
Physic vows to cure savage lesions completely
if the juice is mixed with wine and barley meal,
but if you mingle the juice with barley flour
and apply it thus like a plaster to a pain
(if you believe the doctors), any sort of pustule is cured.
From such great gifts the English call this herb
(as they properly should) Bishopswort.

1.25 Myrtle, *Myrtus communis* L.

Now Myrtle holds the farthest reaches of the northern side,
Myrtle, as pleasing to lovely Venus as Laurel is to Phoebus,
sitting in a bed level with the earth (so that it may love the waters).
For although you see other beds level with your knees
(lest, if you spot or smell the herbs nearby, it be a chore

1.25 MIRTVS / **Myrtle** *Source unknown*

2 *Cf.* Virgil, *Ecloga* 7. 62; Pliny 12. 3 5 *Cf.* Peter of Blois, *The Later Letters of Peter of Blois*, no. 30 (ed. Revell, 163)

Sit tociens curuasse labor) quantumque decoris
Hinc habeant dictis non credas, aspice, credes!
  Ergo mouet mirtus uenerem, dat namque calorem
Mulcentem, quamuis algenti nata palude.
Dulcis amatori, quamuis gustus sit amari,
Multa facit mirtus. Faciat cum multa, libello
Prouidus e multis tandem uix pauca reponam.
Mirti cum ptysana decoccio iuncta sinatur
Ebullire, sed hiis succum plantaginis adde.
Hec coquito donec pars tercia sola supersit;
Hinc dissintericos, hinc curabis ciliacos.
Quod si forte uelis audax grauius medicamen,
Poma simul ponas quercus, fiatque necesse
Tormina sedari. Dabit ergo medela salutem,
Terminus hic uite si non statuatur ab illo
Qui statuit uitam. Lateri finis boreali
Hic datur, et finem libet hic donare libello.

6 quantumque] quacumque *S* 7 credas] credens *P* 8 ergo] hoc *S* colorem *P* 9 algenti] agenti *S* 10 gustus sit] sit gustus *P* 11 faciat] sanat *S* 12 e] est *S* 13 cum] est *S* ptysana] tisana *T* : pusa *S* sumatur *T* 14 addas *T* 16 dissiniericos *S* cyliacos *P* 21 lateris fini borialis *S*

to bend the knees so often) and you might not believe my words
about how beautiful they are from here, look, believe!
Thus Myrtle moves the sexual appetite, for it bestows
a soothing heat, though born in a chilly fen.
Sweet to the lover, although bitter to the taste,
Myrtle does many things. Since it does many things, I will
carefully add to my book, at last, a few out of the many.
Let a decoction of Myrtle, with barley-water added,
be allowed to boil, but add to these some Plantain juice.
Cook these down until a mere third part remains;
with this you'll cure the dysenteric, with this the coeliac.
But if by chance you boldly wish a stronger remedy,
put oak apples in as well, and the pains should,
out of necessity, subside. Therefore this cure will offer health,
if the end of life is not here decreed by Him who decrees
all life. An end is given here to the northern side,
and here I'm pleased to grant an end to this little book.

2 PROLOGVS SECVNDI LIBRI

Clio, que superum gesta decoras,
Que regum fidibus nomen honoras,
Ex qua perpetuum lumen habetur,
Qua nec qui moritur morte tenetur,
Que iam serta michi clara dedisti
Antiquisque parum supposuisti,
Nunc, si parua potes magnificare,
Res fama tenues perpetuare,
Sic, queso, breuibus gramina stringas,
Vt late radiis carmina cingas.
Cum sit materies dura grauisque,
Leuem uestra paret cura leuemque,
Queque forent rudibus forte perosa
Vestro melle fluant deliciosa!

2.1 MANDRAGORA

Mandragora excelso supereminet inclita lecto,
Iure locanda prius, quas si non ortus haberet
Noster, diuiciis hiis Anglia forte careret.
Cumque sit herbarum princeps, ut homo est animantum,

2 PROLOGVS SECVNDI LIBRI *P* 8v: Prologus secundi libri | *S* 32v: [no title] *First edited by Rigg, 261–2.*

1 superni *S* 8 tenues] times *S* 11 maneries *S* 12 leuem] lenen *corr. e* lemen *S* 13 quemque *S*

2.1 MANDRAGORA *P* 9r: Mandragor (*sic*) | *S* 68r–68v: De Mandragora. Henricus | *T* 99r: Mandragora *First edited by Rigg, 262–4, from P and S.*

Exceptiones (*O* 91v–92r): Mandragora<m> humana[m] per omnia membra imitatur figuram. Vere nouo crines eius frondescent; fine estatis fatiscunt. Asserit quidam quod qui eam uelli audierit moritur ut herba, nisi eam circumfodiunt nectuntque canem, fugientes, ad corpus mandragore; canis esuriens petit escas longius positas; hec ru<m>pitur, moritur ille. Succus huius fronti illinitur; capitis dolorem amputat. Nardino oleo iunctum et auri infusum dolorem curat. Preterea sume scripulum de pede dextro, de manu dextra tantumdem, puluis inde factus cum mero tritus et bibitus per septem dies podagram sanat, tumorem sedat. Contractos neruos reuocat uncia corporis trita et oleo perfusa; contractis membris succurrit. Item scripulum de corpore in aqua calida prodest donare caduco. Eius sarticulum collo suspenditur egri, sicque filadericum quidam fidunt superatum.

1 excello *P* 3 diuiciis] duricias *S* 4 animatum *S*

2 Prologue of the Second Book

O Clio, you who beautify the deeds of gods,
you who honour the name of kings upon your lyre,
from whom eternal light is granted,
by whom the dead are not bound by death,
who have already given me splendid garlands
and placed me but a step below the ancients,
now, if you can make the small things great,
and prolong a passing thing with fame,
tie up these herbs, I pray, in briefer words,
so you may gird my poems from afar with rays.
Since the matter is so hard and heavy,
may your care effect it smooth and light,
and may that which might displease the rude
flow, delicious, with your honey!

2.1 Mandrake, *Mandragora officinarum* L.

Illustrious Mandrake stands high in an elevated bed,
rightly found in the foremost place. If our garden did not
have these, perhaps England would lack these riches:
Since it is the prince of herbs, as man is over animals,

2 PROLOGVS SECVNDI LIBRI / **Prologue of the Second Book** *Original*
1–2 Horace, *Odes* 1. 12, 1–6; Horace, *Ars poetica* 83–5 4 *Cf.* Ambrose, *De benedictionibus patriarcharum* c. 9 (PL 14. 686D)

2.1 MANDRAGORA / **Mandrake** *Pseudo-Apuleius no. 131, 'Effectus herbae mandragorae' (pp. 222–5)*

Principis hec princeps imitatur corpore corpus,
Quippe pedes pedibus, crus crure, uerenda uerendis,
Ilibus ilia, pectore pectora, gutture guttur,
Et caput atque manus capitis manuumque figura.
Pro digitis pes atque manus radice tenentur,
At ceruice sitos uideas frondescere crines.
Vere nouo crescunt, estatis fine pauescunt,
Vtque ferunt multi (non hoc tamen assero firme),
Si quis eam uellens, si de gremio genitricis
Audierit uelli, quod homo moriatur ut herba.
Hanc circumfodiunt nectuntque canem, fugientes,
Mandragore ad corpus; canis esuriens petit escas
Longius appositas; hec rumpitur, occidit ille.
Hec que sit uel qualis, habes; quid possit, habeto:
Mandragore succus capitis sedare dolorem
Dicitur et scitur, si frons illo liniatur.
Nardino succum iungas oleo memoratum;
Infundens auris poteris curare dolorem.
Preterea scrupulum sumas tibi de pede dextro
Deque manu dextra scrupulum; puluis tibi fiat
Inde meroque dehinc tritus puluis bibitusque
Per septem luces celeri sanare podagram
Prouentu poterit—sedabit quippe tumorem—
Contractosque simul neruos ad se reuocabit
Corporis egregii si sumitur uncia, sumptam
Si tribules oleo, si perfundas tribulatam;
Vnguen contractis ualet hoc succurrere membris.
Necnon mandragore scrupulum de corpore sumas;
Hunc in aqua calida prodest donare caduco;
Sic poteris rabidi uicium depellere morbi.
Eius sarticulum collo suspenditur egri,
Sicque philactorium quidam fidunt superatum.

5 hec] hoc *S* 7 ylibus *P* illia *S* gucture guctur *S* 9 pes] pedes *P* 10 at . . . uideas] et ceruice solent fructu *T* 11 uere nouo] ut enouo *P* etatis *S* 12 multi *om. P* 13 si de] fide *S* gnitricis *S* 16 canis *om. S* 17 hec] hoc *S* 18 hec] hoc *S* 20 illo] illa *P* : inde *T* 21 iungas] iungens *ST* 22 infundens auris] auribus infundens *T* 23 scripulum *S* summas *P* 24 scripulum *S* 26 septem] uii *P* sanare] curare *P* 27 prouentum *T* 29 uncia] unica *S* 30 tribulos *S* perfundas] confundas *S* : *add.* si *T* 31 unguem *S* membris] morbis *T* 32 scripulum *S* 34 rapidi *S* 36 philactorium *T*] filadelium *P* : fila clerium *S* : filacterium *Rigg* superatam *T*

this prince in body imitates the body of the other prince,
to wit, the feet with feet, leg with leg, genitals with genitals,
hips with hips, chest with chest, throat with throat,
and head and hands by the shape of head and hands.
In place of digits the feet and hands are made of roots,
but observe that the hairs found on the head grow out as leaves:
they grow anew each spring, and fade away at summer's end.
And as many relate (though I don't assert this firmly),
if someone digs it up and should hear it being torn
from its mother's womb, that man may die just like the herb.
They dig around it and, running away, bind a dog
to the Mandrake's body; the hungry dog goes for some food
placed far away; the herb is plucked and the dog is slain.
You know what this is and of what kind. Learn what it can do:
Mandrake juice is said and known to calm
a headache, if the forehead is rubbed with it.
Add the aforesaid juice to oil of nard;
by pouring it in you can cure an earache.
Beyond that, take a pinch from the right foot
and a pinch from the right hand; make a powder
from them and then grind the powder into wine;
when drunk for seven days it can, with quick result,
cure gout; to be sure, it will alleviate the swelling.
This likewise will recall pulled tendons to each other,
if an ounce of the splendid body is obtained, if you pound
it with oil once obtained, if you rub it on once pounded;
this ointment is able to help strained limbs.
Also, take a pinch from the Mandrake's body;
it is good to give this in warm water to an epileptic,
and thus you can remove the suffering of rabies.
A little patch of it is hung from a sick man's neck,
and some claim that like this it is better than an amulet.

5 *Cf.* Ovid, *Met.* 15. 89; Martial, *Liber Spectaculorum* 9. 6 (ed. Coleman, 83) 9 *Cf.* Ovid, *Met.* 4. 269, 14. 292 10 *Cf.* Ovid, *Met.* 4. 395 13 *Cf.* Juvencus, *Evangeliorum libri quattuor* 1. 198 (ed. Huemer)

2.2 ELLEBORVM ALBVM

Frondes ellebori reuerendas aspice sacri!
Scripserunt multi tante de uiribus herbe:
Solam grandiloquis Ypocras canit hanc afforismis,
Vtque sit elleborum Philo docet accipiendum.
Hoc Themeson celebrauit idem, nec Plinius ingens
Transiit ingentem. Multum se preparet, inquit,
Sumere qui tantum sine pena uult medicamen,
Et prius humectis corpus bene temperet escis,
Nec comedat sero qui sumet mane; serena
Claraque sit feruensque dies et libera uentis.
Sic igitur curam qui non despexerit istam
Elleborum sumat, sed pultibus antea coctum
Aut lenti mixtum; sic dixit non nociturum.
Ast alii dicunt succo ptysane sociandum
Et sic sumendum uel mulsa paneue coctum.
Hoc senibus, pueris, timidis, tenerisque uetamus,
Nec nisi dimidiam fortes sumant sibi dragmam
aut pocius scrupulos, nam uis est maxima, binos.
Sic igitur uarios humores extrahit illud,
Sic ueteres pellit morbos renouatque salutem;
Sic melancolicos, insanos atque caducos,
Sic iuuat ydropicos, in principio tamen istos.
Sic etiam lepram, tetanum fugat atque podagram
Sic uertigo tibi, licet inueterata, peribit.
Sic quod curatur limphaticus ipse probatur;
Sic tremulos firmat rediuiuaque tormina curat.
Sic stomachi morbis, tussi, ueteri sciasique,
Sic et quartanis febribus licet inueteratis
Prodest eximie. Temptans testabitur eque.
Elleborum quoque suppositum depellit abortum,
Sternutamentum contractum nare mouebit,

2.2 ELLEBORVM ALBVM *P* 9r–9v: Eleborus | *S* 58v–59r: De Elleboro albo. Henricus
2 multi tante *transp. S* uiribus] uerbis *S* 3 canis *P* achorismis *P* 4 elebori *S* Philo] *scripsi*, pylo *P* : pilo *S* decet *P* 5 temison *S* celebarum *S* 6 preparat *S* 9 sereno *P* 10 et *om. S* 11 despexeris *P* 12 sumat] summas *P* pultibus] cultibus *S* 13 leni *S* 14 ptysane] pusane *S* 15 multa *S* 16 tumidis *S* uitamus *S* 17 sument *P* 19 extrahet *S* 21 mellancolicos *P* 22 idropicos *S* 23 tetranum *S* 24 perhibit *S* 26 rediuiuaque] rediuiua *S* 27 ueteris *S* 29 testatibus *S*

2.2 White Hellebore, *Veratrum album* L.

See the praiseworthy fronds of holy Hellebore!
Many have written about the powers of so great an herb:
eloquent Hippocrates sings of this alone in his aphorisms
and Philo teaches that Hellebore should be taken.
Themison praised it as well and great Pliny did not pass
over this great herb. He says: Let him prepare himself well
who wishes to take medicine only without suffering,
and let him first temper his body well with moist foods,
nor should he eat late who takes it in the morning;
let the day be clear and calm, hot, and free of wind.
So therefore let him who would not despise that cure
take Hellebore, but cooked before with pottage or mixed
with lentils; he said it would do no harm like this.
But others say it must be mixed with barley broth,
and must be taken thus or cooked with mead or bread.
We forbid this to the old, young, fearful, and weak,
nor should even the strong take more than half a dram,
that is to say, two scruples, for its power is very great.
In such a way, therefore, it draws out various humours,
thus it pushes out old diseases and renews your health;
thus it aids the melancholic, insane, and epileptic,
and the dropsical (but those still in the beginning).
Thus it also sends fleeing leprosy, tetanus, and gout,
so also your dizziness, however old, will pass away.
So it is proven that a frantic patient is cured,
it stabilizes the palsied, and cures returning stomach pains.
In such a way it is especially good for stomach diseases,
a cough, and for old sciatica, so also for quartan agues,
even persistent ones. One testing it will testify the same.
Hellebore, as a suppository, also expels a foetus.
It will push out sneezing stuck up in the nose,

2.2 ELLEBORVM ALBVM / **White Hellebore** *Macer, 'Elleborus albus', 1774–1832*
3 Hippocrates, *Aphorisms* 4. 13–16, 5. 1 5 Pliny 25. 48–61

Cumque caput purget nimirum lumina purgat.
Mixtum cum lacte muscis datur exitiale,
Admixtum pulti datur insuperabile muri.

2.3 ELLEBORVM NIGRVM

Elleborum subit elleboro, nigro subit album,
Nec color hos solus diuersificat quia distant
Quod candens sursum purget nigrumque deorsum,
Quod candens sit forte nimis, mediocriter atrum,
Quod candens rarum sit, quod uulgare sit atrum.
Conueniunt quod feruescat, quod siccet utrumque.
Conueniunt quod in hiis gradus illis tercius extat.
Conueniunt quod lente datum medicatur et illud
Insanis sed et ydropicis ualet atque podagris,
Et uarios bibitum morbos leuat articulorum:
Miram sumit opem sumens paraliticus illud.
Extrahit acceptum coleras et flecma per aluum.
Lenit duricias eius cataplasma nociuas;
Tollit idem lepram, maculas, scabiem cataplasma.
Surculus infixus radicis sitque remotus
Post geminas luces collo; syringia delet.
Ydropicus tumor hoc fugiet si forte farinam,
Ordea quam dederint, iungas. Depellit abortum
Si supponatur, purgat quoque menstrua. Surdis
Auribus auditum reddit si sit prius illis
Inpositum, sic post biduum triduumue remotum.
Dentem curabis si coxeris hoc in aceto
Sicque diu dente teneatur in ore dolentis.
Plinius ellebori nigri iussit dare dragmam,
Vt non sit nimium, tenerum quod promouet aluum.
Rusticus inde boum—quid rides?—pectora curans
Pretulit hanc letus caris merito speciebus.

32 purget] purgat *P* 34 ammixtum *S*

2.3 ELLEBORVM NIGRVM *P* 9v–10r: Eleborus albus (*sic*) | *S* 59v–60r: De Eloboro nigro. Henricus

2 diuersificat *corr. e* diuersificant *S* discat *P* 4 nimis] minus *P* 8 medicatur *corr. e* medicabitur *P* illud] istud *P* 11 mira *S* sumit] sumis *P* sumens] sumat *P* illud] istud *P* 12] flegma *S* 13 chataplasma *P* 14 cathaplasma *P* 15 inflixus *S* radici *P* 16 siringia *S* 17 ydropicis *S* 18 dederant *P* 20 prius] pilus *P* 22 curabit *S* cocceris *S* 23 dentem *S* 25 teneram *S* 27 pertulit *S*

and since it purges the head, it doubtless purges eyes.
When mixed with milk it is given as deadly poison to flies,
and mixed in pottage it is given unconquerably to a mouse.

2.3 Black Hellebore, *Helleborus niger* L.

Hellebore looks up to Hellebore, the White looks up to Black,
nor does colour alone distinguish them, because they differ
in that the White purges in front and the Black behind,
because the White acts excessively, the Black in moderation,
because the White is rare and the Black is common.
They agree that each is heating and each is drying.
They agree that the third degree of these is seen in those.
They agree that, given with lentils, it heals the insane
but is also good for those with dropsy and with gout.
When drunk, it lessens different diseases of the joints:
a paralytic, taking it, consumes a marvellous power.
When eaten, it draws out bile and phlegm through stool.
A plaster of it eases harmful hardenings;
the same plaster removes leprosy, blemishes, and mange.
Let a sprout of the root be applied to the neck
and removed after two days; it destroys sores.
A dropsical swelling will flee this if, perchance,
you add the flour which barley provides. It expels a foetus
if used as a suppository, and it also purges menstrual courses.
It returns hearing to deaf ears if first inserted in them
and thus removed after two or three days.
You will cure a toothache if you should cook this in vinegar
and hold it thus awhile on the tooth in the patient's mouth.
Pliny ordered a dose of a dram of Black Hellebore,
(so that it is not too strong), which promotes a gentle stool.
The farmer, curing cows' chests with this,—Why are you laughing?—
carried this propitiously, as is proper for precious spices.

2.3 ELLEBORVM NIGRVM / **Black Hellebore** *Macer, 'Elleborus niger', 1833–58*
4–5 *Cf.* Pliny 25. 48–61 16 *Cf.* Pliny 25. 53 24 *Cf.* Pliny 25. 54 26 Horace, *Satires* 1. 1, 69–70 26–27 *Cf.* Pliny 25. 47

2.4 AZIMVM

Mox azimum surgit quod uulgus dicere sueuit
'Cancrum': non dulcis gustu, non splendida uisu,
Non leuis tactu, sed gustu cum sit amara
Fit stomacho dulcis. Sit quamuis aspera tactu
Matrici lenis fit. Et hec, non splendida uisu,
Splendida uesano per quam dementia turpis
Aufugit et splendor discretus adest racionis.
Huic igitur rutam iungas, iunctas macerabis,
Cum uino potum dabis amenti maceratas,
Et mox uesanum fieri mirabere sanum.
Menstrua purgare, partum solet accelerare.
Nec iam formosis concedit gloria solis!

2.5 PASTINACA

Sunt pastinace species tres, altera maior,
Altera uero minor, quam plebs dixit 'sceruuisam';
Tercia sed species 'siluatica' dicitur esse.
Prima facit medicis; medians tantum ualet escis.
Tercia quid ualeat? Sitis inclemencia dictat.
Hec quia sit pastu bona 'pastinaca' uocatur.
Si pastinace semen uino societur
Ictus compescit quos biceps scorpius egit.
Sic etiam uentris tumor effugiet muliebris

2.4 AZIMVM *P* 10r: Azimum | *S* 43v–44r: Herba azimi. Henricus poeta

Exceptiones (*O* 92r): Acinum, quod uulgus cancrum dicit, que licet sit amara, stomaco tamen dulcis est, licet aspera tactu, matrici tamen lenis, licet non splendida uisu, splendida tamen uesano, quia dementiam pellit. Ex hac et ruta simul maceratis cum uino pocio hec amentem sanum reddit. Menstrua purgat, partum accelerat.

1 azymum *P* 2 cancrum] canor *P* uisa *S* 7 auffugit *P* 8 iunctam *S* 10 et ... sanum *om. S* 11 pratum *S* 12 nec] ne *S* concedat *P*

2.5 PASTINACA *P* 10r–10v: Pastinaca | *S* 76r: [no title]

2 sceruuisam] ceruisam *P* 4 medicans *S* 5 ualet *S* sitis *bis P* : suis *S* ducat *S* 6 pastu bona *transp. P* 7 societur *corr. e* sociatur *P* : solidetur *S* 8 yctus *P* 9 mulieris *P*

2.4 ? Ragwort, *Senecio jacobaea* L.

Ragwort soon comes up, which the people used to call
cancrum, not sweet to taste, nor splendid to see,
nor smooth to touch, but although it is bitter to taste,
it becomes gentle to the stomach. Although it is harsh to touch,
it becomes easy on the womb. This herb, not splendid to see,
is splendid for the insane: vile dementia flees from it,
and the distinguishing excellence of reason returns.
Therefore mix Rue with this, boil them once mixed,
and give them once boiled to a madman to drink with wine,
and soon you will marvel that the insane has become sane.
It is good for purging menstrual courses and hastening birth.
Glory is no longer granted to beautiful things alone!

2.5 Parsnip:

1) Parsnip, *Pastinaca sativa* L.
2) Skirret (*Sium sisarum* L.), or Caraway root (*Carum carvi* L.)
3) Wild Carrot, *Daucus carota* L.

There are three kinds of Parsnip, one larger,
another smaller, which the crowd has labelled 'skirret,'
but the third variety is called 'wild carrot.'
The first serves doctors, and the second is only good for food.
What is the third good for? The discomfort of thirst explains.
Because this is good to partake it is called the 'Parsnip.'
  If the seed of Parsnip is added to wine it restrains
the wounds which the two-headed scorpion makes.
So also will the tumour of a woman's belly flee,

2.4 AZIMVM / **Ragwort** *Source unknown*

2.5 PASTINACA / **Parsnip** *Macer, 'Pastinaca,' 1264–84*

Quo mulier morbo quasi pregnans esse uidetur.
Hoc semen cancris, tritum cum melle, medetur.
Decoque radices multu; decoccio talis
Asmaticos ueteres et uentris tormina curat.
Large sumpta mouet uenerem suspensaque collo
(Vt dicunt) poterit testes curare tumentes.
Dicunt preterea quia si quis uescitur illa
Aut secum tulerit sic cuncta uenena fugabit.

2.6 CARVI

Stat carui sexto paupercula nomine lecto.
Est cerefoliis uirtute, colore, figura
Consimilis: carui uis acris et ignea ualde
Est, cerefoliis uis acris et ignea ualde;
Est carui foliis—est ceruleus color illis—
Ceruleus color hiis. Foliorum summa minutim
Cesa uides illis; sic cesa uidebis et istis.
Ergo mouet uenerem, locium deducit abundans,
Menstrua deducit. Sapor est gratissimus illi;
Perdit enim precium carui presente cimino.

2.7 DRAGANTEA

Te neque transierim, licet infameris odore,
Herba draganteam quam Greci sed colubrinam
Dicunt Romani. (Non immuto colubrinam.)

12 multu] *scripsi*, multa *PS*   15 poterit] *scripsi*, poteris *PS*   17 secum] semen *S*

2.6 CARVI   *P* 10v: Carui | *S* 49r: De Carui. Henricus | *T* 93v: Cerifolio (*sic*)

Exceptiones (*O* 92r): Carui uirtute, colore, figura cerefoliis consimilis est, enim utrique uis acris et ignea ualde, color ceruleus. Foliorum summa his cesa uides. Mouet uenerem, locium deducit habundans carui, menstrua solum. Sapor est gratissimus illi, perdit enim pretium carui presente cuminum.

1 stat] etat *S*   2 cerifoliis *P*   figura] sapore *T*   4 cerifoliis *P*   5 illi *P*   6 ceruleus] *incipit* cel *et canc. P*   minuta *P*   7 cesa uides illis] istis cesa uides *P*   sic] sit *S*   8 ergo mouet] promouet *S*   habundans *P*   10 cuminum *S*

2.7 DRAGANTEA   *P* 10v–11r: Sypentaria / Dragantea / Columbrina | *S* 56r–56v: De Dragancia. Henricus

2 draganceam *S*   calubrinam *S*   3 dicunt . . . colubrinam *om. P*

by which disease the woman seems as if she were pregnant.
The seed, when ground with honey, is good for ulcers.
Cook the roots with milk and this decoction
cures long-time asthmatics and belly aches.
Taken plentifully, it kindles love, and hung from your neck
(as they say) it will be able to cure swollen testicles.
Moreover, they say that if someone consumes it
or carries it with him, he will send all poisons packing.

2.6 Caraway, *Carum carui* L.

In the sixth bed stands the Caraway, very poor in name.
It is similar to Chervil in strength, and colour, and shape:
the force of Caraway is very pungent and hot,
the force of Chervil is very pungent and hot;
the colour of Chervil's leaves is dark green, dark green
the colour of Caraway's leaves. You see the ends of leaves
cut minutely for these; you'll see them cut thus in those.
Therefore it kindles love, draws out urine in abundance,
and brings out menstrual courses. Its flavour is very pleasing;
however, Caraway loses value when Cumin is present.

2.7 Dragon Arum, *Dracunculus vulgaris* Schott

I should not pass you by, although infamous for odour,
the herb which Greeks call *dragantea* but Romans
colubrina. (I don't recommend *colubrina*.)

2.6 CARVI / **Caraway** *Source unknown*

2.7 DRAGANTEA / **Dragon Arum** *Macer, 'Colubrina', 1728–65*
1 Strabo 217

Dicunt quod similis pelli surgat colubrine
Vnde uenena ferunt experti uincere posse,
Quod si quis trita tantum radice sit unctus
Fertur ab incursu serpentum currere tutus
Sumptaque cum uino medicatur morsibus harum.
Hec et multa potest; tibi multis pauca reponam:
Ex succo puro line lumina melleue mixto;
Sic caligo fugit, morbi fugiunt oculorum.
Et caligo perit si ter denis tibi sumas
Cum granis puscam; radix quoque proficit assa.
Si iungas oleo magne semen colubrine,
Infundens auri, sic succurres pacienti.
Naribus hanc infer cum lana: polipus exit.
Radicum puluis iunctus cum melle fugabit
Tussim, sanat et (hoc experto, credo) catharrum;
Sic emoptoicos iuuat, humida pectora siccat:
Hec radix assa facit et decoccio sumpta.
Cum uino radix ciet urinam ueneremque,
Quod si forte talo gelidus tibi pernio sedit
('Mulam' plebs, a 'pernicie' sic dicimus illum),
Hunc coniuncta frequens huius decoccio curat.
Quid quibus in membris det habes; quid corpore dicam:
Rodentem cancrum solet huius rodere succus;
Radix coniuncta maculas depellit aceto.
Hec uulnus sordens purgat, syringia curat.
Si cum melle tamen sociata brionia detur
Hocque parata modo fagedenica uulnera sanat.
Quod si nare trahat pregnans ipsius odorem
Floris dum marcet, deponere fertur abortum,
Vel si sit radix tibi tantum subdita, matrix.

4 similis] simul *S* 6 iunctus *S* 8 horum *P* 9 multis pauca *transp. S* 11 sic] seua *S* 12 et] hocue *S* summes *P* 13 granis] generis *S* 14 oleo] oculo *S* 15 succurrens *S* 16 hanc infer] infer eam *P* 17 uictus *S* 18 hic *S* crede *S* catarrum *S* 19 omoptoycos *P* siccat] sanat *P* 20 sumpta] curat *P* 23 mulam] muleon *P* 25 quid[1]] quod *S* quid[2]] quod *P* 27 coniuncto *S* 28 hec] *scripsi*, hoc *PS* siringia *S* 29 si cum] sicut *S* 30 fagedonica *P* sanat] curat *P* 32 abhortum *S* 33 tibi tantum *transp. P*

They say that it grows in the manner of snake skin,
wherefore the experts claim it can conquer poisons,
but if someone is rubbed with only the ground root,
he is said to escape safely from serpents' approach,
and when drunk with wine it cures their bites.
It does these and many things. I'll tell you a few of many:
anoint the eyes with its juice, pure or mixed with honey;
thus cloudiness and diseases of the eyes depart.
The cloudiness also vanishes if you take vinegar-water
with thirteen seeds; the baked root is also beneficial.
If you mix the seed of mighty Dragon Arum with oil,
and pour it in the ear, you thus will help the patient.
Insert this in the nose with wool and a polyp departs.
The powdered root, when mixed with honey, will chase away
a cough and clean out a catarrh—I believe this, having tried it.
In such a way it aids blood-spitters and dries out humid chests:
the toasted root and a decoction, when drunk, effect these things.
The root with wine brings out urine and semen,
but if perchance there settles on your ankle an icy chilblain
(the people call it *mule* and we name it thus from 'calamity'),
a decoction of this can cure it, when frequently applied.
  You have its gifts for parts; I'll say what it grants the body:
its juice is apt to gnaw at a gnawing tumour;
the root when added to vinegar clears up blemishes.
It purges a filthy wound and cures sores.
Yet if bryony is added, mixed with honey,
prepared like this it heals gangrenous wounds.
But if a pregnant woman draws in her nose the odour
of this flower when it's drooping, it's said to expel a foetus,
or if the root alone is taken as a suppository by you, O womb.

2.8 SAXIFRAGA

Vt 'frangens petram' dixerunt petrosilinum,
Sic et saxifragam quia 'frangit saxa' uocamus.
Hiis igitur iunctis et nodellis cerasorum,
Hec in aqua calida tribues petram pacienti.
Vtilius nullum dicunt medici medicamen,
Sed teneram tantum rapit ista petram pacienti.
Sed teneram rapit ista petram que, dura morando
Si fuerit, duro duram conuellito ferro.
Necnon saxifragam febrientibus esse salubrem
Quidam uiderunt qui scriptis uisa dederunt.

2.9 VIOLA

Purpurea ut uiola, ut rosa roscida, candida sicut
Lilia uirgo prius mater describitur esse.
Et nitor et nidor uiole uiget insuperatus
Et uiror atque uigor sempiternus uehemensque
Iungitur inde rosis formosaque lilia uobis.
 Frigida uis illis perhibetur et humida primo
Esse gradu, tres et species, que flore probantur,
Nam sunt purpurei, sunt albi suntque nigelli.
Quam magnis, rex magne Deus, uel paruula ditas!
Vt Iustus scripsit medicus: si forte plicata
Sit ceruix ictu, lingue perdatur ut usus,
Des ergo uiolam cum Bachi munere tritam;
Postea, si capitis pars dextra plicata sit ictu,
Hanc plante pedis attritam subnecte sinistri,

2.8 SAXIFRAGA *P* 11r: Saxifraga | *S* 91v: De Saxifragia. Henricus

Exceptiones (*O* 91v): Saxifraga saxa frangit ut petroselinum. His iunctis et nodellis cerasorum, hec in aqua calida tribues petram patienti. Nichil ad hoc utilius dum petra tenera est; febrem eciam pellit.

1 petrosillinum *S* 2 frangat *S* 3 cunctis *S* 4 hec] hoc *S* calera tribules *S* 5 dicunt medici *transp. P* 6 sed . . . pacienti *om. P* tantum] *scripsi*, eam *corr. ex* iam *S* 7 ista] illa *P* 8 duro duram *transp. P* 10 uasa *S*

2.9 VIOLA *P* 11r–11v: Lilia (*sic, post* Vio *exp.*) | *S* 102r–102v: De Viola. Henricus

1 uyola *P* cadida *P* 3 uyole *P* 9 rex] rerum *P* uel] et *P* 12 uyolam *P* 13 dextera *S*

2.8 Great Burnet Saxifrage, *Pimpinella major* L.

Just as they named Parsley from 'breaking stone'
so we also call this Saxifrage because it 'breaks up rocks.'
Therefore, having mixed these with cherry pits,
give them in warm water to one suffering with the stone.
The doctors say that no medicine is more useful,
but it takes from the patient only the soft stone.
It takes the soft stone which, if it should become hard
through delay, you should dislodge the hard stone with hard iron.
And certain people, who put observations in writing,
have seen that Saxifrage is salubrious for the feverish.

2.9 Sweet Violet, *Viola odorata* L.

Purple as the Violet, bedewed as the Rose, and white
Like the Lily: so is the first virgin mother described.
Both the beauty and odour of Violet thrive unmatched,
and its greenness and vigour, eternal and powerful,
are joined to Roses and to you, O beautiful Lilies.
  Its power is said to be cold and moist in the first degree
and the three varieties, which are indicated by the flower,
are purple, and white, and nearly black.
O God, great king, with what great gifts do you enrich even tiny things!
As Justus the physician wrote: if perchance the neck
is bent by a blow so that use of the tongue is lost,
then give Violet ground up with Bacchus's gift,
and afterwards, if the head's right part is bent back by a blow,
bind this, ground up, under the foot's left sole

2.8 SAXIFRAGA / **Great Burnet Saxifrage** *Source unknown*

2.9 VIOLA / **Sweet Violet** *Macer, 'Violae,' 1342–94*

1–2 'Sanctae Mariae assumtio, sequentia' (*Lateinische Hymnen des Mittelalters*, ed. Morel, no. 162, p. 99) 2 *Cf.* Strabo, 'De Rosa,' 392–428 12 *Cf.* Ovid, *Remedia amoris* 803

Hoc econuerso facias si leua plicetur:
Os resilit sermoque redit, res mira relatu!
Vlcera curabit capitis melli sociata;
Olfactu capitis grauitas et crapula cedet.
Huius radicem mirre sociato crocoque:
Hec oculos inflamatos reddit tibi puros.
Herba uirens uiole morbos ex sanguine natos
Aut colera rubea, costis, pulmone uel ipso,
Curat si mixto tibi sumitur amne recenti;
Sic bibitum fugat infantum suspiria, tussim.
Contere coniuncto radices eius aceto:
Splen bibite siccant, uel si spleni superaddas.
Matricis prodest elixatura tumori
Si foueatur ea; cerotis addita curat
Ani fissuras (Greci dicunt 'ragadias').
Hanc et aceto addas; poteris fugare podagras.
  Partibus hec tribui; tribuam medicamina toti:
Purpuream perhibent uiolam curare caducos,
Quod pueris fit precipue, si detur in amne.
Sic ualet anginis si mel iungas et acetum.
Per cataplasma uigens queuis collectio cedit.
Pustula si tibi sit, semen cum melle fugabit.
Vis eciam uiole clarissima dicitur esse
Candentis; uiole radix habeatur in ore
Vt transglutetur succus tibi sepius iste;
Vulneris infestum sic dicunt sistere fluxum
Quam gliquiricie uim Plinius asserit esse.
Quod nisi tederet sicut de flore rosarum
Hinc oleum fieri scripsissem quod fugat auris
Infusum sonitus capitisque caloribus obstat.
Infrigidat corpus, dat sompnum, destruit unctum
Vel bibitum uermes uentris, capitis quoque furfur.
  Scripsissem fieri siropum sic: insere partem
Mellis aqueque duas fialas uiole quoque flores;
Rori quindenis hoc pone diebus in umbra;
Sic tibi sit siropum. Plenum coclear tibi sumes
De siropo qui pergis iter; rideto calores.

15 facies *S*   19 mire *S*   21 uyole *P*   22 coctis *S*   23 ampne *P*   26 bibitis *S*   siccas *S*   27 tumorem *P*   28 ea] cum *add. P*   29 Greci] grati *S*   32 uyolam *P*   33 fit] *scripsi*, sit *PS*   ampne *P*   35 cathapla *P*   uigens] iungens *P*   collectio] decoccio *P*   36 postula *S*   37 eciam uiole] uiolarum eciam *P*   41 uim] inde *S*   44 coloribus *S*   45 infrigdat *S*   46 uel] et *P*   48 fialas] fiole *S*   49 rori] non *S*   50 sic tibi sit] sit tibi *S*   syropum *P*   51 syropo *P*   ridete *P*

and do the opposite if the left part is bent:
the mouth springs back and speech returns, a marvel to relate!
When mixed with honey it will cure ulcers of the head;
by smelling it, heaviness of the head and drunkenness will depart.
Blend its root with Crocus and with Myrrh:
this causes inflammations of the eyes to clear.
The green leaves of Violet cure diseases born from blood
or from red bile, from the ribs or the lung itself,
if you take it when mixed with fresh water;
drunk thus it chases away gasping and a cough in infants.
Grind its roots when joined with vinegar:
when drunk, or applied to the spleen, they dry up the spleen.
A boiled mixture is good for a tumour of the womb
if it is washed with it; added to wax plasters it cures
cracks on the anus (the Greeks call them *ragadiae*).
Add this also to vinegar and you can chase away cases of gout.
  I've given medicines for the parts, now I'll offer them for the whole:
they relate that purple Violet cures epileptics
(which happens especially to boys) if it is given in water.
Thus it's good for tonsillitis if you add honey and vinegar.
Any hard gathering yields to this in a plaster.
If you have a pustule, it will flee the seed in honey.
The most famous power of Violet is said to belong
to the white variety; the root of this Violet should be held
in the mouth, so that you often swallow its juice;
they say it thus checks the dangerous haemorrhage of a wound,
a power which Pliny says belongs to Liquorice.
And if it were not wearisome I should write that from this,
just as from Rose blossoms, an oil is made, which when poured
into the ears blocks tinnitus and hinders fevers of the head.
It cools the body, grants sleep, and in an ointment or when drunk
destroys stomach worms, as well as scurf upon the head.
  I should have written that a syrup is made like this:
place a portion of honey and Violet flowers in two cups of water;
place this in the dewy shade for fifteen days,
and thus you will have a syrup. If you're going on a journey,
take a spoonful of the syrup and you will laugh at fevers!

29 *Cf.* Isidore, *Etym.* 4. 7. 39

2.10 ROSA

'Nunc, Herato, que magna canis, ipsis quoque magnis
Fis maior, sic parua canas ut maxima fias.'
Sic ego. Sic Herato, percurrens pollice cordas
Vmbriferoque uagos lauro redimita capillos:
'Non ignara fui, dum perscribens in amorem
Gramina digrediens miro splendore locares,
Hec agressurum te cominus. Ergo fideli
Non infida meo, que dicas ordine dicto.
At rosulam nunc ipsa canam. Dic, candide Macer,—
Sic tibi Tempe uacent, sic astra canora resultent—
Dic tibi de rosula si quid uideatur amena.'
  Sic Dea. Sic Macer: 'Florum flos esse uidetur,
Quod forma pariter precedat odoreque flores.'
'Dic et, Stabe, precor. Sic non grauis irruat ymber,
Non fera girouaget pegaseos incola fontis,
Dum per amena tui lustras uestigia Macri.'
Sic Dea. Sic Stabus: 'Sic ui, sic uincit odore
Flores, ut merito florum flos esse feratur.'
  Tum Dea: 'Quandoquidem tanto sanxistis honore
Veris uterque decus digno donabo decore
Veris et ipsa decus; nec enim, que confero uobis,
Non potero conferre michi? Rosa, sic superasti
Flores puniceo uultu rutiloque colore
Vt superes aurum, superes gemmas superesque
(Non tamen inuideant superi!) uaga lumina celi.
Sic, rosa, sic superas flores et odoris honore
Vt superes mirram, superes nardum superesque
(Inuideant licet Eoi) noua balsama (uicti).
Gallia quid species querat, quid et Anglia felix
Indis inuideat? ('Si non hoc tempore cedat,

2.10 ROSA *P* 12r–12v: Rosula | *S* 87r–88r: De Rosa. Henricus *First edited by Rigg, 264–8.*
1 Herato] eraco *P* canis] cauens *S* 3 Herato] eraco *P* 4 police *S* umbriferoque] umbricoque *P* uagos] *Rigg*, uagens *P* : magos *S* redimita] reduncia *S* 5 fui] *Rigg*, sui *P* : diu fui *S* 6 digrediens] pregrediens *P* 7 accgressurum *S* 8 dicat *S* 9 ipse *S* 10 Tempe] tempore *S* resultant *P* 11 dic] quod *S* tibi] quid *P* 12 sic[1]] dic *P* sic Macer] si mater *P* 13 procedat *S* 15 gira uaget *S* pegaseios *S* 16 tui] tantum *S* 17 deam *S* 19 tum] *Rigg*, cum *PS* quandoquidem] quando quam *S* 20 donabo decore *transp. P* 23 colore] decore *P* 24 superes[1]] superasti *P* superesque] superosque *P* 25 coli *S* 28 uicti] ritu *S* 29 querat] curat *S* quid[2] *om. S* 30 inuideant *P* hoc] hec *P* cedat] cedet *P*

2.10 Rose, family *Rosaceae* L.

'Erato, you who sing great things, as you are greater than those
great things, now sing of small things so that you may be the greatest.'
And so I spoke. Erato, with her thumb strumming the strings
and with her wandering hair wreathed in shady laurel, spoke thus:
'I wasn't unaware that, when you were writing songs on love
and in a digression placed herbs in wondrous splendour,
you would approach this subject closely. Therefore, not unfaithful
to my faithful servant, I will dictate in order what you should say.
But I will sing now of the Rose myself. Speak, splendid Macer,
so Tempe may be free for you and the singing stars resound,
speak, if anything seems pleasing to you about the little Rose.'
  So spoke the goddess. Macer said, 'It seems the flower of flowers,
because it surpasses flowers equally in appearance and in scent.'
'Strabo, I pray, speak too, and thus let no heavy shower fall,
let not the fierce dweller of the Pegasean spring wander far,
while you tread in the pleasant steps of your Macer,'
said the goddess. Strabo said, 'It so surpasses flowers in virtue
and in scent that it is rightly said to be the flower of flowers.'
  Then the goddess: 'Since you both confirmed spring's glory
with such great honour, I myself will endow spring's glory
with worthy grace, for indeed, can I not confer on myself
what I confer on you? O Rose, you have so surpassed
the flowers with your crimson face and ruddy colour
that you surpass gold, surpass jewels, and surpass—
but don't let the gods be jealous!—the wandering lights of heaven.
Thus, Rose, you so surpass flowers with the honour of your scent
that you surpass Myrrh, surpass Nard, and surpass
(though Easterners may envy) fresh Balsam (they're conquered).
Why should France seek spices, and why should blessed England
envy Indians? ('If it should not yield at this time,

2.10 ROSA / Rose *Macer, 'Rosa',* 776–807

15 *Cf.* Ovid, *Met.* 1. 512 17–18 Strabo 400–401 29 *Cf.* Henry of Huntingdon, *HA* 9. 53 (p. 694)

Tempore, pro!, cedat, cum nunquam balsama cedant!').
  Flos rosule marcet, uis nullo tempore marcet:
Puluis habet quod flos habuit—uigor equus utrique.
Huius opes et opus colliria multa requirunt;
Infrictus puluis langoribus obuiat oris.
Si caleat stomachus, caleant si uiscera, prosit.
Fluxum matricis, fluxum conterminat alui;
Vt reliquos ignes, sacros exterminat ignes.
Omnis trita recens feruores destruit omnes;
Mitigat ipsa recens si mulse mixta bibatur.
  Vis Henrice, tibi ius? Nam tibi fama rosatum
Predicat usque oleum distingui.' 'Quomodo fiat?'
'Floris quod rubeum fuerit discerpito talis;
Vncia sub libra leuis iungatur oliui.
Hec soli solum septem suspende diebus
In phyala, nisi Palladii deliret acumen.
Hoc oleum iam nunc roseum noua nomina sumit.'
Sic Dea. Sic et ego: 'Quid et hoc oleum ualet, oro?'
Namque ualere scio; quid, nescio.' 'Me licet,' inquit,
'Cum Pindo Parnasus et Aonie Aganippe
Graminibus stupeant remorantem, non tamen ibo
Donec et ista scias: uentrem mollire probatur;
Hoc foti feruor stomachi solet alleuiari;
Hoc dolor, hoc feruor capitis curatur. Aceto
Coniunctum purgat uulnus repletque profunda.
Combustis prodest, palpebras mollit, et aufert
Mire suppositum pruritus interiorum.
Cetera pretereo, nec enim numerare fauillas
Proderit Ethneas nec glauci prorsus harenas.'

31 pro! cedat] *Rigg* : procedat *PS* 32 marcet²] cedet *P* 33 equs *S* utrique] *Rigg*, uterque *P* : utrumque *S* 35 infrictus] *Rigg*, infricitus *P* : in fructus *S* oris] horis *S* 36 prosit] prodest *S* 37 conteriat *S* 39 feruore *S* 41 ius] *Rigg*, uis *PS* 43 discrepito *S* 44 iungatur] mergatur *S* 45 soli solum] *Rigg*, sibi soli *P* : soli solus *S* 46 phyala] fiola *S* deliret] *Rigg*, delirat *PS* 48 sic *bis et exp.* sic *S* 49 ualore *P* me] cum *P* 50 Aganippe *S*] Paganippe *Rigg*, paganipeus *P* 52 et *om. P* 53 foti] formi *S* 55 repletque] repelletque *S* 56 conbustis *S*

oh, it may yield in time, since the Balsams never yield!')
  The Rose's flower withers; its power never withers.
Its powder has what the flower had: the strength is equal for each.
Many eye salves request its power and assistance;
ground into a powder it resists ailments of the mouth.
If the stomach and the innards are hot, it is of benefit.
It fully stops the flux of the womb and the belly's flux;
it extinguishes Holy Fire like other fires.
Every fresh Rose, when ground, destroys all fevers;
when fresh, it is soothing if mixed with mead and drunk.
  Henry, do you want the juice? For rumour is ever proclaiming
to you that Rose oil is distinguished.' 'How is it made?'
'Separate whatever is red from such a flower,
and let an ounce of smooth olive oil be added in a balance.
Hang these things in the sun for only seven days
in a glass, unless the wit of Palladius has gone astray.
This oil, now 'oil-of-Rose,' acquires a novel name,'
the goddess said. I now spoke thus: 'And what good is this oil, I ask?
For I know it's good, but I don't know why.' 'Although,' she said,
'Parnassus and Pindus, and Aganippe of Aonia,
might wonder at me delaying over plants, yet I won't depart
until you know these things as well: it's proven to soften the belly,
the burning of a stomach can be eased if warmed with this,
and by this oil an ache or fever of the head is cured. When mixed
with vinegar it purges wounds and fills their hollow parts.
It's good for burns, softens eyebrows, and marvellously dispels
an itching of the insides when taken as a suppository.
I pass over other cures, for it will do no good to count
the sparks of Etna or the sands of the deep blue sea.'

50 *Cf.* Virgil, *Ecloga* 10. 11–12

2.11 LILIVM

Formosis equanda rosis se lilia tolli
Poscunt laude pari. Tollantur laude parili
Et si splendori roseo iungantur, honore
Splendescunt simili similes; monstremus honores
Hiis. Flores herbasque simul nidore, nitore
Deuincunt omnes; hii uincunt omnia flores—
Magnus uterque uiget, magne uires utriusque.
Frigida sanguineis, niueis quoque frigida uis est;
Vsturis igitur preclare subuenit ignis
Radicis bulbus, qui gignit lilia, coctus
Lente sub prunis et iuncto tritus oliuo;
Plus oleum prodest roseum si iungitur illi.
Hunc quoque cum uino coquito, coctum tere, tritum
Clauis apponas; aderit lux tercia, soluas.
At floris succus maturat turgida pusque
Atque litus fertur sudorem sepe mouere.
Effugat elixus et cerotis bene mixtus
Hic bulbus rugas uultus maculasque pudendas,
Lichenasque premit furfurque simul faciei.
Necnon porcino pingui coctus uel oliuo
Reddit rite pilos membris ustis rediuiuos.
Quem si cum uino, potes purgare cruorem
Per uentrem, poteris sic et prodesse lieni.
At neruis tritus sectis cum melle medetur.
Exprimito succum foliorum, mel et acetum
Addito, sic coquito sed mellis sint et aceti
Particule bine, memorati quinque liquoris:
Hoc siccat plagas, extirpat et ueteratas.
Ex eius foliis morsus sanabitur anguis
Elixis ac inpositis, bulbusue lyeo

2.11 LILIVM *P* 12v–13r: De rosis (*sic*) | *S* 66r–66v: De Lilio. Henricus
3 et] hec *P* 4 monstramus *P* 5 hii *S* nidore] odore *P* 8 frigida uis est] facta uisque *S* 9 ustruis *S* preclaris *S* 10 cottus *P* 11 prunis] primis *S* 12 oleum] oculum *S* iugitur *P* 14 aberit *P* 15 turida *P* 16 littus *P* 17 efugat *S* ellixus *P* 18 rugas] et *add. S* 19 lichorasque *P* ferturque *P* 20 coctus] coitus *S* 21 ustis] iustis *P* reduuiuos *S* 22 quem] quod *S* pargare *S* 23 lyeni *P* 24 tritus sectis] strutis tritus *P* 25 mel et] melque *S* 26 coquito] quoquito *S* 30 elixis] exilis *P* ac] at *S* bublusue *P* lieo *S*

2.11 Lily, family *Liliaceae* L., probably *Lilium candidum* L.

The Lilies, comparable to beautiful Roses, demand that they
be held with equal praise. Let them be held with equal praise,
and if they are joined to rosy splendour, similar flowers
shine out with similar honour. Let us show them honours!
They overcome all flowers and herbs at once in odour
and in beauty; these flowers conquer everything,
for each is great and strong and the powers of each are great.
The force is cold in the blood red ones, cold for the snowy white,
and therefore the bulb of the famous root which brings
forth Lilies, when cooked with prunes and lentils
and ground and mixed with oil, heals a fire's burns;
it is of greater benefit if oil-of-Rose is added to it.
Cook this down as well with wine, grind once cooked, and apply
it ground to warts; you'll dissolve them after three days pass.
But the flower's juice softens swellings and pus,
and, when rubbed on, it is often said to provoke a sweat.
The bulb, when boiled and mixed well into wax plasters,
chases off wrinkles and shameful spots from your countenance,
and destroys at once impetigo and scales on the face.
Moreover, when cooked with pig fat or with olive oil
it rightly brings back hair again to burnt limbs.
And if you drink it with wine, you can purge blood
through the belly and thereby you can benefit the spleen.
Ground up with honey it's good for severed sinews.
Press the juice of the leaves, add honey and vinegar,
and cook it thus, but make sure there are two parts each
of honey and of vinegar, and five of the aforesaid juice:
this dries out wounds, eradicating even older ones.
By its leaves, when boiled and applied, a snake bite
will be healed, or the bulb, when mixed with wine

2.11 LILIVM / Lily *Macer, 'Lilium', 808–42*

Conditus et bibitus uenando uenena fugabit,
Huius autem uirtus fungi tollet tibi uirus.
Lilia tanta queunt, nec pauci tanta probarunt.

2.12 CELIDONIA

Clarificans spacio celidonia stat duodeno.
Plinius hac dicit quod pullis mater yrundo
Lumina cecatis, quamuis sint eruta, reddat.
Hec illa ueniente uenit, cedente recedit,
Indeque nomen habet quia Greco more 'chelydon'
Ista uocatur auis. Succum florentis in ere
Iunctum melle coquas dum spumam perdat et inde
Crassiciem quamdam mellis decoccio sumat.
Vtilius nichil est oculis caligine pressis.
Trita iuuat dentes, maculas cataplasmate delet.
Radicem terito, trite iungatur anetum:
Hictericis uino sic iunctum proficit albo.

2.13 PIGMENTVM

Hic quam 'pigmentum' uulgus uocat herba subintrat
Sicque uocant illam que gratum mixta saporem
Potibus attribuit, quo possint iure uocari
Altera iam pigmenta tibi si mel simul addas,
Nimirum cum melliferis apibus uideatur
Dulcis. Lac iungas foliis et uasa perungas:
Hoc solet examen tenerum retinere iuuamen.

31 uenando uenena *S*] uirus uenando *P*   32 autem] item *S*   uirus] uires *P*   33 queunt] conuenit *S*

2.12 CELIDONIA   *P* 13r: Celidonia | *S* 51r–51v: De Celidonia. Henricus

2 hanc *S*   puluis *S*   4 credente *S*   5 quia] quod *P*   Greco] grato *S*   chelydon] thelidon *P*   6 succus *S*   7 spumiam *P*   9 pressus *S*   10 cathaplasmate *P*   11 terito] trito *S*   acetum *P*

2.13 PIGMENTVM   *P* 13r–13v: Pigmentum | *S* 80v–81r: De Pigmento. Henricus

Exceptiones (*O* 92r): Pigmentum herba uulgo dicitur eo quod potibus mixta gratum saporem tribuit, adeo quod melle addito altera pigmenta habeantur. Nec mirum cum apes ita oblectet ut si lac foliis iungas et uasa perungas, examen retineatur.

3 attribuant *S*   7 tenere *S*

and drunk, will chase off poisons by hunting them down,
and its power will remove a mushroom's poison from you.
Lilies can do such things, nor are they few who have proven them.

2.12 Celandine, *Chelidonium majus* L.

Shining bright in the twelfth plot stands Celandine.
Pliny says that with this a mother swallow brings eyes back
to her blinded chicks, even if they were torn right out.
It comes with her arrival and goes when she's departing,
and from her takes its name because that bird in Greek
is called the *chelydon*. Cook the flower's juice, mixed with honey,
in a copper pot until it loses the froth and then let
the decoction take on a thickness like that of honey.
Nothing is more useful for eyes weighed down with cloudiness.
When ground it aids the teeth and in a plaster erases spots.
Grind up the root and add Dill to it when ground:
add it to white wine like this and it benefits the jaundiced.

2.13 ? Meadowsweet, *Spiraea ulmaria* L.

The herb which the people call 'piment' creeps in here
and thus they name that herb which, mixed in drinks,
bestows a pleasing flavour, so that they could rightly
now be called your 'second piment' if you add honey too,
since it surely seems sweet to the honeybees.
Blend milk with its leaves and rub on hollow places:
this test is apt to preserve a tender youthfulness.

2.12 CELIDONIA / **Celandine** *Macer, 'Chelidonia', 1690–1708*
2–3 *Cf.* Pliny 15. 89–90

2.13 PIGMENTVM / **? Meadowsweet** *Original*
6 Macer 1645–6

2.14 VETONICA

Cestron aue, quam uetonicam dixere Latini!
Quot uires quantasque tibi Natura creatrix
Vni contribuit, mea quas non sufficit omnes
Tradere mens scriptis, nec sufficit omnibus omnis!
Egregie fracto capiti contrita medetur.
De foliis tritis aut elixis cataplasma
Factum lesuris uiciisque preest oculorum;
Constringit lacrimas hec mansa uel hausta nociuas,
Quod si cum ruta sit eodem pondere iuncta
Et tepida sumatur aqua caligo fugatur.
Sanguis enim nocuus per subteriora relabi
Sic solet ex oculis et libertas reparari.
Commixtus roseo succus fundatur oliuo
Auribus, ast puluis cocto cum melle ligatus
Preualet empicis, curat suspiria, tussim,
Sicque ualet stomacho. Purgatur uomica dira
Hac si cum tepida sumas et pectus eadem;
Cum mulsa mollit uentres emoptoicisque
Prodest cum pusca. Ventris fugat una dolorem
Vncia cum calide ciatis potata duobus.
Splen iuuat atque iecur decoccio tocius herbe.
Vncia iungatur ciatis bis bina uetusti
Cum trinis uini; uiginti quatuor illis
Grana iuga piperis que consociata terendo
Potes sicque potes renum purgare dolores.
Ruptis cum mulsa prodest puluis foliorum,
Vrine prodest lapidique stereque cadenti.
Pondere necne fabe puluis cum melle uoretur
Post cenam quo sic stomachus cito digerat escas.
Per partes quid agat dixi. Per tota quid edam:
Si datur ydropicis cum uino melleque prodest;
Sanat et ydropicos si sit potata frequenter

2.14 VETONICA *P* 13v–14r: Bethonica | *S* 99r–99v: De Vetonica. Henricus
1 betonicam *P* 2 quot] quod *S* 3 omnis *S* 4 tradere] scriptis *add. P et canc.* 6 cathaplasma *P* 9 si cum] sicut (*exp.*) sicut *P* 11 enim] et *P* nocuis *S* 13 comixtus *S* 14 ast] et *S* 16 purgantur uomita *P* 17 hanc *P* 18–19 cum . . . emoptoicisque / prodest . . . dolorem] cum mulsa mollit uentris fugat una dolorem *S* (*as one line*) 18 mollit *bis P* 19 una] uita *P* 20 callide *P* duobus] diebus duabus *S et* diebus *exp.* 22 bis bina uetusti] quaterna uenisti *S* 23 uiginti quatuor] xxiiii^{or} *P* 24 terendo] te'pdo (?) *S* 28 uoretur] moretur *S* 29 digerit *P* 31 idropicis *P* 32 pota *S*

2.14 Betony, *Betonica officinalis* L.

Hail *cestron*, whom the Latins have called Betony!
O how many and how great the powers Nature the Creator
granted to you alone, all of which my mind cannot
suffice to put in writing (nor does any mind suffice for all)!
  Ground up, it excellently heals a fractured skull.
A plaster made from the ground or boiled leaves
is good for injuries or vices of the eyes;
when eaten or drunk it restrains harmful tears,
but if it is blended with the same weight of Rue
and taken in warm water, cloudiness is driven off.
Harmful blood, moreover, is thus apt to be removed from eyes
through the lower parts and freedom will be renewed.
Let the juice, when mixed with oil-of-Rose, be poured
into the ears; or its powder, mixed and cooked with honey,
prevails over blood-spitters, cures asthma and a cough,
and thus it's good for the stomach. Dangerous vomit is purged
if you take this in warm water, and similarly the chest;
with mead it softens bellies and with vinegar-water
it's good for spitters of blood. One ounce, when drunk
with two spoons of hot water, removes a stomach pain.
A decoction of the entire herb helps the spleen and liver.
Let four ounces be mixed with three spoons
of old wine; add twenty-four grains of Pepper
to these and drink this, once mixed by grinding,
and thus you can purge your kidney pains.
The powder of the leaves in mead is good for ruptures,
good for urine, the stone, and for the falling womb.
So let a bean's weight of powder be eaten with honey
after dinner so the stomach may quickly digest the food.
  I said what it does for parts. I'll relate what it does for the whole:
if given with wine and honey it's good for those with dropsy;
it also heals the dropsical if an ounce of the aforesaid,

2.14 VETONICA / **Betony** *Macer, 'Betonica', 429–91*
2 *Cf.* Lucretius, *De rerum natura* 1. 629

Vncia predicte ciato calide sociata;
Vncia preterea cum uino sumpta tepenti
Hictericos curat. Febre si uexabitur eger
Vnaquaque die plantaginis uncia binis
Addita uetonice tepida contrita bibatur
Antea quam punctus febrienti frigoris assit.
Obstat cum uino large potata ueneno,
Semen precipue, quod si desit, dabis herbam.
Plinius istarum radicum sumere dragmas
Bis binas iussit cum mulsa: sic uomitum dat
Quo (uelut elleboro) malus humor flecma recedit.
Plinius inde iubet uiridem fecisse coronam
Circa serpentes: nunquam transire ualebunt
Ipsam, sed proprio morsu pugnaque peribunt.
Plinius hac dicit cum uino sepius hausta
Quod color ascendat iuuenilior et renouetur.
Plinius inquit eam qui gestat nec medicamen
Huic oberit nocuum, nec cum medicamine carmen.
Antidotis Menetamus eam iubet omnibus addi
Namque iuuat stomachum, magis herbis omnibus, una.

2.15 FRAGA

Area que sequitur spaciantibus optima gustu
Fraga libare iubet. Nec uultu pulcrior alter
Illis fructus erit, nec gustu dulcior alter.
Scimus ab expertis, locium nil prouocat eque;
Scimus ab expertis, nil menstrua prouocat eque.
'Quid tibi liuor erit, mea cum nec gramina cedant

33 ciaco *P* 34 tepenti] repenti *S* 35 yctericos *P* 37 betonice *P* 40 si desit] desit si *S* 42 mulsa sic] multa sit *S* 43 uelud *P* eloboro *S* flecma recedit] flegmaque cedit (*corr. e* cedait) *P* 44 choronam *P* 46 proprio morsu *transp. P* pungnaqua *P* perhibunt *S* 47 hac] *scripsi*, ac *P* : hanc *S* 48 remouetur *S* 52 herba *S*

2.15 FRAGA *P* 14r: Fraga | *S* 63v: De frago (*corr. ex* fraga). Henricus | *T* 96v (*lines 2 and 5*): Fra

Exceptiones (*O* 92r): Fraga nil adeo locium prouocat uel menstrua.

1 spacientibus *S* *lines 3–4 transp. S* 3 gustu dulcior *transp. S* 6 nec] nunc *P*

mixed with a spoonful of hot water, is frequently drunk;
that ounce, moreover, when taken with hot wine,
cures the jaundiced. If one is sick and vexed by fever
every day let an ounce of Plantain, when added to two
of Betony and ground up in warm water, be drunk
before the sting of a chill comes upon the feverish patient.
When drunk abundantly with wine it hinders poison,
especially the seed, but if it's lacking, give the leaves.
Pliny orders you to take four drams of these roots
with mead: in such a way it causes vomit by which
(as if by Hellebore) the wicked humour phlegm departs.
Pliny orders that a green chaplet be made from it
to encircle serpents: they'll never be able to move
beyond it, but will die by their own bite and sting.
Pliny says that when this is often drunk with wine,
a more youthful colour arises and is renewed.
Pliny says that no harmful medicine, nor any charm
with medicine, should hurt one who is carrying this.
Menemachus orders this added to every antidote,
for alone it helps the stomach, more than all other herbs.

2.15 Strawberry, *Fragaria vesca* L.

The plot which follows commands those wandering through
to sample Strawberries, the best in taste. No other fruit will be
more beautiful to see than these, no other more sweet to taste.
We know from experts that nothing brings out urine so well;
we know from experts that nothing brings out a period so well.
'Why are you envious, since my shoots do not grow

50 *Cf.* Pliny 25. 84

2.15 FRAGA / **Strawberry** *Source unknown*
7 *Cf.* Ovid, *Met.* 103–104

Arboribus quarum pulcherima fraga uidentur
Vt fructu fructus, folium foliis superare,
Ni populo figmenta ferant pigmenta parantes?'

2.16 PVLEGIVM

Pulegium tanti constare ferunt apud Indos,
Hic quanti piper. O uirtus mira Tonantis,
Dans aliis alias persoluere mutua terras
Quo sit ut una domus sociandus partibus orbis!
Puleium calet et siccat: gradus est in utroque
Tercius. Exusti gingiuis proficit egris
Puleii puluis; sumptus cum melle probatur
Pectoris humores uiscosos attenuare,
Et cum reddiderit tenues solet adnichilare.
Cum tepido tussim compescit; nausea cedit
Et morsus stomachi sumpta in pusca uel aceto.
Iuncta nigram uino coleram fugat, addita spleni
Cum sale proficiet, cum uino menstrua ducit,
Prouocat urinas; sic extrahit ipsa secundas.
Apponas uiridem: sedabit rite podagram
Et solet (aut lente) tepide permixta polente
Quosuis feruores, quosuis curare tumores.
Hec et multa dabis si mel; si sal dabis illi,
Vnguine contractum potes isto flectere membrum.
Cerotis addes, papulas de corpore tolles.
Elixatura si corpus sepe tepenti
Pulegii ablueris, pruritum non pacieris.
Si febre uel casu subito defecerit eger
Quod solet a medicis dici 'malfacio,' tritum
Iungatur ualido puleii gramen aceto:
Naribus apponas egri, releuabit odore.
Obstat cum uino serpentum pota uenenis.

7 quare *S* pulcerrima *P* 8 fructu] fructum *S* 9 ne *S* parantes] per artes *S*

2.16 PVLEGIVM *P* 14r–14v: Pulegium | *S* 84v–85r: De pulegio. Henricus

1 puleyum *P* yndos *P* 4 sociandis *corr. e* sociandus *P* 7 pulei *S* melli *S* 9 redierit *S* anichilare *P* 11 in] cum *S* pusca] *scripsi*, pasca *P* : pascua *S* 14 sic] sed et *S* 18 dabis] *scripsi*, dabit *PS* 20 crotis *S* 21 si *om. S* tepenti] repenti *S* 22 puleii *P* 23 casu subito *transp. P* 24 malfacio] uinafactio *S* tritum] talis trita *et exp.* talis *P* 25 pulei *P* : pulegi *S* 26 releuabit] *scripsi*, reuelabit *PS* 27 pota] potata *post corr. P* ueneno *S*

into those trees whose most beautiful strawberries seem
to outshine fruits with fruit and leaf with leaves,
unless those making pigments also make figments for the crowd?'

2.16 Pennyroyal, *Mentha pulegium* L.

They say that Pennyroyal is worth as much among the Indians
as Pepper is over here. O marvellous virtue of the Thunderer,
who grants that some lands pay equal returns to others
so the world is united in its parts like a single house!
Pennyroyal heats and dries: the degree in either is third.
The powder of roasted Pennyroyal is good
for painful gums; when taken with honey it's proven
to thin out viscous humours of the chest,
and though it could render them thin, it's apt to destroy them.
With warm wine it restrains a cough, and nausea and gripes
depart from it when drunk in vinegar-water or vinegar.
Mixed in wine it chases off black bile, applied with salt
it will benefit the spleen, with wine it leads out menses,
and it brings out urine; in such a way it draws out afterbirth.
Apply it green: it will properly settle gout
and is apt to cure any fevers and swellings
when thoroughly mixed with warm barley porridge (or lentils).
It will grant these and many things if you add honey; if you add salt
to it, you can flex a sprained limb with this ointment.
Add it to wax plasters to remove pimples from the body.
If you should often wash your body with a warm
elixir of Pennyroyal, you will not suffer itching.
If a patient should grow faint from a fever or the sudden fall
which is usually called *malefactio* by physicians,
let the ground leaves of Pennyroyal be mixed with strong vinegar,
apply it to the patient's nostrils and he'll be revived by the odour.
When drunk with wine it hinders serpents' poisons.

2.16 PVLEGIVM / **Pennyroyal** *Macer, 'Pulegium', 626–77*
1–4 Strabo 300–326

2.17 SERPILLVM

Serpillum, quod serpat humi, dixere poete
Puleiique modo siccare, calere probarunt.
Hanc melli iungas et aceto sicque cruentum
Iactantes sputum celeri uirtute iuuabis.
Hanc acri coque cum uino, tundens et oliuo
Cum roseo, capitis frontem mulceto dolentis;
Vnguine presenti, succurres rite dolenti.
Cum uino iecoris fertur sedare dolorem;
Splen iuuat electo si iuncta bibatur aceto;
Sic ualet urinis, sic curat tormina uentris.
Combusti fumus serpentinum genus omne
Et quoduis animal uirus dans ore fugabit,
Quod miscere cibis solet inter pascua pastor
Vt si forte sopor fessum premat huius odore
Vermibus a nocuis tutus liberque quiescat.
Hinc et Virgilius: 'fessis messoribus estu
Allia serpillumque herbas contundit olentes.'
Potum pestiferos iuuat, appositum quoque, morsus.

2.18 PIPERA

Et piperam memorare libet que plurima dumis
Subditur, effetis siluarum nata sub umbris.
Hanc tamen et noster non dedignatus habere

2.17 SERPILLVM *P* 14v: Serpillum | *S* 94r–94v: De Serpillo. Henricus
2 puleique *S* probarunt *corr. e* probabuirunt (?) *P* 3 iunges *S* 4 sputum] sumptum *S* iuuabis] curabis *P* 5 coque] quoque *S* tundes *S* 6 mulceto] *scripsi*, linito *S* : mulcedo (?) *corr. e* mulcebo *P* dolenti *S* 7 unguine . . . dolenti *om. S* 11 conbusti simus *S* serpentinum] *scripsi*, serpillum *exp.* serpentium *P* : serpentum *S* genus] iuuat *P* 12 quoduis] quamuis *S* animal] aliud *P* 13 cibus *S* intra *P* pastor] messor *add. P s.l.* 16 hin *S* mestoribus *S*

2.18 PIPERA *P* 14v–15r: Pipera | *S* 81r: De Pipera. Henricus | *T* 101v: Pipera
Exceptiones (*O* 92r): Pipera et dumis effetis plurimum <subditur> ramorum multitudine. Flore **** ****ur, flore exiguo, et denso. Vis eius est: uulnera mundat, sanat, colorat.
1 libet . . . dumis] quam plurima libet durit *T* 2 effectis *S* siluare *S* nata] uitia *S*

2.17 Wild Thyme, *Thymus serpyllum* L.

The poets called it *serpillum*, for it snakes upon the ground,
and they proved it dries and heats like Pennyroyal.
Add this to honey and vinegar, and in such a way
you'll assist those expelling bloody sputum by its speedy strength.
Cook this in vinegar and, grinding with oil-of-Rose,
dab it on the brow of an aching head;
while the ointment's present, you'll surely help the patient.
When drunk with wine, it's said to settle a pain in the liver;
it helps the spleen if mixed with excellent vinegar and drunk.
In such a way it's good for urine and heals stomach gripes.
The smoke of this, when burnt, will chase away the entire
serpent race and any creature which emits poison from its mouth.
A shepherd in his pastures is wont to mix this in his food
so that, if drowsiness perhaps weighs down his tired body,
by its odour he may stay safe and sound from harmful worms.
So Virgil says of this: 'for reapers faint with heat
she pounds her savoury herbs, Garlic and Thyme.'
When drunk or also applied it helps destructive bites.

2.18 Lesser Burnet, *Pimpinella saxifraga* L.

And it is pleasing to recall the Burnet which is often found
below the bushes, born beneath the sleepy forest shadows.
Yet even our garden has not disdained to hold this

2.17 SERPILLVM / **Wild Thyme** *Macer, 'Serpillum', 1325–41*
15 *Cf. Psalmi Turonenses* xxii. 32 (ed. Orth) 16–17 *Cf.* Virgil, *Ecloga* 2. 10–11; *cf.* Virgil, *Georgica* 4. 30–32

2.18 PIPERA / **Lesser Burnet** *Strabo, 'De Agrimonia', 359–68*

Ortus, in exculta docuit mansuescere terra.
Paruam magna quidem ramorum copia uestit,
Flos niueus, flos exiguus, flos undique densus,
Cuius si uires queras paucis tibi subdam:
Vulnera mundat, mundaque sanat, sana colorat.

2.19 BENEDICTA

Iam licet inuictam tetigisse tibi benedictam,
Philosophi tamen auriculam dicunt leporinam.
Nomina uirtuti plebs, philosophia figure
Comparat. Hanc igitur docte docti uocitarunt,
Doctius indocti. Quid enim benedictius illa
Vulnera que sordent purgat, purgataque sorde
Carne replet, repletaque carne colore perornat?
Quid tibi furtiue preest iniuria gutte
Saucia diuinam si contigerit leporinam?

2.20 CONFERBA

Qui dedit omne bonum cur graminibus tot eandem
Vim dederit quidam dubitant. Dubitare uetabo,
Quatuor humores cum sint et quatuor illos
Res uarient; humor, frigus, calor ariditasque
Corporibus uarie dominantur. Nam modo solus

4 exculta] exisita *S* 5 parua mangna *T* 6 niueus] minus *S* : uinens *T* indique *S* 7 cuius] huius *T* subdam] soluam *T* 8 mundaque] uulnera *ST* colerat *S*

2.19 BENEDICTA *P* 15r: Benedicta | *S* 46v–47r: De Benedicta. Henricus

Exceptiones (*O* 92r): Benedicta que et auricula leporina uulnera purgat, carne replet, colorat, guttam expugnat.

2 aurictam *S* 3 uirtutis *S* 4 igitur] ergo *P* uocitarum *S* 6 sordent] sorde *S* 7 perornat] colorat *P* 8 tibi] sibi *S* preest] *scripsi*, prodest *PS* gurte *S*

2.20 CONFERBA *P* 15r : De conferba siue consolida | *S* 55r–55v: De Conferba. Henricus

Exceptiones (*O* 92r): Conferba cum frustis carnis in aeno decocta, conglutinat illa. Membris luxatis, contusis prodest. Oxigaro iuncta stomacum curat. Splen iuuat, os nodat, tussim fugat, intima curat.

1 dedit] cedit *S* 2 uetabo] uocabo *S* 3 et] cum *P*

and has taught us how to tame it in cultivated earth.
A great number of branches clothes its little shape,
as does a white flower, a tiny flower, a flower packed in on all sides,
whose virtues, if you ask, I will give you in a few words:
it cleans wounds, heals once cleaned, and adds colour once healed.

2.19 Avens (Herb Bennet, Hare's Ear), *Geum urbanum* L.

It's fitting now to mention invincible Herb Bennet,
yet the philosophers call it Hare's Ear.
The crowd matches names to ability, but Philosophy to shape.
Therefore the learned have named this in a learned fashion,
the unlearned more learnedly. For what more blessedly purges
those wounds which are fouled, and fills them, purged of foulness,
with new flesh, and adorns them, once filled with flesh, with colour?
What can the sickly injury of furtive gout inflict
upon you if it should touch divine Hare's Ear?

2.20 Comfrey, *Symphytum officinale* L.

Some people question why He who granted every good
would give the same power to so many herbs. I will forbid
them to be in doubt, since there are four humours and four things
will affect them: moisture, cold, heat, and dryness
rule over bodies in varied ways. For now one alone

2.19 BENEDICTA / **Avens** *Source unknown*
8 *Cf.* Strabo, 'De Abrotano,' 97

2.20 CONFERBA / **Comfrey** *Pseudo-Apuleius no. 59, 'Herba Confirma' (pp. 112–13)*

Horum regna tenet, modo regnant alter et alter,
Nunc tria iuncta simul. Sed iam si quatuor ista
Corregnare uelint mors improuisa subintrat.
Hiis igitur uariata modis cum corpora constent,
Ista michi ualuit; tibi nil medicina ualebit;
Profuit ista tibi; michi prodesse uidebis
Hanc. Plures cause morbo tribuuntur eidem,
Herbe quod uariis pro corporibus uarientur.
Preterea quia non omnis fert omnia tellus,
Si careas istis, ad idem uesci licet illis.
Nam mire conferba uigens in uulnera pugnat.
Fama refert carnis si frusta coquantur aeno
Plura quam hec fient. Istam si concoquis, unum,
Quod, nisi credideris, temptes inpune licebit.
Fertur item membris fieri conferba salubris
Luxatis uel contusis, quod sepe probatur.
Corporis hec regem stomachum si iuncta bibatur
Oxigaro curat regnique potencia durat,
Splen iuuat, os nodat, tussim fugat, intima sanat.

2.21 VIOLA <HYEMALIS>

Viginti uiole uisis genus aspice pulcre!
Hoc 'hyemale' uocant quia, cum natale colatur
Diuinum, nasci teneros mirabere flores.
Predictis uiolis equant flores hyemales
Et uirtute pari solet utraque magnificari,
Sed foliis magis ista patet, magis illa uirescit.

6 horum regna tenet] regnat horum que *P* regnant] regnat *S* 8 corregnare] cum regnare *S* inprouisa *S* 9 igitur] ergo *P* 10 michi ualuit] ualere michi *P* 11 profuit] prosint *S* 12 hac *P* cause] *scripsi*, causas *S* : causa *P* morbo *om. S* 16 pungnat *P* 17 refert carnis] referre solet *S* frustra coquentur aino *S* 18 quam] quod *P* istam] unum *P* unum] istam *P* 21 probarunt *P* 22 hoc *S* iuncta] cuncta *S* 23 oxigare *P* 23–24 regnique ... durat / tussim ... sanat *transp. P*

2.21 VIOLA <HYEMALIS> *P* 15r–15v: Viole | *S* 102v: De Viola. Henricus

Exceptiones (*O* 92r): Viole hiemales circa natale diuinum florent, predictis uiolis pares habet flores parem uirtutem, sed foliis magis ista patet, magis illa uirescit.

1 gens *S* accipe pulchre *P* 2 yemale *P* conatur *S* 3 mirabile *S* 4 uiolis equant] *scripsi*, uiolis equantur *P* : equat uiolis *S* 6 ista] illa *P*

holds dominion over them, now one or the other reigns,
now three joined together at once. But if those four should wish
to rule now as one, unexpected death arrives.
Therefore, when varied bodies agree in these ways,
this medicine was effective for me, none will be effective for you,
that one was good for you, you'll see this one is good for me.
Many causes are attributed to the same disease,
because herbs differ according to different bodies.
Moreover, because not every soil produces all things,
if you lack these, you're allowed to eat those for the same disease.
  For example, powerful Comfrey works wonderfully in wounds:
as rumour relates, if bits of meat are cooked in a brazen pot
more than these will come out. If you cook with Comfrey, only one,
and if you don't believe it, you're free to try with impunity.
Comfrey is likewise said to be salubrious for limbs
when dislocated or bruised, a thing which is often proven.
If added to *oxigarum* and drunk this cures the stomach,
the body's king, and strengthens the powers of his kingdom,
helps the spleen, closes the stomach, cures a cough, cleans the insides.

2.21 Winter Violet, *Viola hiemalis* L.

Having seen twenty, observe the lineage of handsome Violet!
They call this one the Winter Violet for you will marvel
that its tender flowers are born when Christmas is celebrated.
These winter flowers are equal to the aforesaid Violets
and either can be glorified with equal virtue,
but the former is larger in the leaves, and the latter is greener.

22 *Cf.* Quintus Serenus 299–300; Strabo 334

2.21 VIOLA <HYEMALIS> / **Winter Violet** *Original*

2.22 BASILISCA

Proximus extollit locus inmensam basiliscam,
Viribus inmensam, mediocri corpore pulcram,
Cuius si uires queras—nec sit tibi magni
Forma uigore carens—uires ex nomine pensa.
Effundit uirus solo flatu basiliscus.
Vires grata graui basilisca rapit basilisco
Et pote uires possunt hoc uincere uirus.
Hinc pensare licet: cum sic maiora repulset,
Cetera que facili perimat uirtute uenena?
Que si tanta potest, cur tantis amplius addam?

2.23 ABROTANVS

Abrotanus 'tot habet uires quot fila comarum,'
Stabus ait. Calet et siccat, <illi> gradus hiis est
Tercius, ac semen feruencius esse probatur.
Abrotano panis micas et coctana iungas,
Amne coquas; oculis si feruor uel dolor insit,
Hec simul apponas feruorque dolorque recedent.
Abrotani penitus decoccio sumpta iuuabit
Et neruos omnes et causas pectoris omnes.
Sic quoque disnoycos, sic tussim sedat anhelam,
Sic prodest lumbis, sic uulue sumpta querelis,
Sic sciasim curat, sic mire menstrua purgat,
Sic ualet urine, sic uiscera mundat habunde,
Sic et lumbricos uentris potata necabit.
Omnibus hiis prodest crudum uinoque cohaustum.

2.22 BASILISCA *P* 15v: Basilisca | [not in *S*]

Exceptiones (*O* 92r): Basilisca herba quodlibet uenenum pote[n]tur pota expugnat, cum eciam basilisci uenenum deuincat qui solo flatu uirus effundit, unde et nomen habet.

1 extollit locus inmensam] *scripsi*, inmensam extollit locus *P* 5 effundit *corr. ex* effundat *P* 8 sit *P*

2.23 ABROTANVS *P* 15v: Abrotanum | *S* 34r–34v: [no title]

1 quot] cum *P* fila] *scripsi* (*cf.* Strabo 98), sit *P* : filia *S* comarum *om. P* 2 ayt *P* illi] *scripsi*, *om. PS* hiis] hic *S* 3 ac] hac *P* 4 iungens *S* 5 ampne *P* 6 hoc *P* recedunt *P* 9 dysnoycos *P* sedat anhelam] sanat hanelam *S* 12 sic . . . sic] sic . . . si *S* 14 crudum *om. P* uinoque] uino ue *P* coactum *S*

2.22 Autumn Gentian/Felwort, *Gentiana amarella* L.

The following plot bears aloft immense Autumn Gentian—
immense in powers and beautiful in its middling body.
If you should ask its powers (nor should its shape lacking strength
seem worth much to you), judge its powers from its name.
The basilisk pours out poison with its breath alone.
Pleasing Gentian takes the powers from the painful basilisk
and its powers in a potion can overpower this poison.
And so you may ask of this, since it thus repels the greater
poisons, what others might it prevent with an easy power?
And if it can do such things, why should I add more to them?

2.23 Southernwood, *Artemisia abrotanum* L.

Strabo says that Southernwood 'has as many powers
as strands of hair.' It heats and dries and has the third
degree in these; its seed is proven to be hotter.
Add crumbs of bread and figs to Southernwood
and cook in water; if a burning or a pain is in the eyes,
apply these together and the burning or pain will depart.
Taking a decoction made wholly out of Southernwood
will help all sinews and all problems of the chest.
When taken thus it also settles eye diseases, a panting cough,
is beneficial for the groin, and for problems of the womb,
thus it cures sciatica, thus marvellously purges menstrual courses,
thus it's good for urine, thus cleans the insides thoroughly,
and drunk in such a way it will eradicate all stomach worms.
It's good for all these things when eaten raw and drunk in wine.

2.22 BASILISCA / **Autumn Gentian** *Source unknown*
5 *Cf.* Isidore, *Etym.* 12. 4. 6–9

2.23 ABROTANVS / **Southernwood** *Macer, 'Abrotanum', 31–51*
1–2 Strabo 98

Abrotanum socies amni; sic des febrienti
Antea quam punctus rediuiui frigoris assit
Aut oleo quo decoquitur sibi membra perungas.
Abrotani nidor serpentes effugat omnes,
Atra uenena premit potu; stirpesque refixas
Et spinas retrahit uel per se siue peruncutm.
Plinius hac uenerem testatur posse uenire
Si sub puluino sit subdita nocte uirili;
Hoc cunctis ueneri nocuis obsistere scribit.
Cedet et abscedet gutte fastus sociatus
Abrotano, quia perniciem fert perniciei.

2.24 TANETICVM

Taneticum quid commemorem, licet acrius ora
Mordeat exterius, lenem conferre medelam
Pectoris interius? Nec solum pectora purgat
Sed simul omne latens quod celant pectora curat.
Hinc quoniam tibi tam breuibus tam multa notaui,
Cum non pauca queat, paucis contentus abibo.

2.25 LIGVSTICVM

Finis in aduentum postrema ligustica surgunt.
Tercius hiis gradus est siccandi siue calendi;
A Ligurum terra sumpsisse ligustica nomen
Tale putant quidam quod copia presit ibidem.
Maior radicis uis est et seminis illi:

15 ampni *P*   das *P*   18 nidor *corr. ex* uideor *S*   19 stipesque *P*   21 hanc *S*   uenerem] ueneri *S*   22 si sub] *scripsi*, si uel *P* : simul *S*   23 ueneris *corr. e* ueneri *S*   24 guste *S*

2.24 TANETICVM   *P* 16r: Senecion (*sic*) | [not in *S*] | *T* 106r: Taneticum
Exceptiones (*O* 92r): Taneticum pectus et quelibet interiora purgat.
1 saneticum *P*   4 set *T*   pectora] corpora *T*

2.25 LIGVSTICVM   *P* 16r: Ligustica | *S* 67r–67v: De Ligustico. Henricus
1 liturtica *P*   3 a Ligurum] *scripsi*, aligurum *P* : alligure *S*   sumpsere *P*   ligustica *add. P s.l.*] liturtica *P* : locustica *S*   4 presidet *P*

Add Southernwood to water; give it like this to one who suffers
a fever before the bite of a returning chill arrives,
or rub his limbs with the oil in which it was cooked.
The odour of Southernwood will drive away all serpents,
and in a drink it expels deadly poisons; it draws out
splinters and thorns either by itself or in an ointment.
Pliny claims that sexual desire can be achieved with this
if it is placed beneath the man's pillow at night,
and he writes that it hinders all things harmful to sex.
The arrogance of gout will yield and depart when mixed
with Southernwood, for it brings destruction to destruction.

2.24 ? Tansy, *Chrysanthemum vulgare* (L.) Bernh.

Why should I recall that Tansy, although it rather bitterly
gnaws the mouth on the outside, confers a gentle cure
for the chest on the inside? Not only does it purge the chest
but it cures at one time every secret which the chest conceals.
Since I have noted for you so much about this in such brief words,
although it does no few things, I'll depart content with just a few.

2.25 Lovage, *Levisticum officinale* Koch

The Lovages rise up at very last, with the arrival of the end.
Their degree is third in drying and in heating;
some think that Lovages received this name from the land
of the Ligurians because a great amount is present in that place.
A greater power is in its root and seed:

21–23 *Cf.* Pliny 21. 162 24–25 *Cf.* Strabo 97

2.24 TANETICVM / **Tansy** *Source unknown*

2.25 LIGVSTICVM / **Lovage** *Macer, 'Ligusticum', 882–906*
3–4 *Cf.* Isidore, *Etym.* 17. 11. 5

Hec stomacho ualet inflato coniuncta lyeo;
Sic mouet urinas, sic purgat menstrua uelox,
Sic uariis prorsus morbis ualet interiorum.
Hoc igitur potu uis digestiua iuuatur.
Proficit eximie colicis uel mansa uel hausta
Vel si radicum fuerit decoccio sumpta.
Nec tamen hec colicos elixatura iuuabit
Solos sed dictis medicabitur omnibus ista.
Tota uenenatis hec morsibus herba medetur
Si bibitur contrita prius uinoque soluta;
Partem contrite si nectas desuper herbe.
Omnibus antidotis semen iungi statuerunt
Digestibilibus, quod inest huic stiptica uirtus.
Hanc Stabus retulit (nec semper uera referre
Ipse potest Stabus) 'tenebras inferre gemellis
Orbibus' et laudes aliorum 'laude mereri.'
Hinc igitur sunt qui dubitant an dixerit ex se
Tanta uel ex alio, sed plura uolumina uoluens
Inuenio nullum qui talibus astipuletur;
Inuenio multos qui tale quid infitiantur.

6 hec] hoc *S* ualet *om. S* lieo *S* 7 mouent *S* 8 morbus *S* 11 uel] et *P* 12 hec] hoc *S* 13 dictis] dulcis *P* meditabitur *S* istis *P* 15 si bibitur] scribitur *S* 18 digestibilibus] que uentrem soluunt *P* huic stiptica] hec stipica *P* 21 laude] inferre *P* 22 hinc] hic *S* dubitent *S* 24 inuenio] reperio *S* 25 inuenio] reperio *S* quid] a *add. P et exp.* inficientur *P*

When mixed with wine, this is good for a swollen stomach;
in such a way it forces urine, thus hastily purges menses,
and thus is wholly good for various internal diseases.
Therefore digestive power is aided by this drink.
It especially profits the bilious either eaten or in a drink,
or if a decoction of the roots should be consumed.
Yet this elixir will help not only the bilious
but it is curative for all the aforesaid things.
This entire herb is a remedy for poisoned bites
if it is drunk, first ground and then dissolved in wine;
grind a part of the herb if you are binding it on top.
They ordered that the seed be added to all antidotes
promoting digestion, for an astringent power belongs to it.
Strabo related (nor can even Strabo always relate
true things!) that 'it brings shadows to the twin orbs'
and that it 'earned praises from the praise of others.'
So there are those who doubt whether he said such things himself
about this or if it came from another, but leafing through many books
I find no one who agrees with such things,
while I find many who deny this very thing.

20–21 Strabo 231–4

3 PROLOGVS IN LIBRO TERTIO

Corporum quedam docet esse sana
Phisice splendor, docet egra quedam;
Terciam partem uenerem fatetur.
Graminum promptus uigor ista sanat;
Ista conseruat, meliorat illa.
Ergo non parui, tibi, lector, ortus,
Ergo non parui tibi sit libellus,
Alter amplectens gremio tot herbas,
Alter herbarum reserans triumphos.
Editus Phebo titulis earum
Non mori sollers homini dedisset,
Fulminis iactu nisi corruisset
Vidit et nouit titulos earum.
Phebus hiis causas uidet atque noscit,
Prius absconsas radiisque monstrat.
Has et inspexi, didici, notaui.
Crede mortali. Moritura tempnis?
Crede splendoris Domino perhennis.

3.1 DIPTANNVS

In uiridi claustro uexillum tollit ab austro
Diptanum renitens uultu, renitencius actu.
Hec simul omnibus una sequentibus eminet herba,
Vnde prehit sceptrumque uehit splendore superba.
Istam Virgilius (nec fingunt cuncta poete)

3 PROLOGVS IN LIBRO TERTIO *P* 16r–16v: Prologus in libro tertio | *S* 32v–33r: [no title] *Edited by Rigg*, 269–70.

1 corpora *P* 3 uenerem] uentrem *S* fatetur] facetus *P* 4 graminum] carminum *S* 5 ista . . . illa *om. S* 6 paruius *S* 7 ergo] hoc *S* 8 alter . . . herbas *om. S* 9 reserans] referens *P* 10 Phebo] *Rigg*, phebi *P* : plebo *S* titulus *P* 11 solers *S* 12 fluminis *S* coruisset *S* 14 Phebus] plebus *S* 15 prius] premitus *P* radiisque] radiis *P* monstrat] *Rigg*, modo *P* : monstrant *S* 16 has] *Rigg*, hos *PS* 17 temnis *P*

3.1 DIPTANNVS *P* 16v: Diptanus | *S* 56v–57r: De Diptanno. (Macer *canc.*) Henricus

1 austro] alto *P* 2 dyptannum *P* retinencius *S* 3 eminet] et enim *S* 4 premit *P* septrumque *S* 5 fingunt] fugiunt *P* cuntta *S*

3 Prologue of the Third Book

The splendour of Medicine teaches
that some bodies are healthy and some are sick;
it confesses the third part is sexual activity.
The ready vigour of plants heals the sick;
it preserves the former and improves the latter.
So, reader, don't let the garden seem cheap to you,
nor let this book be of little worth to you—
one enclosing in its bosom so many herbs,
the other revealing the triumphs of the herbs.
The skilful son of Apollo would have granted
that, by their glories, man would not die,
if he had not fallen, struck down by lightning,
for he saw and knew their glories.
Apollo sees and knows in them the causes,
first hidden, and reveals them with his rays;
I've inspected, learned, and written them down.
Believe a mortal. Do you despise what will die?
Trust in the Lord of eternal splendour.

3.1 Dittany of Crete, *Origanum dictamnus* L.

Dittany takes up the standard on the emerald cloister's
southern side, bright in appearance, even brighter in performance.
This one herb stands over all her followers at once,
wherefore she bears the sceptre and goes forth, proud, in splendour.
Virgil wrote (and poets don't make up everything!)

3 PROLOGVS IN LIBRO TERTIO / **Prologue of the Third Book** *Original*

10 *Cf.* Ovid, *Met.* 2. 642–8; Isidore, *Etym.* 4. 3. 2   14–15 *Cf.* Henry of Huntingdon, *HA* 10. 40 (p. 776)

3.1 DIPTANNVS / **Dittany of Crete** *Original*

5–11 Virgil, *Aeneid* 12. 411–15

Scribit ab Enea temerato uulnere magno
Alcius infixam mox extraxisse sagittam
Arte manuque tua iuuenum que corda sagittis
Traicis ignitis, tenerorum mater Amorum.
Ergo docet uates ferrum, quod forcipe tangi
Vulnere non possit, diptanno posse uocari.
Quod cum tanta queat, qui tantis amplius addet?
Huic similem fatear que, cum peperisse Gigantes
Nullius esse putat, simiam peperisse putatur.
Nam nil absque modo—nec et ipsa modestia—prodest.

3.2 FENICVLVM

Quid tibi, feniculum, quid dignum laude feremus,
Gracia cum laudem, res uerba supergrediatur?
Corpore terrigenas poteris equare Gigantes:
Cetera turba subit, uix pubetenus, mediantes.
Corpore tanta nites, animis melior renitescis,
Que uino armaris solo, pressura uenenum:
Sic uiro uirus, sic pesti pestis haberis.
Te Greci 'maratrum,' medici siccum calidumque
Dicunt esse gradu (quod temptauere) secundo.
Hanc comedit serpens oculos caligine tergens,
Vnde putauerunt, tandemque putata scierunt,
Humanis hanc luminibus mire medicari.
Ergo radicum succus melli sociatus
Lumina fert oculis, atra caligine mundis.
Rursum si premitur uiridi de semine succus
Soleque torretur, certum medicamen habetur
Vt tollas uarios qui tollunt lumina morbos,

6 scribit] *scripsi*, scribitur *P* : scrip *S* 7 alterius infixa *S* 8 manuque] manu *S* sagictis *S* 9 tractis *S* 10 ergo] hoc *S* uatos *P* ferre *S* 11 dyptanno *P* 13 hunc *S* 14 simiam peperisse putatur] peperit te symia sima *P* 15 nichil *P* et *om. P*

3.2 FENICVLVM *P* 16v–17r: Feniculum | *S* 62r–63r: De Feniculo. Henricus
2 gracia] hec ratia *S* supergrediatur *corr. e* supergrediantur *P* 3 terrigena poteras *P* 5 nites] uires *S* melior] maior *S* renitesces *P* 6 que] quod *S* 7 uirus] uinus *S* habebis *S* 8 martrum *S* 9 tenatuere *P* 10 tergens] purgans *P* 12 meditari *S* 14 mundus *S* 15 uiridis *P* 16 terretur *P* 17 que *S*

that Dittany soon had extracted from Aeneas an arrow
thrust rather deeply in a large and festering wound,
by your art and hand, O mother of gentle Cupids,
you who pierce young hearts with fiery arrows.
Therefore the poet teaches that a blade, which cannot be removed
from a wound with forceps, can be summoned forth by Dittany.
And since it can do such great things, who can add more to them?
I should confess this similar to her who, when she thinks begetting
the Giants was nothing, is thought to have begotten an ape.
For nothing—not even modesty itself—can benefit without
moderation.

3.2 Fennel, *Foeniculum vulgare* Gært.

What thing worthy of praise, O Fennel, can we bring to you,
when your grace surpasses praise, the subject surpasses words?
You could equal the earth-born Giants in size:
the rest of the crowd submits, scarcely children, halved in size.
You shine out, so great in body, and shine again, even greater in spirits,
you who, armed with wine alone, will overwhelm venom:
you are thus considered a poison's poison, thus a plague to a plague.
The Greeks call you *maratrum* and physicians say that you
are dry and hot in the second degree, which they have tested.
A serpent eats this herb to clean its eyes of cloudiness,
so they have thought—and knew at last the things they thought—
that this marvellously medicates a human's eyes.
Therefore the juice of its roots, when mixed with honey,
brings light to the eyes, clean of murky fogginess.
If, on the other hand, the juice is squeezed from the fresh seed
and dried out in the sun, it's considered a certain medicine
for you to remove the various ills which take away the sight,

9 *Cf.* Henry of Huntingdon, *HA* 11.25 (p. 802)   13–14 *Cf.* Ovid, *Met.* 1.151–62

3.2 FENICVLVM / Fennel *Macer, 'Feniculum', 678–710*
3 *Cf.* Ovid, *Met.* 1.151–62   7 Henry of Huntingdon, *De gemmis* no. 29, 2 (ed. Black, 84)

At melius rute cum succo felleque galli
Melleque feniculi succus si iungitur eque
Indeque sint oculi pacientis sepe peruncti.
Auribus infusus uermes perimit tibi succus;
Cum uino pulmonis adest iecorisque saluti,
Radix sicque datur nutrici copia lactis.
Semina cum uino lateris sedare dolorem
Pota solent; dat et hoc herbe decoccio sumpta.
Radicum uino uel aqua decoccio sumpta
Vesice morbis et nefreticis tribuatur.
Herba cum uino sedatur nausea sumpta;
Cum limpha feruor stomachi solet attenuari.
Vrinas maratri uel menstrua coccio soluit,
Aut si trita super pecten tantum religetur.
Renibus in ptysana radix hec cocta ualebit,
At uino decocta potest tenuare dolores
Fomento nimios quos profert uirga uirilis
Aut si coniungas oleo uirgamque perungas.
  Partibus ista dabit, per totum uero tumores
Apposita aut ictus iuncto sedabit aceto;
Ydropicos radix cum uino pota iuuabit;
Sic semen bibitum te, sacra Venus, renouabit.
Tradunt serpentem maratri iuuenescere gustu,
Non sanum minus esse seni comedendo uideri.

3.3 ANETVM

Sede sedens patria letum lasciuit anetum,
Semine nata patris semenque datura paternum
Progenies ut progenie renouata nouetur

18 rute] ritte *P* 19 si iungitur] subiungitur *S* 20 pacientes *S* peruncti] permitti *S* 21 periment *S* 22 iecorisque] iecoris *S* 23 nutrici] *scripsi*, nutriti *S* : marieti (?) *P* 24 dolores *S* 25 hoc *om. S* 26 radicum . . . sumpta *om. S* 27 morbus *S* tribuetur *S* 30 urinas] uestras *S* soluit] sedat *P* 31 petten *P* 32 tysana *S* 34 fomente *P* nimios quos] niueos quo *S* 35 at *S* oleo] oculo *S* 36 ita *S* 37 ait *S* iuncta *P* 38 pota] iuncta *P* 40 maratri] mater *S* 41 non sanum] hocque senen (?) *S* seni] senem *S*

3.3 ANETVM *P* 17r–18r: Anetum | *S* 39r–40r: De Aneto. Henricus
1 sede] fede *S* lectum *S* 2 paternum] patum *S* 3 ut] aut *P* nouetur] medetur *P*

but better still if Fennel juice is blended in equal measure
with juice of Rue, a rooster's bile, and honey too,
and then the patient's eyes are often treated with this ointment.
When poured into the ears the juice kills worms for you;
with wine the root is good for health of lung and liver,
and in such a way an abundance of milk is given to a nurse.
The seeds, when drunk with wine, are apt to soothe a pain
in the side, and taking a decoction of the herb does this as well.
A decoction of the roots, when taken with water or with wine,
is prescribed for diseases of the bladder and for nephritics.
Nausea is settled by this herb, when taken with wine;
a burning of the stomach can be alleviated by it, taken with water.
A potion of *maratrum* releases urine or menstrual courses,
or if it's merely ground and tied upon the pubic region.
This root, when cooked in barley water, will benefit the kidneys,
and boiled down in wine, used in a compress, it can reduce
excessive pains which the manly rod brings forth,
or if you mix it well with oil and rub it on the rod.
  It will give these things to parts, but for the whole,
when applied and mixed with vinegar it will soothe tumours or stings;
the root, when drunk with wine, will help the dropsical;
the seed, when drunk like this, will refresh you, holy Venus.
They say a serpent grows young again by the taste of Fennel
and that it seems to be no less healthy for an old man to eat.

3.3 Dill, *Peucedanum graveolens* Benth.

Cheerful Dill makes sport while sitting in his father's seat,
a progeny now born from father's seed and ready to produce
a fatherly seed to be made anew by progeny renewed

3.3 ANETVM / **Dill** *Macer, 'Anethum',* 395–428
1–22 *Cf.* Claudian, *De raptu Proserpinae* 1.248–51; Boethius, *De cons. phil.* 3 met. 9

(Atque aliquis frustra radici ficus aneti).
Forte sequens annus madido si profluat austro
Pende feniculum dum pendere tendet anetum;
Has facie similes similis natura creauit,
Semen dissimile quas dissimiles reserabit.
Te, nisi credideris, reddent exempla fidelem:
Sic fiunt fluuii nebule, nebule quoque nubes,
Hocque modo nubes nix fiunt nixque lapillus.
Ex yle fiunt elementa, sed ex elementis
Sunt elementata. Licet hec et retro reflectas,
Et genus in speciem, species in subteriora
Pertransire uides et retransire. Patescit
Cognita uis lippis: homo semen, auis fuit ouum,
Postmodo puluis erunt. Sic mutant quelibet esse.
Ceruinum cornu tritum quasi semina sparge:
Hinc apium surgit; dans ozyma densius equo
Telluri coeat micas horretque probatas.
Frumenti granum fieri lolium doluerunt
Cultores sed et hoc conuerti non doluerunt.
Hactenus hec. Calidum siccumque probatur anetum;
Scribitur esse gradus huic ex utroque secundus.
Hec oculis prodest et obest nam tollit eorum
Feruores contrita prius coniunctaque radix;
Sepius adbibitum nocet illis et genitale
Tollit iter, siccans humorem seminis intus.
Flos oleo coctus medicabile reddit anetum
Tam capitis morbo quam natis frigore causis;
Tensuras mollit neruorum, frigora tollit
Vuaque si crudo turgens humore grauetur,
Puluis conbusti suspendit seminis uuam,
Radicumque cinis (qui creditur acrior esse).
Sueuit habundanter dare lac decoccio sumpta
Quod, ciatos eius tepide tres si bibat eger,
Sic stomachi uarios poterit depellere morbos,
Cuius ad indicium ructus demonstrat apertum

4 atque] at *P* ficus] fiscus *P* 5 si profluat] superfluat *P* 6 feniculi *S* pendere tendet] carpere tendit *S* 7 has] hac *S* similis] simul *S* 8 reseranda *S* 12 ile *S* 13 elementa *S* reflectes *P* 15 patescunt *P* 16 uis] ius *S* semine *S* 17 postmodum *S* 18 ceruiccum *S* tectum *S* semine *P* 19 ozyma] oxima *S* 20 creat *S* micas] urticas *S* 21 locum *S* 23 actenus *S* 24 utraque *S* 27 adhibitum *P* 29 aneti *P* 31 tollit] pellit *P* 34 radicumue cisum *S* 36 sciatos *S* 38 demonstrat *corr. e* deptmonstrat *P*

(and someone would in vain plant figs for dill root!).
Perhaps if, in the following year, a wind blows from the balmy south,
fennel will hang while dill is preparing to hang;
a similar nature created these similar in appearance,
and a dissimilar seed will reveal them to be dissimilar.
Examples will make you a believer, if you don't believe.
In such a way do streams turn into mists, and mists to clouds,
and in this manner clouds turn into snow and snow to hail.
From primal matter elements are made, but from the elements come
the 'elementated.' Granted, you may turn these things back again:
you'll see genus transform into species, species into lower classes,
and then pass right back again. A power known even
to the half-blind grows clear: man was a seed, a bird was an egg,
afterwards they will be dust. Thus all things change their essence.
Scatter powdered deer's horn as if it were seed:
from this Celery grows; Basil, growing more thickly than proper,
breeds on the ground and shudders at the specks produced.
The farmers lament that wheat seed turned into Cockle
but they do not lament that Cockle has turned back again.
Enough of this. Dill is proven to be hot and dry;
its degree is said to be second in either of these.
It both benefits and harms the eyes, for the root,
first ground and applied, takes away their heat.
If drunk too often it harms the eyes and destroys the genital path,
drying the moisture of semen from within.
The flower cooked in oil makes Dill into a medicine
both for a head disease and for problems born from cold;
it soothes pulled tendons, removes your chills,
and if a swollen uvula is burdened by a bloody humour,
the powder of the burnt seed lifts the uvula,
as do ashes of the root, which is believed to be more powerful.
Taken as a decoction, it's been apt to give milk in abundance
and, if a sick man drinks three teaspoons of it warm,
it thus could conquer various diseases of the stomach.
As proof of this, belching reveals that the stomach's mouth

12–13 William of Conches, *De philosophia mundi* 22 (PL 172: 49); Bernardus Silvestris, *Cosmographia*, Megacosmus 4. 7 (ed. Dronke, 118) 16 Horace, *Satires* 1. 7. 3 17 *Cf.* Henry of Huntingdon, *HA* 11. 23, 39–40 (p. 800)

Os stomachi simul et uentum cessisse nociuum;
Hoc eciam potu sedari nausea scitur.
Singultus assum feruens quoque semen aneti
Olfactu cohibet si sepius olfacit eger.
Cum tepida tritum si quis potarit anetum
Intestinorum uentrisque doloribus obstat
Hocque frequentanti digestio crebrior extat.
Vrinę potu, matrici fit bona fotu
Coccio radicis. Membri curare uirilis
Vulnera posse cinis infusus creditur illis.
Apponas emorroydis medicabile semen
Sed prius hoc uras; hinc condilomata soluas.
Preterea cinis extantes in uulnere carnes
Radicis rodit, serpencia uulnera tollit.

3.4 FEBRIFVGA

Febrifugam delere febrem quis nominis huius
Nesciat auditor? Quis magni nesciat illud
Nominis (et merito) quod febres delet acerbas?
At dubitant, nec enim medici nunquam dubitarunt,
Quo sit in antiquis hec nomine consita libris,
Cum centhauree speciem quidam fateantur
Maiorem quidamque negent—sub iudice lis est;
Hanc arthemisiam cum quidam confiteantur
Eptaphilos aliique negent—sub iudice lis est;
Cum sint qui proprio uel horum nomine dictam

39 ceciuisse nocumen *S*   43 portarit *P*   45 hecque *P*   frequentati *S*   astat *S*   46 fit *corr. e* sit *P*   fotu] potu *S*   47 radicum *S*   49 emoroydis *S*   50 condilemata solues *P*   51 in uulnere] *scripsi*, inuoluere *P* : in uulnera *S*   52 radicum *S*   serpenticia *S*

3.4 FEBRIFVGA   *P* 18r: Febrifuga | *S* 63r: De Febrifuga, Henricus | *T* 96r–96v: Febrifuga

Exceptiones (*O* 92v): Febrefugia eo quod febrem fuget dicta est. Hanc quidam centauream maiorem uocant, quidam uero artemesiam, eptaphilos.

1 nominum *P*   eius *T*   2 magni] quis *add. et exp. S*   3 meriti *S*   acerbos *S* 4 at] an *S* : hinc *T*   enim *om. S*   nunquam *om. T*   5 que *T*   consita] tonsito *P* : conscita *T*   libris *corr. e* libros *P*   6 centauree *S* : centaure *T*   8 artemisiam *P* : arthemesiam *T*   9 heptafilos *P* : ethaphilos *T*   10 cum sint] et sunt *T*   uel] uero *S* : non *T*   dicam *S*

has opened at the same time that the harmful wind has ceased;
nausea is also known to be settled by this drink.
Hot seed of Dill, when roasted, also restrains hiccoughs
by its smell if the patient often sniffs it.
If someone should drink Dill ground with warm water,
he may stop pains of the intestines and the belly
and by using this frequently a swifter digestion is created.
A decoction of the root in a drink is good for urine, and in a wash
becomes good for the womb. The ash is believed to cure
wounds of the male member if poured over them.
Apply this medicating seed to haemorrhoids,
but burn it first, and with this you will dissolve the boils.
The ashes of the root, moreover, gnaw flesh away that's
sticking in a wound, and takes away serpents bites.

3.4 Feverfew, *Chrysanthemum parthenium* Bernh.

Who doesn't know, when hearing its name, that Feverfew
fights fevers? Who doesn't know it has a famous name
(and rightly so) because it foils fierce fevers?
But doctors are in doubt (for they've never not had doubt!)
by what name it should be found in ancient books,
since some claim it is a larger type of Centaury
and some deny (the case is still in court);
since some reply that this is the Artemisia
heptaphilos and some deny (the case is still in court);
since there are some who assert it's called by its own name

3.4 FEBRIFVGA / **Feverfew** *Source unknown*
7, 9, 11, 13 Horace, *Ars poetica* 78

Confirment, sunt qui renuant—sub iudice lis est,
Vtque sit ingenium lectoris acucius et sic
Quod querat dubitans et adhuc sub iudice lis est.

3.5 NIMPHEA

Quinta libro detur que morbis mille medetur.
Quippe datur quinto, notissima nomine, lecto,
Nomine quod taceo quod 'millemorbia' uersus
Si non horreret, nec nostra Talia taceret.
Nomine nunc opus est alio. Species solet ergo
Nimphee dici. Vulgus 'fyalam' quoque dicit.
Quantum conferba plagis hec preualet herba
Inque modo rute dat ocellis lumen acute,
Nec plus diuinam fera gutta cauet leporinam
Nec magis urget ea gelidum uirus basilisca,
Proficit et mire! Sed quid temptem numerare
Cum numero careant uires tam nobilis herbe?

3.6 ASARVM

En, habitans paucis asarum consurgit in ortis
Quod, cum sit rarum, sit tanto magis michi carum.
Feruet et exsiccat—gradus illi tercius extat;

11 cor firment *P* : confirmant *T* sunt] sicut *S* 12 accucius *P* et] hec *S* sic] sit *PS*

3.5 NIMPHEA *P* 18r–18v: Nimphea | *S* 63r–63v: De Febrifugo. Henricus (*incorrectly repeated from 3.4*)

Exceptiones (*O* 92r): Millemorbia species solet nimphee dici a uulgo fiola. Plagis preualet ut conferba, lumen acuit ut ruta, guttam extinguit ut leporina, uirus urget ut basilea.

1 quanta *S* misse *S* 3 millemorbea *S* 4 si] et *S* nostram *P* 6 nymphee *P* fiolam *S* 8 lumine *S* 9 nec . . . leporinam / nec . . . basilisca *om. S* 11 sed] *scripsi*, si *PS* tempten *S* 12 cum] dum *P* careant] creauit *P*

3.6 ASARVM *P* 18v–19r: Asarum | *S* 44v–45r: De Asaro. Henricus

1 en habitans] inhabitans *S* 2 fit tantum *S* caris *P*

or by theirs, and some who deny (the case is still in court).
And like the reader's wit, this may be rather sharp, and so
because the doubter asks, the case is even still in court.

3.5 Figwort, *Scrophularia nodosa* Pursh.

Let the fifth herb in the book appear which cures a thousand ills.
To be sure, it's found in the fifth bed, very well known in name,
a name which I keep silent because if poetry does not dread
millemorbia, our Thalia would not keep silent.
Now we need another name. Therefore it is accustomed
to be called a variety of Figwort, and commoners call it *fiala*.
This herb prevails over wounds as well as Comfrey,
and in the manner of sharp Rue grants vision to the eyes.
Neither does harsh gout fear divine Hare's Ear more,
nor does Gentian expel a chilling poison more than this,
and this is wonderfully effective! But why should I attempt to count,
when the powers of so noble an herb are numberless?

3.6 Hazelwort/Asarabacca, *Asarum europaeum* L.

Look here! The Hazelwort which lives in few gardens
springs up, and since it's rare, it's so much dearer to me.
It heats and dries: its grade stands out as third;

3.5 NIMPHEA / **Figwort** *Source unknown*
8 *Cf.* Ovid, *Remedia amoris* 801–802

3.6 ASARVM / **Hazelwort** *Macer, 'Asarum,' 1532–68*

A medicis asarum, uulgo 'uulgago' uocatur.
Prouocat urinam stipatam flecmate grosso,
Yctericos sed et ydropicos, sciasim quoque sanat.
Pota eciam iecori fit certa medela dolenti;
Menstrua pota uocat, uuluas decoccio sanat,
Et uomitu uelud elleborum precordia purgat.
  Quomodo detur habes; egri circumspice primum
Etatem, corpus, uires, tempus, regionem:
Etatem, plus namque decet iuuenique uiroque
Atque minus senibus puerisque dari medicine;
Corpus, nam duris et pinguibus est tribuenda
Amplius ac teneris multo minus et macilentis;
Vires, nam ualidis multo magis attribuatur,
Debilior sic debilibus medicina medetur;
Tempus, namque diem calidam uult pocio talis
Sicque serena dies uentisque carens relucescat.
Si regio presens sit frigida plus dabis illi
Quam si sit feruens; sic hanc, sic quamlibet herbam,
Des que dat uomitum. Communiter omnibus ista,
Nunc asaro proprie tribuam documenta medele:
De foliis eius sumes triginta recentis,
Nocte mero forti facias tota macerari,
Quo macerata mero sunt mane terendo resolue.
Tunc olus excoctum cum porci carne recenti
Da prius egroto satis et uini satis albi—
Hoc uulgago modo tandem potetur ab egro.
Sufficit hic numerus foliorum fortibus; ipsum
Comminues ut uis, etas et tempora poscunt.

5 flemmate *S* 6 et *om. S* 9 uomitum *P* elloborum *S* 11 religionem *S* 13 dari] decet *P* 14 tribuendis *S* 15 ac] at *S* 16 attribuetur *P* 17 sit *S* 19 uentrisqus carnes renitescat *S* 20 si] sic *P* 21 quaslibet herbas *P* 22 dat] dant *P* comuniter *S* 25 mero] uino *P* facies *S* 26 mero] uino *P* 27 holus *S* recentis *S* 29 uulgato *S*

it is called *asarum* by physicians and *vulgago* by the vulgar.
It calls forth urine blocked up by heavy phlegm,
but also heals the jaundiced, dropsical, and sciatica as well.
When drunk it also becomes a sure remedy for an aching liver;
a decoction, drunk, brings out menses and it cleans the womb;
it purges the diaphragm through vomit just like Hellebore.
You know how it is given; examine first the patient's
age and body and strength, the weather, and the region:
age, for it is more suitably given as a medicine to a youth
and a man and less so to the elderly and to boys;
body, for more must be given to the tough and fat
and much less to the tender and the lean;
strength, for it is prescribed much more for the powerful,
and so a weaker medicine is a cure for the weaker;
weather, for a potion like this demands a warm day,
so let the day shine out, calm and free of wind.
If your present region is cold, give more to him
than if it were warm; in such a way should you give this
or any herb which causes vomiting. These rules are common to all,
so now I'll give healing instructions specific to Hazelwort:
take thirty of the leaves of the herb when fresh,
steep them all at night in strong, unwatered wine, and blend them
in the morning by grinding with the wine in which they're boiled.
Then give it first to the invalid as a vegetable
cooked with enough fresh pork and enough white wine;
in such a manner should the patient at last drink Hazelwort.
This number of leaves is good for the strong;
diminish it as strength, age, and weather demand.

3.7 MACEDONIA

Inter odoratam uelox Macedonia siluam
Spargitur, infirmis et densa patescit aristis.
Diues, opum nec auara tamen, dare sufficit omni
Expellitque famem, facilis spernitque laborem
Nam per se crescit olerisque modo datur escis.
Hec ab Alexandro nomen quoque nobile traxit.
Corpore diffusas restringere sanguinis undas
Non acri, non difficili, solet uncia gustu.
Hinc, tibi dampnoso si uenter forte dolore
Conturbetur, opem poscas; opus ipse stupescas
Si fomenta super caua uentris cocta repones,
Ramos puleii frondesque papaueris addes.

3.8 YRIS

Flos equatur yris celestis honoribus Yris
Nam uariatur yris flos ut uarius color Yris.
'Ylliricam' quod in Illiria nascatur eandem
Dicunt at gladii nomen de nomine nostri
Extraxere sue rimati signa figure.
Siccat et accendit—gradus est in utroque secundus;
Maior uis huius radici fertur inesse.
Hanc si desicces, per frusta rotunda secato
Siccaque sic ne se contingant: insere filo,

3.7 MACEDONIA *P* 19r: [no title] | *S* 68v–69r: De Macedonia. Henricus

Exceptiones (*O* 92r): Macedonia, id est Alexandria, a plebe ut olus comeditur. Sola sanguinis fluxum restringit. Si ea iuncta puleio et papaueris frondibus uentrem foueas, omnem eius dolorem amputabis.

2 spergitur *S* et] *om. et add. et exp.* nec auara tamen *P* 5 olerique *S* 8 non[1]] namque *P* unica *P* 9 hinc] hic *S* uenter] *scripsi*, uenerit *P* : uentris *S* forte] et aula (?) *S* 10 conturbatur *P* poscat *P* stupescas] reponens *P* (*exp. et add.* stupescas *s. l.*) 11 uentris] mentis *S* cocta] tecta *S* repones] *scripsi*, reponens *PS* 12 addas *P*

3.8 YRIS *P* 19r–19v: Yris | *S* 104r–104v: De Yri. Henricus

1 celestibus *S* 3 Illiria] yllirita *S* 4 at gladii] ad glandis *P* 5 extraxisse *S* rimati signa] sub mota figura *P* 6 secunda *P* 8 si] ut *S* frusta] *scripsi*, frustra *PS* 9 contingat *P*

3.7 Alexanders/Black Lovage, *Smyrnium olusatrum* L.

Swift Alexanders is scattered through the perfumed wood
and opens widely, packed with fragile pods.
Rich, yet not jealous of its wealth, it is good to give to all
and it drives out hunger; easy to cultivate, it despises labour,
for it grows on its own and is given like a vegetable for food.
It also has taken its noble name from Alexander.
An ounce of it can restrain effusions of the blood which pour
from the body, with a taste neither bitter nor difficult.
If perchance your stomach is disturbed by a harmful pain,
ask the aid of this; you yourself will marvel at the effect
if you place it cooked, as a compress, on hollows of the stomach,
and add branches of Pennyroyal and Poppy leaves.

3.8 Iris, *Iris pseudacorus* L.

The flower Iris is equal to the heavenly honours of the rainbow
for the flower Iris varies like the varied colour of the rainbow.
They call this plant *Illyrica* for it is born in Illyria
but they have also taken its name from the name
of a *gladius*, examining the aspects of its shape.
It dries and it heats—the grade for each is second;
its greater power is said to be within the root.
If you want to dry this, cut it in round pieces, and dry them out
so they do not touch each other: insert them on a string

3.7 MACEDONIA / **Alexanders** *Strabo, 'De Cerfolio', 235–47*
1 Strabo, 'De Lybistico', 229

3.8 YRIS / **Iris** *Macer, 'Iris', 1456–88*
3 Isidore, *Etym.* 17.9.9–10   4–5 Strabo 217–18; *cf.* Isidore, *Etym.* 17.9.83

Sicco inserta loco suspendantur sed in umbra,
Sic suspensa potes (aliter siccare nequibis).
Hec sompnum dant cum uino, tussim quoque sedant.
Puluere cum uino sumpto precordia ledens
Egreditur sanies; cum mulsa puluere sumpto
Eicies coleras; puluis coniunctus aceto
Tormina sedabit; sic sumpta uenena fugabit.
Idem cum uino sumptus prodesse probatur
Spleni, contractis uel quouis frigore lesis.
Idem cum uino tardancia menstrua purgat
Radicumque steras mollit decoccio duras.
Hec cum clysterio si diffundatur in anum
Optima fit sciasis (nisi fallunt scripta) dolori.
De radicibus hiis tibi mixto melle probabis
Vnguen quod seuas trahit expellitque secundas.
'Hee quid sunt?' Dicam. Matris uescitur in aluo
Pellicula puer; hanc rumpit nascens genitumque
Hec quasi sit partus sequitur festina secundus,
Que nisi festinet uel mors festina subintrat
Vel dolor inmodicus quem coccio dicta repellit.
Ipsa locis infixa cauis syringia curat,
At puluis melli sociatus uulnera siccat
Carneque si fuerint sine carnibus ossa replebit.
Radicum puluis duplus coniungitur harum
Necnon ellebori, pars cocto tercia melli,
Quo uultus papulas ualido cataplasmate pellas,
Quo careat cultus feda lentigine uultus.

10 incerta *S* suspendatur *P* 11 nequibit *P* 12 somnum dat *P* cum] in *S* uino] sed *add. et exp. P* sedat *P* 16 uenera *P* 18 contritis *P* frigdore *P* 19 tardancia *corr. e* tradancia *P* 20 radicisque *P* 21 hec] hoc *S* clysterio] disterio *S* diffundantur *P* 22 fit] sunt *P* fallant *P* 23 potabis *S* 25 sint *S* 29 quam *S* 30 siringia *S* curat] purgat *S* 32 repellit *P* 33 radicis *P* 34 ellibori *S* cocto] toto *S* 35 cathaplasmate *P*

and let them hang, inserted, in an arid place, but in the shade,
and drink it when hung up like this (you cannot dry it otherwise).
These pieces with wine grant sleep and settle a cough.
By means of its powder, drunk in wine, harmful bloody matter
departs the diaphragm; by the powder drunk in mead
you will expel bile; the powder mixed with vinegar
will settle gripes, and thus it will chase off swallowed poisons.
The same thing taken in wine is proven to benefit
the spleen and sprains, or injuries from any chill.
The same, in wine, purges tardy menstrual courses
and a decoction of the roots softens a hardened cervix.
If this is injected into the anus with a clyster
it's excellent for sciatic pain, unless the writings lie.
Prepare for yourself an ointment, mixed with honey,
from these roots, which draws out and expels harsh afterbirths.
'What are they?' I will say: a child is nourished on a thin skin
in the belly of the mother; it breaks this while being born, and the skin
quickly follows the begotten child as if it were an 'after-birth.'
If it does not come out quickly, either hasty death or serious pain
creeps in, which the aforesaid decoction repels.
Applied to hollow places, this cures fistulae,
but its powder, mixed with honey, dries out wounds and will fill
them up with flesh, if the bones should be lacking flesh.
Two parts of the powder of these roots are also mixed
with Hellebore, and a third part with boiled honey,
and by this strong poultice you'll banish pimples from the face,
and a face, when treated with this, may escape the vile spots.

3.9 YREOS

Sunt yreos et yris similes ut nomine, uultu,
Vt tyma et tyme similes ut nomine, gustu.
A medicis yreos et yris uirtute uidentur
Consimiles et dissimiles paulisper habentur.
Rarior est et carior est postrema priore,
Gracior est et latior est maiorque nitore.

3.10 MENTA

Sic quoque menta gradu feruet siccatque secundo.
Instillata ualet cum melle doloribus auris;
Lingua dolens illa curatur sepe fricata
Raucisonamque solet uocem rehibere canori.
Addere lac mammis superaddita tritaque sueuit,
Roborat et stomachum, uomitum quoque comprimit hausta.
Hac eciam pota digestio tarda iuuatur;
Hac et lumbrici stomacho fugiunt inimici
Ac super hec morbos curabit testiculorum
Si foueantur aqua qua cocta prius fuit herba,
Ac emoptoycis iuncto succurrit aceto.
Trita canis morsus, superaddita cum sale, sanat
Potaque cum sapa partum solet accelerare.
Si mente succus matrici subditur ante
Quam coeat, mulier coeat satis, haud paritura.
Caseolos succus prohibet putrescere mente
Vel si mixtus uel uiridis superadditur herba.

3.9 YREOS *P* 19v: Yreos | *S* 105v: De Yreos. Henricus

Exceptiones (*O* 92r): Yreos et yris sunt consimiles ut thima et thime, nisi quod rarior et carior est postrema priore, gratior et [que] latior est maiorque nitore.

1 uoltu *P* 2 tyme] tymum *S* 3 yreos et yris] et iris yreos *P* uidentur *corr. e* medentur *P*

3.10 MENTA *P* 19v–20r: Menta | *S* 70r–70v: De Menta. Henricus

1 sic] cic *S* quoque] et *add. S* 4 raucisonam] auri suam (?) *corr. ex* aurisonam *P* rehibere] cohibere *P* conari *S* 5 addere] reddere *S* trita *S* 6 compremit *P* 7 eciam pota] quoque potata *P* 8 hanc *S* stomachi *P* inimici *corr. ex* inimuci *P* 9 ac] at *S* hoc *S* curabis *P* 11 ac] at *S* iuncto] *scripsi*, iuncte *P* : uinco *S* 12 sanat] purgat *P* 13 solet accelerare] festinat anelum *S* 15 haud] *scripsi*, hanc *PS* 17 si *om. S* uel²] si *add. P*

3.9 Yreos (fictional plant) or *Iris florentina* L.

Yreos and Iris are as alike in name and appearance
as garden Thyme and wild Thyme are alike in name and taste.
Yreos and Iris seem to doctors to be similar in virtue
and are considered only slightly different.
The latter is rarer and dearer than the former,
and it is more beautiful, larger and stronger in odour.

3.10 Mint, genus *Mentha* L.

So Mint also heats and dries in the second degree.
When dripped in with honey, it's good for earaches;
an aching tongue is cured if often rubbed with this
and it is apt to restore a hoarse voice into song.
When ground and applied it can add milk to breasts,
it strengthens the stomach, and when drunk it represses vomit.
Slow digestion is also aided by this when drunk;
wicked worms flee the stomach with this herb
and, moreover, it will cure diseases of the testicles if they
are washed with the water in which the herb was first cooked;
when blended with vinegar it brings aid to spitters of blood.
Ground and applied with salt it cleans dog bites
and drunk with wine must it is apt to speed up birth.
If Mint juice is taken as a suppository to the womb before sex,
a woman may have sex to satisfaction and won't conceive.
The juice of Mint prevents cheeses from putrefying
either when mixed in or if the green herb is applied on top.

3.9 YREOS / **'Yreos'** *Source unknown*

3.10 MENTA / **Mint** *Macer, 'Mentha', 1569–84*
4 Strabo 287

3.11 ABSINTHIVM

Absinthii ingentis uis feruida siccaque fertur:
Primum prima gradum tenet atque secunda secundum.
Plinius immensis hanc effert laudibus auctor,
Scribens temporibus Romanos rite statutis
Absinthii succum solitos donasse bibendum
Victori claro uictrici sede locato
Quam quadrigarum currus sublimus habebat.
Cuius erat precium, seruatrix herba, salutis
Que constat precio preciosior omnibus una.
Hec igitur claros oculos cum melle parabit
Liuoremque fugat qui luminis obsidet orbem.
Hec auris cum felle bouis sonitum remouebit;
Liberat obstrusas cocte uapor unicus aures;
Hiis tumidis sanie cum melle terens superadde;
Sic quoque sub lingua poteris curare tumorem.
Subdita dat sompnum capiti, dat sompnum odore
Herbam supponi si non presenciat eger.
Cerotis mixtus nigros reddet cinis eius
Crines si ceruix sit eo non raro perunct a.
Destruit anginam cum nitro melleque iuncta.
Huic iungatur yris: sic pectora lesa iuuabit.
Vt bene curet epar societur Gallica nardus
Quoque modo prodest stomacho, melius tamen isto
Si fuerit pluuie claro decocta liquore
Et sic aerio frigidata, bibatur, aperto;
Sic stomacho gratissima fit, sic temperat aluum;
Pellit lumbricos, delet cum gramine morbos,
Sic dolor inmodicus sedatur—crede probatis!

3.11 ABSINTHIVM *P* 20r–20v: Absinthium | *S* 35v–36r: [no title]

2 atque] ergo *P* 3 autor *P* 4 romanos *corr. e* romauos *S* statutis *corr. e* statutos *S* 5 succum solitos *transp. P* solitos] *scripsi*, solito *PS* 6 uictrici] *add.* sullimia habebat *et exp. S* 7 cursu *S* sublimus] sullimia *corr. e* sullima *S* 8 cuius] quid *S* 9 que] quod *S* precio] preciis *S* 10 hec igitur] hanc ergo *S* 11 liuoremque] humoremque *S* 12 hec] hoc *S* cum] melle *add. S* 12 sonuritum *P* renouebit *S* 13 unicus] inusus *S* 14 hiis tumidis] hoc tumidus *S* 16 capiti *om. S* sompnum²] *scripsi*, sompnos *P* : *om. S* odorem *S* 17 egre *S* 18 mixtus *om. S* 19 raro] racio *S* 20 angina] *scripsi*, angwinam *corr. ex* anginam *P* : anguina *S* mixto felleque iunta *S* 21 huic] hunc *S* iris *P* pectore *S* iuuabit] mirabis *S* 22 curat *S* 23 stomacho] sint *S* ista *corr. ex* isto *P* 25 aerio] *scripsi*, aereo *P* : aerieo *S* frigidata] infrigidatur *S* 26 fit] sit *S* temperet *S* 28 sic] si *S* *ll.* 29–30 *om. P*

3.11 Wormwood, *Artemisia absinthium* L.

The power of mighty Wormwood is said to be hot and dry:
the first has the first degree and the second has the second.
The author Pliny extols this with mighty praise,
writing that the Romans, at properly established times,
were accustomed to give Wormwood juice to drink
to the famous winner seated in the victor's chair,
which used to be at the famous chariot course.
A protective herb, its value was in health which,
alone, is considered more valuable in price than anything.
Therefore with honey this will clear up the eyes
and chase off discolouration that besets the eyeball.
With cow's gall this will remove ringing in the ears;
the steam alone from this, when cooked, clears obstructed ears.
Grind with honey and apply it to those swollen with bloody pus;
in such a way you can also cure a tumour under the tongue.
It gives sleep when placed beneath the head, and gives sleep
by its odour if the patient doesn't wish the herb to be placed beneath.
Its ash, when mixed in plasters of wax, turns hair
to black if the neck is not rarely rubbed with it.
It destroys tonsillitis when mixed with Soda and honey.
Add Iris to this, and thus it will help an injured chest.
So that it cures the liver well, let Gallic Nard be added
and in this manner it's good for the stomach,
yet better than that if it should be cooked down
in clear rainwater and drunk, chilled thus in the open air;
like this it's very pleasing for the stomach and soothes the bowels.
It forces out worms, destroys disease with its leaves,
and thus an excessive pain is settled. Believe these proven things!

3.11 ABSINTHIVM / **Wormwood** *Macer, 'Absinthium', 52–114*
3–9 *Cf.* Pliny 27.7

Amplius, herba recens oleo si forte coquatur
Sic eciam stomachum crebro iuuat unguine fotum.
Amplius, huic rutam coniungas salque piperque;
Hec contusa mero decoctaue des licet egro;
Sic stomachi crudus, sic noxius exiet humor.
Splen lesum sibi coniuncto sanabit aceto,
Splen durum mollit melli iunctum cataplasma.
In lini panno si circumcinxeris illam
Inguinis ingentem cohibet curatque tumorem.
Prouocat urinam, producit menstrua potu.
Huic igitur nardum, medicis quam Gallia profert,
Coniungas, coniuncta teras, contrita resoluas
Mulsa; precipue medici sic menstrua purgant,
Subdita uero steram desiccat, menstrua soluit.
  Partibus hec dat, et hec toti: contrita recentes
Plagas herba iuuat, pruritus coccio sanat,
Mel si coniungas sugillatis ualet herba.
Fungorum uirus coniuncta repellit aceto,
Destruit inuisam uino coniuncta cicutam
Sicque uenenatos morsus tibi quoslibet aufert.
Hanc apio soli dabis yctericis sociatam;
Huic siler et nardus et acetum consocientur,
Hec mala qui delere uolet fastidia potet.
Nausea uero maris illum uexare nequibit
Qui uino mixtam cautus presumpserit illam.
Efficit a tineis tutam qua ponitur archam.
Mutua, scriptor, habe: quo sit macerata resolues
Incaustum uino; sic mures scripta cauebunt.
Acri cum uino trita se quilibet ungens
Non metuet pulices musceque fugantur odore.

30 fotum] *scripsi*, focum *S*   31 huic] *scripsi*, hoc *P* : hic *S*   rutam] uictam *S*   32 mero] uino *P*   des] deus *S*   34 sanabis *P*   35 durum] dicuntur *S*   mollit] lenit *P*   cathaplasma *P*   36 circumcinxerit *S*   37 inguinis] iungimus *S*   curatque] dolorem *add. et exp. P*   timorem *S*   39 huic] hinc *S*   40 resoluas] recentes *S*   *ll. 41–43 om. S*   44 herba] erga *S*   46 si coniungas] sius iungas *S*   47 inuisa *P*   48 quolibet *S*   49 soli] cum *add. P*   ycticis sonatam *S*   53 presumserit *P*   55 scriptorum *S*   quo] que *P*   *ll. 57–58 om. S*

What's more, if the fresh herb is cooked, in oil perhaps,
it also helps the stomach which is rubbed frequently with this ointment.
What's more, add Rue and salt and Pepper to this;
you should give these, ground or cooked with unmixed wine, to the patient,
and thus a bloody and harmful humour of the stomach will depart.
It will heal an injured spleen when vinegar is added to it,
and, as a plaster mixed with honey, it softens a hardened spleen.
If you should bind it round with a linen cloth
it restrains and cures a great swelling of the groin.
In a drink, it calls forth urine and brings out menstrual courses.
Therefore mix with this the Nard which Gaul provides
physicians, grind it up once mixed, and dissolve in mead
once ground; in such a way especially do doctors purge menses,
but as a suppository it also dries the cervix and releases menses.
It gives those things for parts, and these things for the whole:
the ground herb aids recent wounds, a decoction heals itching,
and if you add honey, the herb is good for bruises.
When mixed with vinegar it repels the poison of mushrooms,
when mixed with wine it destroys the hated Hemlock,
and thus it takes away from you any poisonous bites.
Give this to the jaundiced when blended with only Celery;
let Sermountain and Nard and vinegar be mixed with it
and let him drink these who wishes to remove foul distaste.
In fact, seasickness won't be able to bother him
who shall have prudently taken this mixed in wine.
It renders a coffer in which it's placed secure from moths.
Hey, scribe, take my advice: compound an ink with wine
in which this herb was boiled, so mice will fear your writings.
Whoever anoints himself with this, ground up in vinegar,
will not fear fleas and flies will fly from its odour.

3.12 BALSAMA

Balsama scribantur multo lustrata decore;
Balsama scribantur grato dilecta sapore;
Balsama scribantur que precellant et odore.
Hoc et 'terralis' solet atque 'sisimbria' dici.
Hinc faciet succum procurator febrientum,
Cuius aqua scrupulos calida geminos det anhelis;
Quod si uesice dolor aut stranguria subsit,
Cum uino succum dabis et morbos releuabis.

3.13 RAPHANVS

Perdere uis cancrum? Sumas ranam religesque
Ad cancrum; totam cancer sic hauriet illam
Vt stupeas siccam uix pellem mane manere.
Qua dempta raphani radix urinaque uacce
Flosque siligineus cancri robur omne necabunt.
Vulnus sic sanes ut cetera uulnera sanas,
Quod facient caulis rubeus griasque rubescens
Quam 'uarenca' uocant. Canabum coniunge simulque
Yrigeron, qui senecion uocitatur, et herbam
Absinthii; herbarum quinque hec medicina uocatur.
At quoniam multas docui multasque docebo
Vulnera que sane purgant purgataque curant,

3.12 BALSAMA *P* 20v: Balsama | *S* 45v: De Balsamo. Henricus | *T* 91r: Balsama

Exceptiones (*O* 92r): Balsamum que et terralis et sisimbria dicitur, decore, sapore, odore grata. Hec pota febrem pellit. In aqua calida anhelis succurrit. In uino dolorem uesice et stranguiria curat.

1 balsamum scribatur *S* 2 grata *T* 3 precellantur *S* 4 hoc] hoc *corr. ex* hec *P* : hec *T* sysimbria *P* : simbria *T* 5 facit *S* succum] sinct' (?) *S* febricienti *P* : februlentum *T* 6 dat *PT* hanelis *ST* 7 aut] an *P* strangria *S* 8 succum *corr. e* succus *P* reuelabis *P*

3.13 RAPHANVS *P* 20v–21r: Rafanus | *S* 85r–86r: De Raphano. Henricus

1 summas *P* 2 cancer *om. P* illam] alam *S* 3 uix pellem] *lacuna et add.* est *S* 4 urinaque] firmaque *corr. ex* urinaque (?) *S* 5 necabunt] uexabunt *S* 6 sic] tunc *S* 7 girasque *S* 8 uarenca] uuarena *S* canabum] cauabunt *S* 9 qui *corr. e* quam *P* : que *S* herba *P* 10 quinque] .V. *P* hec *om. S* 11 at] *scripsi*, aut *PS* 12 sanie *P*

3.12 Horsemint, *Mentha longifolia* (L.) Huds.

Horsemint is described as illumined with great beauty;
Horsemint is described as beloved for its pleasing flavour;
Horsemint is described as excellent too in odour.
It is also apt to be called *terralis* and *sisimbria*.
Have a caretaker of the feverish make a juice from this,
and let him give two scruples of it in hot water to gaspers;
but if kidney pain or painful urination occur,
give the juice with wine and you'll relieve these vices.

3.13 Horseradish, *Armoracia rusticana* Gaertn. Mey & Scherb.

Do you want to remove a tumour? Take a frog and tie
it to the tumour; the tumour will drink up the whole frog so that
you'll marvel that just a dry skin remains in the morning.
After this is removed, a Horseradish root, the urine of a cow,
and the flower of wheat will kill all the tumour's strength.
You'll thus clean out a wound as you clean other wounds,
just as red Cabbage and the rose madder which
they call *varenca* will do. Add cannabis and also
yrigeron, which is called Groundsel, and the leaves
of Wormwood; this is called the Five-Herb Medicine.
  But since I've taught and will teach many herbs
which surely purge wounds and cure them once they're purged,

3.12 BALSAMA / **Horsemint** *Pseudo-Apuleius no. 106, 'Herba Sisimbrium' (p. 189)*

3.13 RAPHANVS / **Horseradish** *Source unknown*
1–3 *Cf.* Quintus Serenus 114, 668, 782, 912

Quaslibet aut dictas aut dicendas sociabis,
Hanc tamen eximiam facilemque uocant medicinam.
Si tamen hic queras, que sint prorsus pociores
Ad coniungendum curanti uulnera, dicam.
Gratis grata feram, precio preciosa carebunt.
Herbarum matrem sumas agrimoniamque;
Istis buglossam cum sanicla sociabis;
Sinula, terrestre piretrum iungantur et elna,
Nec plantago tibi deerit, nec lanceolata;
Querito fabiculam secus amnes atque ruuetam.
Ortus conferbam, portulacam dabit ortus,
Acidulam tibi prata, nemus piperam generabit;
Hiis 'uictoriolam' quam plebs uocat adde, sed equi
Omnia ponderis hec, canabum duplum simul atque
Herbam quam dicunt 'reginam' siue 'melandram'.
Hiis igitur iunctis duo, sed contraria, iunge
(Nam si forte uelis ut duret uulnus apertum)
Consolide minus omnibus hiis sed ponito done
Dimidium pondus respectu prepositarum.
At cito si sanare uelis, addens tibi tantum
Consolide quantum primarum, iunge parumper
Done. Sic igitur iunctas uinoque solutas
Frigentes de luce bibat sed nocte calentes.
Nil plage religes; potu sanabitur eger.
  Hic nullus dolor est, nullus timor, ergo beatum
Predico predictas qui nouit et agregat herbas.
Viginti solet herbarum hec medicina uocari.
Preterea raphanus quacientem uiscera tussim
Aut fugat aut mollit uentrisque animalia tollit.

13 dictas] discas *S*   14 exinimiam *P*   15 prorsus] pocius *S*   pociores *corr. e* poares (?) *S*   17 carebit *S*   20 peretrum *S*   21 lancealata *S*   22 querito] quod rite *S*   ampnes *P*   25 uictoriolam] nucerciolam (?) *P*   adde *om. S*   26 atque] aque *S*   31 prepositam *S*   36 potu] ponet *S*   37 hic dolor est nullus *P*   40 rafanus *S*

add what you will of those already described or still to come,
yet they call this an excellent and easy medicine.
But if you now ask, 'Which, in short, are the better herbs
for a physician binding wounds?,' I will say.
I'll bear pleasing things to the pleasing; the precious are priceless.
Gather the Mother of Herbs and agrimony,
then mix Ox-Tongue with these and Sanicle;
let Curled Mallow, Pellitory, and Elecampane be blended in,
nor should you lack the Greater and the Ribwort Plantain;
seek out the little bean found next to waters and brambles.
The garden will give Comfrey, the garden will give Purslane,
Sorrel the fields will produce for you, and Pimpernel the woods;
add to these the herb which the people call *victoriola*,
but an equal weight of all of these, and twice as much
of cannabis, as well as the herb they call *regina* or *melandra*.
So after these two, albeit contrary, things are mixed,
then mix (if perhaps you should wish the wound to remain open)
less of Comfrey than all the others and add half the weight
of *dona* with respect to the aforesaid herbs.
But if you wish to heal quickly, add as much of Comfrey
as of the first ingredients and mix in an equal amount
of *dona*. So let him drink these mixed like this and dissolved
in wine, chilling it in the day but heating it at night.
You'll leave no wound; the patient will be healed by this drink.
There is no sorrow here, no fear, and therefore I proclaim
him happy who knows and collects the aforesaid herbs.
This is usually called the Medicine of Twenty Herbs.
What's more, Horseradish chases off or soothes a cough
which shakes the insides and removes animals in the belly.

3.14 RADIX

Iure subest raphano que 'radix' dicitur herba:
Vim quoque consimilem gerit hec sed paulo minorem,
Consimilem gustu sed paulo debiliorem,
Hec tamen urine fertur preclara mouende.
Pectora confortat, corroborat interiora,
Vnde supradictam comedentes tempore Martis
Hiis aminiculis producunt tempora mortis.

3.15 ENVLA

'Enula, que tibi uis, quam uulgus nominat elnam?'
'Vis michi feruescens et uis michi contigit humens;
Primo prima gradu uiget atque secunda secundo.'
'Enula, quanta potes, nisi nulla potes, manifesta.'
'Puluis radicum prodest cum melle mearum
Inflatis aut ortomicis, tussique et anhelis,
Et meus et rute succus ruptis medicatur.
Nefreticos foliis cum uini nectare coctis
Et radice iuuo sciasim superaddita cruri.
Coccio uero mei stipatum commouet aluum;
Tam leuiter mouet urinam quam pellit abortum;
Menstrua tam leuiter purgat quam pectora sanat.'
'Turpe loquax mulier! Vates odere loquaces!'
'Cum non pauca queam, paucis contenta recedam.'

3.14 RADIX *P* 21r–21v: [no title] | *S* 86r: De Radice. Henricus

Exceptiones (*O* 92r): Radix herba raphano uritute et gustu consimilis, sed paulo debilior. Vrinam mouet, pectus confortat et interiora, unde et tempore Martii salubriter comeditur.

1 rafana *S* 2 quoque] que *S* gerit *bis P* hoc *S* paula *S* 3 consimilem] et similem *S* sed] super *S* paulo] parum *P* rebiliorem *S* 4 hec] hoc *S* 6 tempora *S*

3.15 ENVLA *P* 21v: Enula | *S* 60r–60v: De Enula campana. Henricus *Edited by Rigg, 270–71.*

1 uis] ius *S* 2 uis] ius *S* 3 atque *om. P* 4 potes²] potest *S* 6 inflatis aut ortomicis] inclatis diptonoicis *S* anelis *S* 7 meus] mens *S* 8 nefreticos] nec *cum lacuna S* 9 et radice] at *cum lacuna S* iuuo] uino *S* 10 uero mei] uel mel *S* commouet] mollitat *S* 13 loquax] loquar *P* uates] *Rigg*, nates *P* : uaces *S* odore *P* loquaces] loquacos *P* 14 queam] quedam *S* contenta] contempta *S*

3.14 Radish, *Raphanus sativus* L.

The herb called Radish rightly follows Horseradish:
it also bears a similar power, but lesser by a little,
a similar taste, but weaker by a little,
yet it is labelled excellent for the bringing out of urine.
It strengthens the chest, reinforces the insides,
so those who eat the aforesaid herb in the time of Mars
put off their time of death with these auxiliaries.

3.15 Elecampane, *Inula helenium* L.

'O Elecampane, whom the crowd calls *elna*, what is your power?'
'A heating power and a moistening power belong to me;
the first is strong in the first degree, the second in the second.'
'Elecampane, reveal how much you can do, unless you can do nothing.'
'The powder of my roots with honey is good for the bloated
and those with orthopnoea, for a cough and for gaspers,
and my juice and that of Rue are medicine for ruptures.
I help those with kidney disease by my leaves cooked in
nectar of the vine, and sciatica when my root's applied to the leg.
A decoction of me, in fact, clears constipated bowels;
it both moves urine gently and expels a foetus,
it purges menstrual courses as easily as it cleans the chest.'
'You foul-mouthed woman! Poets hate chatterboxes!'
'Although I can do no few things, I will depart content with a few.'

3.14 RADIX / **Radish** *Source unknown*
6 *Cf.* Claudian, *In Eutropium* 2. 567 (ed. Hall, 188)

3.15 ENVLA / **Elecampane** *Macer, 'Enula', 1489–1502*
13 *Cf.* Horace, *Satires* 1.9, 33–4

3.16 ALTEA

Alteam dixere patres quia frondibus alta est;
Alteam dixere simul quia uiribus alta est.
Fertur et 'euiscum' quia contrahitur quasi uisco
Radix, quod uulgus corrumpens dixit 'ybiscum.'
Hanc malue speciem quosdam dixisse recordor.
Hec prodest emoptoicis, lapidi quoque sumpta
Vesiceque ualet morbis pellitque secundas.
Coccio cum uino dissentericos releuabit.
Cocta prius radix porcino adipi quoque iuncta
Matrices reprimit tumidas sanatque dolentes;
Hoc eciam tepida confert decoccio fotu.
Flos mulsa coctus uel cum uino bene tritus
Fit scrophis, fit quassatis anoque salubris.
Hec et multa ualet; sic flos et uulnera purgat:
Vulnera cocta prius cum melleque trita replebit
Que caua sunt, si sepe tamen superadditur herba.
Mollit duricias sic deflectitque rigores.
Iuncta adipi radix fugat apostemata dura.
De foliis oleo coctis fiat cathaplasma
Vt sic pestiferos morsus conbustaque curet
Potaque cum pusca poterit delere uenena.
Forti cum uino solidatum semen oliuo
Leni coniunges maculasque salutifer ungues.

3.16 ALTEA *P* 21v–22r: Althea | *S* 37v–38r: De Altea. Henricus
1 quia] quod *P* 2 quia] quod *P* 4 ybiscum] ubiscum *P* 5 hanc] hac *S* dixere *P* 6 emptoysis *S* 7 uesiceque] uesice *S* morbus *S* 8 disintericos *S* 9 porcino *om. S* 10 tumudas sanabit *S* 11 hoc] hec *P* tepido *S* decoccio] *add.* flata *et. exp. P* focu *S* 13 scrosis *S* squassatis *S* 15 repellit *P* 18 apostema datur *S* 20 pectiferos *S* 21 potaque] pota *S* 23 coniungens *P* ungens *P*

3.16 Marsh Mallow, *Althaea officinalis* L.

The elders called this herb *altea* for the altitude of its leaves;
they also called it *altea* because it is ultimate in powers.
It's also called *eviscus* because the root is sticky as if
with viscous birdlime, but the corrupting crowd call it *hybiscus*.
I recall that some have said this is a type of Mallow.
It's beneficial for the jaundiced, and when eaten it's good
for the stone and bladder diseases, and forces out the afterbirth.
A decoction with wine will relieve the dysenteric.
The root, first cooked and mixed with pork fat,
relieves swollen and heals aching wombs;
the decoction also grants this in a heated compress.
The flower cooked in mead or ground well with wine
is salutary for scrofula, for bruises, and for the anus.
It does these and many things. The flower purges wounds like this:
when cooked first with honey, then ground, it will fill up wounds
which are hollow, but only if the herb is often applied.
It softens hardenings and thus prevents rigidity.
The root, when mixed with lard, keeps hard abscesses away.
Let a plaster be made of the leaves cooked in oil
so that like this it cures destructive bites and burns
and drunk with vinegar-water will be able to vanquish poisons.
You will add the seed, when fortified with strong wine,
to gentle olive oil and healthfully anoint blemishes with it.

3.16 ALTEA / **Marsh Mallow** *Macer, 'Althaea,' 366–94*

3.17 SINVLA

Huc illucque means, remeans quoque, sinula salue,
Nulli certa loco, species clarissima malue!
Hec, quod adest et abest ita quod corrupcio non fit
(Subiecti non signa patent) tellureque clausa
It, redit, intrat, abit, erratica malua uocatur.
Quicquid habent malue, prestat sed forcius ista,
Ergo canam quid malua queat: quia molliat aluum,
'Maluam' dixerunt et laudibus excoluerunt.
Vrina coctam capiti superaddito maluam;
Hec lauacro turpes acoras furfurque repellit.
Tranquillat dentes radix adiuncta dolentes.
Ipse cacostomacham Sextus Niger asserit illam
Atque Diascorides; tamen interioribus esse
Sumptam sicut olus confirmat uterque salubrem;
Sic et uesice testantur eam medicari.
Duriciasque steras mollit decoccio malue.
Intestina iuuat, matricem subdita curat
Et reddet sanum si tantum subditur anum.
Sumpta uenenosos ut olus reprimet tibi potus.
Dixit abortiuam Thebanus Olimpius ipsam
Anseris huic si detur adeps uulueque premantur.
Egylopas foliis expelles cum sale tritis.
Puncturis apium succus ualet eius oliuo;
<Decoctis eius foliis si iungis oliuum>
Deleri sacer ignis eo cataplasmate sueuit.
Illud idem combusturis bene subuenit ignis.
Affirmat Diascorides malue salicisque
Contritis foliis melius ciciusque cruentum
Vulnus curari quam coniunctis preciosis.

3.17 SINVLA *P* 22r: Sinula | *S* 94v–95r: De Sinula. Henricus
1 quoque] *scripsi*, que *PS* 2 carissime *P* 3 hec] hoc *S* et] uel *P* 5 it] id *S* erratura *P* 6 malue *om. S* prestat] *scripsi*, prestant *PS* sed] si *S* iste *S* 7 canan *S* 8 excoluerunt] hiis coluerunt *S* 9 urinam *S* 10 hec] hoc *S* achoras *P* repelles *S* 11 transquillat *S* 12 cachostomacham *P* 13 dyascorides *P* 15 testatur *P* meditari *S* 16 steras] *scripsi*, stera *P* : stere *S* 18 tantum] tamen *S* 19 repremit *P* 21 huic] hoc *P* uulueque] *scripsi*, wuluaque *P* : uuluaque *S* premantur] sequuntur *S* 23 apum *P* oliuo] *scripsi*, olyuum *P* : oliuum *S* 24 decoctis . . . iungis] *conieci* (*cf. Macer 1987*), *om. PS* 25 cathaplasmate *P* 27 dyascorides *P*

3.17 Mallow:
1) Curled Mallow, *Malva verticillata* L.
2) High Mallow, *Malva sylvestris* L.

Hail, Curled Mallow, travelling hither and thither, and returning,
fixed in no sure position, the most famous species of Mallow!
Because this herb comes and goes so that no corruption occurs
(signs do not appear on the patient) and moves close to the earth,
returns and enters and exits, it is called the Curled Mallow.
Whatever Mallows have, this one offers it, but stronger still,
so I'll sing what Mallow does: because it mollifies the bowels,
they called it Mallow and have honoured it with praises.
Apply Mallow cooked in urine to the head:
this, as a wash, repels foul ulcers and scaly skin.
The root, when applied, becalms aching teeth.
Sextus Niger himself, and also Dioscorides, assert
that it's upsetting to the stomach; yet each confirms that,
when eaten as a vegetable, it's healthful for the insides;
they also state that in such a way it cures the bladder.
A decoction of Mallow softens hardenings and the cervix.
As a suppository it cures the womb, aids intestines,
and makes the anus healthy if inserted alone.
When eaten as a vegetable it will stop poisonous drinks for you.
Olympius the Theban called it abortifacient
if goose grease is added to it and pressed upon the womb.
You'll banish tear-duct tumours with the leaves ground with salt.
Its juice with olive oil is good for bee stings;
<if you mix olive oil with its boiled leaves,>
by this plaster Holy Fire is apt to be destroyed.
The same thing rightly helps burns from a fire.
Dioscorides affirms that a gory wound is cured more properly
and more quickly by the crushed leaves of Mallow and willow
than with the addition of expensive ingredients.

3.17 SINVLA / **Mallow** *Macer, 'Malva',* 1962–92
7–8 *Cf.* Isidore, *Etym.* 17. 10. 5

Auctores perhibent alii quod malua potenter
Conquassata iuuet adipi commixta uetusto.
Omnia malua potest et sinula forcius ista.

3.18 PIRETRVM

Sinula si nulla superari creditur herba
Preter terrestre piretrum (quod et Anglia diues
Esse problema refert) rem tollere quomodo tantam
Arida sufficiat ieiune formula Muse?
Hec quoniam piretro similem dat mansa saporem
Inque gradu quarto similem dat sicca calorem,
Nomina pro meritis speciosa tenet speciei.
Vix species melior, sed tantum rarior herba est,
Nam quecumque facit species, facit herba. Canamus
Ergo quid piretrum faciat: si frigidus humor
Excruciet dentes, hoc masticet oreque uoluat
Aut gargarizet mixto qui languet aceto;
Sic et sedabit tumefactam flecmate linguam,
Sic uue prodest humoris pondere presse,
Sic eciam multis medicaminibus ualet oris.
Ex oleo quo decoquitur renes superunge,
Hoc iuuat: ante febris motum corpus superunges.
Hoc iuuat: hinc sudor si uis ut perfluat unges.
Hoc iuuat: ungatur paraliticus unguine tali.
Hoc iuuat, ungantur si membra stupencia sepe;
Hoc iuuat, ungantur si frigescentia sepe.
Hoc iuuat, ungatur si tetanus unguine tali,

32 sinulia *S*

3.18 PIRETRVM *P* 22r–22v: Piretrum | *S* 79v: De piretro terestri. Henricus

Exceptiones (*O* 92v): Piretrum terrestre sapore et uiribus omnino equatur piretro speciei, et eodem modo utendum est eo ut predicto.

1 si] uel *S* 2 terestre *S* 3 esse] ut *P* probleuma *P* refert] dedit *S* 4 arrida *S* Muse] cause *S* 5 hec] hoc *S* manca *S* 6 quarto similem *transp. P* 8 est *om. P* 10 quid] quod *S* piretrum faciat] *scripsi, transp. P* : peretrum faciat *S* 11 excruciat *S* macticet *S* 13 flenmate *S* 17 superungues *S* *l. 18 om. S* 19 paraliticos *P* 20 ungatur *S* si] sepe *add. S* *l. 21 om. S* 22 thetanus *S*

Other authors relate that Mallow, once strongly
beaten and mixed with old fat, will be helpful.
Mallow can do all these things and Curled Mallow more strongly still.

3.18 Pellitory:
1) Pellitory, *Anacyclus pyrethrum* D.C.
2) Pellitory-of-the-Wall, *Parietaria officinalis* L.

If Curled Mallow is thought to be surpassed by no herb
apart from Pellitory-of-the-Wall (which even wealthy England
claims to be a riddle) how can the dried-up formula
of our meager Muse suffice to take up such a subject?
Since it, when eaten, gives a flavour similar to Pellitory
and, dry in the fourth degree, provides a similar heat,
it has for its merits the beautiful name of a spice.
The spice is scarcely better, but the herb is merely rarer,
for whatsoever the spice does, the herb accomplishes.
So let us sing what Pellitory can do: if a cold humour
is torturing the teeth, let him who is suffering chew this
and roll it in his mouth, or gargle it mixed with vinegar;
thus also will it soothe a tongue swelled up with phlegm,
thus it is beneficial for a uvula swollen by the weight of moisture,
thus also is it good in many medicines of the mouth.
Anoint the kidneys with the oil in which it's cooked,
and it helps this: anoint the body before the onset of a fever.
It helps this: rub with this if you want sweat freely to flow.
It helps this: have a paralytic rubbed with such an ointment.
It helps this: if benumbed limbs are often rubbed with it;
it helps this: if cold ones are often rubbed.
It helps this: if a neck-cramp is rubbed with such an ointment,

3.18 PIRETRVM / Pellitory *Macer, 'Pyrethrum',* 2086–2108
4 Strabo 248–9

Hoc iuuat et piretrum si tritum iungis oliuo.
Hoc iuuat: hinc morbis quos predixi superunctis
Proficit et piretrum sumptum cum melle caducis;
Sic eciam soluit morbum qui membra resoluit.
Hoc piretrum species hoc et piretrum facit herba.

3.19 CENTAVREA

Cum centauree species minor agnita multis
Et species maior pateat uix cognita paucis,
De nota tibi nota canam. Siccare secundo
Atque calere gradu (nisi fallunt scripta) probatur.
Melle sibi iuncto caligine lumina mundat.
Qui sciasim patitur mire decoccio prodest
Illius et sanum reddet subiecta per anum;
Hec eadem neruis fomento proficit egris
Sanguine contracto, compescit et ipsa dolorem.
Ista recens plagas conglutinat herba recentes,
Pellit abortiuum, deducit menstrua succus
Illius, expellit medicamina seua per aluum.
Hinc eciam presses autumpni tempore succum
Et desiccatum feruenti sole reponas,
Vt reddat morbos quos diximus ante salubres.

3.20 MARRVBIVM

Marrubium medici, quam dicunt 'prassion' Argi,
Tradunt esse gradu calidam siccamque secundo.
Marrubii succus cum uino melleue iunctus

23 iungis] soluis *S* olyuo *P* *l. 24 om. P* 24 morbis] *scripsi*, morbus *S* 26 soluit] ducit *S* 7 hoc . . . hoc] hec . . . hec *P*

3.19 CENTAVREA *P* 22v: Centhaurea | *S* 50v: De Centaurea. Henricus
2 congnita *P* 7 annum *S* 8 neruis] unus (?) *S* 12 per] ab *S* 15 quod *S*

3.20 MARRVBIVM *P* 23r: Marubium | *S* 69r–69v: De Maurubio. Henricus
1 maurubium *S* prassion Argi] passio nardi *S* 2 tradunt] tradcucunt *add.* morbi *et exp. S* callidam *P* 3 maurubii siccus *S*

and Pellitory helps this if you blend it, ground, with olive oil.
It helps this: it benefits diseases (which I named before) when rubbed
with this, and Pellitory taken with honey is good for epileptics;
in such a way it also removes the disease that enervates the limbs.
Pellitory the spice does this as does Pellitory the herb.

3.19 Centaury, *Centaurium erythraea* Rafn.

Since the smaller type of Centaury is known to many
and the larger type appears known to scarcely few,
I will sing known things to you about the known. It's proven
to dry and heat in the second degree, unless my books deceive.
With honey added to it, it cleans the eyes of cloudiness.
A decoction of it marvellously helps someone who suffers
from sciatica and received into the anus makes it healthy;
this same herb in a poultice benefits tendons ailing
with diminished blood, and it restrains the pain.
This herb, when fresh, binds up recent wounds,
forces an abortion, its juice leads out menstrual courses,
and expels bad medicines through the stool.
You may also press the juice from this in autumn's season
and place it out to dry in the burning sun so that
it brings the ailments we named before back to health.

3.20 Horehound, *Marrubium vulgare* L.

Physicians relate that Horehound, which the Greeks
call *prassion*, is hot and dry in the second degree.
The juice of Horehound, when blended with wine or honey,

3.19 CENTAVREA / **Centaury** *Macer, 'Centaurea,' 1709–27*
3 *Cf.* Ovid, *Ex Ponto* 4. 19

3.20 MARRVBIVM / **Horehound** *Macer, 'Marrubium,' 1437–55*

Prodest debilibus caligine. Conditus idem
Naribus aut auri iuuat has illamque dolentes,
Aut si cum roseo diffunditur intus oliuo.
Seminis aut herbe ptysicos decoccio mire
Pectoris et morbos iuuat huic si iungatur yris.
Sic ualet asmaticis, tussi laterisque dolori.
Huius item siccus hec proficit omnia succus:
Expellit partus, expellit et ipsa secundas.
Marrubium melli iunctum cito uulnera purgat,
Taliter et carnem que rodunt ulcera curat.
Yctericis nari iniectus ualet, ac nocet illis
Qui uel uesica uel renibus excruciantur.
  Antidotum sic conficiunt dyaprassion inde:
Quatuor unceolas assumunt yreos, addunt
Tres prassii, ficus, calmenti puleiique,
At gemine ysopi, squille pinusque nucelli.
Octo predictis unam miscent fenugreci
Ad mediumque coqunt in aqua, sed postea iungunt
Tantundem mellis, proiectis scilicet herbis
Mel et aquam postremo coqunt, sic spissa capescant.
Hoc mire tussim, pulmonem, pectora purgat
Si duo ieiuno coclearia uel tria dones.

3.21 SCLAREGA

Viginti uisis uiridis sclarega uidetur!
A medicis dulci calde conferre putatur
Et uires et odorati fermenta saporis.
Dat rauco sclarega sonum clarissima clarum
Sed nec pulmoni nec uisceribus fit inepta.
Hec et multa potest que uel tacuere scientes
Vel non nouerunt (nec cuncta sciunt sapientes).

5 has] hos *S* 6 diffundas *S* 7 tysicos *S* 8 iungitur *P* 10 idem *P* 11 et ipsa expellit *S* 12 maurubium *S* uulnerat *S* 14 ac] at *P* 15 renibus] naribus *P* excruciatur *S* *ll. 16–25 om. S* 22 tantundem] *scripsi*, tantumden *P* tussim] et (?) *add. P*

3.21 SCLAREGA *P* 23r: Sclarega | *S* 93r: De Sclarega. Henricus

Exceptiones (*O* 92v): Sclarega dat dulci calide uires et odorati fermenta saporis. Vocem clarificat, pulmoni et uisceribus prodest.

2 medici *S* calde] colore *P* 4 claris *P* 5 nec ... nec] non ... nec *S* fit inepta] refragatur *S* 7 mouerunt *P*

is good for those weak from dizziness. The same thing inserted
in the nose or ear helps the former and those aching in the latter,
or if it is poured inside with oil-of-Rose.
A decoction of the seed or herb helps in an amazing way
consumptives and chest diseases if Iris is added to it.
In such a way it helps asthmatics, a cough, and a pain in the side.
Its juice, when dried, likewise profits all these things:
it forces out a foetus, and also expels the afterbirth.
Horehound mixed with honey quickly purges wounds,
and in such a way it heals flesh that ulcers gnaw upon.
Injected in the nostril, it's good for jaundice, and it's harmful
to those who are suffering in the bladder or the kidneys.
They compose from it the antidote *dyaprassion* like this:
they take four ounces of Yreos, and add
three of Horehound, fig, Catnip, and Pennyroyal,
but two of Hyssop, Sea-Onion, and pine nut.
They mix one ounce of Fenugreek to the aforesaid eight
and cook it down in water by half, but then they add
the same amount of honey, that is, they at last cook honey
and water with the herbs thrown in, so that they make it thick.
This marvellously purges a cough, the lung, and chests
if you give two or three teaspoons when fasting.

3.21 Wild English Clary, *Salvia verbenaca* L.

Having seen twenty, green Clary appears!
It is thought by physicians to confer by a gentle heat
both its virtues and drinks of a savoury odour.
Most famous Clary gives clear voice to the hoarse,
but it is not without use for the lungs or the innards.
It can do these and many things which experts have kept quiet
or did not know (for wise men do not know all things).

16–25 Constantine, *Opera* 1.205

3.21 SCLAREGA / **Wild English Clary** *Strabo, 'De Sclarega', 275–83*

3.22 SCLAREGA MAIOR

Sclarege sclarega subest latissima late:
Quamuis hec passim campis superextet et ortis,
Huius enim succus niuee cum lacte capelle
Pectora percurat cureque potencia durat.

3.23 NEPTA

Quis reputet neptam (nisi cordis egenus!) ineptam,
Cui sane mentis non sit magni calamentis?
Tercius in sicca ui uel calida gradus huic est.
Cum lepre species 'elephanciasis' uocitetur
Quod maior morbis elephasque animalibus extat,
Hanc in principio magne potus calamentis,
Humida siccando, curat sociata lyeo.
Sic cure iecoris, lateri prodest et anhelis
Quos dicunt Greci 'asmaticos.' Valet ictericorum
Et stomachi morbis Bachi contrita liquore.
Perdit singultus quacientes uncia uultus.
Cum mulsa totum corpus sudore resoluit;
Ex oleo quo decoquitur linies febrientem
Sicque fricans frigus, febrem quoque, sepe repelles.
Contritam uiridem sciasis superadde dolori
Sicque uirens pellem reddit siccando salutem.
Pota uel apposita festine menstrua purgat;
Pota uel iniecta lumbricos enecat atque
Omnibus in membris cum melle et cum sale uermes.
Morsus pestiferos superaddita, trita medetur;

3.22 SCLAREGA MAIOR *P* 23r: [no title] | *S* 93r: De sclarega maiore. Henricus

Exceptiones (*O* 92v): Est sclarega minor [*sic*] cuius succus cum lacte niuee capelle pectus optime curat.

2 hortis *S* 4 pecora *S*

3.23 NEPTA *P* 23r–23v: Nepita | *S* 73v: De Nepta. Henricus

1 corde *S* 3 ui *om. S* 4 specie *P* 5 morbis] in orbis *S* extent *S* 6 hanc] hunc *S* 7 lieo *S* 8 lateret *S* anelis *S* 10 liquere *P* 11 uncia] *scripsi*, unica *PS* 12 multa *S* 14 fricans] fugans *P* frigus] et *add. P* quoque *om. P* repelles] resoluit *P* 15 superaddere *S* dolore *P* 16 uirens] urens *S* 18 pota] *add.* uelume (?) *et canc. P* iniecta *corr. ex* iniectam *P* enecat] enodat *P* *ll.* 20–21 *transp. P*

3.22 True Clary, *Salvia sclarea* L.

The largest Clary comes after large Clary.
Although it stands out everywhere in fields and gardens,
its juice, in fact, when mixed with the milk of a white goat
thoroughly cures chests and strengthens the powers of a cure.

3.23 Catnip, *Nepeta cataria* L.

Who could imagine Catnip inept (unless devoid of heart!),
and who of sane mind does not think this is mighty Calamint?
Its degree is third in power dry or hot.
Although the type of leprosy is called *elephantiasis* because
it is larger than diseases and the elephant larger than animals,
a drink of mighty Catnip, when mixed with wine,
cures this at its start by drying out moist things.
Thus it's good for care of the liver, for the side, and for gaspers
whom Greeks call 'asthmatics.' It's good for diseases
of the jaundiced and the stomach when mixed with Bacchus's drink.
An ounce of it destroys hiccoughs shaking the face.
With mead it liberates the entire body from sweat;
anoint a feverish person with the oil in which it's cooked
and rubbing thus you'll often repel a chill as well as a fever.
Apply this ground, when fresh, to a sciatic pain
and thus the green herb brings health by drying the skin.
When drunk or applied it quickly purges menstrual courses;
when drunk or injected it kills stomach worms
and worms in all the members with honey and with salt.
When ground and applied it cures destructive bites;

3.22 SCLAREGA MAIOR / **True Clary** *source unknown*
3 *Cf.* Quintus Serenus 197, 312

3.23 NEPTA / **Catnip** *Macer, 'Nepeta,' 592–625*
1 Henry of Huntingdon, *HA* 11. 14 (p. 792)

Pellit cum uino uirus. Superaddita nigras,
Trita, cicatrices purgat redditque nitorem,
Quod uino cocte melius faciet cataplasma.
Eius serpentes dicunt auertere fumum;
Pota potens nepta fit amaro pestis amori.
   Antidotum post inde parant dyacalamentis:
Hii sumunt tres unciolas nepte piperisque,
Puleii et sisileos et petrosilini,
At geminas apii, cimini, ligusticos; addunt
Vnam gyngiberis; hec omnia melle resoluunt.
Cor lenit, stomachum soluit, curat pituitam
Pectoris atque iecur, splen, petram, menstrua soluit.
Prolongat spacium uiuendi pluribus annis.

3.24 PORTVLACA

'Andraginis' Danais, sed 'portulaca' Latinis,
Vulgo 'pes pulli' que dicitur, humida friget,
Vnde febrem curat quam 'causon' Grecia dicit
Trita super stomachum si ponitur, herbaque mansa
(Aut succus dat idem) solet et lenire calorem
Si sumas ut olus. Solet ergo mansa uel hausta
Sanguinis hec fluxum, uentris quoque stringere fluxum.
Auferet hec igitur estate commesta calorem.
Est emoptoycis non raro commesta salubris
Ac uentrem mollit cum uino. Cum sale prodest
Vesice; dentes dabit hec non esse stupentes.

21 uirus] tyneas (!) *P*   23 faciet] *scripsi*, facit *PS*   cathaplasma *P*   24 eius] diccint (?) *add. et exp. P*   euertere *P*   25 nepte *S*   amaro] amate *S*   *ll.* 26–33 *om. S*   26 dyacalamentis] *scripsi*, dyacamalentis *P*

3.24 PORTVLACA   *P* 23v–24r: Portulaca | *S* 81r–81v: De Portulaca. Henricus | *T* 101v: Portulaca

1 andragini *S*   danays *P*   3 dixit *P*   4 si ponitur herbaque mansa] uiridis si ante ponatur *T*   herbisque *S*   5 linire *S*   6 summas *P*   olus] oliis *S*   7 hec] hoc *S*   fluxit . . . fluxit *S*   8 hec] hoc *S*   comesta *P*   calorem] salubris *P*   9 est . . . salubris *om. P*   10 at *P*   uino] et *add. S*   11 hec] hoc *S*   stupientes *S*

with wine it forces poison out. When ground and applied
it clears up blackened scabs and brings back whiteness,
but a plaster of it, cooked in wine, will do this better.
They say that snakes avoid its smoke;
when drunk, potent Catnip is a plague to bitter love.
Then they prepare from it the antidote *dyacalamentum*:
they take three ounces of Catnip and of Pepper,
of Pennyroyal, laserwort, and Parsley,
but two of Celery, Cumin, and Lovage; they add
one ounce of Ginger, and mix all these things with honey.
It soothes the heart, loosens the stomach, cures mucus
in the chest, and releases the liver, spleen, stone and menses.
It prolongs the length of life for many years.

3.24 Purslane, *Portulaca oleracea* L.

The herb which is called *andrachne* by the Greeks, but Purslane
by the Latins, and 'Chicken Foot' by the crowd, is moist and cold,
wherefore it cures the fever that Greece calls *causon*
if it is placed ground upon the stomach. The herb, when eaten
(or the juice provides the same), is also apt to soothe a fever
if you take it as a vegetable. Therefore when eaten or drunk
it can restrain a flow of blood and the belly's flux
and so, when eaten, it takes the summer's heat away.
When eaten, not rarely is it healthful for blood-spitters,
and with wine it softens the belly. With salt it benefits
the bladder and will prevent the teeth from going numb.

26–33 Pseudo-Oribasius 1. 129 (*Physica S. Hildegardis*, 139)

3.24 PORTVLACA / **Purslane** *Macer, 'Portulaca', 748–64*

3.25 SEMPERVIVA

Hic, inuicta uires que semperuiua uocaris
Barba uocata Iouis, domuum gratissima tectis,
Plinius acidule similem te iudicat esse
Nam fugit accidule (que pratis et secus amnes
Crescere multa solet) tumor ex oculis cataplasma,
Ac uisus hilarat succus capitisque dolori
Proderit antiquo roseo permixtus oliuo,
Qui dolor est Greca dictus 'cephalargia' lingua.
Auribus expressus si succus funditur eius
Auditum reparat, sonitum fugat atque dolorem.
Hec genus omne solet uentris restringere mire
Fluxus cum uino potata comestaue sepe.
Menstrua sic sistit, lumbricis seua rotundis.
Frigentem dicunt calidam sedare podagram
Si cataplasmetur sociata terendo polenta
Vel fuerit tantum foliis cooperta uirentis.
Cum uino uariis solet hec obstare uenenis;
Vt perhibent quidam, qui secum gesserit ipsam,
Letali non appetet hunc uel scorpius ictu.
Appositam fugiunt sacer ignis et herpeta rodens.
Proficit ulceribus que serpunt ustaque sanat.
Hec quoque, barba Iouis, potes et tibi tercius extat
Frigenti sicceque gradus, qui constat et illi.

3.25 SEMPERVIVA *P* 24r: Semperuiua | *S* 45r–45v: De Barba Iouis. Henricus poeta
1 hec *P* inuicta] in uita *S* uocatur *P* 2 youis *P* donum *P* testis *S* 3 Plinius acidule similem] perdimus accidule que pratis et secus silerem *et exp.* que pratis et secus *S* acydule *P* 4 acydule *P* ampnes *P* 6 ac] aut *P* hilarat] hylarat *corr. ex* hyalarat *P* 7 antiquos *S* olyuo *P* 8 qui] quod *P* dolor *corr. e* color *P* dictus] cela *add. P* 8 cefalargia *S* 11 hec] *scripsi*, hoc *PS* genius *S* 13 lumbricus *S* retundit *S* 14 fringentem *S* 15 cathaplasmetur *P* polente *S* 16 coapta *S* 17 solet hec] ualet hoc *S* 18 gestant *S* istam *S* 19 appetit *P* 21 sperunt *S* 22 hec] hoc *S* youis *P*

3.25 Houseleek, *Sempervivum tectorum* L.

Here, unconquered in powers, you who are called Live-Forever,
known as Jove's Beard, most pleasing on the roofs of houses,
Pliny concludes that you are similar to Sorrel
for an eye tumour flees a plaster of Sorrel (which likes
to grow abundantly in meadows and next to water),
and the juice, when mixed well with old oil-of-Rose,
revives the sight and should benefit the headache
which is called *cephalalgia* in Greek.
If its juice, pressed out, is poured into the ears
it repairs the hearing and chases off ringing and pain.
It's apt to restrain in an amazing way every type
of stomach flux when often drunk with wine or eaten.
Thus it stops menstruation and is deadly to roundworms.
They say that since it's cold it soothes hot gout if applied
in a plaster, blended with barley-meal by grinding,
or if it should be covered with only the green herb's leaves.
With wine this is apt to hinder various poisons;
as some relate, if a person should carry this with him,
even a scorpion won't approach him with its lethal sting.
The Holy Fire and gnawing herpes flee this when applied.
It's good for ulcers which spread and it heals burns.
You can do these things as well, Jove's Beard, and the third degree
in cold and dry is known in you, which also occurs in the other.

3.25 SEMPERVIVA / **Houseleek** *Macer, 'Acidula',* 711–42
3 *Cf.* Pliny 25. 162

4 LIBER QVARTVS

Bina profundi
Sidera celi,
Splendida Phebe
Phebus et ingens,
Omnibus eque
Pregrediuntur.
Sic quoque scriptis
Bina preesse
Iure putantur
Omnibus eque
Phisica sanans,
Ethica saluans.
Cetera Phebo,
Cetera Phebe,
Sidera fulgent,
Sic quoque scriptis
Ante relatis
Cetera florent
Tempora rite
Solque sororque
Lumine miro
Cuncta gubernant,
Noctibus illa,
Lucibus ille,
Quod nisi lucis,
Quod nisi noctis
Tempus habetur.
Nec minus istis
Cetera plane
Scripta coherent,
Phisica carnis,
Ethica mentis,
Saluificatrix,

4 LIBER QVARTVS *P* 24r–24v: Liber Quartus | *S* 33r: [no title] *Edited by Rigg*, 271–2.
1 bina] sina *S* 2 sydera *P* 4 Phebus] plebus *S* 8 preest *S* 11 sonans *S* 15 sydera *P* 16 sic quoque scriptis *om. P* 20 sororque] sorique *S* 21 lumina *S* miro *corr. e* mire *P* 22 cuncta gubernant *om. P* 25 quod nisi] quin *S* 26 quod nisi] quin *S* 30 cohercent *S* 33 saluicatrix *S*

4 The Fourth Book

Twin stars
of deep heaven,
shining Phoebe
and mighty Phoebus,
advance equally
before all things.
So also in writings
two things
are rightly thought
to surpass all equally:
healing Physic
and saving Ethics.
The stars gleam,
some with Phoebus,
some with Phoebe,
so also in writings
reported before,
other times
duly flourish,
and sun and his sister
govern all things
with wondrous light,
she by night,
and he by day,
unless this time belongs
to light, unless this time
belongs to night.
No less than these,
other writings
clearly agree:
the saviours are
Physic for the flesh,
Ethics for the mind—

4 LIBER QVARTVS / **The Fourth Book** *Original* (*Cf.* Boethius, *De cons. phil.* 1 met. 7)
1–6 *Cf.* Boethius, *De cons. phil.* 1 met. 7, 1–4   13–15 Boethius, *De cons. phil.* 2 met. 2, 4; Horace, *Carmina* 2. 16. 3–4

Que nisi carnis,
Hec nisi mentis
Cura tenetur.

4.1–2 <IACINCTVS ET NARCISSVS>

Dum tibi res magno modicas ornamus honore,
Tot labor est, inquis, herbas plantare librosque
Tot legisse grauat; magis euitare labores
Hos aliosque libet. Tibi dum respondeo paucis,
Ni labor est, audi, piger, indignissime uita,
Si quicquid labor est uitas et uiuere uita
Ne cures aliquid. Quis enim uiuit, nisi curet,
Aut quis curantem nescit sentire laborem?
Quod si res homini labor est, natura uolatus
Vt uolucri, Salomone ipso testante, labora,
Insta, perquire, planta, lege, disce, doceto!
Si labor est, modicus labor est, uictoria magna est
Vincere pugnantes morbos presentibus herbis.
   Hic igitur, Iacincte, nites; Narcissus adheret—
Nunc flores, olim pueri—tu natus Amiclis,
Hic Elicone satus. Te durus contudit error,
Hunc leuis destruxit amor—te discus amantis,
Hunc species fontis. Te morti demere frustra
Et deus et medicus et amans temptabat Apollo.
Hunc tam mirifice quem copia fecit egere
Flebat et Echo grauis. Te florem fecit Apollo,

34 que nisi] quin *S* 35 hec] que *P*

4.1–2 <IACINCTVS ET NARCISSVS> *P* 24v–25r: [no title] | *S* 33v–34r: [no title] | *T* 100r (*only lines 25–29*): Narcisus *First edited by Rigg, 273–5.*

Exceptiones (*O* 92v): Iacinctus flos est ceruleus uulnera curans, contusa et luxata sanans. Narcisus flos est roseus feruores reprimens. Si capud inde laues, febres extinguit acutas.

1 dum] quot *P* 2 iniquis *S* 3 legisse] tetigisse *P* grauant *S* 4 hos aliosque libet] *Winterbottom*, hosque libet alios *P* : hos aliquosque libet *S* dum] dura *P* respondeo] resplendeo *S* 5 ni] nil *P* indignissima *S* 10 ut] et *P* Salamone *P* 11 insta] in ista *S* 12 est[3] *om. S* 13 pungnantes *P* 14 hic] hinc *P* nites] uires *S* Narcissus] *Rigg*, narciscus *P* : narticus *S* adheret] adher *S* 15 Amyclis *P* 16 Elycone *P* 17 amantes *P* 18 morti] fonti *P* 19 temptabit *S* 20 quem] quam *S* 21 flebit *P* Echo] etho *S*

the former if care is not kept
of the flesh, the latter
if care is not kept of the mind.

4.1–2 Hyacinth, *Hyacinth orientalis* L. and Narcissus (Daffodil), *Narcissus pseudonarcissus* L.

While we adorn small things for you with great honour,
it's a burden, you say, to plant herbs and to have read
so many books, and you would rather avoid
these and other tasks. Now I reply to you in few words:
if it's not too hard, listen up, lazybones, most unworthy of life,
if you avoid whatever's work and fail to live so you don't
have to care for anything. For who is alive, but that he cares,
and who is unaware that the one caring feels the effort?
But if labour is essential to mankind, as flight is the nature
of a bird (as Solomon himself testifies), then work,
press on, inquire, plant, read, learn, and teach!
If it's an effort, the effort's small, and it's a mighty victory
to overcome battling diseases with the present herbs.
  Here, then, you gleam, Hyacinth; Narcissus stands close by—
now flowers, once boys. You were born at Amyclae;
he was born on Helicon. A hard error crushed you;
smooth love destroyed him: you, your lover's discus;
him, the beauty of the spring. Apollo—a god and physician
and lover—tried in vain to snatch you from death;
sad Echo mourned him whom abundance so astonishingly
made needy. Apollo made you, and pitying Echo

4.1–2 <IACINCTVS ET NARCISSVS> / **Hyacinth and Narcissus** *Original*
1 *Cf.* Virgil, *Georgica* 3. 290; Strabo 75 9 *Cf.* Eccles. 6: 7 9–10 Prov. 30: 18–20; Wisd. 5: 11 20 Ovid, *Met.* 3. 466

Hunc miserans Echo. Te ceruleum dedit ictus,
Hunc roseum flammata Venus—decor equus utrique
Floribus in uariis fuit, et dolor equus utrimque.
  Vulnera Iacinctus, periit quia uulnere, curat;
Feruores alius reprimit feruore peremptus.
Contusus contusa iuuat luxataque sanat,
Ast hic quem Veneris feruens extinxit acumen,
Si caput inde lauas, febres extinguit acutas.
Corpore formosos quia preradiauit uterque,
Corpore deformes maculas abradit uterque.
  Vos igitur pueri, si carmine gloria fame
Queritur atque datur per uos quesita poete
Gloria, per uatem data uobis fama uirescet,
Dum Stacio Thebe, Maroni Pergama stabunt,
Nisus et Eurialus, Dymas dum uiuet et Opleus.

4.3 SINAPIS

Tercia stat sinapis; preciosior hec numeratur
Inter eas quas Pitagoras numerat preciosas:
In quarto feruere gradu siccareque fertur.
Maxima uis eius in semine scribitur esse.
Plinius in musto cum semine precipit eius
radices poni, quarum cum suxerit omnem
Vim Bachus, capiti pronunciat esse salubre
Potatumque oculos, fauces, stomachum quoque seruat.
Hanc tere cum ficu rasumque caput superadde:
Huic qui letargum patitur medicina probata est
Vnguendoque pedes hiis sepe fricare ualebit.

22 Echo] etho *S*   24 equs utrumque *S*   25 uulnera . . . uulnere] uulnere . . . uulnera *PT* quia] que *S* : nunc *T*   26 alius] aliis *T*   27 contusos *P*   laxataque *S*   28 ast] at *P* extinxit] extrinxus *S*   29 laues *S*   *ll. 30–31 transp. S*   30 formosus *P*   preradiant *S* 34 gloriam *P*   36 Dymas dum] diuasdum *S*   uiuet] *Rigg*, uiuit *P* : iuuet *S*   Opleus] emplaus *P*

4.3 SINAPIS   *P* 25r–25v: Sinapis | *S* 96r–96v: De Sinapio. Henricus

1 synapis *P*   numeratur] minuatur (?) *S*   3 feruere] fuere *S*   4 uis] *add.* fertur *et canc. P*   eius] est *S*   5 cum] in *S*   6 quorum *S*   7 bacus *S*   pronuncciat *P*   salubrem *P*   8 oculis *P*   10 patitur] patet *S*   *l. 11 om. P*   11 unguendoque] *scripsi*, unguendo *S*

made him, into a flower. A blow made you deep blue,
inflamed Venus made him rosy—equal was the beauty for each
in different flowers, and equal the grief for the one and the other.
Because he perished by a wound, Hyacinth cures wounds;
the other, destroyed by hot passion, represses fevers.
The bruised one helps bruises and heals battered limbs,
but he, whom the burning dart of Venus killed,
allays sharp fevers if you wash your head with it.
Because each outshone the beautiful in body,
each washes away ugly blotches from the body.
Therefore, boys, if you seek the glory of fame in song
and the poet's glory sought by you is granted,
the fame given you through the poet will stay green,
as long as Thebes will stand for Statius, and Troy, Nisus
and Euryalus stand for Virgil, as long as Dymas and Opleus live.

4.3 Mustard, *Brassica alba* L. or *Sinapis alba* L.

Mustard stands third: it is counted as rather precious
among those herbs which Pythagoras counts as precious:
it is said to heat and dry in the fourth degree.
Its virtue is described as greatest in its seed.
Pliny orders that its roots be placed in wine must
with its seed, and when Bacchus has sucked up
all their power, he proclaims it's healthy for the head
and, when drunk, also preserves the eyes, throat and stomach.
Grind this with a fig and apply it upon a shaven head:
this is a proven medicine for one who suffers lethargy,
and it will often be good for rubbing their feet in an ointment.

23 Ovid, *Met.* 3. 482; *cf.* Pliny 21. 128 25–31 *Cf.* Pliny 21. 128–9 32 *Cf.* Martial, *Liber Spectaculorum* 15. 1 35–36 *Cf.* Virgil, *Aeneid* 9. 176–223; Statius, *Thebaid* 10. 347–448

4.3 SINAPIS / **Mustard** *Macer, 'Sinapi', 1139–1200*
2 *Cf.* Pliny 20. 236, 24. 156–60 5 *Cf.* Pliny 20. 240

Si tepide iungas tritam uersesque palato
Ad solem, capitis depellet flecma nociuum.
Sternutamentis hanc admiscent sapientes
Nam per eam capitis strictura resoluitur omnis.
Exprimito succum sinapis de caule tenello,
Quem siccum mandendo diu denti medicatur.
Vocales uenas lenit, sensus quoque semen
Exacuit; sic uiscosi humores tenuantur.
Confortat stomachum, sedat suspiria, uentrem
Commouet; urinam, lapides et menstrua purgat.
Infuso facies oleum de semine lumbis
Vtile contractis stupidisque iuuabile neruis.
Fumus uero stere causas iuuat atque caducis
Proficit. Hoc adipi melliue terendo iugatum
Sanat alopicias et scrofas sepe fricatum;
Acri cum uino lepras restringit inunctum.
Hoc mansum tumidos sanare solet febrientes
Antea quam morbus rapiat poterisque uenena
Tollere serpentum, superaddens hanc et acetum;
Mansa uetat seuos precordia ledere fungos.
Vt Menemacus ait sinapis cataplasma docebo:
Semine cum sinapis iungatur candida mica
Panis; sint sinapis gemine, pars tercia panis.
Hiis ficus siccas, mel, acetum iunge secundum
Quod poscent etas uel morbus, nam sinapismus
Acrior esse solet quo mel uel ficus habundat;
Lenior esse solet quo uel panis uel acetum.
Hoc cataplasma uigens in multis sepe probatur
Quod rapit inmensos languores atque uetustos.
Hoc stomachi morbos pellit tussimque ptysimque,
Hoc humor capitis siccatur, lumina ledens,
Pulmonumque simul stillando concaua replens.
Hoc sciasis splenisque tumor iecorisque fugatur
Sicque graues cause soluuntur et inueterate.

12 tritum *P* uertesque *P* 13 depellit *P* fegma *S* nocumen *S* 16 exprimendo *S* siccum synapis *P* tenello] reuello *S* 17 quem] *scripsi*, quod *PS* succum *S* madendo *S* denti] tenti *S* 19 tenuantur] renunciantur *S* 22 faciet *S* 23 neruis] membris *P* 24 uere *S* 25 adypi melleue *P* 27 inunctum] munitum *S* 28 sole *S* 30 serpentem *S* 32 meneacus *S* synapis cathaplasma *P* docebo *om. S* 33 iugatur *P* 35 mel] uel *P* 39 hoc] hec *S* cathaplasma *P* 40 langores *S* *l. 41 om. S* 43 pulmonisque *P* 44 splenisque] plerumque *P* yecorisque *P* 45 ineterate *S*

If you mix this, ground, with warm water and roll it on your palate
toward the sun, it will repel harmful phlegm from the head.
The wise men take this as snuff,
for every hardening in the head is released by it.
Press Mustard juice with tender Cabbage,
and chew it a while when dry to cure the teeth.
It soothes the vocal chords, the seed also sharpens
the senses, and in this way viscous humours are reduced.
It strengthens the stomach, settles asthma, and moves
the belly; it purges urine, stones, and menstrual courses.
Make an oil from the seed which, as an infusion,
is useful for pinched loins and helpful for numb tendons.
The smoke aids problems of the cervix and benefits
the epileptic. By grinding this, when mixed with grease or honey,
it cures hair loss and scrofula when rubbed on often,
and in an ointment with vinegar it holds back leprosy.
When eaten, this is apt to heal the swollen and the feverish
before the disease takes hold, and you shall be able to take away
the poison of snakes by applying this and vinegar;
when eaten, it forbids wicked fungi from harming the diaphragm.
I'll teach you a Mustard plaster as Menemachus has described it:
blend white bread crumbs with Mustard seed,
and let there be two parts Mustard and a third of bread.
Add dried figs to these and honey and vinegar
according to the demands of age or sickness, for *sinapismus*
is apt to be sharper according to how much honey or figs abound
and is apt to be more gentle according to how much bread or vinegar.
This plaster is often proven strong in many ways
because it takes away cases of faintness old and great.
It forces out stomach diseases, a cough, and consumption,
and this dries the moisture of the head that hurts the eyes,
while also filling the hollows of the lungs by a dripping action.
Sciatica and swelling of the spleen and liver are exiled by this
and in such a way serious and long-lasting cases are resolved.

4.4 ERVCA

Erucam synapi similem quis nesciat esse?
Tercius huic gradus est in ui feruente, secundus
In desiccando. Si sumitur digerit escas,
Egerit urinas, tussim fugat. Vtilis ipsa
Fit pueris: cum melle cutis maculas fugat omnes;
Splendet eo cultus, liber lentigine uultus;
Hac maculas lino nigras cum felle bouino.
Radicem prius elixam ualideque subactam
Ossa superpono confractaque reficit illa
Tritaque cum uino predicte semina dono
Hiis quos pestiferos ictus affligere noui.
Scripta canunt uatum (nec fingunt omnia uates!)
Hanc stimulare tuos, Venus insaciabilis, ignes.
Mira canam (nec ficta tamen): coniuncta lyeo
Largiflue duros dat contra uerbera sensus.
Sunt condituris gratissima succus et herba,
Vt Greci perhibent (qui digne singula censent).

4.5 LACTVCA

Hanc cum lactucis calidam gelidis sociabis,
Lactucis etenim uis frigida constat et humens,
Vnde leuat nimios superaddita, trita calores
Mansaque prestat idem. Dat sompnum, prouocat aluum
Atque semen bibitum cum uino comprimit aluum.
Sompnia uana premit, lac fert lactuca redundans,
Vtilis et stomacho non lota commesta probatur.
Luminibus quidam perhibent hanc esse nociuam.

4.4 ERVCA *P* 25v–26r: Eruca | *S* 61r–61v: De Eruca. Henricus
1 sinaperis *S* 2 huic] hoc *P* ui *om. S* 3 digerit] *scripsi*, egerit *PS* 5 pueris] prius *S* cutis maculas *transp. S* fugat *om. S* omnis *S* 7 lino *canc. P* 9 superpono] *scripsi*, superpone *P* : suppono *S* confractaque] contracta et *S* reficit] *scripsi*, reicit *PS* 13 hanc] hec *P* Venus *om. S* 14 lieo *S* 16 gratissimus *S*

4.5 LACTVCA *P* 26r: Lactuca | *S* 61v, 65r–65v: De Lectuca. Henricus
1 sociabis] sanabis *S* 2 lactucis] iactusis *S* frigida] facta *S* 3 nimios] niueos *P* colores *P* 5 atque ... aluum *om. S* 6 premit] prestent *S* redundas *P* 7 loca *S*

4.4 Rocket, *Eruca sativa* Mill.

Who doesn't know that Rocket is similar to Mustard?
Its grade is third in heating power, and in drying
second. If it is eaten it digests foods,
brings out urine, and chases a cough away. It is useful
for boys. With honey it drives off every blemish of the skin;
a face nourished with this shines out, free of spots:
I smear black blemishes with this and cow's bile.
I apply the root, first boiled and strongly beaten,
to bones, and it restores the broken ones,
and I give the seeds of the aforesaid herb, when ground with wine,
to those whom I have known to suffer from destructive blows.
The poets' poems relate (nor does every poet lie!)
that this stimulates your fires, insatiable Venus.
I'll sing some marvels (yet not untrue!): when mixed with wine
it abundantly grants a hearty resistance to blows.
The juice and the leaves are most pleasing in condiments,
or so the Greeks relate (who worthily judge all things).

4.5 Lettuce, *Lactuca sativa* L.

You will bring together hot Rocket with chilly Lettuces,
for a cold and humid power is discerned in Lettuces,
by which it lightens excessive fevers when ground and applied,
and when eaten bestows the same. It gives sleep, moves the bowels,
and the seed drunk with wine stops the bowels.
Lettuce suppresses empty dreams, brings out overflowing milk,
and eaten unwashed is proven useful for the stomach.
Some relate that this is harmful for the eyes.

4.4 ERVCA / **Rocket** *Macer, 'Eruca', 1016–36*
1 *Cf.* Virgil, *Aeneid* 1.565 14 Ovid, *Fasti* 4.267

4.5 LACTVCA / **Lettuce** *Macer, 'Lactuca', 765–75*
6 *Cf.* Ovid, *Met.* 11.614

4.6 SATVREIA

Et satureia gradu sicca est et feruida quarto.
Hanc Argi 'timbram' dicunt. Puluis sociatus
Melli uel sumptus cum uino pectora purgat,
Protinus humorem pellens per sputa tenacem.
Tormina cum uino compescit sumpta tepenti
Si large bibitur—res hec certissima scitur.
Nausea sedatur si uino trita bibatur;
Promouet urinam, producit menstrua, purgat
Viscera, pellit abortiuum, pregnantibus obstat
Nam partus (non mansa modo sed subdita) tollit.
Letargus scitur contrarius esse frenesi,
Nam sompnum uetat hec, sompno grauat hic pacientem;
Hic pressus sompno timbram distendat aceto
Et caput inde fouens morbum soluet pigritantem.
Timbra mouet uenerem sumpta in uino uel in ouo
Aut si largiflue uiridis uel sicca bibatur;
Quod si cum uino, pipere et melli socientur
Accendit Veneris nimis et corroborat ignes,
Hinc est a satiris merito satureia uocata.

4.7 NASTVRCIVM

Septima stant orto nasturcia feruida, quarto
Sicca gradu, quare uenerem siccando cohercent
Sicut ruta solet si semina sepe bibantur.

4.6 SATVREIA *P* 26r–26v: Saturegia | *S* 92v: De Satureia. Henricus
1 et[1]] at *P* quarto *om. P* 2 hanc] *om. S* argiui *S* tymbram *P* 3 pectora] menstrua *S* 4 protinus humorem] pro cuius humore *S* sputa *corr. e* sumpta *S* 6 hec] est *P* scitur] scriptis *P* 7 nausea *corr. e* nausisea *S* 11 frenasi *S* 12 sompnum] sompnos *P* uetat] necat *S* hic] hoc *P* 13 hic] hoc *S* tymbram *P* distendat] descendit *S* 14 soluit *P* 15 tymbra *S* mouet] et *add. S* uenerem *om. P* in[1] *om. S* 16 aut] at *S* uiridis *om. P* uel] et *P* 17 pipere] *scripsi*, piper *PS* melli] *scripsi*, *om. P* : mel si *S* 18 Veneris] uerius *P* coroborat *S* 19 huic *P* Satiris] saturis *S* uocatur *S*

4.7 NASTVRCIVM *P* 26v: Nasturcium | *S* 72v: De Nasturcia. Henricus
1 orto] quarto *S* feruida] frigida *P* 2 quare uenerem] queritur uenerendo *S* cohercet *P*

4.6 Savory, *Satureia hortensis* L.

And Savory is dry and hot in the fourth degree.
The Argives call it *tymbra*. As a powder added
to honey, or drunk with wine, it purges chests,
constantly driving out thick moisture through the sputum.
When drunk with warm wine it restrains gripes
if it is drunk in quantity—this thing is known to be most certain.
Nausea is settled if it is ground and drunk with wine;
it moves urine, leads out menstrual courses, purges
insides, forces an abortion, and hinders pregnancies,
for it takes away the foetus (not eaten, but as a suppository).
Lethargy is known to be the opposite of frenzy:
the latter shuns sleep, the former burdens the patient with sleep;
let the one burdened by sleep soften Savory with vinegar
and, washing his head with it, he'll dissolve the sleepy disease.
Savory incites lust when taken with wine or an egg,
or if it is drunk abundantly, whether green or dry;
but if these are blended with wine, Pepper, and honey,
it excessively kindles and strengthens the fires of Venus,
hence it is rightly named Savory after the satyrs.

4.7 Cress, *Nasturtium officinale* L.

Hot Cress stands seventh in the garden, dry in the fourth
degree, and because of this it restrains lust by drying,
just as Rue is accustomed to, if the seeds are often drunk.

4.6 SATVREIA / **Savory** *Macer, 'Satureia', 843–69*
19 *Cf.* Isidore, *Etym.* 17.9.42–3

4.7 NASTVRCIVM / **Cress** *Macer, 'Nasturtium', 988–1015*

Si prurigo caput, si fedent ulcera, iunges
Anseris huic adipem uiciumque fugabis utrumque,
At succus crines fertur retinere fluentes,
Fusus in aure solet dentis delere dolorem.
Si coquis aut herbam capre cum lacte recenti
Aut semen, tepido curabis pectora potu,
Aut semen tussim sumptum cum melle retundit.
Linchenas succus curat cum melle perunctus.
Cum tepida semen contritum pondere dragme
Hocque modo bibitum duratum prouocat aluum.
Splen reprimit semen si iunctum detur aceto;
Cum uino perimit lumbricos, pellit abortum.
Herbam uel semen cum polline iunge et aceto;
Hec sciasi superadde graui: medicina probata est.
Sufficit herba recens fermento iuncta terendo
Delere antracas (bona que plebs ulcera dicit),
Incipit et cura mollire furunculus ista:
Emittit saniem cum qua dolor ipse recedit.
Obstat serpentis cum uino sumpta uenenis;
Solus odor posite carbonibus effugat illos.

4.8 AMEOS

Hic ameos lecto stat, amabile gramen, ameno:
Frondibus alta nimis, uix nascitur alcior illa
Inter eas quas cogit yemps inuisa perire.
Semina parua uides per que rediuiua resurgit,

4 capit *S* fetent *P* iungens *S* 5 huic] hoc *P* : huic *corr. ex* adhuic *S* adypem *P* fugabit *P* 6 at] ad *P* 9–10 aut . . . potu / aut . . . retundit] aut semen tussim sumptum cum melle retundit / aut semen tepido curabit pectora potu *P* 11 linchenas . . . perunctus *om. S* 12 tepido *S* 17 scyasim superat *P* 19 anturcas *S* que] quas *S* 20 mollit forunculus *P* 21 emittit . . . recedit *om. S* ipse] *scripsi*, ipsa *P* 22 sumptum *P* 23 effudat illas *S*

4.8 AMEOS *P* 26v–27r: Ameos | *S* 38r–38v: Herba Ameo. Henricus

Exceptiones (*O* 92v): Ameos alte crescit, semina habens parua per que resurgit, calore suo febrem cotidianam extinguit. Omnibus morbis ex frigiditate uenientibus obsistit. Vrine, lateri, renibus apta.

1 hic] sic *P* amicabile *S* 3 quas] aquas *S* hyems *P* 4 uidens *S* rediuiua] *add.* perire *S*

If itching or ulcers befoul your head,
mix goose fat with this and you'll chase off either vice,
while the juice is said to preserve your flowing hair,
and poured into the ear is apt to remove a toothache.
If you cook either the greens or the seed in fresh goat's milk,
you will cure chests with this warm drink,
or the seed when taken with honey drives out a cough.
The juice with honey, as an ointment, cures skin eruptions.
A dram's weight of the seed, ground with warm water,
and drunk in this manner loosens constipated bowels.
The seed represses spleen if is given mixed with vinegar;
with wine it kills worms and expels a foetus.
Blend the herb or seed with flour and with vinegar;
apply these to a serious sciatica, for this is a proven medicine.
The green herb, blended with yeast by grinding, is sufficient
to destroy carbuncles (which the people call 'good ulcers'),
and by this cure the boil begins to soften:
it emits bloody pus with which that pain recedes.
Taken with wine it hinders a serpent's poisons;
the mere odour of it, when placed on coals, chases them away.

4.8 Giant Hogweed, *Heracleum mantegazzianum* L.

Here Hogweed stands, a delightful herb, in its charming bed:
with very high branches, a taller herb than it is scarcely found
among those that hated winter forces to die.
You see the small seeds by which it leaps up, reborn,

4.8 AMEOS / **Giant Hogweed** *Source unknown*

Sed uis grandis inest per quam preciosa patescit,
Nam solet innato gelidas temerare calore,
Vnaquaque die uexantes corpora febres.
Prelia magna uides, sed quo maiora uidentur,
Herbe uincentis tanto est uictoria maior.
Morbis preterea quibus est frigus ueniendi
Causa comesque grauis simul omnibus obuiat una:
Vrine grata <est>, lateri bona, renibus apta,
Pectoribus prudens sed et hiis (ne singula narrem)
Omnibus, ut dictum est, quibus algor causa manendi est.

4.9 PSILLIVM

Psillia frigida sunt. Quam frigida? Res probat ipsa:
Cum late campi niue candescunt boreali,
Tunc assume niuis modicum faciesque trociscum;
Hunc in seminibus relocabis graminis huius.
Cum late campi fundentur lampade Phebi
Inuenies modicum niue perdurante trociscum,
Tam bene frigentem frigencia psillia seruant.
Deprehensum est igitur quod morbos enecat herba
Qui nimio ueniunt conseruanturque calore,
Vt febres alia uexantes corpora luce,
Vt podagram nimio feruore suo cruciantem,
Vt capitis morbum grece 'cephalargia' dictum.
'Et que talia sunt?' Quid nunc per singula curram?

5 gradis *P* 6 galidas *S* colore *S* 8 quo] coque *S* uidentur] minoris *P* 10 morbus *S* 12 est] *scripsi, om. PS* 13 et] in *P*

4.9 PSILLIVM *P* 27r: Psilium | *S* 83r–83v: De Psillio. Henricus | *T* 105v: Spillia (*lines 8–12*)

Exceptiones (*O* 92v): Psillia frigida esse hinc probantur: sume in hieme modicum niuis trociscum et in seminibus psillii pone; nec poterit solis feruore resolui, tanta est herbe frigiditas. Constat igitur quod morbos calidos enecat, ut febrem tercianam, podagram calidam, cephalargiam.

1 sillia *S* 2 lacte *S* boriali *S* 4 hunc] hanc *P* relocabit *P* 5 lacte *S* funduntur *P* 8 depremum *S* : deprensum *T* igitur *om. T* enecat] enodet *P* : enecet *T* 9 qui] quod *S* : que *T* nimio . . . calore] nimion ueneunt conseruantur quaque *T* 10 alia] ternas *T* 11 suo] scio *P* : suos *S* cruciantem] truciorem *P* : traciantem *T* 12 cefalargia *S* : sephargia *T* 13 curris *P*

but a mighty power is in them by which it is clearly precious,
for by its innate heat it can destroy
the chills and fevers vexing bodies every day.
You see great battles, but however great they may seem,
greater still is the victory of this conquering herb!
Moreover, it can hinder on its own all diseases for which a chill
is the cause of onset and a burdensome companion:
it's pleasing for urine, good for the side, fitting for kidneys,
skilled for chests, and for all those cases (lest I narrate
every one), as it is said, in which a chill is the cause of persistence.

4.9 Fleaseed (Psyllium Plantain), *Plantago psyllium* L.

The Fleaseeds are cold. How cold? This fact proves it:
when the fields are widely white with winter's snow,
then gather a little snow and make a pill;
place it within the seeds of this plant.
When the fields are broadly lit by Phoebus's lamp,
you'll find the little pill of snow remains,
so well do cooling Fleaseeds preserve a chilly thing.
Therefore it's revealed that the herb destroys diseases
which begin and are preserved with excessive heat,
like fevers plaguing bodies on every other day,
like gout which tortures with its excessive burning,
like the head disease called *cephalalgia* in Greek.
'And what's that?' Do I have to cover every single thing?

4.9 PSILLIVM / **Fleaseed** *Source unknown*

3 *Antidotarium Nicolai* 157–63 5 *Cf.* Silius Italicus, *Punica* 1. 193; Henry of Huntingdon, *HA* 12. 8, 48 (p. 818) 13 *Cf.* Sedulius, *Carmen paschale* 3. 358

4.10 CORIANDRVM

Ecce saporiferum subit et superest coriandrum!
Frigida uis huius austeraque noscitur esse,
Vt Galienus ait, per quod depellere uentris
Lumbricos solet et tineas uel condita uino
Vel si preualido confecta bibatur aceto.
Semen aque iunctum uentrem stipare solutum
Fertur sepe datum, quod si febris ante tremorem
Hinc tria grana uoras alterna febre carebis;
Fertur idem quod prestet item si mane prius quam
Sol surgat ceruicali supponitur egri.
Vua cum passa mel iungas et coriandrum:
Ista prement uarios sic associata tumores;
Precipue tumidos potes hinc testes leuiare.
Huic fabe succo medicatur iuncta farina
Scrofis et fugit hoc emplastro pustula queuis.
Argenti spume cerusam contere, tritis
Consocia succum coriandri, iunge et acetum,
Quatuor hiis roseum tandem sociabis oliuum.
Hoc sacros ignes preciosum dissipat unguen
Hincque tumor calidus cedit. Confeccio tanta
Ni tibi sit facilis, iungatur succus aceto
Aut si frumenti panis mundissima mica
Iungitur huic succo sedat quoscumque calores.
Xenocrates totidem dixit tardare diebus
Menstrua predicte quot grana uorant mulieres.
Si tibi pauperies piper aufert, sumito semen
Istius, carui, nasturcia, petrosilinum;
Hec tibi consimilem poterunt conferre saporem.

4.10 CORIANDRVM *P* 27r–27v: Coriandrum | *S* 54v–55r: De Coriandro. Henricus
1 saporiferum *corr. e* saporiferam *P* : soporiforum *S* et superest] frigidum *P* 3 quod] quem *S* 4 lubricos *P* 5 prebando *S* 7 si *om. P* 8 trita *S* uoras] mors *S* carebri *S* 10 surgit *P* seruicali *S* 12 sic associata] siccas sociata *S* 15 emplaustrum postula *S* 19 unguem *S* 20 hincque] hinc *S* 21 ne *S* 22 fermenti *P* 23 iunge *S* 24 Xenocrates] et senocrates *S* 27 istius] illius *P* nastrucia *S*

4.10 Coriander (Cilantro), *Coriandrum sativum* L.

Behold, the tasty Coriander follows and is superior!
Its power is known to be both cold and dry,
as Galen said, and by means of this he liked to force out
stomach worms and tapeworms if it were drunk,
either kept in wine or prepared in the strongest vinegar.
The seed, when added to water and often given, is said
to stop a runny belly, but if you eat three grains
of this before a fever's tremor, you'll avoid a tertian fever;
it also is related that it provides the same thing if, before
the sun comes up, it's placed below the patient's pillow.
Mix Coriander and honey with a raisin:
when mixed like this, these subdue a variety of swellings;
you can especially alleviate swollen testicles with this.
When flour is mixed with the juice of this seed it cures
scrofulous sores and any pustule flees from this plaster.
Grind white lead with silver dross and blend
these when ground with Coriander juice, also adding vinegar;
and at last you can add oil-of-Rose to these four things.
This precious ointment demolishes Holy Fire completely
and a hot swelling departs from it. If so great a recipe
does not come easily to you, then mix the juice with vinegar
or if the purest crumbs of wheaten bread
are added to this juice, it settles any fevers whatsoever.
Xenocrates once said that menstrual courses are delayed
by as many days as seeds of the aforesaid herb that women eat.
If poverty has taken Pepper from you, gather the seed
of Coriander, Caraway, Cress and Parsley;
these will be able to give a similar flavour to you.

4.10 CORIANDRVM / **Coriander** *Macer, 'Coriandrum', 957–87*

4.11 LVPINVM

Iamque premens uinum sua concutit arma lupinum
Thebeum pulsura deum, granaria secum
Ampla ferens ubi tela ferox austera locauit.
Huius enim quisquis presumpserit acre legumen
Fecundi calices non cogent esse disertum,
Non stricta facient in paupertate solutum,
Nec timido uires nec egenti cornua tradent.
Absinthii frutices et prassion atque lupinum
Eque miscentur et mulsa conficientur
Et sic lumbrici per amara fugantur amari.

4.12 FENVGRECVM

Insilit in cetum, mollire studens, fenugrecum;
Duricias mollit collecturasque resoluit;
Si tamen alteam, maluam quoque iunxeris illi,
Quas bene sola domat melius sociata domabit.
Semen item lini cum polline iungitur illi:
Non encathisma restabit ad hoc cataplasma.
Cum fenugreco caulem tundas et aceto:
Molliet artheticos gratum cataplasma dolores
Et poterit seuam saltem lenire podagram.

4.11 LVPINVM *P* 27v: Lupinus | *S* 68r: De Lupino. Henricus

Exceptiones (*O* 92v): Lupinum amarum est. Qui huius legumen post gustauerit tutus erit ab ebrietate. Cum absinthio et prassio, uino confectum lumbricos pellit.

2 tebeum *S* 3 locauit *corr. e* locabuit *P* 4 presumserit *P* legumen] lyea *P* 8 passion *S* 10 fungantur *S*

4.12 FENVGRECVM *P* 27v–28r: Fenugrecum | *S* 63r: De Fenugreco. Henricus | *T* 96r: Fenigrecus

Exceptiones (*O* 92v): Fenugrecum duritias mollit collecturasque resoluit melius cum altea et malua. Item semen lini cum polline, iunctum fenugreco, hoc agit. Item fenugrecum cum caule et aceto cataplasma artericos dolores mollit, podagram lenit.

2 collecturasque] et collecturas *T* 3 si . . . quoque] si tres maluarum species tu *T* unxeris *S* 5 ite *T* iungimus *P* 7 encatisma *corr. ex* enacatisma *S* : encatesma *T* prestabit *T* ad] ex *T* cathaplasma *P* 7 cumque fenigreco *T* 8 atericos *S* gratum] istud *T* cathaplasma *P* 9 et . . . podagram *om. S*

4.11 Lupin, *Lupinus albus* L.

Now Lupin, bearing down on wine, strikes her blades together,
ready to repel the Theban God; she carries full granaries
with her where she fiercely keeps her biting weapons.
For whosoever should take up its bitter bean,
bountiful chalices will not force him to be loquacious,
nor will they release him into binding poverty,
nor will they give courage to the meek or horns to the needy.
Let the fruits of Wormwood with Horehound and Lupin
be equally mixed and consumed together in mead:
thus bitter worms are put to flight by bitter beans.

4.12 Fenugreek, *Trigonella foenum-graecum* L.

Fenugreek, striving to soften, charges into the fray;
it softens hardenings and loosens bound up places;
but if you should add to it Mallow and Marsh Mallow,
it will conquer better, mixed, what it conquers well, alone.
Linseed, likewise, is added to it with flour:
a swollen eyelid won't resist against this plaster.
You should grind up Cabbage with Fenugreek and vinegar:
this pleasing plaster will soften arthritic pains
and will be able at least to soothe a savage gout.

4.11 LVPINVM / **Lupin** *Source unknown*
1 Ovid, *Met.* 1. 143 5–6 Horace, *Epistulae* 1. 5. 19–20 7 *Cf.* Ovid, *Ars amatoria* 1. 239; Ps. 68: 32–3 10 *Cf.* Pliny 22. 155

4.12 FENVGRECVM / **Fenugreek** *? Pliny 24. 184–8*
1 *Cf. Ilias Latina, passim* 5–6 *Cf.* Pliny 20. 251 7–9 *Cf.* Pliny 20. 88

4.13 PAPAVER

Miconius stat tredecimus, quod Roma 'papauer'
Dixit, ui gelida siccaque uigens speciesque
Tres habet: hic albet, rubet hic flos, pallidus ille est.
Carior est albus namque ex huius capitellis
Conficiunt opium: cesa cute, cum capitella
Lacte fluunt, lac uero fluens cocleis capientes,
Siccum conseruant, claris aptum medicinis.
Sunt qui, tundentes cum lacte suo capitella,
Inde simul pressum siccant in sole liquorem.
Huic uis magna datur, primo tamen impar habetur;
De specie rosea iocundum sompniferumque
Conficiunt oleum, tundentes sperma minutum.
Tercia dat species reliquarum more soporem.
Elixatura languens cuiuslibet harum
Si foueat faciem, uel si bibat ipse tepentem,
Confert optatum, nisi mors sit proxima, sompnum.
Eius de foliis factum cataplasma subactis
Curabit fauces tumidas. Potuue ciboue
Aut cantu aut estu uel frigore reddita si sit
Aspera uocalis uena, hoc cataplasma leuabit.
Namque sacros eciam iunctum discriminat ignes.
Huius item semen cum uino tussibus obstat,
Constringit uentres fluxusque premit mulieris.
'At candens quid agit?' Melli iungatur aqueque:
Hec conseruetur quasi mel decoccio spissa,
Vene uocalis bene reumatismata siccans,
Dans sompnum tussimque premens aluumque cohercens.
'Scis opium quam prestet opem?' Nam, nominis extat
Et fame ingentis. Roseo iungatur oliuo,
Hinc caput ungatur: capitis dolor hiis superatur,
Dant grate sompnum. Si fila croci redolentis

4.13 PAPAVER *P* 28r–28v: Papauer | *S* 77r–77v: De Papauere. Henricus

1 miconius] siconius *S* tridecimus *S* 2 uigens] iungens *S* 3 albet] albus *S* 4 carior est] cariorque *S* 5 opium] oleum *S* capitello *P* 7 siccum] sicli *P* 8 capitello *P* 10 datur] *add.* quod in *et exp. P* 13 mor *S* soporem] *scripsi*, saporem *PS* (*cf. Macer 1053*) 15 faciem] at *add. S* repentem *S* 17 cataplasma] *add.* curabat *et exp. P* 18 curabat *P* 19 cantu] tantu *P* frigora *S* 21 discriminat] discermn*et S* 23 constringet *S* 24 agis *P* *l. 25 om. P* 28 scis opium] cysopium *S* prestet *S* exstat *S* 31 filia crocis *S*

4.13 Poppy, *Papaver somniferum* L.

Miconius stands thirteenth, which Rome calls Poppy,
strong in its powers cold and dry. It possesses three varieties:
this one is white, this flower is red, and that one is yellow.
The white is more precious since they make opium
from its seedpods: having cut the skin, when the seedpods
flow with milky juice, they capture the flowing juice
with spoons, and preserve it dried, suitable for famous medicines.
There are those who grind the seedpods with their juice
and dry the liquid pressed from these together in the sun.
A great power is in the second, yet it's held unequal to the first;
from the red variety they manufacture an oil, both pleasing
and inducing sleep, by grinding the tiny seed.
The third variety grants sleep just like the other two.
If you treat a listless person on the face with an elixir
of any of these, or if he drinks it warm,
it confers a superior sleep, except when death is near.
A plaster made of its ground up leaves
will cure a swollen throat. If the vocal chords are made rough
from drink or food or from singing or eating
or from a cold, this plaster will relieve it,
and in fact, when mixed, it also removes the Holy Fire.
Its seed with wine likewise hinders coughs,
restrains the belly, and forces out a woman's flux.
  'But what does the white one do?' Blend it with honey and water;
let this decoction be kept as thick as honey,
drying well a rheumatism in the vocal cords,
giving sleep, forcing out a cough, and restraining the bowels.
'Do you know what help opium provides?' Yes, it has
a great name and great fame. Add it to oil-of-Rose,
then rub the head with it: these overwhelm a headache
and they agreeably give sleep. If you add threads of odorous Saffron

4.13 PAPAVER / **Poppy** *Macer, 'Papaver', 1037–86*
28–29 Ovid, *Ars amatoria* 2.637; Henry of Huntingdon, *HA* 11.22, 2 (p. 796)

Predictis socies, infunde doloribus auris.
Sume opium, coniunge crocis, cape lac mulieris:
Hiis iunctis calidam sedabis rite podagram
At solum solo sompnum largitur odore.

4.14 GIT

Git cornute, tuos depromit Musa triumphos!
Quatuor aduersis in celum cornibus audes
Tendere, collectis in summam uiribus arcem,
In qua grana locas mirum latura saporem.
Hic in pane sapor panem longe meliorat
Et causa effectum preciosa parat preciosum.

4.15 GAZARA

Gazara uero quid est, namque herba putatur et arbor?
Arbor namque potest herbas imitata uocari
Consimilisque potest herba arboribus reputari.
Quicquid eam reputes, magnos lenire dolores
Interius positos mira uirtute sueuit.
Radicem tritam si uino consociabis
Mox uomitus trahit ingentes morbumque repellit.
Nec tamen hanc facies—nam grandior est medicina—
Ni uideas non posse alias prodesse medelas.

33 summe *P* opium *bis S* crocum *P* 34 rite] recte *P* 35 aut *P*

4.14 GIT *P* 28v: Gith | *S* 64r: De Git. Henricus

Exceptiones (*O* 92v): Git, .iiii. aduersis cornibus elatis, oritur in summo, grana miri saporis habens qui panem ualde meliorat.

1 git] gyth *P* depromat *S* triumfos *P* 2 celum] telum *S* audax *P* 3 tendere] tandem *P* 4 qua] mea *P* 6 et causa *om. P* preciosum] precia *corr. e* precii *P*

4.15 GAZARA *P* 28v: Gazara | *S* 63v–64r: De Gazara. Henricus | *T* 96v: Gazara

Exceptiones (*O* 92v): Gazara arbor et herba putatur. Interiores dolores mire lenit. Radix uino iuncta uomitus ingentes trahit morbumque repellit. Difficilis est tamen medicina.

1 uero *om. P* quid *om. S* herba] barba *S* 4 quidquid *P* 5 uirtuteque *P* 6 radicem . . . consociabis] radicem tritam cum uino iungita potum *T* 7 mox] *add.* ge (?) *P* uomitum *T* morbosque *T* 8 nec] non *S*

to the aforesaid things, pour it into aching ears.
Take opium, mix well with Crocus, and add a woman's milk:
with these united you'll properly settle a fiery gout
but it grants sleep alone by its odour alone.

4.14 Git/Nigella, *Nigella sativa* L.

O horn-bearing Git, the Muse calls forth your triumphs!
You dare to reach towards heaven with your four
opposing peaks, the powers gathered in the highest citadel,
in which you place grains which will grant a marvellous flavour.
In bread this flavour improves the bread by far
and a precious cause brings about a precious effect.

4.15 Knotweed, family *Polygonaceae* L.

But what is Knotweed, since it's reckoned a herb and a tree?
For it can be called a tree which imitates herbs
and it can be considered a herb which is similar to trees.
Whatever you consider it, it is accustomed to soothe
with marvellous virtue great pains found on the inside.
If you will blend the ground root with wine,
it soon forces great vomiting and repels disease.
Yet you should not use this—for the medicine's quite strong—
unless you see that no other cures will avail.

4.14 GIT / **Git** *? Pliny*
1 *Cf.* Pliny 27. 121 5–6 *Cf.* Pliny 19. 167–8

4.15 GAZARA / **Knotweed** *Source unknown*

4.16 PIONIA

Pioniam perhibent calidam siccamque secundo
Esse gradu speciesque duas testatur habere.
Mas maior speciesque minor sit femina dicta:
Maioris radix, quasi palmis longa duabus,
Grossa est ut digitus; radix diuisa minoris
Cernitur in plures radices. Hec sociata
Vino post partum purgare steras bene sueuit,
Vtraque uero fugat scotosim (capitis dolor hic est).
'Quomodo sumetur?' Vino decoccio detur,
At si pionie iungantur amigdala trita
Splen, iecur et renes hiis cum mulsa releuabis;
Sic igitur fluxus alui, sic menstrua sistit.
Vesice stomachoque ualet decoccio pota;
Neffreticos iuuat, infantum sic calculus exit,
Sic iuuat hictericos, at semina pota frequenter
Quas inferre solent pressuras sompnia delent.
Pionie petito ter quinque rubencia grana;
Hiis uino tritis matricis subdito fluxus.
Pionie petito totidem liuencia grana;
Hiis poteris uarios matricum pellere morbos,
At radix pueris prodest suspensa caducis,
Vt Galienus ait, annorum circiter octo.
Conspexit puerum sic conualuisse caducum:
Decidit illa semel, collo disiuncta gerentis,
Decidit ille simul colloque reiuncta iacentis,
Erexit puerum. Galienus uero probare
Rem cupiens, iterum radicem dempsit et ille
Concidit; apposuit rursum, surrexit et ille.
Tanto auctore fuit uis herbe cognita tante,
Et Diascorides cunctis hanc esse caducis
Scripsit si bibitur uel si suspenditur aptam.

4.16 PIONIA *P* 28v–29r: Pionia | *S* 80v: De Pionia. Henricus

1 pyoniam peribent *P* 2 haberi *P* 4 duobus *P* 8 scotasim *S* 9 uino] cocte *S* 10 pyonie *P* iungatur amigdola *S* 11 cum] in *P* releuabit *P* 12 flexus *P* 14–15 neffreticos . . . exit / sic . . . frequenter] neffreticos iuuat hictericos at semina pota frequenter *P* (*as one line*) : neusticticos *S* infantum] *scripsi*, *om. P* : infantulum *S* 17 pyonie *P* quinque] .V. *P* *ll. 18–19 om. S* 19 pionie] *scripsi*, pyonie *P* 23 puer *S* 24 illa *om. S* gerentis] iacentis *P* 25 decidit *corr. e* dedcidit *S* : decedit *P* reuncta recentis *S* 26 puer *S* 27 dempsit] pressit *P* 28 considet *S* rursus *P* 29 autore *P* 30 et Diascorides] ipse Dyascorides *P* cunctis] coniunctis *S*

4.16 Peony, *Paeonia officinalis* L.

They claim that Peony is hot and dry in the second
degree and it is said to have two varieties.
The male is called the larger type and the female the smaller:
the root of the larger is as long as two palms,
as fat as a finger; the root of the smaller is seen to be
divided into many roots. When mixed with wine,
this is well accustomed to purge the cervix after birth,
but either type chases away *scotosis* (this is a headache).
'So how is it taken?' Let a decoction be given with wine,
but if bitter almonds are blended with Peony, you will
relieve the spleen, liver, and kidneys by these in mead;
so it settles diarrhoea in such a way, so also menstrual courses.
A decoction when drunk is good for the bladder and stomach;
it aids nephritics, and thus the stone in infants goes away,
thus it helps the jaundiced, but the seeds drunk frequently
remove the pressures that are apt to bring on dreams.
Seek out three times five red seeds of Peony;
help the flux of the womb with these ground up in wine.
Seek out just as many green seeds of Peony;
with these you can defeat several diseases of the womb.
The root hung from the neck, as Galen says, is beneficial
for boys of about eight years with epilepsy.
He observed that an epileptic boy improved this way:
once the root fell off, separated from the wearer's neck,
he at once fell down, and when it was put on his neck again,
it roused the boy. But Galen, desiring to prove the case,
again pulled the root away and the boy fell down;
he then attached it again, and the boy got up.
The power of so great an herb was discerned by so great an author,
and Dioscorides wrote that this is suitable for all epileptics
if it is drunk or worn suspended from the neck.

4.16 PIONIA / **Peony** *Macer, 'Paeonia', 1605–40*

4.17 AQVILEIA

Quatuor ut constans aquilis 'aquileia' uocatur;
Pulcrior argento sic 'argentilla' uocatur.
Non argentille color est argenteus atqui
Purpura cedit ei. Mire gramen, specie
'Herba puellaris' pulcherima iure uocaris,
Et tribus ex causis: uel quod te forma uenustet,
Vel quia fecundas reddis gustata puellas
Vel quia mansum oris semen meliorat odores.

4.18 VERBENA

'Verbenam' quam Roma uocat 'statillina' grece
Et perysterion yerabotanumque uocatur.
Ex hac componi quidam iussere coronam,
Compositam capiti aptari aptamque ualere
Dixerunt ipsi causa quacumque dolenti.
Si succus tepidus uoluatur in ore medetur
Oris uulneribus, sed idem decoccio prestat;
Ore diu tenta putredo repellitur oris.
Plinius hanc auctor pronunciat esse salubrem
Visceribus, lateris morbo nocuisque querelis
Pectoris et causis iecoris, ualideque mederi
Pulmonum uiciis hanc asserit ille ptysique.
Herba, trahens nomen foliis de mille, iugata
Vetonice necnon uerbene ponderis equi,
Hec in aqua dentur quos calculus anxius angit.
Vtilius nullum (michi crede!) dabis medicamen.

4.17 AQVILEIA *P* 29r: Aquilegia | *S* 41r: De Aquileya. Henricus

Exceptiones (*O* 92v): Quatuor ut constans aquilis 'aquileia' uocatur; purior argento sic 'argentilla' uocatur. Non argentille color est argenteus, at purpura fecundat uel <quia os redo>lens facit.

1 aquileya *P* 2 pulcrior] purior *O* 3 non] nam *P* atqui] at *O* 4 purpara *P* 5 pulcerrima *P* 6 formam *S* 7 gestata *P*

4.18 VERBENA *P* 29r–29v: Verbena | *S* 100r–101r: De Verbena. Henricus

2 peristerion *P* 4–5 compositam ... ualere / dixerunt ... dolenti] apponi capiti causa quacumque dolenti *P* (*written as one line*) 5 quascumque *S* 9 autor *P* 10 lateris ... querelis] lesis morbo lateris nocuisque *S* 12 pulmonis *P* ptisique *S* 13 melle *S* 16 medicinam *S*

4.17 Columbine, *Aquilegia vulgaris* L.

Columbine's called *aquileia* as if similar to four eagles;
more beautiful than silver, it's thus called *argentilla*.
The colour of *argentilla* is not of silver but rather
a purple colour is granted to it. O marvellous herb, most beautiful
in appearance, you are rightly called the 'girl's herb'
for these three reasons: either because appearance makes you beautiful,
or because once eaten you make girls fertile,
or because the seed when eaten improves odours of the mouth.

4.18 Vervain, *Verbena officinalis* L.

The plant which Rome calls Vervain is called in Greek
statillina and *perysterion* and *hierobotanum*.
Some have ordered a chaplet to be woven from it,
and woven to be fitted to the head, and they said
that when fitted it's good against a pain with any cause.
If the warm juice is rolled inside the mouth, it medicates
oral wounds, but a decoction offers the same;
festering of the mouth is repelled by it held in the mouth a while.
The author Pliny announces that this is healthful
for the vitals, a disease of the side, harmful complaints
of the chest, and problems of the liver, and he asserts
that it's a strong cure for vices of the lungs and consumption.
Let the herb which takes its name from a thousand leaves,
when added to Betony and to Vervain in equal weight,
be given in water to those whom the vexing stone vexes.
You'll give no more useful medicine, believe me!

4.17 AQVILEIA / **Columbine** *Original*
2 Marbode of Rennes, *Liber decem capitulorum* c. 4, 35 (ed. Leotta and Crimi, 42)

4.18 VERBENA / **Vervain** *Macer, 'Verbena', 1859–1902*
9–12 *Cf.* Pliny 26. 37–8 13 *Cf.* Quintus Serenus 693, 813 15 Virgil, *Aeneid* 10. 89

Talia per partes. Quid toto corpore dicam?
Herba recens uulnus conglutinat addita, trita
Mitigat hictericos cum uino pota dolores;
Pestiferos uino trita et superaddita curat
Morsus (bis binis si sit renouata diebus)
Quartanasque febres foliis cum quatuor ipse
Si potentur aque cum tot radicibus aufert,
Ternas uero febres ternis radicibus atque
Ternis cum foliis nondum se febre mouente
Moreque buglosse (nisi nolis credere scriptis)
Conuiuas hilares inter conuiuia reddit.
Hanc herbam gestans, 'Quid agis?,' si querat ab egro,
Si languens bene respondet, tibi spes bona sistit;
Si male, spes absit nam mortis signa patescunt.
Plinius hanc laudare magos nimis asserit herbam
Nam perhibent cunctos ipsam disperdere morbos.
Vnctus ea quorum cupies sis nactus amores;
Quod pociare petas, quodcumque petas pocieris.
Sed licet hec Natura potens dare pluraque possit,
Non, nisi temptarim quod celem, credere possim.

4.19 MEV

Meu quoque diureticum dicunt. Quas res tibi dicam
Diureticas queris? Locium quecumque lacescunt.
Hec et nefreticos innato grata calore,
Tam uirtute ingens quam pauper nomine, curat.
Huius Alexander uires docet et Galienus
Herbarumque michi ne cedat gloria soli,
Has ab Alexandro perquiras et Galieno.

18 uulnus] nullus *S* 19 mitigat] libet *S* hyctericos *S* potata *P* 20 curat] morsus *S* 21 morsus] mordet *S* binis] biniis *corr. e* binos *P* 23 potantur *P* aqua *S* aufert] atque *P* *l. 24 om. P* 26 more *P* boglosse *S* 27 hylares *S* conuiua *S* 29 bona] bene *P* sistit] subdit *S* 30 patescunt *post corr. P*] fatescunt *PS* 33 capies *P* sic *S* 34 pociare] ponare *S* 35 sed] set *S* hec *om. P* 36 non] nec *S* quod] quid *P*

4.19 MEV *P* 29v–30r: Meu | *S* 70v: De Meu. Henricus

Exceptiones (*O* 92v): Meu quoque diureticum est. Diuretica dicunt queque locium lacessent. Neufreticos calore suo curat.

1 dureticum *S* 2 querit *P* locum *S* quocumque lacescit *P* 3 hoc *S* nefreneticos *P* innata *S* colore *S* 5 huius] hoc *S* Alexander] *scripsi*, Allexander *P* : Alexandrum *S* 7 Allexandro *P*

So much for the parts. What can I say for the entire body?
The fresh herb when applied binds up wounds, when ground
and drunk with wine it soothes the pains of jaundice,
when ground with wine and applied it cures
pestilential bites (if it's replaced every four days),
and it takes away quartan fevers if water
is drunk with four leaves and as many roots.
But it takes away tertian fevers with three roots
and three leaves so long as the fever does not leave,
and just like Ox-Tongue (unless you refuse to believe the books)
it renders companions at their banquets happy.
If one holding this herb inquires of a patient, 'How are you doing?',
and if the invalid responds well, good hope is prepared for you;
if poorly, hope may be lost for the signs of death are clear.
Pliny claims that magicians greatly praise this herb
for they relate that it destroys all diseases.
Anointed with it, you can attain the embraces of those whom you desire;
seek what you would acquire, and acquire whatever you seek.
Although mighty Nature could give these things and more,
I couldn't believe it, unless I should seek what is kept in the dark.

4.19 Spignel, *Meum athamanticum* Jacq.

They also say that Spignel is diuretic. Do you ask what things
I name as diuretic for you? Anything that moves the urine.
This is pleasing with an innate heat and cures the nephritic,
as great in virtue as it is poor in name.
Alexander and Galen teach its powers
and lest the glory of herbs be granted to me alone,
ask Alexander and Galen about them.

31–34 *Cf.* Pliny 25. 106 34 Ovid, *Met.* 7. 683 35 *Cf.* Horace, *Satires* 2. 1. 51; Boethius, *De cons. phil.* 3 met. 2, 1–2 36 *Cf.* Ovid, *Ex Ponto* 2. 4. 5

4.19 MEV / **Spignel** *Source unknown*
1 *Cf.* Pliny 20. 253

4.20 CIPERVS

Diureticum peribent ciperum siccumque secundo
Feruentemque gradu. Puluis ciperi ualet oris
Vlceribus; stomachum confortat debilitatum.
Petras confringit, iuuat ydropicos satis haustum,
Namque per urinas humores purgat aquosos.
Dixit Apollodorus consumi posse lienem
Ex ciperi fumo si sepius ore trahatur.
Asserit hic idem, quod pellere possit abortum
Si mulier foueatur aqua qua coxerit ipsum.
Dixit Appolodorus, fumo si fumiget eius
Se sanus, fiet leuior uel firmior idem.
Alarum uiciis succus commixtus oliuo
Subuenit; humores desiccat sepius haustus,
Cui trito ualidum si coniungatur acetum
Vlcera que serpunt, necnon conbusta, iuuari.
At ciperi solus puluis melliue coherens
Vlcera sordida, uulnera putrida purgat inherens.

4.21 VALERIANA

Viginti uisis, ualidis tibi ualeriana
Frondibus assurgit que strictum corpus obumbrans;
Verticibus latis crispata, cacumine magno
Semina parua locat. Dicamus ualeriana

4.20 CIPERVS *P* 30r: Cipperus | *S* 52v–53r: De Cipero. Henricus

1 ciperu *corr. e* ciperum *S* succumque *S* 3 conformat *P* debilitatum] debile potum *S* 4 petram constringit *P* 6 dicit *S* consummi *P* lienum *P* 7 ex ciperi fumo] illius fumus *P* trahitur *P* 8 asserit . . . abortum] dicit Appollodorus ciperui quod pellat abortum *S* 10 dicit *S* si fumiget] subfumiget *S* eius] illo *P* 11 fiet] fit *S* 12 alacrum *S* uiciis succus *transp. P* olyuo *P* 13 haustum *S* 14 tritum *P*

4.21 VALERIANA *P* 30r–30v: Valeriana | *S* 97v–98r: De Valeriana. Henricus | *T* 106r–106v: Valeriana

Exceptiones (*O* 92v): Valeriana ualidis assurgit frondibus que strictum corpus obumbrans uerticibus latis crispata cacumine paruo semina parua locat. Valeriana multa ualet. In uino trita et bibita febrem acutam soluit. Preterea guttam et magnos sanat liuores superaddita.

1 uisis] uisi *S*

4.20 Cyperus, *Cyperus longus* L.

They relate that Cyperus is diuretic and hot and dry
in the second degree. The powder of Cyperus is good
for ulcers of the mouth and it soothes a weakened stomach.
It breaks up stones and, when drunk enough, aids the dropsical,
for it purges watery humours through the urine.
Apollodorus said that spleen can be consumed
by Cyperus smoke if it is often inhaled through the mouth.
The same author also asserts that it can expel a foetus
if a woman foments herself with the water in which it cooked.
Apollodorus said, if a healthy man should fumigate himself
with the smoke of Cyperus, he'll become more nimble or robust.
The juice, when mixed with olive oil, assists with vices
of the armpits; when drunk it often dries out humours,
and if strong vinegar is mixed with this, when ground,
he said that ulcers that spread, as well as burns, are helped.
But the powder of Cyperus, alone or mixed with honey,
purges rotting ulcers and putrid wounds by sticking in them.

4.21 Valerian, *Valeriana officinalis* L.

Having seen twenty, Valerian rises up before you,
overshadowing with strong branches and straight body;
curly in its spacious crowns, it places tiny seeds
inside a mighty summit. Let us call that herb Valerian

4.20 CIPERVS / **Cyperus** *Macer, 'Cyperus', 1585–1604*

4.21 VALERIANA / **Valerian** *Source unknown*

Que ualeat, nam multa ualet! Tere, ponito tritam
In uino, positam preme, compressam bibe, solues
Hac bibita febrem que corpora soluit acute.
Preterea seuam leni medicamine guttam
Et magnos paruo liuores tempore sanat
Si superaddatur morbis. † Hec (morbus et hostis) †
Tam facili cura mala rite grauissima curat.
Ergo neget liuor te, ualeriana, ualere
Et nichil impendat medicis quod amara rependit.

4.22 BORAGVM

Boragum nostri quam 'mellisoffilos' Achiui
Dicunt. Hec apibus cunctis est gracior herbis,
Cui si lac iungas et earum uasa perungas
Non fugient: remanere solent per eam fugientes.
Luminibus prodest cum melle, ut Plinius inquit,
Mansa diu dentis cladem reparat comedentis,
Cuius si uiridis decoccio rite bibatur
Asmaticos, dissintericos iuuat et cyliacos
Antiquos; iuuat emptoycos ortobnoicosque.
Cum sale trita solet uiciis succurrere fedis.
Femina sanatur decocto cum sale succo;
Illius cocte decoccio menstrua purgat,
Et sic fotorum morbos leuat articulorum.
Herba canis morsus superaddita cum sale curat
Et fugit hoc potu; fugit hec inflacio potu.
Trita solet ueteres compescere cum sale strumas.

5 quod *S* tere *om. T* 7 febres que corbora soluunt *P* acutam *ST* 8 seuam] ceuam *S* : senem *T* 10 morbis] morbo *T* morbus] morbis *corr. e* mobis *T* 13 nichil impendat] *scripsi*, nichil in pendat *P* : nichili pendat *S* amara] amata *S*

4.22 BORAGVM *P* 30v: Melissa | *S* 47r: De Borago. Henricus

1 boragum] pan rogum *P* quam *om. P* melissofillos *P* 2 hec] hoc *S* herbis *corr. ex* erbi (?) *et add.* herbis *in mg. P* 6 mansa] causa *S* commedentis *S* 8 asmatericos *P* yliacos *S* 9 anticos *S* emptoycos] *add.* antiquos *P* : et yliacos antiquos *S* ortobnoycosque *P* 10 fedis] sedis *S* 11 decocte *S* 12 cocte] et fote (?) *P* 13 fetorum *S* 14 erba *P* superaddita] fraudita *S* 15 potu²] *scripsi*, potum *P* : furtu *S*

which is good, for it is very good! Grind it, place it ground
in wine, press it placed, drink it pressed, and with this drunk
you will dissolve the fever that dissolves bodies sharply.
Moreover, this gentle medicine cleans the savage gout
and large bruises in a small amount of time
if it's applied to these diseases. By such an easy remedy
it justly cures these gravest evils, the disease and the enemy.
Therefore envy denies that you, Valerian, are strong
and that which returns bitterness pays out nothing to the doctors.

4.22 Balm, *Melissa officinalis* L.

Our people call the herb Balm which the Greeks
call *mellisophilos*. It's more pleasing to bees than any other herb,
and if you add milk to it and anoint their hives
they will not flee: those fleeing are apt to stay because of it.
With honey it is beneficial for the eyes, as Pliny says;
when chewed a while it repairs decay of the eater's teeth,
and if a decoction of fresh Balm is drunk regularly
it helps those with asthma, dysentery, and persistent coeliac disease;
it also helps blood-spitters and those with orthopnea.
When ground with salt it's apt to aid foul vices.
A woman is cleaned by the juice cooked down with salt;
a decoction of this, when cooked, purges menstrual courses,
and in such a way relieves diseases of joints as a poultice.
The herb, applied with salt, cures the bite of a dog
and it flees from this in a drink; the swelling flees from this drink.
When ground with salt it's apt to curb old scrofulous sores.

12 Marbode, *De ornamentis verborum* III, 4 (ed. Leotta and Crimi, 4)

4.22 BORAGVM / **Balm** *Macer, 'Barrocus', 1641–63*
5 *Cf.* Pliny 21. 150

Auxilium presens apium fert ictibus herba
Cuspide si tangat mox istius ictus acerba.
Sic morsus quos uespa mouet uel aranea curat.

4.23 ARISTOLOGIA

Aristologie tres sunt, hec namque rotunda est,
Hec uero longe radicis, tercia grece
Nomen habet 'clematis' que longa est, apta medele:
Apcior est clematis, aptissima uero rotunda.
Omnes uim siccam pariter calidamque ministrant;
Primo prima gradu uiget atque secunda secundo.
Hanc et yrim melli si dulci iungis amaram,
Gingiuas ungas, dentes putredine mundas.
Hec in aqua splen duratum laterisque dolorem,
Asmaticos et pleureticos si frigida curat;
Hec in aqua uentris fertur lenire dolorem;
Hec in aqua diram sedat potata podagram;
Hec in aqua febres mire compescere fertur;
Hec in aqua spasmis super omnia subuenit hausta;
Hec in aqua morbum curat potata caducum;
Hac in aqua leuior sic fit paraliticus arens.
Cum uino morsus curat potata malignos;
Cum uino sumptis solet opungnare uenenis;
Cum uino tardas educit sumpta secundas;
Cum uino nimios singultus sedat et aufert;
Cum pipere et mirra putredine purgat ab omni.
Fistula curatur sancte radicibus herbe
Si bene purgatis loca morbi concaua, farcis.

17 presens] et *add. P* apum *P* ictibus] morsibus *P* erba *P* 18 suspide *S* istius] ictus *S* 19 si *S* uespera *S* arena *S*

4.23 ARISTOLOGIA *P* 30v–31r: Aristologia | *S* 42r–42v: De Aristologia. Henricus
1 aristologiie 3s *P* rotunda] *scripsi*, rotunde *PS* est *om. P* 3 medele] est *add. P* 5 omnes *corr. ex* opmnes *S* uim] inde *S* calidaque *S* 6 prima primo *S* 7 dulcis *S* amaram] *scripsi*, amarem *P* : amaris *S* 8 unguas *S* *ll.* 9–10 *om. P* 10 frigida] *scripsi*, frigora *S* 11 hec] hoc *S* 13 compes *S* 14 spasmis] spacius *S* subuenit *om. S* 16 hac] *scripsi*, hec *PS* sic fit] *scripsi* (*cf. Macer* 1420), sit agit *PS* 17–18 cum ... malignos / cum ... uenenis] cum uino morsus sumptis solet appugnare uenenis *S* (*as one line*) 18 appungnare *S* 20 sedat] linit *S* 21 pipere] uino *P* omni] ortum *S* 23 purgatis] curatis *S* *ll.* 29–30 *om. S*

The herb brings ready aid to bee stings
if it quickly touches the sting with its bitter point.
In such a way it cures the bites which wasps or spiders cause.

4.23 Birthwort/Dutchman's Pipe, genus *Aristolochiaceae* L.

The Birthworts are three, for this one is round,
but this one has a long root, and the third has the name
clematis in Greek, which is long and good for medicine:
clematis is quite suitable, but the round is best of all.
All of them equally provide dry and heating powers;
the first is strong in the first degree, the second in the second.
If you blend this bitter plant and Iris with honey sweet
and smear it on the gums, you'll clean the teeth of rottenness.
This herb in water, if it's cold, cures a hardened spleen,
a pain of the side, asthmatics and pleuritics,
in water it is said to soften a stomach pain,
imbibed in water it allays the wicked gout,
in water it's said to restrain fevers in an amazing way,
when taken in water it aids spasms better than any other,
when drunk in water it cures the falling disease,
by this in water a thirsty paralytic is thus made lighter.
When drunk with wine it cures malignant bites,
with wine it's apt to conquer swallowed poisons,
if drunk with wine it removes a delayed afterbirth,
with wine it settles and removes excessive hiccoughs,
and with Myrrh and Pepper it purges every putrefaction.
A fistula is cured by the roots of this holy herb
if you purge it well and fill the vice's hollow places.

4.23 ARISTOLOGIA / **Birthwort** *Macer, 'Aristolochia', 1395–1436*

Pisces trita necat (sed mixta calce) rotunda,
Hanc ideo terrestre patres dixere uenenum.
At longam formare mares cum carne bouina
Vulue post coitum subiectam Plinus inquit.
Cetera longa tibi patrat simul atque rotunda,
Longa tamen uirtute nequit certare rotunde,
Vnde ferunt quod si desit quandoque rotunda
Tantundem longe sumas tibi dimidiumque.
Infantes fumo laudabilis exhilarantur;
Demonium clare fumus fugat et fugit herbe.

4.24 PALMA CHRISTI

Quod solet 'herba fera' uel 'palma Dei' uocitari
Formosum gramen formoso nomine uulgus
Sancte Marie solet appellare sigillum.
Nomen habet dignum quia fulget pulcra statura,
Pulcrior effigie, pulcerrima uero colore.
Nomen habet dignum quoniam dulcedine fructus
Eximia et modica superat dulcissima gustu.
Hec et pigmentis fertur gratissima gratis
Ni figmenta <ferant> artem querentibus illam
Qui pigmenta parant. Eius, uenerabile gramen,
Nomen habes, que sola parit sine patre patremque
Cuius (nil timidus) preconia transeo, quippe
Que parit et mater patris <est> et filia, namque
Qui paritur matris pater est et filius, ergo
Virgo parens, generans Deus est et homo generatus,
Progenies matris sine patre, prius sine matre,
Cuius odos premit omnimodos et uincit odores
Et superat quosquos—reserat uer dapsile—flores.

30 rotunda] *scripsi*, rotunde *P* 31 sumas tibi] tibi summas *P* 32 infantes] in fauces *P* exhilaratur *S* 33 fugit] fuget *S*

4.24 PALMA CHRISTI *P* 31r–31v: Palma Christi | [not in *S*] | *T* 102r–102v (*lines 1–3, 8*): Palma Christi uel Dei

Exceptiones (*O* 92v): Herba fera uel palma a uulgo Sancte Marie sigillum appellatur, merito precellit statura, magis effigie magisque colore, odore uero alios uincit odores. Hec pigmentis gratissima, gustu dulcissima. Venerem eciam cohercet.

1 quod] que *T* 8 pingmentis *T* fertur] herba *T* 9 ferant] *scripsi*, *om. P* (*cf.* 2.15, 9 *supra*) 13 est *om. P* 16 prius] patris *corr. e* prus (?) *P*

The round variety, ground up and mixed with chalk, kills fish,
therefore the elders used to call this plant 'land poison.'
But Pliny says the long variety creates male children
if inserted, mixed with beef, into the womb after intercourse.
The long variety, and the round as well, do other things for you,
yet the long cannot contend with the round's ability,
for which reason they say that if you ever lack the round,
take for yourself the same amount of the long and half again.
Infants are gladdened by the smoke of this praiseworthy herb;
the smoke of this famous herb scares a demon away and it flees.

4.24 St Mary's Seal (Solomon's Seal), *Polygonatum multiflorum* L.

The common people like to call this beautiful herb,
which is often labelled 'wild herb' or 'Palm of God,'
by the beautiful name of St Mary's Seal.
It has a worthy name since it gleams with noble form,
quite beautiful in shape, but most beautiful in colour.
It has a worthy name since the fruit, with a sweetness
both extraordinary and moderate, excels with sweetest taste.
This is also deemed most pleasing of all in pleasing paints,
if those who produce the dyes aren't telling lies
to those who seek their skill! O venerable seed, you have
the name of her who alone, without a father, begot the father
whose praises I (unfearful) am passing over. To be sure,
she who gave birth is both mother of the father and daughter,
for He who was begotten is father of the mother and her son,
therefore a virgin mother, the generating God and generated man,
progeny of a mother without father, first without a mother.
Its odour surpasses and excels all kinds of other odours
and shows up any flowers, as luxuriant spring reveals.

24 *Cf.* Pliny 25. 98 26–27 Pliny 25. 97–8

4.24 PALMA CHRISTI / **St Mary's Seal** *Original*

11–16 *Cf.* Augustine, Sermon 217, c. 1 (ed. Fuertes Lanero) 15 Sedulius, *Carmen Paschale* 1. 323

4.25 SAVINA

Vltima procedit, que multas uiribus herbas
Precedit, sauina uirens siccansque calensque
Tercius huic gradus est. Hanc dicunt 'brateon' Argi.
Nominis hec noti uerbellis corpus obumbrans
Predurum duris, foliis densata pusillis,
Grande cacumen habet quod uix spiramina uenti,
Vix radius solis, uix unda sonis penetrabunt.
Hec tactu modico nimios dispergit odores
Et Bachum gustu predulcem reddit amaro.
Huius iure nouo uertigo uetusta lauetur
Herbaque tymporibus et fronti cocta ligetur.
At mel sauine si dulce iugatur acerbe
Antracas uincit, bona que plebs ulcera dicit;
Sic humens uulnus, sic sordens expiat ulcus.
Ipsa facit faciem cerotis mixta nitentem;
Frigore nata graui leni feruore coartat.
Menstrua deducens, mulieribus apta probatur,
Apta probatur item tumido que protrahat aluo
Effetos fetus, quod agit si subdita fiat
Matrici matris uel pota frequenter lyeo.
Cinnama si desint sauine ponere duplum
Congnita non notis iubet Oribasius equans.

4 <EPILOGVS I. PALMES ET LACTERIDIS>

Tedia ni tulerint cernenti gramina centum,
Iam theatrum pete, sed modicum, medio quod in orto
Suspicies. Baiula subnixus arundine palmes,

4.25 SAVINA *P* 31v: Sauina | [not in *S*]
19 effetos] *scripsi*, effectos *P* 20 matrici] *scripsi*, matricis *P* pota frequenter] *scripsi* (*cf. Macer 498*), leuiter pota *P* 21 cinnama] *scripsi*, cinama *P* ponere] *scripsi*, pondere *P* 22 iubet Oribasius] *scripsi*, iubetque Orbasius *P*

---

4 <EPILOGVS I. PALMES ET LACTERIDIS> *P* 31v–32r: [no title] *First edited by Rigg*, 275–6.
Exceptiones (*O* 92v): Lactea lacteridis qua nulla uirentior herba est uentrem soluit acute.
1 tulerint] *add.* que or *et. canc. P* 3 suspicies] *Rigg*, suspicis hic *P*

4.25 Juniper, *Juniperus sabina* L.

The final herb, which excels many herbs in powers,
steps forth, green Juniper. Drying and heating,
its degree is third. The Greeks call this *brateos*.
This plant of famous name, overshadowing a very hard body
with hard little whips, dense with tiny leaves,
has a lofty top which scarcely gusts of wind,
scarcely rays of sun, and scarcely waves will penetrate with sound.
This, at the lightest touch, disperses mighty odours
and makes a wine most sweet with its bitter taste.
Let a chronic vertigo be washed with its fresh juice
and tie the cooked herb to the temples and the brow.
But if sweet honey is added to bitter Juniper
it conquers carbuncles, which the people call 'good ulcers';
in such a way it resolves a humid wound or a vile ulcer.
When mixed in wax salves, it causes a face to glow;
born from heavy cold, it restricts with a gentle heat.
It's proven good for women, bringing out the menstrual courses,
and it's also proven useful in that it draws a dead foetus
out from a swollen belly, which it does if put into
the mother's womb as a suppository or often drunk with wine.
Oribasius, balancing the known with the unknown,
orders you to take two parts of Juniper if Cinnamon is lacking.

4 Epilogue 1
1) Vine, *Vitis vinifera* L.
2) Squirting Cucumber, *Ecballium elaterium* A. Rich.

If the one hundred herbs do not already bore the viewer,
now seek out the theatre, though small, which you'll admire
in the middle of the garden. A Vine, propped up by a supporting stake,

4.25 SAVINA / **Juniper** *Macer, 'Sabina', 492–506*
6 *Cf.* Ovid, *Met.* 1.552

---

4 <EPILOGVS I. PALMES ET LACTERIDIS> / **Epilogue 1** *Source unknown*

Circumquaque situs summoque cacumine tandem
Pulcre contiguus, dedit ut sint frondea tecta
Porticus et uitis. Cancella zaphirea dicam
Aut galeam ueris, nam uernus palmes odorans
Condit eos, uarii quos stipant undique flores?
Hos inter uolitat, numidarum nube uagantum,
Lactea lacteridis, que semine fertur aeno,
Lactea lacteridis, qua nulla inmicior herba,
Lactea lacteridis, que uentrem soluit acute.
Rarescente die, gelidos iam promouet ortus
Vesperus et fessos requiei dedicat artus.

4 <EPILOGVS 2>

Hec super herbarum michi laude ferebat Apollo,
Nec puduit uatis, nec te Normannia bellis,
Rex Henrice, tenet, nec enim liuor probitatem,
Optima corrodens, tibi deserit incomitatam,
Sed te qui rodunt dentes molasque retundunt,
Dumque premunt gratis, te uix dignante, premuntur.
At ne uana putes nos hic commenta tulisse,
Autores si uis istorum noscere, scripsi
Quod Phebus Pheboque satus, quod Olympius autor,
Quod Themeson, quod Apollodorus cecinere, Sorores,
Siue quod excellens Ypocras, diuinitus eger,
Quod Prodymus, quod Crisipus, et quod Plinius ingens,
Quod memorat Iustus, quod diuinat Galienus,
Et quod Xenocrates quem philosophia uenustat,
Quod Catho, Pittagoras, Palladius asseruere,
Quod Stephanus, quod melliti Mellicius oris,

4 situs *corr. e* sitis *P* 6 uitis] *Rigg*, uita *P* zaphireaus *P* 7 nam] *conieci*, que *P, Rigg* 8 uarii *corr. e* uary *P* stipant] *Winterbottom*, spicant *P, Rigg* 9 nube] *Rigg*, iube *P* 10 aeno] *Rigg*, et eneo *P* 11 qua] *Rigg*, que *P* inmicior] *Rigg*, mencior *P*

---

4 <EPILOGVS 2> P 32r: [no title] *First edited by Rigg*, 277–9.

1 hec] *Rigg*, nec *P* Apollo] *scripsi*, appollo *P* 3 Henrice] *Rigg*, enrice *corr. ex* enridere *P* (Henricus *in mg.*) 7 commenta] *Rigg*, commensa *P* 8 si uis] *Rigg*, que uelis *P* 10 Themeson] *Rigg*, temeseon *P* 13 dyuinat *P* 16 quod] *Rigg*, qud *P*

growing all around, and finally touching prettily at the highest peak,
has caused the portico and Vine to become
a leafy ceiling. Should I call it a sapphire lattice
or the helmet of spring, for the perfumed Vine of spring
conceals those whom varied flowers surround on all sides?
Among these is flying, with a cloud of wandering nomads,
milky Caper Spurge, which is begotten from a bronze seed,
milky Caper Spurge, than which no herb is more ungentle,
milky Caper Spurge, which dissolves the stomach sharply.
While daylight grows scarce, the evening now stirs
the start of cold and gives up these tired bones to sleep.

4 Epilogue 2

Apollo brought these poems to me on the praise of herbs,
and the poet was not ashamed; nor does Normandy
hold you in wars, King Henry, nor indeed does envy,
which gnaws the best, leave your prowess unaccompanied,
but those who bite you blunt their teeth and molars,
and while they freely oppress, they're oppressed (you scarcely notice).
But lest you think that we have brought here falsehoods,
if you wish to learn their authors, I have written
what was sung by Phoebus, Phoebus's son, by Olympius the author,
by Themison, by Apollodorus, by the Sisters,
or what was sung by eminent Hippocrates, divinely sick,
by Prodymus, Chrysippus too, and by the mighty Pliny,
what Justus mentions, what Galen has foretold,
and what Xenocrates, whom philosophy adorns,
what Cato, Pythagoras, and Palladius asserted,
what Stephen, what Mellitius of the honeyed mouth,

5 *Cf.* Virgil, *Georgica* 4. 61–2 13–14 *Cf.* Ovid, *Ibis* 11; *cf.* Pseudo-Virgil, *Culex* 204–205 (ed. Fairclough); Strabo 392

---

4 <EPILOGVS 2> / Epilogue 2 *Original*

9–20 Pseudo-Dioscorides, 'Quod natum Phoebus docuit' (in Marcellus Empiricus, ed. Niedermann and Liechtenhan, 2. 624–7)

Asclepiusque, pater medicine, splendidus autor,
Quod Dyascorides, quod Philo, quod Menetamus,
Quod Macer nitidus, Macrique pedissequa Stabus,
Nota quod ignotis iubet Oribasius equans
Siue alii quos fama uirens florente corona
Lucescente manu caua circum tympora cinxit.

17 splendidus] *Rigg*, spendidus *P*   20 orbasius *P*

and Asclepius, father of medicine, a splendid author,
what Dioscorides, what Philo, what Menemachus,
what polished Macer, and Macer's follower Strabo,
what Oribasius orders, matching the known to the unknown,
or what others teach, whom fame, green with a flowering crown,
has girt with shining hand around their hollow temples.

21–22 *Cf.* Ovid, *Met.* 2. 27; Virgil, *Aeneid* 9. 808

5 <PROLOGVS LIBRI QVINTI>

O tibi si placeant nostrorum carmina florum,
Aut saltem nisi displiceant, plasmator eorum,
Indefectiuis paradysum floribus ornans,
Cui rosa martirii, cui lilia uirginitatis,
Cui uiole mitis bene sunt redolencia mentis,
Vita beata, uigor uite, medicina uigoris,
Principium rerum, uegetacio, finis earum,
Cui, ludens Veneremque fugans et gramina plantans,
Ter nitui, quarto quadratum texo libellum,
In quo uulgares recito ter quatuor herbas,
Tot species, totidem gemmas totidemque lapillos,
Nec postrema duo medicamentis aliena
Iudico, ni uatem Phebus deludit Apollo.
Hic michi florigeris ter cinxit tympora sertis:
'Nunc magis ut deceat, hiis gemmas insero,' dixit,
'Gemmas preclaris interpellabo lapillis:
Quantus splendor inest predictis, tanta potestas.
Serta decora gerens, pro sceptro dextra tenebit
Diuinas, quas uulgus habet nec iudicat, herbas.
Que magis ut placeant, Orientis aromata iungam:
Talia serta meis et talia sceptra ministro.'

5 <PROLOGVS LIBRI QVINTI> P 32v: [no title] *First edited by Rigg, 277–9.*
8 cui] *Rigg*, qui *P* 9 ter nitui] *P*, seruitui *Rigg* 10 recito] *Rigg*, renito *P* 13 deludit] *Rigg*, diludit *P* 14 ter *corr. ex* terer *P* 16 interpellabo] *Rigg*, intercellabo *P* 20 ut] *Rigg*, nec *P*

5 Prologue of the Fifth Book

O, if the songs of our flowers are pleasing to You,
or if, at any rate, they don't displease You, their creator,
who decorated Paradise with unfailing flowers, You,
to whom the Rose of martyrdom, to whom the Lilies of virginity,
to whom the Violets of a gentle mind smell so sweet, You,
a happy life, the force of life, and medicine of the force,
the beginning of things, their growth, and their end, You,
for whom I strove three times, playing with, and fleeing Venus,
and planting herbs, and for a fourth I've woven a squared book,
in which I recite three times four of the common herbs,
as many spices, and as many gems and stones.
(I do not judge the last two foreign to medicine,
nor does Phoebus Apollo play his poet false.)
He bound my temples thrice with flowering garlands:
'So it may be more pleasing now,' he said, 'I'll insert gems in these,
and I'll intersperse the gems with precious stones:
how much splendour, and what great power, lies in these!
Your right hand, bearing beautiful garlands for a sceptre,
will hold godlike herbs, which the people have and do not understand.
And that they may be more pleasing, I shall add aromas of the East:
Such garlands I provide my servants and such sceptres too.'

5 <PROLOGVS LIBRI QVINTI> / **Prologue of the Fifth Book** *Original*
1–2 Pseudo-Ovid, *De medicamine aurium* 1–2 (ed. Lenz) 2 *Cf.* Bernardus Claravallensis, *Tractatus de gradibus humilitatis et superbiae* 3. 12 (PL 182. 948) 4–5 *Cf.* Ovid, *Ars amatoria* 2. 115–16; Isidore, *Etym.* 17. 9. 17–19; Bernard of Cluny, *De contemptu mundi* 1. 177 (ed. Pepin, 22); Alexander Neckham, *De laudibus divinae sapientiae* 5. 105–106 (ed. Wright, 442) 7 Henry of Huntingdon, *HA*, Prologue (p. 6); *Anglicanus ortus*, Prose Prologue, line 1 9 Henry of Huntingdon, *De contemptu mundi* (*HA* 618) 14 *Cf.* Statius, *Achilleid* 1. 611 15–17 Henry of Huntingdon, *De gemmis* (ed. Black) 18 Henry of Huntingdon, *HA* 10. 40, 13–14 (p. 776)

5.1.1 PLANTAGO

Omnipotens tibi perpetuos Natura uigores
Contribuens, plantago, solo plantauit in omni
Communique bono. Non urbs, non uicus egenus,
Querentique leuis occurrit callibus ipsis.
Huius sunt gemine species: est altera maior,
Altera uero minor que 'lanceolata' uocatur.
Vtraque magna uiget, magne uires utriusque,
Que tamen est maior precii maioris habetur.
Hanc 'arnoglossam' quam quasi lingua sit agni
Grecia docta uocat signum rimata figure.
Tercius huic gradus est in ui sicca frigidaque.
Pellitur ex oculis succo plantaginis unctis
Et tumor et feruor; sedatur hoc dolor auris.
Hinc lane succum coniungas: ulcera sanat
Que faciem circa nares et lumina turpant;
Hoc cathaplasma nouem debes reparare diebus.
Ore diu tentus iuuat omnia uulnera succus;
Dentibus attrita gingiuas sanguine plenas
Et tumidas reprimit dentisque doloribus obstat
Scrofaque non oritur collo gestantibus illam,
Iam uero natam superaddito cum sale curat.
Fert emoptoicis (qui uomunt rite cruorem)
Per se subsidium, melius si iungis acetum.
Sic bibitus prodest ptisicis, si uero per anum
Inicias fluxum stringit dissintericorum,
Vel si sicut olus coquis hanc et sal et acetum
Vel si predictis lens sit commixta coquendo
Et dissintericos melius iuuat et ciliacos.
Prodest predictis eius decoccio causis
Vel semen potum cum uino, sic quoque prodest
Vesice si potetur renumque dolori;
Vesice quoque cum passo succus ualet eius.
Si succo tepido uentrem foueas dolor exit;

5.1.1 PLANTAGO *D* 192r: De Plantagine (*lines 57–64*) | *P* 32v–33v: Plantago, Lanceolata, Arnoglossa

2 plantago *corr. e* plantabo *P* 3 egenus] *scripsi*, egesat *P* 13 tumor] *scripsi* (*cf. Macer* 225), timor *P* 17 omnia] *scripsi*, omnis *P* 21 yam *P* 28 siliacos *corr. e* ciliacos *P* 30 semen *corr. e* semel *P*

5.1.1 Plantain:
1) Greater Plantain, *Plantago major* L.
2) Ribwort Plantain, *Plantago lanceolata* L.

All-powerful Nature, who bestowed perpetual strength
on you, Plantain, planted you in every soil
and for the common good. Neither city nor town is lacking
and, easy to find for the seeker, it grows in the very roads.
There are two varieties, for one is Greater,
but the other smaller, which is labelled Ribwort.
Each is great and strong, great the powers of each,
yet that which is larger is worth a higher price.
Learned Greece, appropriating name to shape,
calls this *arnoglossa*, as if it were 'lamb's tongue'.
Its degree is third in a dry and cooling power.
Both swelling and burning are beaten from eyes, when they're
anointed with the juice of Plantain, and an earache is soothed by this.
Add the juice of this to wool: it cleans the ulcers
which befoul the face around the nose and eyes;
you ought to let this plaster work for nine whole days.
The juice held in the mouth a while helps all wounds,
and ground up with the teeth it restrains gums which flow
and are swollen with blood, and stops pains of the teeth,
nor does scrofula affect those wearing it from the neck,
but when applied with salt it cures it once it's formed.
It brings to the haemoptic (those who regularly vomit blood)
relief all by itself, and better still if you add vinegar.
When drunk like this it's good for consumptives, but if injected
through the anus it restrains the flux of dysentery,
or if you cook it like a vegetable with vinegar and salt,
or if lentils are mixed well with the said ingredients by cooking,
it helps the dysenteric even more, and those with troubled bowels.
A decoction of Plantain helps the aforesaid cases
or the seed when drunk with wine, so also is it good
for the bladder and for kidney pains if it is drunk;
its juice, with raisin wine, is beneficial for the bladder.
Pain departs if you foment the belly with its warm juice;

5.1.1 PLANTAGO / **Plantain** *Macer, 'Plantago', 196–266*

Potatum duras depellit sperma secundas;
Matricis fluxus cum lana ius iuuat eius.
Si porcina uetus anxugia consocietur,
Sic tumefacta nimis quamuis durissima sedat;
Parotidas uulnusque recens iuuat hoc cataplasma.
Acri cum uino superaddita, trita, iuuabit
Quos uel longa facit uia uel saxosa dolere.
  Partibus ista dedit; subdam medicamina toti:
Adiuuat ydropicos decocta comestaque sepe;
Proderit asmaticis ita succurretque caducis.
Tres uini cyatos trinis radicibus eius,
Tres et aque iungas coniunctaque sic bibat eger
Febris in accessu cui dat lux tercia nomen
Quartaneque ualent numero donata quaterno.
Quartanis eciam succus ualet unicus herbe:
Ante duas horas accessus sepe probatum est.
Fluxum constringit superaddita, trita, cruoris;
Oui cum lacrimo ualide succurrit adusto;
Vulnera cum melle iuuat humida, sordida purgat.
Sic siccare refert maiorem Plinius autor
Vt possit seruare uelud cauteria corpus.
De sola librum scripsit Themeson luculentus
In quo preclaris celebrauit laudibus illam.
  Antidotum salubre dyarnoglossa fit inde:
Sumat qui guttam uolet extirpare caducam
Arnoglossam, castoreum, lasar, opoponacem,
Sauinam, dentes et equi, simul et sagapinum.
Hiis iunctis eque mellis quod sufficit adde
Inque modum nucis hanc luna crescente det egro
Et decrescente, uenerem uinumque cauenti.
† Pous † eciam tremulus probat et lunaticus istum.

34 sperma *corr. e* spermas *P* 40 uel[1]] *scripsi*, ue *P* dolere] *scripsi*, dolore *P* *ll.* 45–46 *transp. P* 46 tercia] *add.* lu *et canc. P* 48 succus] *scripsi*, sucus *P* 51 lacrimo] *scripsi*, lacrima *P* 57 antidotumque *D* saluberre *P* diarnaglossa *D* 58 que *P* 59 arnaglossam *D* clasar opopanacem *P* 63 decrescentem *P* 64 eciam] et *D* prob*erat* (?) *P*

the seed, when drunk, forces out blocked afterbirth;
its juice in wool can help the flow of the womb.
If old pig grease is mixed with it, in such a way
does it diminish a serious swelling, even if very persistent;
this plaster helps abscesses or a recent wound.
When ground up with vinegar and applied, it will give help
to those whom a long or rocky road has caused to ache.
  It grants these cures to the parts; I'll add medicines for the whole:
when cooked and eaten often it aids the dropsical;
it should benefit asthmatics thus and will aid the epileptic.
Blend three spoons of wine with three spoons of its roots
and three also of water, and mixed thus, let the patient drink
at the onset of the fever named from the third day's light,
and when given four in number they're good against the quartan.
The juice alone of this herb is also good for quartan fevers:
this is often proven within two hours of the onset.
Ground up and applied on top, it restrains a flow of blood;
it greatly helps with burnt chalazae of an egg;
with honey it aids moist wounds and purges filthy ones.
So Pliny the author says that Greater Plantain dries
so that it preserves the body just like cauterization.
Distinguished Themison composed a book on this alone
in which he celebrates it with outstanding praise.
  The healthful antidote *dyarnoglossa* is made from it:
let him who wants to eradicate the malady of epilepsy
take Plantain, castoreum, laserwort, and opoponax,
Sage and horse's teeth as well, with Sagapenum.
With all these blended equally add enough of honey as is needed
and give it, shaped like a nut, to the patient while the moon is waxing,
and have him shun intercourse and wine while it is waning.
A shaky and a lunatic † pulse † also proves that.

53 *Cf.* Pliny 25. 80

5.1.2 VRTICA

Te contingentes digitos urtica perurens
Nomen habes dignum sed 'acalife' Grecia dicit,
Vnde patet nimio quod sis dotata calore.
Nam nare positus succus foliumue cruorem
Elicit, at nimis electum cupiens retinere
Vrtice succo frontem linit et premet illum.
Vt Galyenus ayt, cape succum seminis eius:
Defluuium capitis hoc sepe fricando iuuabit;
Ore diu tentus tumide medicabitur uue.
Si fuerit sumptum semen cum melle iugatum
Pleureticos <et> pulmones et pectora purgat,
Pellit pulmonum frigus, ueterem quoque tussim
Et uentrem tumidum iuuat, at si semine grato
Forte cares agit hec puluis melli sociatus
Aut uiridis succus cum uino sepe receptus,
Splenque tumens radix cum uino trita iuuabit.
Illius semen colicis cum melle medetur;
Sudorem mouet ex oleo decocto perunctis
Sumptaque sicut olus decoccio molliet aluum.
Si teneram claudit uuluam matrix nimis humens
Et grauis, urtice foliis contacta resurget,
At si cum mirra supponas menstrua purgat.
Prouocat urinam si cum mulsa bibis amplam
Potaque cum uino podagris ualet arteticisque
Aut oleo cocta foueas si membra frequenter.
  Per partes quid agat dixi; per tota quid edam:
Adiuuat hictericos cum uino sumpta frequenter;
Cancros, parrotidas, luxata, canis quoque morsus
Cum sale de foliis factum cathaplasma iuuabit
Et carnem reparat que dissociatur ab osse;
Humores eciam premit hoc cataplasma nocentes.
Si trite uinum coniungas melque piperque
Sicque bibas Veneris uires reparare ualebis.
Si quadrupes Veneris motus perferre recusat

5.1.2 VRTICA *D* 192r: De Ortica (*ll.* 22–5, 27–30, 36–7) | *P* 33v–34r: Vrtica

1 digitos] *scripsi*, digittos *P* 2 habes] *scripsi*, habet *P* acalife] *scripsi*, acalite *P* 3 nimio *add. in mg. P* sis] *scripsi*, sit *P* 11 et^1] *scripsi*, *om. P* 17 colicis] *scripsi*, collericis *P* 18 decocto] *add.* d *et canc. P* 24 artericisque *D* 27 yctericos *D* 28 parotidas *P* 29 cataplasma *D* 30 reparat] reperat *P* 33 Veneris] uenis *P*

5.1.2 Nettle, *Urtica urens* L.

O Nettle, burning the fingers which touch you,
you have a worthy name but Greece calls you *acalife*,
from which it's clear that you're endowed with a mighty heat.
For the juice or a leaf placed in a nostril draws out blood,
but if you wish to check blood that's drawn out excessively,
smear the brow with Nettle juice and this will restrain it.
As Galen declares, take the juice of its seed:
by often rubbing this on it will keep hair from falling out,
and held in the mouth awhile it will cure a swollen uvula.
If the seed should be eaten when mixed with honey,
it purges the pleuritic, as well as lungs and chests,
beats out a chill in the lungs, and helps a chronic cough
or a distended belly, but if perhaps you lack this pleasing seed,
the powder added to honey does these things
or the fresh juice taken often together with wine,
and the root, ground up in wine, will help a swollen spleen.
The seed of Nettle with honey heals the colicky;
it causes sweating in those anointed with its decocted oil,
and a decoction eaten like a vegetable will soften the stool.
If an overly humid and heavy womb shuts up a tender
cervix, when touched with Nettle leaves it will revive;
take it as a suppository with Myrrh: it purges menses.
It forces urine if you drink a lot of it with mead,
and drunk with wine it's good for gout and arthritis
or if you frequently rub the limbs with it when cooked in oil.
  I've said what it does for the parts; I'll give that for the whole:
it helps the jaundiced when taken frequently with wine;
a plaster made of the leaves and salt will help
your tumours, abscesses, sprains, and the bites of dogs,
and repairs the flesh which has separated from the bone;
this plaster also represses harmful humours.
If you add wine and honey and Pepper to it, when ground,
and drink it thus, you can revive the powers of Venus.
If a heifer refuses to hearken to the call of Venus,

5.1.2 VRTICA / Nettle *Macer, 'Urtica', 115–60*
34 *Cf.* Ovid, *Amores* 2. 10. 36

Illius foliis uuluam tetigisse memento.
Vrtice semen, Sextilis tempore lectum,
Pixidibus sapiens thesaurum seruat opimum.

5.1.3 IVSQVIAMVM

Antidotum nam iusquiamon sic conficietur:
Iusquiami, piperis, confire, petrosilini,
Agarici, absinthii, prassi, costi, siselei
Atque aloe dragmam poscit, postremo quaternas
Gingiberis dragmas, soffroaci quoque denas
Et mel quod satis <est>; caput hoc uertigine curat,
Vim cerebri memorem mira uirtute reducit,
Si tamen ista grauant leuiora feremus egenis.
  Seminis illius compescere succus inunctus
Viscosum reum calidumque potest oculorum.
Hic perimit uermes si diffundatur in aures
Sicque potest uariis obstare doloribus harum.
Eius radicis decoccio fiat aceto:
Ore tepens tentum denti medicabitur egro.
Seminis illius obolus semenque iugatum
Myconis dabis in mulsa, gratum medicamen
Hiis qui forte spuunt causa quacumque cruorem
Et sic matricis fluxus restringere fertur.
Semen cum uino cataplasmatum ualet eque:
Mammas et testes scito percurare tumentes.
Et quia iusquiami uis frigida constat et ualde,
Contritis foliis eius adiunge polentam:
Sic podagram calidosque potes lenire tumores;
Vulneribus fusus curabit uulnera succus.
Iusquiamum dicunt Romani 'caniculatam.'
Nobis herba nimis multis accepta medelis,
Emplastris, solet antidotis dari preciosis,
Sed cum tres species eius sint semine note—
Hoc etenim candet, rubet hoc illudque nigrescit—
Alba magis, rubicunda minus, nil efficit atra.

37 thezaurum seruet *P*

5.1.3 IVSQVIAMVM *P* 34r–34v: Iusquiamum

1 iusquiamon *corr. ex* iusquiammon *P* 6 est *om. P* 17 causa] *scripsi*, carisa *P* 20 tumentes] *add. P supra* tepentes 21 constat et ualde] *scripsi*, ualet constat *P* (*cf. Macer 1934*)

remember to touch her vulva with Nettle's leaves.
A wise man preserves the seed of Nettle, gathered
in the time of August, as a rich treasure in his medicine chest.

5.1.3 Henbane, *Hyoscyamus niger* L.

The antidote *iusquiamon* shall be made like this:
it calls for a dram of Henbane, Pepper, Comfrey and Parsley,
of Mushroom, Wormwood, and Leek, Cost, and Laserwort,
and Aloe, and afterwards four drams
of Ginger, as well as ten of *soffroacus*, and as much
honey as is needed; this cures the head of vertigo,
brings back, by marvellous virtue, the brain's power of memory,
but if these are costly, we'll bring cheaper things to the needy.
The juice of Henbane's seed in an ointment is able
to restrain a hot and viscous rheum of the eyes.
This destroys worms if poured into the ears
and in such a way it can stop their various pains.
Let a decoction of its root be made with vinegar:
warmed and held in the mouth it will heal an ailing tooth.
You'll give an *obolus* of its seed, when mixed
with Poppy seed in mead, a pleasing medicine
for those who for any reason might be spitting blood,
and in such a way it's said to check the flow of the womb.
The seed in a plaster with wine is equally as good:
know that it thoroughly cures swollen breasts and testicles.
And because the power of Henbane is agreed to be very cold,
add barley-meal to its ground-up leaves:
in such a way you can allay gout and fiery tumours;
poured into wounds, the juice will cure those wounds.
The Romans call Henbane *caniculata*.
The herb is very popular among us in many medicines
and in plasters, and is apt to be given in costly antidotes,
but since its three varieties are distinguished by the seed—
for this one's white, this is red, and that one's rather black—
the white does more, the ruddy less, the black does nothing at all.

5.1.3 IVSQVIAMVM / **Henbane** *Macer, 'Iusquiamus', 1933–61*
17 *Cf.* Macer, 'Porrum', 510–11

5.1.4 CERIFOLIVM

Ignea uis cerifoliis exundat et acris.
Te, uertigo ferox, eius decoccio sanat,
Si tamen inde caput pacientis sepe lauetur
Et simul herba tepens frontes et tympora cingat,
Potaque cum uino lateris curare dolorem
Sic poterit si trita super latus additur herba.
Hec quoque sumpta frequens aceto commouet aluum,
Excitat uomitum; cum uino sumpta mouebit
Menstrua uel locium; si pectine trita ligetur
Herbaque potetur nil urinam mouet eque.
Lumbricos tineasque in aceto pota repellit;
Virgine cum cera ualet huic anxugia iuncta
Parotidas curare frequens et quosque tumores
Tritaque melle frequens cancris sanare probatur.
Si coquis hanc oleo frigus fugit unguine tali.
Elleboro nimium sumpto fortissima restat
Et multis aliis multum preciosa medetur.

5.1.5 LAPAPHVM

Herba subest lapaphi quam plebs dici 'paradellam.'
Hec est que pueris urtice spicula lenit.
Hec uirtus feruens austeraque dicitur esse,
Illius ergo tepens decoccio proderit auri;
Gargarizata leuat uuas dentisque dolorem.
Radices uino coque contritas, superadde
Et scrofis et parotidis, curabis utrumque.
Et scrofas radix collo suspensa fugabit
Mansaque confortat stomachum uentumque nociuum
Ructibus expellit; ut olus stringit tibi uentrem.
Pota iuuat dissintericos, sanat cyliacos;
Illius decocta diu radix in aceto
Ingentes splenis premit addita sepe tumores;
Stringit aqua iuuenem petram. Nec nota tacebo:

5.1.4 CERIFOLIVM *P* 34v: Cerifolium
11 repellit] *scripsi*, superabit *P* 12 huic] *scripsi*, hoc *P* 16 elleboro] *scripsi*, elleboris *P*

5.1.5 LAPAPHVM *P* 34v–35r: Lapatium
1 dicit] *add.* fugit *s.l. et canc. P* 3 hec] *scripsi*, hoc *P* 14 aqua] *scripsi*, aque *P*

5.1.4 Chervil, *Anthriscus cerefolium* (L.) Hoffm.

A fiery and a bitter power abounds in Chervil.
A decoction of it heals you, fierce vertigo,
if a patient's head is often washed with it and, at the same time,
the warmed herb is wrapped around his forehead and temples;
when drunk with wine, it thus should be able to cure a pain
of the side if the ground herb is applied upon the side.
Taken frequently with vinegar it also moves the bowels
and forces vomit; when taken with wine it will move
menstrual courses or urine; if it is ground and tied
to the groin and the herb is drunk, none moves urine so well.
When drunk in vinegar it repels stomach and tapeworms;
when fat is added to this with virgin wax it can
frequently cure abscesses and any tumours and,
when ground with honey, it's proven to heal cancers frequently.
If you cook this in oil a chill flees such an ointment.
Very strong, it counteracts an overdose of Hellebore
and, most precious, it medicates many other things.

5.1.5 Dock or Sorrel, family *Rumex* L.

The herb Dock comes next, which the people call *paratella*.
This is the herb which soothes Nettle's spines for boys.
This is said to be hot and dry in virtue,
therefore a warm decoction of it should benefit the ear;
when gargled it relieves uvulas and dental pain.
Cook the ground up roots in wine, apply this
to scrofula and abscesses, and you will cure either one.
The root hung from the neck protects from scrofula
and when chewed it strengthens the stomach and expels
a harmful wind with belching; as a potherb it restrains your belly.
When drunk it helps the dysenteric, and heals the coeliac;
its root, cooked down a lengthy time in vinegar
and then applied, often reduces giant tumours of the spleen;
with water it checks the newer stone. I won't stifle the facts:

5.1.4 CERIFOLIVM / **Chervil** *Macer, 'Cerefolium', 928–46*

5.1.5 LAPAPHVM / **Dock** *Macer, 'Paratella', 1993–2014*

Pruritum scabiemque tepens decoccio sanat
Vel si decocte radicem conteris uncto,
Quod cicius facit et melius sibi sulfure iuncto.

5.1.6 SENECION

'Senecion' quod sit quasi cano tincta colore
Dicunt; 'yrigeron' a Grecis dicitur ipsa.
Senecion mire uis frigida dicitur esse;
Eius radices medicorum respuit usus.
Plinius ut docuit, si dentem uis medicari
Hanc circumfodias sine ferro moxque dolentem
Tange tribus uicibus et ter spuat eger ad herbam;
Pone loco quo cepisti: sic crescat ut herba.
Potari quidam, quia suffocare bibentem
Posse putant, prohibent, quos contra Plinius autor
Quod cordis uiciis uentrisque doloribus obstet
Yctericisque et uesice si sumpta lyeo
Potetur prosit pluresque ait. Ista probarunt.
Potaque cum uino curat precordia, sedat
Tormina, quod faciet si tincta uoretur aceto.
Floribus et foliis tunsis infundito uinum,
Testiculis tumidis anoque tepencia ponas,
Quod si thus addas predictis uulnera queuis
Curabis neruosque simul cathaplasmate tali;
Hoc eciam faciunt herbe triti capitelli.
Cum sale trita solet preduras spargere strumas.
Inuentu facilis muris, ortis, thabulatis,
Preualet in grauibus facili medicamine causis.

5.1.7 MAVRELLA

'Strignum' Mirmidone, 'maurellam' uero Latine
Dicunt. Maurelle uis extat frigida ualde,
Eius enim capitis cataplasma iuuare dolorem

5.1.6 SENECION *P* 35r: Senecion
10 prohibent] *scripsi*, perhebent *P*

5.1.7 MAVRELLA *P* 35r–35v: Maurella

a warm decoction heals itching and the mange
or if you grind the root of it when cooked in oil,
which it does faster and better with sulphur added to it.

5.1.6 Groundsel, *Senecio vulgaris* L.

They call it Groundsel because it seems as if it's dyed
with a greyish colour; it's called *erigeron* by the Greeks.
The power of Groundsel is said to be amazingly cold;
physicians customarily reject its roots.
As Pliny has taught, if you wish to cure a tooth,
dig Groundsel up without iron and next touch the aching tooth
three times and have the patient spit three times at the herb;
put it in the place where you picked it: so let it grow as an herb.
Some forbid this to be drunk, since they think it's able
to suffocate the drinker, and against them the author Pliny
says that it blocks vices of the heart and stomach pains
and benefits the jaundiced and bladder if it's drunk,
taken with wine. They have proven these things.
Drunk with wine it cures the diaphragm, settles gripes,
and it will do this if it's soaked in vinegar and consumed.
Pour wine onto its crushed flowers and leaves
and place it, warmed up, on swollen testicles and the anus,
but if you add Frankincense to the aforesaid you'll cure
any wounds and tendons as well with such a plaster;
the ground seedpods of the herb also accomplish this.
Ground with salt it can dissolve the hardest scrofulous tumours.
Easy to find on walls, in gardens, or between the floorboards,
it prevails over difficult cases with an easy medicine.

5.1.7 Black Nightshade, *Solanum nigrum* L.

The Myrmidon's *strignum* is called *maurella* in Latin.
The power of Nightshade is on record as very cold,
for a plaster of it is believed to aid a headache;

5.1.6 SENECION / **Groundsel** *Macer, 'Senecion', 1664–89*
1 *Cf.* Isidore, *Etym.* 17. 9. 53   5–8 *Cf.* Pliny 25. 167   23 Quintus Serenus 299

5.1.7 MAVRELLA / **Black Nightshade** *Macer, 'Maurella', 1918–32*
1 *Cf.* Isidore, *Etym.* 9. 2. 75

Creditur; egilopis simul obstat perniciosis;
Auriculis succus sensim diffunditur eius.
Panem, sal, strignum contrita fugare uidebis
Parotidas. Succus subiectus menstrua purgat
Eius; prurigo fugit et perit illita succo.
Si uis ut fugiant sacer ignis et herpeta mordax,
En, medicamen adest medicamine forcius omni!
Maurelle foliis contritis iunge polentam,
Argenti spumam, cerusam oleumque rosatum
Iungito predictis: mirum cathaplasma stupebis.

5.1.8 YSATIS

'Ysatis' a Grecis, a plebe 'gaysno' uocatur,
Optima uulneribus, tinctoribus utilis herba;
Ex huius foliis factum cathaplasma sacratum
Vulnera, magna <licet>, conglutinat atque cruorem
Stringit eorundem. Nec decipit hoc medicamen:
Quemuis feruorem premit et quodcumque tumorem.
Isatin egregiam miscens albumen et oui
Et maculis ignique sacro succurrere fertur
Melleque confectum sordencia uulnera purgat.

5.1.9 CYNOGLOSSA

Salue, munificum munus, cynoglossa, deorum,
Salue, certa salus! Sic te Greci sapientes,
Roma 'canis linguam' uocat, ambo uocant preciosam,
Nam canis ut medica lambendo uulnera lingua
Sanat, sic multos tua curat gracia morbos.

5 succus] *add.* subiectum *P*

5.1.8 YSATIS *P* 35v: Ysatis
4 licet] *scripsi* (*cf. Macer 1769*), *om. P*

5.1.9 CYNOGLOSSA *D* 192r: De Cinoglossa id est Lingua canis | *P* 35v: Cinoglossa
1 cinaglossa *D* 3 canit *D* 5 curat] sanat *P*

it likewise hinders dangerous tear duct tumours;
its juice is poured slowly into the ears.
You'll see that bread, salt, and Nightshade, ground up,
chase abscesses away. Its juice as a suppository purges
menstrual courses; an itch, smeared with the juice, departs and dies.
If you wish for Holy Fire and biting herpes to flee,
look, a medicine stronger than any medicine is here!
Add barley-meal to ground Nightshade leaves
and add silver dross, white lead, and oil-of-Rose
to them: you'll be amazed at the marvellous plaster.

5.1.8 Woad, *Isatis tinctoria* L.

Woad is called *isatis* by the Greeks, *gaysno* by the people,
the best herb for wounds, and useful too for dyers;
a sacred plaster made from its leaves
binds together wounds, however large, and restrains
their blood. Nor does this medicine disappoint:
it settles any fever and whatsoever swelling.
Mixing famous Woad and egg white
is said to help both blemishes and the Holy Fire,
and prepared with honey it purges filthy wounds.

5.1.9 Hound's-Tongue, *Cynoglossum officinale* L.

Hail, *cynoglossa*, generous gift of the gods,
hail, sure health! The wise Greeks call you this,
Rome calls you Hound's-Tongue, and both name you as precious,
for as a dog, like a doctor, cleans wounds by licking
with its tongue, so your influence cures many ailments.

5.1.8 YSATIS / **Woad** *Macer, 'Gaisdo', 1766–73*

5.1.9 CYNOGLOSSA / **Hound's-Tongue** *Source unknown*
2 *Cf.* Martial, *Ep.* 2. 91. 1

Ipsam paralisim cum uino pota repellis
Mirificumque malum mira uirtute reuellis.
Antidotumque salubre dyacynoglossa fit ex te:
Vnciolam, cynoglossa, tui costique crocique,
Iusquiami simul et spice iungunt geminasque
Mirre, opii, libani. Predictis tres superaddunt
Aristologie, post hec selinon lasarisque
Ana dimidiam, piperis sex grana decena.
Hiis bene contritis mellis quod sufficit addunt:
Hec oculos ualide lacrimosos pocio siccat,
Hec oculos ualide detergit sanguinolentos,
Hec oculos ualide solet alleuiare dolentes,
Hec capitis ueterem ualet adnichilare dolorem.

5.1.10 LOLIVM

Quam Grecus 'lolium' uocitauit Roma 'nigellam.'
Cum sale, cum raffano superaddita, trita fugabit
Zernas atque lepras. Semen quod lilia prebent
Adiunctum lolio purgamentisque columbe
Et sulfur scrofas delebunt cocta lyeo;
Sic apostema, sic queuis dura resoluet.
Mulsa cocta, croco thurique iugata, fugabit
Te, sciasis. Pariens si se suffumiget illa
Ventris onus leuius ciciusque reponere fertur.
Vlcera que pascunt carnes cancrosque refringit.

6 paralisin *D*   8 dyacynoglossa] *scripsi*, diarnaglossa *D* : dyarnoglossa *P*   9 unciolam] yncidulam *P*   cinoglossa *D*   10 et spice] siffice *P*   12 aristologye *P*   lazarisque *P*   14 his *D*   15 hec . . . siccat *om. P*   16 hec] hoc *P*   ualde *P*   17 hec . . . dolentes *om. P*   18 hec] hoc *P*

5.1.10 LOLIVM   *P* 35v–36r: Nigella, Lolium
6 resoluet] *scripsi*, resolues *P*

When drunk with wine you repel paralysis itself
and by an amazing virtue you strip away an amazing evil.
And the salubrious antidote *dyacynoglossa* is made from you:
they add an ounce of you, Hound's-Tongue, of Cost, and Crocus,
likewise of Henbane and Spikenard, and two ounces of Myrrh,
opium, and Incense. They add to the aforesaid things
three ounces of Birthwort, after this just half as much of Parsley
and of Laserwort, and sixty grains of Pepper.
They add to these, ground well, enough honey as is needed:
this potion powerfully dries out weepy eyes,
this powerfully cleans out bloodshot eyes,
this is powerfully apt to soothe your aching eyes,
and this can reduce to nothing an old pain in the head.

5.1.10 Cockle, *Agrostemma githago* L.

The herb which the Greek called *lolium*, Rome called Cockle.
Ground with salt and Horseradish, and applied, it will chase away
impetigo and leprosy. The seed which Lilies offer,
mixed with Cockle, pigeon droppings and sulphur,
will destroy scrofulous sores when cooked with wine;
it will thus dissolve abscesses and thus any hardenings.
Cooked in mead and mixed with Crocus and Incense,
it will fend off you, sciatica. If a mother fumigates herself with it,
it's said to bring out more gently and quickly the burden of the womb.
It breaks apart the ulcers which feed on flesh as well as sores.

9 *Cf.* Ovid, *Met.* 4. 393   8–18 *Cf. Antidotarium Nicolai* 123

5.1.10 LOLIVM / Cockle *Macer, 'Lolium',* 2015–28

5.1.11 CICVTA

In regionibus est funesta cycuta quibusdam;
In nostra pueri comedunt inpune cicutam
Vt uocitent herbam plures uulgi 'benedictam.'
Herba cicuta reis pena esse solebat Athenis
Ac Socrates doctus pena fuit exanimatus.
Hanc si quis calidis bibit in regionibus herbam
Forte recensque merum sumat mortemque fugabit
Sed quam pota nocet tam per cathaplasmata prodest.
Si frontem foliis operis uel lumina succo
Vnxeris illius fugat epiforas oculorum;
Herpeta sic fugiet, sacer ignis sic morietur.
Scripsit Anasialus, si mammas uirgo perungat
Sepius hoc succo (quoniam iuuenilibus annis
Turgescunt), modicas fore, semper stare decenter,
Herbaque trita uirens lac mammis addita siccat.
Si pecten circa cathaplasmes sepe cicuta
Et tu, Venus amans et amarus amor, superaris,
Seminis et fluxus perit omnis. Ea quoque iuncta
Argenti spumis adipique podagra fugatur
Ipsaque sola tamen curat persepe podagram.
Et ne longa tibi generem fastidia longis,
Hac curare potes nocuos quoscumque tumores.

5.1.12 LAPPA

Sed dum Caliope uulgares concinit herbas
Cur lappam taceat qua non uulgarior ulla est?
Corpore magna patet, maior patet in medicina.

5.1.11 CICVTA *P* 36r: Cicuta
3 benedictam] *scripsi*, bene dicam *P* 4 reis] *scripsi*, reos *P* pena esse] *Rigg* (*private conversation*), pre iure *P* 7 sumat] *scripsi*, summat *P* 9 operis uel] *scripsi*, operisue *P* 10 epiforas] *add.* ep *et canc. P* 11 fugiet] *scripsi*, fugit *P* 16 si] *scripsi*, sic *P* 17 tu] *scripsi*, te *P* superaris] *scripsi*, superatur *P* 19 spumis] addit *add. et canc. P* 22 hac *corr. ex* ac *P*

5.1.12 LAPPA *D* 192r: De Lappa | *P* 36r: Lappa
1–2 sed . . . herbas / cur . . . est] nunc igitur quoniam uulgares pandimus herbas / lappa sit in medio, qua non uulgarior herba *D* 3 corpore . . . medicina *om. P*

5.1.11 Hemlock/Herb Bennet, *Conium maculatum* L.

Hemlock, in certain regions, is a deadly plant.
In our land boys eat Hemlock with impunity
so many of the common people call it a 'blessed' herb.
The herb Hemlock was used to punish condemned Athenians
and by this punishment wise Socrates gave up the ghost.
If someone in warmer regions drinks this herb
with, perhaps, some new, unwatered wine, he'll fend off death,
but it's as harmful in a drink as it is beneficial in a plaster:
if you cover the forehead with its leaves or anoint the eyes
with its juice, it chases away blocked tear ducts in the eyes;
in such a way will herpes flee, thus Holy Fire will perish.
Anaxilaus wrote that if a girl anoints her breasts
often with this juice (since they swell in tender years),
they will remain small, and will always stay fittingly erect,
and the green herb ground and applied to breasts dries up milk.
If you often apply Hemlock in a plaster around the groin,
you will be conquered, loving Venus and bitter Love,
and every flow of semen dies away. And with Hemlock
added to silver dross and lard, gout is chased away,
yet Hemlock alone very often cures gout.
And lest I make your boredom long with my lengthy words,
you can cure any harmful tumours with this herb.

5.1.12 Cocklebur, *Xanthium spinosum* L.

But while Calliope is singing of the common herbs,
why is she silent about Cocklebur, more common than any herb?
It is clearly great in body, clearly even greater in medicine.

5.1.11 CICVTA / **Hemlock** *Macer, 'Cicuta', 2029–55*
12 *Cf.* Pliny 25. 154 17 *Cf.* Venantius Fortunatus, *Carmina* 3. 23a, 12 (ed. Leo, 74); Walther, *Proverbia* nos. 2387, 10775, 11058, 17235

5.1.12 LAPPA / **Cocklebur** *Source unknown*

Concinat antracas qua ui depellat acerbas;
Cum sibi 'porcinam' sociat quam plebs uocat herbam
Et sic coniuncto feralia dissipat uncto.
Sit licet ista leuis tamen est medicina salubris.

5 <INTERLVDVM>

Notificans herbas Phebi monitu duodenas
Incepi promissa tibi persoluere, lector.
Quas si prescriptis centum subdas, medicina
Difficiles facile languores quosque iuuabis:
Sic medicis Phebi similis, gratissimus omni,
Orbe legar toto nomenque perenne tenebo!
Hec dum iacto frequens, 'O Phebe!' cocus michi quidam
Subridens, 'pociora tacens, inglorius,' inquit,
'Qui porrum, cepas, caules—uulgaria certe
Sed prorsus <ualde> gratissima—conticuisti.'
Tunc ego: 'Non scriptis escas sed tradimus herbas;
Hec, quia sunt esce, non sunt, proth Iupiter, herbe!'
'An pocius quoniam compilas singula libris
Hec non uidisti? Que nescis conticuisti?'
'Nescio, confiteor. Quis enim simul omnia noscat?
Tu, si quid nosti, refer,' et simul incipit, ecce:

5.2.1 CEPA

'De cepis medici—nec enim per longa morabor—
Diuersi diuersa tenent: auctor Galienus
Flecmaticis aptas, fellicis uero nociuas
Asserit, at Dyaschorides inflare caputque
Conturbare sitimque datas accendere dixit.

4 concinat] ***icet *D* (*illegible in gutter*) qua ui] mire *corr. e* more *D* depellit *D*

---

5 <INTERLVDVM> *P* 36r–36v: [no title] *Edited by Rigg, 280–81.*
7 michi *add.* fidem *et. canc. P* 8 inglorius] *Rigg*, inglor' *P* 9 cepas] *Rigg*, cepe *P* 10 ualde] *add. Rigg, om. P* 16 incipit] *Rigg*, incipis *P*

5.2.1 CEPA *P* 36v–37r: Cepa

Let her sing with what power it destroys harsh, running sores;
let her mix with it the herb that people call 'hogweed,'
and with it mixed like this with oil let her overthrow deadly things.
Granted, it is trifling, yet it is a salubrious medicine.

5 Interlude

'O Reader, I have begun, once admonished by Apollo,
to repay what I have promised, making known twelve herbs.
And if you add these to the one hundred written above,
you will easily aid any difficult maladies with medicine:
thus similar to Phoebus's physicians, most pleasing to all,
I'll be read through the entire world, I'll have an eternal name!'
While I was boasting overmuch, a certain cook smirked and said to me,
'By Phoebus, worthless man, you're quiet about greater matters,
and have also kept silent about Leeks, and Onions, and Cabbage—
vulgar things, to be sure, but by all means very pleasing.'
Then I said, 'We name herbs, not foods, in our writings,
and these, by Jove, aren't herbs, since they are foods!'
'Or could it be, since you plagiarize every little bit from books,
you haven't noticed these? Are you silent on what you do not know?'
'I don't know, I confess. For who can know all things at once?
You—if you know anything—tell.' And he began at once, like this:

5.2.1 Onion, *Allium cepa* L.

'Diverse doctors hold diverse opinions on Onions
(but I will not linger over them long): the author Galen
asserts they are good for the phlegmatic but harmful
to the bilious, and Dioscorides said that, once given,
they puff up and disturb the head and kindle the thirst.

5 <INTERLVDVM> / **Interlude** *Original*

1–2 *Cf.* Martial, *Ep.* 9. 102 8 *Cf.* Virgil, *Georgica* 4. 94 12 *Cf.* Virgil, *Aeneid* 4. 590; Ovid, *Met.* 13. 5 15–16 *Cf.* Job 34: 32–3

5.2.1 CEPA / **Onion** *Macer, 'Cepa,' 1087–1126*

Asclepius sanas ualde pronunciat ipsas
Precipue stomacho soloque creare colorem
Conspectu pulcris. Semper ieiunia cepis
Solue—nec eger eris. Loca si nudata capillis
Sepe frices, reparare comas hac arte ualebis.
Naribus attractus succus purgat caput eius
At succo melli iuncto caligo fugatur.
Femineo lacti coniuncto funditur auri;
Mane frica dentem semperque dolore carebis
Oris et ulceribus prosunt cum pane comeste,
Et sic os fetens curant, fastidia tollunt.
Succus aqua bibitus subito mutum releuabit.
Dicuntur cepe mollire salubriter aluum;
Menstrua tarda cient seu pote siue comeste
Lesurasque pedum succo pinguique perungas
Galline. Glandes curabis sepe fricando
Intinctis oleo. Qui coctis uescitur illis
Morsus lenificat quos dissenteria donat.
Succus item curat maculas coniunctus aceto;
Si cepe sint contrite melli uel aceto
Hoc triduo sanat morsus cathaplasma caninos.
Cum sale contritas superaddens morsibus anguis
(Ni fallit Dyaschorides) lesum reparabit.

5.2.2 PORRVM

'Extollit Ypocras, medicorum gloria, porrum,
Sepius usus eo. Si succo iungitur eius
Tercia pars mellis, per nares siue per aures
Infusus tepidus caput esse dolens releuabit.
Obsistit capre cum felle doloribus auris;
Prestat idem tepidus si diffundatur in aures.
Admixtum galle porrum thurisque farine
Ac dragmis geminis porrorum seminis, unam
Mirre, si iungas et uino trita resoluas,
Naribus hoc sanguis medicamine sistit inunctis,

10 comas] *scripsi*, conas *P*   ualebis] *scripsi*, ualebit *P*   22 qui] *scripsi*, que *P*

5.2.2 PORRVM *D* 192v: De Porro (*lines 12–14*) | *P* 37r: Porrum
4 infusus] *scripsi*, infundens *P*   7 admixtum] *scripsi*, admixtus *P*

Asclepius pronounced them very sound,
especially for the stomach, and they bring colour
by a mere look at this beautiful herb. Always end fasts
with Onions—you'll never be sick. If you often rub places
naked of hair, by this art you can bring back the hair.
Its juice, taken up the nose, purges the head,
but cloudy vision flees from the juice when mixed with honey.
It is poured, if blended with a woman's milk, into an ear;
in the morning rub your teeth and you will always lack
mouth pain, and eaten with bread they're good for ulcers;
thus they cure a stinking mouth and they remove distaste.
The juice, when drunk with water, will cure the suddenly mute.
Onions are said healthfully to soften the stool;
either drunk or eaten they release late menstrual courses
and you should rub foot injuries with the juice
and chicken fat. You will cure penises by rubbing often
with these soaked in oil. He who eats these cooked
softens the pains which dysentery effects.
Likewise the juice, when mixed with vinegar, cures spots;
if Onions should be ground with honey or vinegar,
this plaster heals dog bites in three days.
Applying these ground with salt to serpent bites
will repair the injury (unless Dioscorides is wrong).

5.2.2 Leek, *Allium tricocum* L.

'Hippocrates, the glory of physicians, extols the Leek,
and often used it. If a third part of honey
is added to Leek juice and poured warm
into the nose or ears, it will relieve an aching head.
It hinders pains of the ear with goat's gall;
it provides the same cure if poured warm into the ears.
If you add a Leek mixed with gall and Incense,
powdered with two drams of Leek seeds
and one of Myrrh, and mix these when ground in wine,
blood ceases from nostrils anointed with this medicine,

28 Latin Dioscorides, 'De cepulla' (10. 2, 229)

5.2.2 PORRVM / Leek *Macer, 'Porrum', 507–48*

Hoc emoptoycis nec quicquid proficit eque.
Humor si capitis stillet quo leditur eque
Pulmo, uox, pectus, tussisque creatur hanela,
Cum ptysana succum porri sorbere memento;
Et succus lacti si iungatur muliebri
Pulmonem recreat, ueteranis tussibus obstat.
Qui lumbos dolet hunc succum uino medicamen
Potet: nil tali melius medicamine dicunt.
Omnibus hiis per se solum prodesse putatur.
Contracte succo uulue curantur eodem
Fecundasque facit gustatum sepe puellas.
Cum sale fracturas solidat; predura relaxat
Atque recens uulnus conglutinat hoc cathaplasma
Et melli iunctum nichilominus ulcera sanat.
Cum uino datur hiis quos morsus leserit anguis
Aut aliud quoduis animal letale uenenis;
Cum mulsa solet hoc fungis obstare comestis.
Porrum preterea crudum leuat ebrietatem,
Sic auget uenerem; mollit perutile uentrem.

5.2.3 CAVLIS

'Caulis romane uocitatur brassica grece.
Scribunt egregie multi de uiribus herbe:
Omnes quod curat caligine lumina scribunt.
Quod de caule canat Catho magnus, Clyo, memento:
Annis sexcentis solo medicamine caulis
Vsos testatur Romanos nam medicine
Ars illis ignota fuit per tempora tanta.
Ipsemet affirmat curare recencia caules
Vulnera, nec ueterana minus cancrosque feroces;
Sed loca seu uino tepido seu ampne lauentur
Vult et quaque die tritum bis ponere caulem.
Neruis contractis urinam censuit aptam

11 quicquid] *scripsi*, quicumque *P* 13 thussisque *D* 14 ptysana] tpisana *D* 22 fracturas] *scripsi* (*cf. Macer 545*), iuncturas *P* 25 anguis] *scripsi*, angwis *P*

5.2.3 CAVLIS *D* 192ra: De Caule. De eodem statim post (*lines 12–13, 31–4*) | *D* 192rb: Item De Caule (*lines 35–40, 45–54*) | *P* 37r–38r: Caulis

8 curare] *scripsi*, cura *P*

nor does anything profit blood-spitters so well as this.
If moisture in the head drips so that the lung, voice, and chest
are injured equally, and a panting cough develops,
remember to swallow Leek juice with barley-water;
and if the juice is blended with a woman's milk
it refreshes the lung and hinders lingering coughs.
Let him who has pains in his loins drink this juice with wine
as a medicine: they say nothing is better than such a medicine.
It is thought that on its own it helps all these things.
Contracted wombs are cured by the same juice
and when eaten it often makes young women fertile.
With salt it mends fractures; this plaster
loosens hardenings and binds a recent wound,
and mixed with honey it nevertheless cleans ulcers.
It is given with wine to those whom a snake bite has injured
or any animal at all that is lethal with its poison;
with mead this can hinder fungi when eaten.
What's more, raw Leeks remove drunkenness,
and like this inflame lust; most useful, it softens the belly.

5.2.3 Cabbage, *Brassica oleracea* L.

'Cabbage, the *caulis* of Rome, is called *brassica* in Greek.
Many write about the powers of this extraordinary herb,
and everyone writes that it cures eyes of cloudiness.
Clio, remember what great Cato sang about the Cabbage:
he says the Romans used Cabbages for six hundred years
as their only medication, for the art of medicine
was unknown to them for such a great time.
He himself affirms that Cabbages cure recent wounds
and old ones no less, as well as ferocious cancers;
but those places should be washed in warm water or wine
and he chooses to apply ground Cabbage twice each day.
He reckoned as fitting for strained tendons the urine

5.2.3 CAVLIS / Cabbage *Macer, 'Caulis,' 1201–63*

Eius qui uiridi uescetur caule frequenter;
Asserit et pueris multam conferre salutem
Vrina tali fuerint si sepe peruncti.
Edocet et scriptis cauli miscere farinam
Ordea quam dederint, cum qua rutam, coriandrum
Salque iubet misceri: mirum cataplasma podagre,
Proficit arteticis, mire siringia tollit,
Sic luxata iuuat uariisque doloribus obstat.
Prebuit has laudes uobis censor Catho, caules.
  Scripsit facundus libris de caule Crisippus
Quo purgare caput succum pronunciat huius
Naribus infusum. Coniunxit alumen aceto
Et caules, corpus contrita redegit in unum
Predictisque fabam se dixit iungere coctam:
Inde lepras simul et maculas ungendo fugabit,
Hinc eciam crines solitus retinere fluentes,
Hinc eciam testes solitus curare tumentes
Et uarios morbos qui per genitalia regnant.
Cum fenugreco tundebat eas et aceto
Et sic arteticos curauit sepe dolores
Et podagre dirum destruxit sepe periclum.
Quodque probauit agens, docuit certissima scribens
Idem, quod si quis uescetur caule frequenter
Auget lac mammis purgareque menstrua scribit;
Adiuuat et stomachum sumptas ut concoquat escas.
Si multum coquitur restringit, si minus ultro,
Dissoluit uentrem, sed crudus sumptus aceto
Splen reprimit semenque datum depellit abortum.
Vncto contriti caules oleumque rosarum,
Hec febris ardores ualide decocta iuuabunt
Si certe religes stomacho membroue calenti.
  At quid melliti dixit Mellicius oris?
Si radix caulis uellatur, postea terram
Sic ne contingat, collo suspensa fugabit
Ex uua morbos omnes, sic namque probauit:
Vel cinis ex caulis qui fit radicibus ustis
Vuam suppositus siccat releuatque iacentem.

17 ordea] *scripsi*, ordeam *P* rutam] *scripsi*, ruttam *P* 20 uariisque] uariis d que *et canc.* d *P* *ll.* 28–29 *transp. P* 29 testes] *scripsi*, terestes *P* 31 tundebat eas] fundebat eos *D* 32 artericos *D* 33 durum *P* sepe] *add.* podagris *et exp. P* 34 agens] egens *P* 36 lac] *add.* p *et exp. P* scribit] dicit *P* 39 sed] si *D* 42 ardores] *scripsi*, ardori *P* 44 oris] *scripsi*, orsi *corr. ex* orbi (?) *P* 45 terram] tritam *P* 49 suppositum *D*

of one who frequently consumes green Cabbage;
he also asserts that it confers great health on boys
if they should often be anointed with this urine.
And in his books he teaches how to mix with Cabbage
the flour which comes from barley, and he orders Rue,
Coriander and salt to be mixed with it: an excellent plaster for gout,
it's good for arthritis, marvellously takes fistulae away,
and thus it helps dislocations and stops all sorts of pain.
O Cabbages, Cato the Censor offered you these praises.
  Eloquent Chrysippus wrote in books about the Cabbage,
where he announced its juice can purge a head
when poured into the nose. He mixed vinegar with alum
and Cabbages, and gathered these, ground up, in one mass,
and said that he added a cooked bean to the aforesaid things.
By anointing with this it will clear up spots as well as lesions,
with this he liked to keep his hair full and flowing,
and with this he also liked to cure swollen testicles
and various diseases that are dominant in the genitals.
He ground up Cabbages with Fenugreek and vinegar
and in such a way he often cured arthritic pains
and often destroyed the fearful pain of gout.
And what he proved by doing, he taught the same and wrote
most certain things, and if one frequently eats Cabbage, it increases
milk in breasts and he writes that it purges menstrual courses;
it also aids the stomach so that it fully cooks eaten foods.
It restrains the stomach if cooked a lot; if less so, the reverse:
it dissolves; but when eaten raw with vinegar
it represses the spleen, and the administered seed expels a foetus.
Cabbages and oil-of-Rose ground up in grease:
these things, cooked down, will powerfully aid a fever's heat
if you firmly bind them to an inflamed stomach or limb.
  But what did mellifluous Mellitius say?
If Cabbage root is plucked in such a way that afterwards
it does not touch the earth, when hung from the neck it chases off
all diseases from the uvula. In fact, it's proven in this way:
even Cabbage ash that comes from the burnt roots,
taken as a suppository, dries out and relieves a falling uvula.

Vncto cum ueteri cineres eius sociati
Et lateris ueteres sanant coxeque dolores.
Lumbricos pellit si ius iungatur aceto
At succus uiridis rauce succurrere uoci
Glutitus fertur; crudus fugat ebrietatem.'

5.2.4 ATRIPLEX

Ista cocus uerbis uehemens sine fine ferebat.
Hec ego: 'Nunc finem facies? Nondumque latrasti
Quascumque audisti nugas?' 'Si sunt mea nuge,
Sunt tua multo magis.' 'Nec enim—non que modo dixi
Nescio.' 'Non notam tibi noui notificoque,
Atriplicem, primoque gradu frigere, secundo
Humectare, canam. Nescis quod molliat aluum?
Soluere duricias nescis clauisque mederi?
Si crude cocteue superponas cataplasma,
Sic scabros ungues, sic sacros destruit ignes.
Nescis coniunctam cum nitro, melle et aceto
Sicque superpositam disperdere sepe podagram?
Semine predicte cum uino sepius hausto
Soluitur yctericus, nisi delirat Galienus.

5.2.5 PETROSILINVM

'Amplius, O liuor, cur scribens petrosilino
Detrahis? An quod sit nostre mirabile genti?
Huius enim uires apio canis esse minores,'—

51 ueterens *P*   52 ius iungatur] coniugatur *P*   53 at] aut *P*

5.2.4 ATRIPLEX *P* 38r: Attriplex *First edited by Rigg*, 282.
1 ista] *Rigg*, esca *P*   7 molliat aluum] *Rigg*, mollit uentrem *P*   10 scabros] *Rigg*, scrabos *P*   11 cum] *Rigg*, nec *P*

5.2.5 PETROSILINVM *D* 192r–192v: De Petrosilino (*lines 14–26*) | *P* 38r–38v: Petroselinum *First edited by Rigg, 282–5, from P.*
1 cur *corr. e* cum *P*   2 detrahis] *Rigg*, detrahiis *P*

Ashes of Cabbage, when blended with old grease,
clean old pains of the side and of the hip.
If the juice is mixed with vinegar it forces out stomach worms
but the juice of green Cabbage, when swallowed, is said
to help a raspy voice, and eaten raw puts drunkenness to flight.'

5.2.4 Garden Orache, *Atriplex hortensis* L.

The cook kept saying these things forcibly and ceaselessly.
I said, 'Will you finish already? Haven't you yet barked out
all the nonsense you have heard?' 'If my words are nonsense,
yours are much more so.' 'No truly—I do not *not* know
what I just said!' 'I know a plant unknown to you, and I make it known,
the Orache, and I'll sing that it cools in the first and moistens
in the second degree. Don't you know that it softens the belly?
Don't you know that it dissolves hardenings and heals warts?
If you apply a poultice of it, when raw or cooked,
in such a way it clears up rough nails and Holy Fire.
Don't you know that, when mixed with Soda, honey and vinegar,
and applied like this on top, it often eradicates gout?
One with jaundice is freed by the seed of the aforesaid plant
when drunk often with wine, unless Galen has gone mad.

5.2.5 Parsley (no. 2), *Petroselinum crispum* (Mill.) Nyman

'O Envy, why do you continue to write critically
about Parsley? Is it that it is a marvel to our race?
For you have sung that its powers are less than Celery.'

5.2.4 ATRIPLEX / **Garden Orache** *Macer, 'Atriplex', 947–56*
1–5 *Cf.* Martial, *Ep.* 8. 3, 11–12; 13. 2, 4–5

5.2.5 PETROSILINVM / **Parsley** *Source unknown*
1–2 Martial, *Ep.* 11. 94, 1–2

Quod quam mendosum sit, ui patefecit erumpens—
'Quatuor antidotis aliis precellere scimus:
Hoc quod Alexander, que dicitur 'aurea,' fecit,
Quodque Mitridates ternis rutilans speciebus,
Quodque 'climax' dicunt cohibens sex dena gradatim,
Et dyamargariton ex omni parte beatum.
In tribus ex istis apponere petrosilinum
(In solo selinon preciosius) est preciosum.
Sepius in uanum corrodas grece libellum?
Iam scripsisse pudet? Malles tacuisse? Notanda
Dic michi. Dic, uates! Que si nescis tibi dicam
Herbarum numerum que splendescunt preciosis
Sepius antidotis. Has bis senas numeraui:
Petrosilinum, iusquiamum, aristologieque,
Post rosa, post yreos, post camedreos apiumque,
Rutaque, pulegium, ligustica, prassion inde
Et maratrum. Dictas dignissimus ordo locauit
Pluribus antidotis primas, sed posteriores
Paucis ponuntur, sic uis descendit earum.
Absinthiique et peonie atque ysopi et calamenti
Nomina subicerem, si non prolixior essem.
Sepe quidem ponunt alias sed sepius istas,
Vnde supercellunt aliis ut sidera gemmis.

5.2.6 ALLIVM

'Nondum latraui quicquid scio: corrue, liuor!
Allia, saluete, diuinum munus, auete!
Allia, uos docti dixerunt 'scordeon' Argi.
Quid super ista canat, uates paupercule, nosti,
Mundi lux Ypocras: pulmonum sepe querelas

6 Alexander] *scripsi*, Allexander *P* 7 ternis] *Rigg*, teris *P* 11 preciosius] *Rigg*, preciosus *P* 12 in uanum] *Rigg*, inunctum *P* grece] *Rigg*, g^{e} *P* 13 malles] *Rigg*, mallas *P* 14 dic uates] *D*, preterea *P et Rigg* 15 splesdescunt *D* 17 aristologiaque *P et Rigg* 19 puleium ligurtica *P* 21 primas] *Rigg*, prime *DP* 22 sic] sed *P et Rigg* 23 pyonie *P* calamentis *P et Rigg* 24 nomina subicerem] uix subiunxissem *P* : uim subiunxissem *Rigg* 25 quidam *P* 26 sydera *P*

5.2.6 ALLIVM *D* 192v: De Alliis (*lines 1–2, 5–6, 22–5, 30–31, 33–7*) | *P* 38v–39r: Allium
Lines 1–8 were first edited by Rigg, 285, from P.

How false this is he made clear by exploding with force:
'We know that four antidotes surpass other antidotes:
this one which Alexander made, which is called "golden",
and that which Mithridates made, gleaming with three spices,
and that which they call "ladder", containing sixty items in steps,
and *dyamargariton*, blessed in every land.
In three of these it is valuable to add Parsley
(in one alone the more precious *selinon*).
Do you often gnaw in vain on the little book in Greek?
Are you now ashamed to have written? Do you prefer to remain silent?
Tell me what ought to be noted—Speak, poet! If you don't know these,
I'll tell you the number of herbs which often gleam
in costly antidotes. I have counted out these twelve:
Parsley, Henbane, and Birthworts,
then Rose and Yreos, then Germander and Celery,
and Rue, Pennyroyal, Lovage, and Horehound,
then Fennel. A most worthy plan has placed
the first named herbs in many antidotes, but the later ones
are placed in few, and so their power diminishes.
And I would add the names of Wormwood and of Peony,
of Hyssop and Catnip, if I were not too long-winded.
To be sure, they often include others, but these most often,
wherefore they surpass the others as stars surpass gems.

5.2.6 Garlic, *Allium sativum* L.

'I've not yet barked out what I know. Envy, go to hell!
Hail, Garlic! Greetings, gift of the gods!
Garlic, the learned Argives called you *scordeon*.
Poor little poetling, you know what Hippocrates,
light of the world, sings about it: when cooked in milk

13 *Cf.* Ovid, *Ex Ponto* 1. 5. 15; 4. 2. 3 14 Horace, *Ars poetica* 141

5.2.6 ALLIVM / Garlic *Macer, 'Allium', 161–95*

Decoctum cum lacte iuuat crudumue comestum.
Serpentis morsum dixit curare comestum
Et nocuos perdi uermes ipsius odore
Atque canis rabidi morsum cum melle iuuare.
Hoc inquit mulsam simul adiungas <et> acetum
Sicque bibas: uentris uermes tineeque peribunt.
Ex oleo cum reste sua coque scordeon: inde
Morsus letales reddes non exitiales;
Hoc corpus circum sanabitur unguine fotum
Et sic uesice dolor et tumor alleuiantur.
Combuste fumo si uulua diu foueatur
Expelles seuas, ipso testante, secundas.
  Hec Ypocras. Quod Pittagoras? Iunctum coriandro
Et uino morbum dispertiet yctericorum;
Affirmat quoque Pittagoras caput inde sanari
Si faba iungitur (hoc et tympora). Plinius inde
Idem confirmat, quod si sit consociatum
Anseris hoc adipi sanat si funditur aurem.
  Talia Pittagoras. Et quod Diocles? Dabit illud
Cum centaurea, sic desiccabitur ydrops.
Idem neffreticis elixum tradere iussit
Incoctumque iuuat pulti sumptumque thenasmon,
Et sibi coniuncto bene contrito suis uncto
Magnos feruores repremit durosque tumores.
  Hec Diocles. Et quid Macer tibi? Multa cauillans
Furaris iactasque tuum imitans alienum!
Elixum pariter tussim, suspiria sedat.
Clarificat uocem si crudum scordeon edas,
Sed magis elixum raucis prodesse probatur.
Illo si frangat ieiunia, uel loca mutans
Vel qui potat aquas infames, sanus abibit.
  Hec Macer. Quid ego? Laudes quoque laudibus addo.
Dico quod impar ei sapor omnis erit speciei,
Si piper addatur longoque tenore teratur.'
  'Ad patinas tandem, frater, girando redisti.
Dii tibi pro meritis dent crebra genimina uitis.'

6 comostum *P* 10 et] *scripsi*, *om. P* 11 tyneeque *P* 19 dyspertiet *P* 23 adypi *P* 24 pitagoras *D* Dyocles *P* 25 centhaurea *P* 28 suis] *scripsi*, si uis *P* (*cf. Macer 191*) 30 tibi] cui *D* 31 ymitans *P* 34 probauit *P* 35 frangas *D* 36 adibit *P* 40 girando *add.* resistit *et canc. P*

or eaten raw, it often helps our lung complaints.
He said that when eaten it cures a serpent's bite,
that harmful worms are ruined by its odour,
and with honey it helps the bite of a rabid dog.
He says you should blend mead and vinegar with this
and drink it thus: stomach and tapeworms will be destroyed.
Cook Garlic with its stalk in oil: with this
you'll render lethal bites no longer lethal;
a body, rubbed all over with this ointment, will be healed
and thus a pain and swelling of the bladder are relieved.
If the womb is warmed a while with the smoke of burning Garlic,
you will expel a harmful afterbirth, as he witnesses himself.
  Hippocrates said these things. What does Pythagoras say?
Added to Coriander and wine it dispels the disease of jaundice;
Pythagoras also confirms that the head will be healed
if a bean is mixed with this (so also the temples by this).
Pliny confirms the same things concerning it, but if it's added
to goose fat it cleans an ear if it is poured in.
  Pythagoras said such things. And what about Diocles?
He will give it with Centaury, so dropsy will dry out.
He ordered it given, boiled, to those with kidney disease,
and when eaten uncooked, in porridge, it helps tenesmus,
and when pig fat is added and ground up well with it,
Garlic represses great fevers and hardened tumours.
  Diocles said this. And what is Macer to you? You mock it all,
then you steal, and aping another, you boast it as your own!
When boiled, it equally settles a cough and asthma.
It clears up the voice if you consume the Garlic raw,
but boiled it is proven to assist sore throats more.
If a man breaks a fast with it, either while changing places
or drinking from notorious waters, he will depart healthy.
  Macer said this. What about me? I'll also heap praise on praise.
I say that the flavour of no spice will equal it,
if Pepper is added and ground for a long time.'
  'At last, brother, you've returned, stumbling, to your stew pots!
May the gods grant you frequent fruit of the vine as your due.'

18–26 *Cf.* Pliny 20. 50–57   41 *Cf.* Ps. 64: 11; Ezek. 36: 30

6 <PROLOGVS LIBRI SEXTI>

Felix qui potuit rerum congnoscere causas,
Precipue quicquid causa salutis erit.
Si non uis aliis, saltem tibi disce mederi:
Te quoque si spernis, cui bene fidus eris?
Arbitror insanos proprie monimenta salutis
Qui didicisse queunt nec didicisse uolunt.

6.1.1 PIPER

Protinus eoas species, celestia dona,
Exequar. Hec tanto studiosius inspice, lector,
Quanto graminibus species presunt speciose.
Principio piperis naturam nobilitemus
Quidque sit ipsius particio discutiamus:
In longum, candens, nigrum diuisio constat.
Nigrum collaudat eque sollers medicina
Fetaque damnoso semper bibitore culina
Vnde quidem cum sit species notissima cunctis
Notificabo tibi scribens incognita multis.
Vim piperis, uim gingiberis similes perhibemus
Vnde tuam, piper, atque suam uim consociemus.
Vtraque quippe solet rebus digne sociari
Que purgant tenerum dira caligine lumen,
Vtraque toracis prodesse persepe querelis;
Vtraque uim iecori digestiuam dat oliuo;
Sedat cum tepido tamen utraque tormina uino
Si lauri foliis uel bachis consocietur.
Cum nitro piperis maculas delet cathaplasma
Et cathaplasmatum dispergit cum pice scrofas.

6 <PROLOGVS LIBRI SEXTI> P 39r: [no title] *First edited by Rigg, 285–6.*
4 si *add. manu recentiore P*

6.1.1 PIPER P 39r–39v: Piper *Lines 1–4 were first edited by Rigg, 286.*
1 species] *Rigg*, specias *P* 15 prodesse] *scripsi*, prodese *P* 16 uim iecori] *scripsi*, uim et gecori *P* 18 bachis] *scripsi*, bachi *P*

6 Prologue of the Sixth Book

Happy is he who can know the causes of things,
  especially whatever will be the cause of health.
If you don't wish it for others, at least learn to heal yourself:
  if you spurn even yourself, to whom will you truly be true?
I properly judge them insane who were able to learn
  the articles of health but did not wish to learn.

6.1.1 Pepper and Ginger:
1) Black Pepper, *Piper nigrum* L.
2) White Pepper, *Piper album* L.
3) Long Pepper, *Piper officinarum* L.)
4) Ginger, *Zingiber officinale* Rosc.

At last I will pursue the eastern spices, heavenly gifts.
Reader, inspect them all the more closely
for how much the beautiful spices surpass the herbs.
To begin, let us ennoble the nature of Pepper
and discuss how it can be differentiated:
its division is agreed to be into Long, and White, and Black.
Skilful medicine heaps as much praise on Black Pepper
as the kitchen, always bloated with that damnable drinker,
and so, since it is indeed a spice known so well to all,
I will inform you in writing of things unknown to many.
  We relate as similar the power of Pepper and power of Ginger,
so let us join its power to yours, O Pepper.
  That is to say, either can be rightly mixed with things
which purge the tender eye of a fearful fog;
either is most often beneficial for thoracic complaints;
either with olive oil bestows digestive power on the liver;
yet with warm wine each settles stomach pains
if it is mingled with the leaves or berries of bay.
A plaster of Pepper with Soda removes blemishes
and as a plaster with pitch it disperses scrofulous sores.

6 <PROLOGVS LIBRI SEXTI> / **Prologue of the Sixth Book** *Original*
1 Virgil, *Georgica* 2. 490 2 Ovid, *Ex Ponto* 3. 9. 24

6.1.1 PIPER / **Pepper** *Macer, 'Piper', 2056–85, and 'Gingiber', 2109–10*
1–2 Virgil, *Georgica* 4. 1–2 4 *Cf.* Virgil, *Georgica* 4. 8 8 *Cf.* Martial, *Ep.* 7. 27. 7, 13. 13. 2 11–12 Macer 2109–10

Quod si sumatur febris piper ante tremorem
Discutiet frigus quod dat periodica febris.
Pestiferos morsus lenit, fastidia tollit.
Stercoris humani puluis coniungitur ustus
Ex equo piperi: cancros nil destruit eque.
Omnes nemo uelit piperis congnoscere uires,
Nam si forte uelit, nec tot nec tanta ualebit.
De tribus efficiunt medici piperis speciebus
Antidotum summi precii quod uersus abhorret:
Vnciolas piperis niuei nigrique gemellas,
Tres uero longi, predictis petrosilini,
Gingiberis, costi, carui, ligurticon unam
Et siler ac ysopi, mellis quod sufficit addunt.
Hiis ita confectis curatur passio queuis:
Res antiqua nimis confectio regis Herodis.

6.1.2 MIRRA

Mirra, datum puero munus mirabile Christo,
Fit medicamentis decus acceptabile summis.
Post piper antidotis nil crebrius additur illa,
Vnde liquet quanti precii sit mirra medenti.
Illius uires multi multas retulerunt
Inque gradu calidam dicunt siccamque secundo.
Flodius affirmat: si uino mirra teratur
Et cathaplasmetur fit mire cura dolorum
Et sic constringit cataractas oculorum
Mixtaque colliriis oculorum uulnera mundat;
Visum clarificat, palpebras lenit et aptat.
Andromachus dixit quod mundet uulnera, guttur,
Pectora, pulmones et pectoris omnia uasa.
Ante febres sumpta febrientes mitigat ipsa
Missaque sub lingua, dum soluitur asperitatem
Lenit in arteriis rauceque fit optima uoci,
At Dyaschorides lumbricos ascaridesque

21 piper] *add.* aque *et canc. P* ante] *add. in mg. P* 29 summi] *add.* spe *et canc. P*
30 unciolas] *scripsi*, unciolam *P*

6.1.2 MIRRA *P* 39v–40r: Mirra
6 calidam] *scripsi*, callidam *P* 8 fit mire] *scripsi*, sic mirre *P* dolorum] *scripsi*, dolorem *P*

But if Pepper is taken before the fever's tremor
it will cut off the chill that an intermittent fever causes.
It soothes poisonous bites and takes away distaste.
Powdered and burnt human excrement is mixed
with an equal amount of Pepper: nothing destroys cankers so well.
No one wishes to learn all the powers of Pepper,
for if he so wishes, he cannot do so many or such great things.
 Physicians make from the three kinds of Pepper
an antidote of very great value which poetry abhors:
they add two ounces each of Pepper Black and White, three of Long,
and to the aforesaid they add one ounce of Parsley,
Ginger, Cost, Caraway, Lovage, of Sermountain,
and of Hyssop, and as much as is sufficient of honey.
With these combined like this, any suffering is cured:
this is the very ancient potion of King Herod.

6.1.2 Myrrh, *Balsamodendron myrrha* Nees

Myrrh, the miraculous gift given to the child Christ,
becomes an adornment pleasing in the greatest medicines.
After Pepper, nothing is added more often than it to antidotes,
from which it's clear how valuable Myrrh is for a healer.
 Many have related its many powers
and they say it's hot and dry in the second degree.
Flodius agrees: if Myrrh is ground with wine
and applied in a plaster it is a marvellous cure for aches;
in such a way it checks cataracts in the eyes,
and mixed in salves it cleans the eyes of wounds;
it clarifies the sight and softens and improves the eyelids.
 Andromachus said it cleans out wounds and the throat,
the chest and lungs, and all cavities of the chest.
When taken before fevers it soothes the feverish
and held beneath the tongue, while it dissolves it softens
scratchiness in the windpipe and is very good for a hoarse voice.
And Dioscorides said in his writings that it drives out

6.1.2 MIRRA / **Myrrh** *Constantine, 'Myrrha', 359*
1 *Cf.* Matt. 2: 11

Atque secundinas scribens expellere dixit
Inque fabe modulum si sit potata iuuabit
Tussim sicque latus, sic pectus curat hanelum;
Intestinorum sic uulneribus medicatur.
Absinthii succo uel rute consociata
Menstrua producit, putridis humoribus obstat.

6.1.3 SPICANARDVS

Spica gradu primo feruens et sicca probatur.
Sunt spice gemine species: hec Indica nardus
Dicitur et miro precellit odoris honore,
Altera uero minor uocitatur Celtica nardus
Et (quoniam Celte sunt Galli) Gallica nardus.
Hec igitur quanto predicte cedit honore!
Lumina, si spice foueat decoccio sepe,
Scripserunt acri prurigine mundificari
Atque pili palpebrarum reparantur eadem.
Dicunt hec nimium cordis sedare dolorem;
Lenit et ipsius renes decoccio purgat.
Sumpta solet uento stomachum uacuare nociuo.
Humores capitis transmissos sepe per uuam
Ad pectus sistit, locium uel menstrua ducit.
Optima uesice, matricem subdita siccat;
Eius fomento stericas decoccio sanat
Duricias. Valet hictericis potata frequenter
Et morsus et puncturas fugat interiorum,
Quod si cum sape sumatur spica liquore
Concitat ipsa tuos, Venus infitiabilis, ignes.

6.1.4 GARROFILVM

Garrofilum gaudent reges inponere prelis;
Garrofilum gaudent summates ferre crumenis.
Confortatiuum nature dicitur omnis

6.1.3 SPICANARDVS *P* 40r–40v: Spicanardus
4 Celtica] *scripsi*, cethica *P* 5 Celte] *scripsi*, cethe *P* 18 puncturas] *scripsi*, pucturas *P* 19 liquore] *scripsi* (*cf. Macer 2194*), honore *P*

6.1.4 GARROFILVM *P* 40v: Garrofilum
1 prelis] *supplet Henrici Danielis 'Aaron'*, frenis *P* 2 summates] *scripsi*, sumates *P*

stomach worms, intestinal worms, and afterbirth,
and if it is taken in the shape of a bean in a drink
it will help a cough, and thus it cures the side and a wheezy chest;
in such a way it heals wounds of the intestines.
When blended with juice of Wormwood or of Rue
it brings out menstrual courses and hinders putrid humours.

6.1.3 Spikenard, *Valeriana celtica* L.

Spikenard is proven hot and dry in the first degree.
There are two kinds of Nard: one is called Indian Nard
and is superior for the marvellous grace of its odour,
but the other is lesser and is named Celtic Nard
and Gallic Nard (since the Celts are Gauls).
Therefore, with what great honour does the latter yield to the former!
They have written that the eyes are cleansed of bitter itching,
if a decoction of Spikenard often washes them,
and that eyelashes are repaired by the same.
They say it settles a serious pain in the heart,
and a decoction of it soothes and purges the kidneys.
When eaten, it can empty the stomach of harmful wind.
It settles the humours of the head which are often passed
from the uvula to the chest, and brings out urine or menstrual courses.
Excellent for the bladder, as a suppository it dries the womb;
a decoction of it in a poultice heals cervical hardenings.
Drunk frequently it is good for the jaundiced
and fends off bites and punctures of the inner organs,
but if Spikenard is taken with liquid of wine must
it stirs up your fires, unspeakable Venus.

6.1.4 Cloves, *Syzygium aromaticum* (L.) Merrill &Perry

Kings rejoice in placing Cloves in their wine presses,
and nobles rejoice to carry Cloves inside their purses.
It is said to be comforting for every nature

6.1.3 SPICANARDVS / **Spikenard** *Macer, 'Spica',* 2182–2203
5 *Cf.* Julius Caesar, *De bello Gallico* 1. 1 20 *Cf.* Ovid, *Ars amatoria* 2. 414

6.1.4 GARROFILVM / **Cloves** *Macer, 'Gariofilus',* 2141–6
1 *Cf.* Boethius, *De cons. phil.* 1 met. 5. 41

Et precii grandis non condescendit egenis;
Dicitur ergo gradu siccare, calere secundo.
Garofili puluis cum uino consociatus
Auget uim memorem cerebri si sepe bibatur;
Sic sumptum iecur et stomachum corroborat ipsum.
Et quo multa breui concludam, cuncta iuuare
Garofilum medici scripserunt interiora
Et, quod mirari possim, cum concitet alui
Vim digestiuam tamen alui fluxibus obstat.
Pondere si dragme cum uacce lacte bibatur,
Cincta Venus fragiles hac arte reuentilat ignes.

6.1.5 CYNNAMA

Cynnama nec possunt uirtutibus exsuperari
Nec possunt gustu dulcedinis equiparari.
Hec species oculos siccando curat aquosos;
Mundat possessum feda lentigine uultum
Hanc si contritam forti superaddas aceto.
Hac specie tussis delebitur atque catharrus;
Hac sumpta curatur epar lociumque redundat.
Humentem stomachum desiccat et adiuuat ipsum
Vt cicius coquat acceptas et digerat escas.
Ydropisis species extat cui 'tympana' nomen
Prebent; hanc reprimit pestem renumque dolorem.
Sic morbum perdit qui nomen ab 'impete' ducit.
Sanant reptilium festine cynnama morsum.
Huius tres medici species dixere periti:
Est harum species aliis subtilior una.
Est preciosa magis * * * * * * * * *
Sed que grossior est fluxus emorroydorum
Si ieiunus aqua tritam potet bene sanat.
Hec querit geminas lautissima pocio dragmas.

5 siccare] *scripsi*, feruere *P*   14 cincta] *scripsi*, cuncta *P*

6.1.5 CYNNAMA *P* 40v–41r: Timiama (*sic*)
1 cynnama] *scripsi* (*cf. line 13*), tymiama *P*

and, great in value, does not stoop to the level of the poor;
therefore it is said to dry and heat in the second degree.
Powdered Clove, when mixed with wine, increases
the brain's power of memory if it is often drunk;
taken thus it strengthens the liver and the stomach.
And so that I might briefly wrap up many things,
physicians have written that Cloves aid all interior matters
and (here's what I could marvel at!) although it hastens
digestion in the belly, yet it hinders the belly's flux.
If a dram's weight is drunk with cow's milk,
Venus, armed with this skill, fans again the weak flames.

6.1.5 Cinnamon, *Cinnamomum zeylanicum* Nees

The Cinnamons cannot be beaten for their powers,
nor can they be equalled for their sweetest taste.
This spice cures watery eyes by drying;
it cleans a face occupied by a nasty mole
if you apply this, ground with strong vinegar.
A cough and catarrh will be destroyed by this spice;
take this and the liver is cured and urine rushes out.
It dries a humid stomach and helps it
to cook and digest eaten foods more quickly.
There is recorded a type of dropsy which they name
tympana; this represses that disease and kidney pain.
Thus it destroys the disease that takes its name from 'attack!'.
The Cinnamons quickly heal reptilian bites.
Learned doctors said there are three varieties of this:
one of these is a more refined spice than the others.
It is more precious [. . .]
but the one that is heavier heals well bleeding haemorrhoids
if a person drinks it, ground in water, on an empty stomach.
This most luxurious of potions demands two drams.

14 *Cf.* Ovid, *Ars amatoria* 1. 362; 2. 480

6.1.5 CYNNAMA / **Cinnamon** *Macer, 'Cinnama', 2147–64*
12 *Cf.* Quintus Serenus 155

6.1.6 CASSIA

Cassia non eadem que cassia fistula confert,
Cassia namque gradu feruet siccatque secundo
Sed Galienus ait quod cassia fistula prestet
Inter utrosque gradus. Calidam nec iudicat ipsam,
Nec frigescentem, nec humentem, neque siccam—
Tanta temperie dedit hanc Natura uigere.
Cassia sumpta iecur confortat, * * * * sterasque
Cunctaque primatum retinencia corpore membra,
At rubeam coleram bene cassia fistula purgat.
Cassia confortat ualide muliebria membra
Eius si tepido sint apozimate fota;
Sanguinis extinguit uim cassia fistula diram.
Cassia uentosas dissoluit rite querelas;
Soluit apostema sic cassia fistula durum
Quod cruor ipse creat, nec quicquid soluit ut ipsa.
Cassia purificans grossis humoribus obstat;
Rumpit apostema bene cassia fistula bucce.
Cassia si ueniat, fugit opilacio uulue;
Gargarizetur si cassia fistula curat
Eque gingiuas, fauces uuasque tumentes
Et melius stringni succus si iungitur illi.
Vix igitur uideas quenam precellit earum
Viribus excelsis eque uires utriusque.
Cinnama Cleopatra, si desit cassia, ponit
At Dyascoride aliter nam cinnama duplat;
Cinnama si desint eadem, te, cassia, ponit.
Elige quem pocius (nam summus uterque) sequaris.

6.1.7 GALANGA

Gratificat gratos galanga salubris odores
Si sit odoriferis commixta recens speciebus,
Nam galanga uetus multas agitata per auras

6.1.6 CASSIA *P* 41r: Cassia
6 uigere] *scripsi*, rigere *P* 24 desit] *scripsi*, desint *P* 26 si] *add.* duplant *et canc. P* 27 summus] *scripsi*, fumus *P*

6.1.7 GALANGA *P* 41r–41v: Galanga

6.1.6 Cassia, *Cinnamomum cassia* Blume

Cassia bark does not provide the same things as Cassia fruit,
for Cassia bark heats and dries in the second degree,
but Galen says that Cassia fruit stands between
both degrees. He does not judge it hot,
nor cooling, nor moistening, nor dry—
Nature grants that it is effective by such moderation.
Cassia bark, when eaten, strengthens the liver, [. . . . .] and womb,
and all members of the highest rank within the body,
but Cassia fruit purges red bile well.
Cassia bark powerfully strengthens feminine parts
if they should be washed with a warming salve of it;
Cassia fruit destroys the harmful power of blood.
Cassia bark properly dissolves windy problems;
thus Cassia fruit dissolves the hard abscess
that blood itself creates, and nothing dissolves like it.
Purifying Cassia bark stops fatty humours;
Cassia fruit breaks up cheek ulcers well.
If Cassia bark arrives, a blockage of the womb departs;
if Cassia fruit is gargled it equally cures
swollen gums and throats and uvulas,
and even better if Nightshade juice is added to it.
So you can scarcely see which one of these excels
the powers of the other with equally lofty powers.
If Cleopatra is missing Cassia, she uses Cinnamon,
but Dioscorides does otherwise, for he doubles the Cinnamon;
if Cinnamon is lacking, Cassia, she uses you.
Choose whom you would rather follow, for either is the best.

6.1.7 Galangal, *Alpinia officinarum* Hance.

Wholesome Galangal grants agreeable odours
if it is mixed, when fresh, with sweet-smelling spices,
for old Galangal and other spices, beaten about

6.1.6 CASSIA / **Cassia** *Constantine, 'Cassia fistula', 346–7, and 'Cassia lignea', 369*

6.1.7 GALANGA / **Galangal** *Macer, 'Galanga', 2125–30*

Et species alie ui deficiunt et odore,
At galanga recens oris commendat odores.
Si stomachus sit flecmaticus corroborat ipsum:
Flecma solet nimium stomachi depellere sumptum.
Hoc prodest colicis, hoc prompte digerit escas,
Renum frigorem fugat accenditque calorem.
Concitat indecorem ueneris stillando calorem.

6.1.8 ZEDVAR

At zeduar stomachum confortat debilitatum
Vnde mouet ructus speciei crebrior usus,
Atque frequens eius fastidia comprimit usus
Nam stomachi ueterem perhibent delere dolorem.
Si ieiunus eam lento commasticet ore
Et sic infectam trahat intus ab ore saliuam,
Ventri lumbricos interficit hec inimicos.
Hanc eciam sumptis scribunt obstare uenenis
Et quod reptilium morsus mire iuuat hausta.
Allia quem faciunt fetorem sumpta repellit
Et uini nimis assumpti depellit odorem.

6.1.9 CIMINVM

Pauci diuini uires nouere cimini
Quamuis sit plebi sapor acceptissimus illi.
Vires innumere sunt sed captus breuitate
De multis non multa tuli que certa notaui.
Vt piper hec species siccare, calere probatur:
Tercius est in eis gradus, illis tercius isti,
Sed distant quoniam piper auget amoris acumen,

8 hoc ... hoc] *scripsi*, hec ... hec *P*

6.1.8 ZEDVAR *P* 41v: Zeduar
9 hausta] *scripsi*, haustum *P* 10 allia] *scripsi*, alia *P*

6.1.9 CIMINVM *P* 41v: Ciminum

by many breezes, are lacking in strength and scent,
but fresh Galangal improves odours of the mouth.
If the stomach is phlegmatic, this improves it:
when taken, it is apt to destroy excessive stomach phlegm.
This is good for the bilious, it readily digests foods,
chases out a chill of the kidneys and kindles their heat.
In drops, it arouses the unseemly heat of sexual desire.

6.1.8 Zedoary, *Curcuma zedoaria* Roscoe

But Zedoary strengthens a weakened stomach,
so repeated use of the spice causes belching,
and its frequent use removes distaste,
for they relate that it destroys an old stomach ache.
If one should chew it slowly, on an empty stomach,
and then swallow the imbued saliva from the mouth,
this kills harmful stomach worms.
They write that this also blocks swallowed poisons
and that, when drunk, it marvellously aids reptile bites.
When taken, it repels the odour that Garlic makes
and removes the smell of drinking too much wine.

6.1.9 Cumin, *Cuminum cyminum* L.

Few have known the powers of divine Cumin,
although its flavour is very pleasing to the people.
Its powers are countless but, seized by brevity, I have related
but a few of the many things that I have observed for certain.
Like Pepper, this spice is proven to dry and heat:
the degree is third in the former, and third as well in the latter,
but they differ in that Pepper increases the prick of love,

10 *Cf.* Virgil, *Aeneid* 11. 845

6.1.8 ZEDVAR / **Zedoary** *Macer, 'Zedoar', 2131–40*

6.1.9 CIMINVM / **Cumin** *Macer, 'Cyminum', 2111–24*

Hec uero species contundit amoris acumen.
Affirmant emoptoicos sedare ciminum,
Si tamen hoc fuerit cum pusca sepius haustum.
Affirmo quod aque si iungatur bene tritum
Pectora, corda, iecur (res est probata) iuuabit.
At quocumque modo sumas qui uiscera uexat
Excludit uentum stomachi iecorisque calorem
Commouet acceptas ut prompte digerat escas
Sumptaque cum uino uirosis morsibus obstat.
Tritum uero fabe cum polline, melle tepenti
Coniuncto, testes poterit curare tumentes;
Sumptum cum mulsa mulieris menstrua sistit.
Efficit exanguem mansum persepe colorem
Et ne uana putes nos hic commenta tulisse,
Verba uide Flacci, 'biberent exangue ciminum,'
Verba uel Ouidii, 'pallentis grana cimini.'

6.1.10 CEROTON

Est ceroton genus in species diuersificatum:
Vna quidem species redolentibus exit ab Yndis
Ast aliam mittunt Arabes et crescit in ortis.
Illa rubens et amara nimis que uenit ab Yndis,
Ista subalba, leuis, exorta nitentibus ortis,
Viribus et distant nam prestat prima secunde
Quantum syderibus Latonia, sidera gemmis,
Gemma rosis, uiole rosulis, uiole saliuncis.
Ergo si tepido potetur trita lyeo
Curat epar languens et splen laterisque dolorem;
Proficit urine, pellens obstancia queque.
Femina languescens si se suffumiget illa
Menstrua purificat uulueque dolor tenuatur.
Si tritam cum melle linas lentigo peribit.
Ex oleo cocta febrientes illine costo:

16 cum *add. s.l. P* 17 tritum *corr. e* tritam *P* 18 poterit] *scripsi*, poteris *P* 20 exanguem] *scripsi*, exangwe *P* colorem] *scripsi*, calorem *P* 22 Flacci] *scripsi*, Flaccii *P* biberent] *scripsi*, bibens *P*

6.1.10 CEROTON *P* 41v–42r: Ceroton

2 quidem *corr. e* quidam *P* 8 gemma] *scripsi*, gemme *P* uiole[1]] si *add. et canc. P*

while this spice beats down love's sting.
They affirm that Cumin soothes blood-spitters
if it should be drunk quite often with vinegar-water.
I affirm that if it is ground well and mixed in water
it will aid the chest, heart, and liver (this is a proven thing).
But however you may take it, it removes the stomach wind
that vexes the interior, and it provokes the liver's heat
so that it digests eaten foods without hesitation,
and when taken with wine it hinders poisonous bites.
But ground with bean meal, and with warm honey
blended in, it should be able to heal swollen testicles;
taken with mead it stops a woman's menstrual courses.
Eaten very often, it brings on a bloodless pallor,
and lest you think we've offered empty statements here,
check the words of Horace, 'Let them drink the bloodless Cumin,'
or the words of Ovid, 'the grains of pallid Cumin.'

6.1.10 ? Carob, *Ceratonia siliqua* L.

Carob is a genus distinguished into species:
one variety comes from the sweet-smelling Indies
but the Arabs send the other and it grows in gardens.
The former, red and very bitter, which comes from the Indies,
and the latter, rather pale and smooth, born of blooming gardens,
differ also in powers for the first is superior to the second
as much as Diana is to the stars, the stars are to gems,
a gem is to Roses, Violets are to Roses, and Violets are to *saliunca*.
Therefore if it is ground into warm wine and drunk,
it cures a suffering liver and spleen and a pain in the side;
it is good for the urine, breaking up any obstructions.
If a weakened woman should fumigate herself with it,
it purifies her period and a pain of the womb is soothed.
If you rub this on, when ground with honey, a mole will vanish.
Anoint the feverish with this cooked in oil-of-Cost:

22 Horace, *Epistulae* 1. 19. 17–18   23 Persius, *Satira* 5. 55

6.1.10 CEROTON / ? Carob *Source unknown*

1 Boethius, *Porphyrii Isagoge*; Isidore, *Etym.* 1. 37. 12   5 *Cf.* Ovid, *Fasti* 5. 11. 543   8 *Cf.* Virgil, *Ecloga* 5. 16–17

Ante febris typum tutos a frigore cernis.
Hec sciasi, trepidis hec proderit unctio membris;
Vulneris antiqui puluis cladem uacuabit.
Lumbricos perimit mulse sociata tepenti;
Dat quod amarus amor uenansque Venus remouentur.

6.1.11 LIQVIRICIA

Vis liquiricie non parua potest reputari,
Vlla nec specie dulcore potest superari.
Illi temperiem tantam Natura ministrat
Vt uix humectans, uix infrigidans neque primi
Esse gradus possit. Cunctis bona, noxia nulli,
Sic igitur genus humanum splendens medicatur,
Alloquitur: 'Sum uestra salus—properate, uenite!
Quosquos pulmo grauans, quos tussis hanela fatigat,
Pectora, guttura, constrictos humecto canales;
Pectora, guttura, duratas expurgo toraces.
Si cum penidiis mea sit decoccio mixta
Et paciens mandat, nil eque pectora mundat.
Ampne cocor, decocta premor compressaque siccor;
Sicca uocor 'chylum,' mundi per climata notum.
Sic iuuo pulmones duros mulcendo rigores
Et species stomacho tam prodest nulla perusto.
Ac instrumentis pulmonis, pectoris ipsa
Quoque modo medeor, nec dulcius ulla medetur,
Nam, non ut costus eructans aloeue fremiscens,
Nec torquendo fero sed demulcendo salutem.'

6.1.12 ALOE

Est aloe species sanctissima: corpore toto
Regnat et humores expellit quosque per aluum.
Hanc acri uino iunges oleoque rosato:

6.1.11 LIQVIRICIA *P* 42r: Liquiricia
1 liquiricie *corr. ex* illic/quiricie (?) *P* 6 medica*tur corr. e* medica*tis P* 7 properate] *scripsi*, properte *P*

6.1.12 ALOE *P* 42r–42v: Aloe
1 est *corr. ex* ast *P*

before the fever takes shape you see them safe from chill.
This ointment should be good for sciatica and shaky limbs;
its powder will clear up the scourge of an old wound.
Mixed in warm mead it destroys stomach worms
and grants that bitter lust and the huntress Venus are removed.

6.1.11 Liquorice, *Glycyrrhiza glabra* L.

The power of Liquorice cannot be considered small,
nor can it be surpassed by any spice in sweetness.
Nature bestows on it such moderation that,
scarcely heating and scarcely cooling, it cannot be
even of the first degree. Good for all and harmful to none,
it therefore splendidly medicates mankind in this way
and says: 'I am your health. Hasten and come!
I moisten whomever the lung burdens, whom a panting cough
fatigues, and chests, throats, and constricted windpipes;
I purge chests, throats, and congested torsos.
If my decoction is mixed with barley-sugar
and the patient eats, nothing cleanses chests so well.
I'm cooked in water, cooked I'm pressed, and pressed I'm dried;
when dry I am called *chylum*, known through the world's climes.
In such a way I help hard lungs by softening hardenings
and no spice is as beneficial for a burning stomach.
And now I myself also heal the channels of the lungs
and chest, nor does any other heal more sweetly,
for—neither like belching Cost nor shaking Aloe—
I don't bring health by torturing, but by softening.'

6.1.12 Aloe, *Aloe vera* L.

Aloe is a most holy spice: it rules the whole body
and expels any humours through the stool.
Blend it with vinegar and oil-of-Rose: by rubbing

6.1.11 LIQVIRICIA / **Liquorice** *Constantine, 'Liquiritia,'* 347
3–6 *Cf.* Ovid, *Met.* 1. 51 7 (*Sum uestra salus*) *Cf.* Augustine, *Confessions* 1. 5 7 (*properate, uenite*) *Cf.* Isa. 55: 1

6.1.12 ALOE / **Aloe** *Macer, 'Aloë,'* 2233–69

Hoc caput et frontem sanes ungendo dolentem;
Vnguen pruritum mire fugat hoc oculorum.
Cum uino retinere pilos quoscumque cadentes
Si cathaplasmere medici dixere periti,
Quam si soluis aqua, superaddens, † sic oculorum
Dolor, † sic naris, sic apostema labrorum,
Sic et liuorem caua circum lumina purgat.
Hanc uino cum melle teras fricataque linguis
Gingiuisque ualet, uiciis simul omnibus oris.
Interiora iuuat iecoris stomachumque caputque
Articulosque simul purgando flecma per aluum;
Prodest ictericis mire purgacio talis.
Illius puluis curabit testiculorum
Vulnera, curabit uentris (res sepe probata)
Sicque recens uulnus putredine mundat ab omni.
Cetera cum soleant soluencia ledere uentrem,
Hanc stomacho multum probat Oribasius aptam
Ledere que nescit—quamuis non soluat acute.
Idem constituit, si flecma uelis coleramque
Expurgare, duas cum mulsa sumere dragmas.
Post cenam pilulas tres eius sumere siue
Binas cum succo caulis nimis utile dicit
Vnaquaque die formatas ut cicer hocque
Non stomachum uexans humores purgat iniquos.
Dicit quod pilulas qui sepius ederit istas
Nesciet ille grauem capitis tolerare dolorem,
Affirmans oculis nichil umquam gracius ipsis.
Idem testatur cum durum largiter aluum
Dissoluisse uolunt geminans pars additur huius,
Vna dyagridii: sic antidotum fit amicum.
Dicunt autores quod partibus hec geminatis
Constet: nam rubet hec preciosa quidem medicinis,
Altera nigrior est medicisque beatior extat.
   Sint satis hec nam de piretro que quantaque possit
Continet ille liber qui centum continet herbas.

8 soluis] *scripsi*, solius *P*   10 purgat *canc. et add.* turpat *P*   17 uentris] *scripsi*, uentri *P*   25 dicit] *add.* esse *P*   26 cicer] *scripsi*, citer *P*   29 tolerare] *scripsi*, tollerare *P*   31 durum] *scripsi*, duram *P*   37 que] *scripsi*, qui *P*

this on you may heal an aching head and forehead;
this ointment marvellously chases off an itching of the eyes.
Learned physicians said that you can keep any hair
from falling if you should apply this as a plaster with wine,
and if you dissolve it in water and apply, it thus purges
† a pain of the eyes, so also abscesses of the nostril and the lips,
so also the darkness found around sunken eyes. †
Grind this into wine with honey: when rubbed it is good
for tongues, gums, and likewise any vices of the mouth.
It helps the interior of the liver, the stomach and the head,
and the joints as well by purging phlegm through the stool;
such a purgative is wonderfully good for the jaundiced.
Powdered Aloe will cure wounds of the testicles,
and will cure those of the stomach (an often proven thing!)
and thus it cleans a recent wound of all putrefaction.
Although other solvent cures are apt to injure the belly,
Oribasius proves that this is very suitable for the stomach,
and can do no harm (although it does not sharply dissolve).
The same author ordered you to take two drams
with mead if you wish to purge phlegm or bile.
He says it's very useful to take after dinner
three pills of this, or two with Cabbage juice,
formed in the shape of a chickpea, every day; this purges
wicked humours without troubling the stomach.
He says that he who rather often takes these pills
will be unable to suffer a serious headache,
confirming that nothing's ever better for eyes than these.
He says that when they wish to have dissolved
a greatly hardened stool, two parts of this are added
and one of Scammony: thus it becomes a friendly antidote.
The authors say that this exists in two varieties,
for one is red and precious, to be sure, in medicines,
the other darker and reckoned better by physicians.

Let this suffice, for that book which contains one hundred herbs
contains, under Pellitory, what things and how many it can do.

6 <INTERLVDVM>

Finieram. Quidam uero, qui tota uerendus
Pectora pubetenus barba contexerat hirta,
Is barbam digitis contrectans, 'Sit licet,' inquit,
'Hoc signum non discendi sed rite docendi,
Quero tamen dubius cur has species duodenas
Quam species alias tractatu condecorasti?
Iste sunt equidem—nec detrecto—preciose.'
Tunc ego: 'Seu Socrates sis uel de gente Crisippi,
Docte pater, uulgo uulgarem ferre poetam
Vota decet: uix has nouerunt, et michi note
Sunt harum uires et nomina, non aliarum.'
Ille sub hec: 'Quod Arabs quondam, quod Serus et Yndus
Inter eos peregrinantes, docuere reponam.'

6.2.1 BALSAMVM

Sunt summi precii prestancia balsama mire,
Sunt et opis summe medicancia balsama mire.
Hec Natura parens summo dotauit honore,
Omnis et hec mundus summo dignatur odore.
  Scribunt ipsa gradu siccare, calere secundo.
Vtilius nichil est oculis caligine pressis.
Sacra diuturne succurrunt balsama tussi
Materiamque grauem disrumpunt perque canales
Pulmonis pellunt; urinam, menstrua ducunt.
Membri natiui mulierum frigiditatem
Subdita percurant et abortum siue secundas.
Hinc epitimatus febrium lenire rigorem
Posse liquor scitur. Si durus hanelitus assit
Huic peragorisat. Posuere tuas medicantes,
Camphora lenis, aquas eque cum balsama desunt.

6 <INTERLVDVM> *P* 42v–43r: [no title] *Edited by Rigg*, 286–7.
3 sit] *Rigg*, sic *P* 9 uulgo . . . poetam / uix . . . note *inv. et corr. P*

6.2.1 BALSAMVM *P* 43r–43v: Balsamum
3 dotauit] *scripsi*, predotauit *P* 10 mulierum] *add.* febrietatem *et canc. P*

6 Interlude

I had finished. But a certain awesome man, who was covered
with a shaggy beard down his entire chest to his privates,
was fondling this beard with his fingers and said, 'Although
this is not a sign of learning, but rightly of teaching,
yet I ask, in doubt, why you have adorned these twelve spices
with a treatise rather than some other spices?
They are precious, to be sure. I won't deny it.'
Then I replied: 'Whether you are Socrates or of Chrysippus's race,
O learned father, it is fitting that a people's poet fulfil
the wishes of the people: they scarcely know these spices.
The names and virtues of these are known to me, but not of those.'
He replied to this: 'I will add what the Arab once taught,
and what the Chinese and Indian, travelling among them.'

6.2.1 Balm of Gilead, *Commiphora opobalsamum* L.

The wonderfully outstanding Balms have the greatest value,
and the wonderfully medicating Balms provide the greatest aid.
Mother Nature endowed them with the greatest honour,
and the whole world thinks them worthy for their odour.
  They write that they are dry and hot in the second degree.
Nothing is more useful for eyes burdened with a mist.
Holy Balms help a persistent cough
and break up heavy matter, forcing through
the pulmonary canals; they bring out urine and a period.
As a suppository they thoroughly cure frigidity
of women's genitals and expel a foetus or afterbirth.
The juice of this, made into a lotion, is known to be able
to allay the severity of fevers. If a heavy gasping occurs,
this is soothing for it. Gentle Camphor, they have applied
your medicating juices just as much when Balms are absent.

6 <INTERLVDVM> / **Interlude** *Original*

1 *Cf.* Martial, *Ep.* 8. 3. 9; Ovid, *Met.* 2. 103 12 (*Ille sub hec*) *Cf.* Virgil, *Aeneid* 5. 394; Statius, *Thebaid* 3. 516 12 (*Arabs . . . Yndus*) *Cf.* Isidore, *Etym.* 17. 8. 1; Isidore, *Versus* xix, 1–2; xx, 1–2 (ed. Sánchez Martín, 229, 231)

6.2.1 BALSAMVM / **Balm of Gilead** *Constantine, 'Balsamus', 356–7*

Carpobalsama sunt fructus quos balsama produnt:
Hunc fructum uertigo ferox, ortomia feruens,
Tussis hanela fugit, timet epilensis acerba,
Pleuresis et sciasis, strangiria, flecma recedunt.
Reptilium morsus ualet hic compescere potus.
Nec mirum si tanta potest * * * * * * * * * * *.
Si deerit fructus eque xilobalsama pones
Dimidiumque equi, nam carpobalsama presunt,
Nec raro medicina frequens xilobalsama poscit;
Suauius hec eadem que carpobalsama donant.
Cum sol feruentes Cancrum tenet atque Leonem
Finditur hoc lignum: de cuius cortice manant
Quadraginta libre uel quinquaginta liquorum.
Isdem persistunt gradibus carpo, xilo, gutta;
Gutta preest, carpum sequitur, xilo cedit utrique
Et 'carpum' fructus, 'xilo' lignum, 'balsama' gutta.

6.2.2 AGARICVM

Agaricum, quod diureticum perhibet Galienus,
Neffreticis et pleureticis fit amabile munus.
Hoc Dyaschorides, hoc Oribasius aiunt
Grossos humores et flecmata stringere potum.
Inflatum tranquillat epar, strangiria cedet
Atque dolor renum. Matricibus ycctericisque
Prodest; cum sapa pulmonis uulnera sanat.
Agaricum laudans, inquit magnus Galienus:
Viscera munda facit, simul opilata resoluit.
Proficit yctericus, ualet epilenticus illo.
Menstrua dat, fugat arteticam sciasimque febremque
Et, quo philosophus concluderet omnia, solus
Addidit: omne latens quod celant corpora purgat.

16 produnt] *scripsi*, edunt *P* 20 hic] *scripsi*, hec *P* 21 *uerba post caesuram desunt* 22 xilobalsama *corr. e* silobalsama *P* 24 xilobalsama *corr. e* silobalsama *P* 25 suauius] *scripsi*, suauis *P* 29 xilo *corr. e* silo *P* 30 xilo *corr. e* silo *P* 31 xilo *corr. e* silo *P*

6.2.2 AGARICVM *P* 43v: Agaricus
5 strangiria] *scripsi*, strangiriam *P* 7 sapa] *scripsi*, sapo *P* 8 inquit magnus] *scripsi*, magnus inquit *P*

Carpobalsama are the fruits that Balms produce:
fierce vertigo, burning orthopnea, and a panting cough
flee from this fruit, the bitter epilepsy fears it,
and pleurisy, sciatica, strangury, and phlegm depart.
It is able to restrain reptilian bites when taken in drink.
No wonder that it can do such things, [........].
If the fruit is lacking, use the same amount of *xilobalsama*
and half again as much, for *carpobalsama* are superior,
and not rarely does medicine repeatedly ask for *xilobalsama*,
which more pleasantly give what the *carpobalsama* grant.
When the sun holds burning Cancer and Leo,
a branch of this is split and from its bark pour
forty or fifty pounds of its juices.
The fruit and branch and gum stand in the same degrees:
the gum is superior, the fruit is next, and the branch yields to both.
The fruit is *carpum*, *xilo* the branch, and *balsama* the gum.

6.2.2 Field Mushroom, *Agaricus campestris* L., or family *Agaricaceae* L.

The Mushroom, which Galen says is diuretic, becomes
a pleasing gift for those with nephritis and with pleurisy.
Dioscorides and Oribasius say that this,
when drunk, restrains thick humours and phlegm.
It soothes a swollen liver, strangury will depart
as does kidney pain. It is beneficial for wombs and for
the jaundiced; with wine must it cleans wounds of the lungs.
Great Galen, praising the Mushroom, said it makes
the insides clean and at the same time loosens blockages.
One with jaundice profits by it and an epileptic improves.
It causes menstruation, chases off arthritis, sciatica, and fever,
and—so that the Philosopher might sum up all things—he alone did add:
it purges every hidden thing that bodies may conceal.

26–28 *Cf.* Boethius, *De cons. phil.* 1 met. 6, 1–2

6.2.2 AGARICVM / **Field Mushroom** *Constantine, 'Agaricus,' 346*

3 Latin Dioscorides, 'De agaricu,' 10. 375; Oribasius, 'De Agarico,' 4. 3

Agaricum dicitur hic mas, hec femina fertur;
Integer est qui masculus est, leuis atque rotundus.
Illa fit, ex frustis grauis, prestancius illo
Inque gradu primo feruet siccatque secundo.

6.2.3 AMOMVM

Dulce Dei donum, mirabile fraglat amomum
Quod quam famosum tam crediderim preciosum.
Hoc igitur famam preciumque meretur odore;
Si non esset odor, reniteret utrimque uigore,
Nam uicium dire solet extirpare podagre
Eius si fuerit tantum decoccio pota,
Sic et nefreticis et sic prodest epilensi.
Subdita si uulue mulieris forte sedentis
Hec decoccio sit, uulue dolor adnichilatur.
Hec et multa potest, que longum multa referre.
Tercius huic gradus est in ui sicca calidaque.

6.2.4 STORAX

Primum storace que sit diuisio dicam:
Hec liquet et sigiam dicunt, aliam calamitam,
Inque gradu primo feruent siccantque secundo.
Hanc mollitiuam digestiuamque probarunt.
Tussis eam ueterana fugit resonansque catarrus
Atque Dyascorides uocem raucam tenuare
Et uuluam perhibet duram tumidamque leuare.
Pectus dat calidum, dat proflua menstrua potum.
Storace sigia quidam perhibent ueniente
Pustula quod queuis cedat scabiesque repente.

14 femina] *add.* femina *et exp. P*

6.2.3 AMOMVM *P* 43v–44r: Amomum

1 mirabile] *Rigg* (*private conversation*), iocunde *P* 8 uulue (wlue) *ante corr. P*] wulue *post corr. P* 9 sit] *scripsi*, fit *P* uulue] *scripsi*, wulue *P*

6.2.4 STORAX *P* 44r: Storax

1 storace] *scripsi*, strorace *P* 7 uuluam *corr. ex* wuluam *P*

This Mushroom is called male, and that one is said to be female;
the one which is masculine is whole, light, and round.
The female, heavy with small pieces, is more valuable than the male;
it heats in the first degree and in the second dries.

6.2.3 Bastard Cardamom, *Amomum xanthoides* Wal.

A sweet gift of God, admirable Amomum is fragrant,
and I should believe it is as valuable as it is famous.
Therefore it merits fame and value for its odour;
if it had no odour, it would shine out everywhere with strength,
for it can extirpate the vice of wicked gout
if only its decoction should be drunk,
and thus it is good for nephritics and for epilepsy.
If perhaps this decoction is introduced to the womb
of a sitting woman, a pain in the womb is destroyed.
It can do these and many things, which would take long to tell.
Its degree is third in powers dry and hot.

6.2.4 Gum Tree, *Liquidambar orientalis* Mill.

First, I will tell you how the Gum Tree is distinguished.
This part is a liquid: they call it *sigia*; the other is *calamita*,
and they heat and dry in the second degree.
They have proven that it is softening and digestive.
An old cough and the whooping cough flee from it,
and Dioscorides relates that it soothes a hoarse voice
and relieves a hard and swollen womb.
When drunk, it warms the chest and causes a period to flow.
Some claim that with the arrival of the *sigia* of the Gum Tree,
every pustule and scab immediately departs.

6.2.3 AMOMVM / **Bastard Cardamom** *Constantine, 'Amomum', 376*

6.2.4 STORAX / **Gum Tree** *Constantine, 'Styrax', 351*

6.2.5 MASTIX

Est mastix species quam quidam 'mastica' dicunt
Affirmantque gradu siccare, calere secundo.
Mastix, quod stomachus caleat, dat ut appetat escas
Et uento nocuo depurgat flecmaque soluit.
Intestinorum necnon epatis stomachique
Apostema grauans rumpit sedatque tumores.
Masticis affectus tristes rumpit medicatus
Cumque oleo roseo stomachum confortat opime
Clarificatque cutem si mixtis bis superungas.
Hec Oribasius. Dyascorides docet autor
Hanc emoptoycis mire tussique salubrem
Hanc. Damasceni dicam decreta Iohannis:
Hec in aqua gelida stomachum confortat et eius
Expiat humores; nichil in calida ualet ipsa.
'Quid Galienus ait?' Si laueris illius ampne
Os sic gingiuis fissis, tumidis, putrefactis
Prodest, ac Cleopatra docet prodesse squinantum
Tantundem. Dicunt alii, cum gutta sit ista
Lenticii, pinee ualet eque aut gumma cipressi.

6.2.6 ANISVM

Fit medicamentis anisi gratissima multis.
Tercius huic gradus est dum siccat dumque calescit.
Humores grossos uentumque fugat stomachalem.
Splen opilatum potu percurat eparque.
Lac mammis, locium, sudorem, menstrua confert.
Assum feruentis constipat tormina uentris.
Naribus iniecto fumo dolor ille recedit
Quem capiti uentus grossus uel reuma ministrat.

6.2.5 MASTIX *P* 44r–44v: Mastix

3 ut] *scripsi*, et *P* 7 affectus] *scripsi*, effectus *P* 9 mixtis *corr. e* mixtus *P* 10 Oribasius] *scripsi*, orbasius *P* 13 hec] *scripsi*, hanc *P* 17 squinantum] *scripsi*, quinantum *P*

6.2.6 ANISVM *P* 44v: Anisium

2 siccat] *conieci*, feruet *P* 5 mammis *corr. e* manus *P* 8 grossus] *scripsi*, gressus *P* reuma] *scripsi*, reum *P*

6.2.5 Mastic, *Pistacia lentiscus* L.

Mastic is a spice which some call *mastica*
and they affirm it dries and heats in the second degree.
Because Mastic heats the stomach, it makes it desire food,
and purges it of harmful wind and dissolves phlegm.
It breaks a heavy abscess in the intestines,
the liver, and the stomach, and represses tumours.
A medicine made of Mastic breaks a sad disposition,
with oil-of-Rose it superbly strengthens the stomach,
and it cleans the skin if you apply this mixture twice.
Oribasius says these things. The author Dioscorides teaches
that this is very wholesome for spitters of blood and for a cough.
I will tell you the teachings of John of Damascus:
in cold water this strengthens the stomach
and repairs its humours; it is no good in hot water.
'What does Galen say?' If you rinse the mouth in Mastic-water,
it is good for split, swollen, and rotten gums,
and Cleopatra teaches that Lemongrass is just as good for this.
Others say that since this is the gum of the Mastic tree,
the gum of a pine or cypress works equally as well.

6.2.6 Anise, *Pimpinella anisum* L.

Anise is very pleasing in many medicines.
It has the third degree when it dries and when it heats.
It chases off coarse humours and windiness from the stomach.
In a drink it thoroughly cures an obstructed spleen and the liver.
It creates milk in the breasts, and urine, sweat and menses.
When roasted, it stops up the pains of a burning belly.
With its smoke inhaled up the nose, that pain departs
which a heavy windiness or catarrh brings to the head.

6.2.5 MASTIX / **Mastic** *Constantine, 'De Mastice', 354*
16 Constantine, 'De mastice' (in *Opera omnia Ysaac*, 2. 81r)

6.2.6 ANISVM / **Anise** *Constantine, 'Anisum', 376*

Ictus uel casus si conturbauerit aurem
Hoc oleo roseo mixto releuabitur auris.
Te puer ales amat; tibi spicula rite ministrat.

6.2.7 GENCIANA

Da ueniam, lector, quod genciana locatur
Versibus, huius enim ueniam michi fama meretur.
Huius opes et opus sollers medicina stupescit,
Nec—licet hec Ypocras neget—experiencia fallit.
Melle et aqua potum uel compositum cathaplasma
Morsum serpentis miro certamine uincit.
Mundificat, tenuat, colat quodcumque nociuum
Splen uel epar generant; simul opilata resoluunt.
Menstrua producens, depellere prompta secundas
Quodque nimis magnum diiudico, pellit abortum.
Tercius huic gradus est dum siccat siue calescit.

6.2.8 EVFORBIVM

Feruida, sicca gradu prestant euforbia quarto,
Antidotis species speciosis dedita multis.
Attenuans, urens, incidens flecmata purgat
Corporis in quocumque loco dampnosa lutescant,
Hec tamen angustat, desiccat discoriatque.
Sed iunguntur ei que frangunt eius acumen:
Bdellius aut asarum uel cinnama, cassia, spica,
Queque ualent alie fortissima lenificare.
Hoc cum melle ualet cataractis oculorum;
Hoc oleo mixtum si distillatur in aures,
Auribus abscedent dolor et sonitus grauitasque,
At depurgat aromaticis sciasim sociatum.
Hoc oleo iunctum dat ut allopicia cedat,
Ac uentrem curat. Medicis tot tantaque patrat.

6.2.7 GENCIANA *P* 44v: Genciana

6.2.8 EVFORBIVM *P* 44v–45r: Euforbium

6 iunguntur] *scripsi*, iungutur *P* 9 hoc] *scripsi*, hec *P* 12 at . . . sociatum] *scripsi*, atque sciam depurgat aromaticis sociatum *P* 13 allopicia] *scripsi*, allopica *P* 14 patrat] *scripsi*, patrant *P*

If a blow or fall should disturb the ear,
the ear will be relieved by Anise mixed with oil-of-Rose.
The Winged Boy loves you and rightly provides you with little darts.

6.2.7 Gentian, family *Gentianaceae* L.

Reader, please forgive the fact that Gentian is found
within these verses, for its fame merits forgiveness for me.
Skilful medicine grows dumb at its influence and effect,
nor does experience deceive—though Hippocrates denies these things!
When drunk with honey and water or made into a plaster
this conquers a serpent's bite in a marvellous struggle.
It cleans, thins out, and soothes whatever harm
the spleen or liver bring about; it also dissolves obstructions.
It brings out menstrual courses, is quick to expel the afterbirth and—
what I consider exceptionally powerful—it expels a foetus.
It has the third degree when it dries or heats.

6.2.8 Spurge, probably *Euphorbia resinifera* Berg.

The Spurges stand out as hot and dry in the fourth degree,
a spice that is added to many valuable antidotes.
By thinning, heating, and cutting, it purges injurious phlegm
in whatever place of the body it grows thick,
yet it reduces, dries out, and destroys it.
These things are added to it which dull its edge:
Bdellium, Hazelwort, Cinnamon, Cassia, and Spikenard,
and whatever others are able to soften the strongest things.
With honey this is good for cataracts of the eyes;
if this is mixed with olive oil and dripped into the ears,
pain and ringing and heaviness will depart from them;
but mixed with aromatics it purges sciatica.
When mixed with oil, this causes balding to depart, and it cures
the stomach. It achieves so many and such great things for doctors.

11 Horace, *Odes* 3. 12. 4

6.2.7 GENCIANA / **Gentian** *Constantine, 'Gentiana', 367*

1 *Cf.* Ovid, *Heroides* 4. 156; *Ars amatoria* 2. 38; *Met.* 11. 132 3 Hildebert of Lavardin, *Carmina minora* no. 46, 9 (ed. Scott); Firmicus Maternus, *Mathesis* 4. 19 (ed. Monat, 2. 183)

6.2.8 EVFORBIVM / **Spurge** *Constantine, 'Euphorbium', 381*

6.2.9 FOLIVM

Et folium feruetque gradu siccatque secundo,
Inter odoriferas species non ultima laude.
Hec stomacho prodest, confortat epar reparatque,
Prouocat urinas inflataque soluere fertur,
Et cathaplasmatum tergit clades oculorum.
Si desit folium ponetur Celtica nardus.

6.2.10 CARDAMOMVM

Nec cardamomi laudes taceantur odori.
Est igitur duplex: istud maius, minus istud,
Vtraque uero gradu siccans et feruida primo.
Corpore si maius, minus est uirtute caloris,
Quoque minus calida est, tanto magis extat odoris.
Maius cum roseo siropo uomitum bene stringit.
Huic aloes lignum iungatur, mastica necnon
Et succus mente: nil flecmata dissipat eque.
Corticibus commixta suis facit alcius illud
Nam cortex est stipticior stomachoque beata.
Corpore que minor est ructura robore maior;
Vim digestiuam iuuat ista, leuat magis illa.

6.2.11 REV

Reu aliud Pontus, aliud parit India; primum
Vilius est. Sunt sicca gradu, sunt feruida primo,
Stiptica sunt et acuta nimis. Stomachum refocillant
Defectum, durum quoque splen epatisque dolorem,
Renes, uesicam, matricem, ypocondria sanant.

6.2.9 FOLIVM *P* 45r: Folium

6.2.10 CARDAMOMVM *P* 45r: Cardamomum
1 taceantur] *scripsi*, tacentur *P* 5 calida est] *scripsi*, calidam *P*

6.2.11 REV *P* 45r: Reu
1 India *corr. ex* insula *P* 3 refocillant] *scripsi*, refocillat *P*

6.2.9 Malabathrum, *Cinnamomum nitidum* Blume

And Malabathrum heats and dries in the second degree,
not last in praise among sweet-smelling spices.
It benefits the stomach, strengthens and repairs the liver,
brings out urine, and is said to dissolve swellings;
in a plaster it clears up injuries of the eyes.
If Malabathrum is lacking let Celtic Nard be used.

6.2.10 Cardamom, *Elettaria cardamomum* L.

Nor should the praises of fragrant Cardamom be overlooked.
Therefore it is double, for one is greater, one is lesser,
but each is dry and hot in the second degree.
If it is larger in size, it is less in the virtue of its heat,
and the less hot it is, so much greater is it in odour.
The larger, with syrup-of-Rose, restrains vomit well.
Let aloeswood be added to this, as well as Mastic
and juice of Mint: nothing loosens phlegm so well.
When mixed together with its pods it does that more strongly,
for the husk is quite astringent and a blessing for the stomach.
The one that is smaller in body is greater in belching strength;
the former helps digestion, but the latter improves it even more.

6.2.11 Rhubarb, *Rheum rhaponticum* L.

The Black Sea produces one Rhubarb and India another; the first
is the cheaper kind. They are dry and hot in the first degree;
they are astringent and very bitter. They revive a weakened stomach
and a hardened spleen, and they heal a pain in the liver,
kidneys, bladder, womb and diaphragm.

6.2.9 FOLIVM / **Malabathrum** *Constantine, 'Lolium' (sic), 361*
2 *Cf.* Venantius Fortunatus, 'Ad domnam Radigundem', 7

6.2.10 CARDAMOMVM / **Cardamom** *Constantine, 'Cardamomum', 347*

6.2.11 REV / **Rhubarb** *Constantine, 'Rheum', 354*

<Vulnera>, singultus <et> hanelitus <inde> iuuantur.
Hec ueteres febres adimunt sistuntque cruorem;
Tam dissinterie quam seuis morsibus obstant;
Acri cum uino faciem lentigine mundant.

6.2.12 EPITIMVM

Epitimum feruere gradu siccareque quarto
Scribunt; hoc ualide * * * * *. Cum sal et acetum
Illi miscentur, dat grossum cedere flecma.
Coccio cum melle succurrit hanelituosis
Et de pectoribus uiscosum flecma repellit.
Menstrua deducit, depellit rite secundas,
Lumbricos perdit atqui opilata resoluit.
Ponitur antidotis uires adhibendo uerendis.

6.2.13 SAGAPINVM

Carmine condignum non transierim sagapinum.
Feruida siccaque uis et tercius est gradus illi;
Expurgat coleram, uiscosum flecma repellit,
Ingerit amissum stomacho uuluaque calorem.
Idropicis prodest; urinam, menstrua promit;
Hoc morsus, tussim, lapides et pectora sanat.
Illius exagium uino coctum bibitumque
Destruit ad plenum, superans, quodcumque uenenum.
Hoc acri uino cathaplasmans lumina curat;
Mixto colliriis oculorum pustula cedit.
Galbana tantundem uel opopanace ualebunt.

6 uulnera . . . iuuantur] *scripsi*, hoc singultus hanelitus minatur *P* 7 hec] *scripsi*, hoc *P*

6.2.12 EPITIMVM *P* 45r–45v: Epithimum
2 *verbum deesse videtur P* 4 hanelituosis] *scripsi*, hanelituosiis *P* 5 de] *scripsi*, qui *P* 7 perdit] *scripsi*, disperdit *P* atqui] *scripsi*, et *P*

6.2.13 SAGAPINVM *P* 45v: Sagapinum
1 sagapinum] *scripsi*, sapiganum *P* 4 uuluaque] *scripsi*, wlueque *P* 6 sanat] *scripsi*, ijuuat (*sic*) *P*

<Wounds> are helped <by this>, as are hiccoughs and wheezing.
The Rhubarbs destroy old fevers and staunch bleeding,
they hinder dysentery as well as savage bites;
they clear a face of spots when mixed with vinegar.

6.2.12 Dodder of Thyme, *Cuscuta epithymum* L.

They describe Dodder of Thyme as hot and dry
in the fourth degree; this powerfully [. . . . . . .]. When salt and vinegar
are mixed with it, it causes thick phlegm to depart.
A decoction with honey helps asthmatics
and repels sticky phlegm from chests.
It brings out a period, properly expels the afterbirth,
and kills stomach worms, however it also loosens blockages.
It is included in awesome antidotes, adding its powers.

6.2.13 Sagapenum, *Ferula persica* Willd.

I shouldn't pass over Sagapenum, so worthy of song.
Its power is hot and dry and it has the third degree;
it purges bile, repels a viscous phlegm,
and replaces heat lost from the stomach or womb.
It's good for those with dropsy, brings out urine and menses,
it cleanses bites, a cough, the stone, and chests.
A measure of it, cooked with wine and drunk,
fully destroys and overcomes any poison whatsoever.
Applying this as a plaster with vinegar cures the eyes;
eye pustules depart from it when mixed in salves.
Galbanum or opoponax are just as beneficial.

6.2.12 EPITIMVM / **Dodder of Thyme** *Constantine, 'Thymum' (sic), 368*

6.2.13 SAGAPINVM / **Sagapenum** *Constantine, 'Sagapinum', 373*

6.2.14 SQVINANTVM

Grata salutiferi recitemus dona squinanti:
Tercius huic gradus est dum siccat dumque calescit.
Idropicos curat decoccio facta squinanti,
At stomachum radix confortat ut appetat escas.
Soluit apostema quod epar congessit humidans
Et uelud urinam sic menstrua, prouocat, aluum.
Mundat epar, renes, uuluam, <frangit> lapidesque;
Sanguinis et fluxum mulieris curat acerbum.

6.2.15 THVS

Thus calet et siccat; gradus est in utroque secundus.
Vim cerebri memorem confortat odore beato.
Origano iunctum qui masticat hoc capitales
Humores per sputa iacit; sic lingua leuatur.
Ouo uel lacte mulieris contere sicque
Lumina clarificat uinoque tepente solutum
Sedabit mammas; emoptoicis nichil eque
Prodest cum uino si potetur uel aceto.
Vulnera consolidant thus, pix et lac et acetum.
Ouum, thus, aloe secte superaddito uene
Siue plagis nimio que manant sanguine; solues
Cum partes coeunt uel idem repetis medicamen.
Thus lacti iungas: ani sic ulcera curat,
Aut quocumque loco fuerint. Curabit adusta
Anseris aut anate aut porci si iungitur uncto.
Si melli socies unguis panaria sanat.

6.2.14 SQVINANTVM *P* 45v: Squinatum
7 uuluam] *scripsi*, wuluam *P* frangit] *scripsi*, *om. P* (*cf. Constantine*, 372)

6.2.15 THVS *P* 45v–46r: Thus
3 hoc] *scripsi*, hec *P* 5 uel] *scripsi*, mel *P* 13 lacti] *scripsi*, lacte *P*

6.2.14 Lemongrass, *Cymbopogon citratus* L.

Let's relate the pleasing gifts of health-bearing Lemongrass:
its degree is third when it dries and when it heats.
A decoction made of Lemongrass cures those with dropsy,
but the root strengthens the stomach so that it desires food.
It dissolves an abscess that a moist liver built up
and it provokes menses and the stool as well as urine.
It cleans the liver, kidneys, womb, and breaks up stones;
it also cures a harsh flow of blood or a woman's flux.

6.2.15 Frankincense, *Boswellia thurifera* L.

Frankincense heats and dries; it has the second degree in both.
It strengthens by its blessed odour the memory in the brain.
He who chews this, mixed with Oregano, gets rid of humours
in the head through his spit; so also is the tongue relieved.
Grind it together with an egg or a woman's milk
and thus it clarifies eyes, or if it is dissolved in tepid wine
it will soothe the breasts; nothing is quite as good
for spitters of blood if it is drunk with wine or vinegar.
Frankincense, pitch, milk and vinegar solidify wounds.
Apply Frankincense, egg and Aloe to a severed vein
or to wounds that flow with excessive blood;
remove when the sides come together, or repeat the same cure.
Add Frankincense to milk: it thus cures ulcers of the anus
or in whatsoever place they should be. It will cure burns
if it is mixed with the fat of a goose or a duck or a pig.
If you blend it with honey it heals pains of the fingernails.

6.2.14 SQVINANTVM / **Lemongrass** *Constantine, 'Squinantum',* 372

6.2.15 THVS / **Frankincense** *Macer, 'Thus',* 2204–32
2 *Cf.* Exod. 30: 34; Lev. 2: 1–2, 15–16; Eccles. 50: 8–9

6.2.16 SQVILLA

Squilla gradu quo thus manet humida spargit et aret.
Egerit et supra et subtus: sic pectora mundat,
Pulmones iuuat, yctericis et hanelituosis
Ydropicisque ualet; epatis uiscosa coartat.
Ad nocuos morsus cathaplasmes hanc in aceto
Et pedibus fissis oleo cannaque iugato.

6.2.17 SILER

Si sileri re nos celebremus carmine uires,
Stat quo squilla gradu? Locium dat, digerit escas,
Strangiriam soluit. Cui tussim suggerit humor
Hanc bibat in uino; sic optima constat hanelis.
Pergendo fractis uel summo frigore tactis
Cum pipere et ualido dat opem sociata lieo.

6.2.18 DRAGAGANTVS

Ponitur antidotis dragagantus sepe probatis,
Lenis enim duri moderatur acumina potus
Humectatque gradu primo frigetque secundo.
Optimus est oculis, tussi, pulmonibus aptus,
Raucisonis aptus, uesice, renibus aptus.
Lenificat lingue lenissimus asperitatem.

6.2.16 SQVILLA *D* 192v: [*lines 5–6, no title, included within poem* De Alliis] | *P* 46r: Squilla
1 manet humida] *scripsi*, manat humidam *P* aret] *scripsi*, arcet *P* 5 nocuos] nocertios *D* cataplasmes *D* hanc] hac *P*

6.2.17 SILER *P* 46r: Siler
1 sileri *corr. e* siteri *P* celebremus] *scripsi*, cebremus *P*

6.2.18 DRAGAGANTVS *D* 192v: De Dragaganto | *P* 46r: Dragagantum
2 durum *D* 4 thussi *D*

6.2.16 Sea-Onion, *Urginea scilla* Steinheil

Sea-Onion dries and heats in Frankincense's degree.
It works both above and below, so that it cleans the chest,
helps the lungs, and is good for the jaundiced, asthmatic,
and dropsical; it forces out viscous humours of the liver.
Apply this as a plaster in vinegar to harmful bites
and mix it with oil and reeds to cure split feet.

6.2.17 Sermountain, *Laserpitium siler* L.

If, in fact, we are celebrating the powers of Sermountain in song,
in what degree does Sea-Onion stand? It brings out urine, digests food,
and relieves strangury. Let him drink this in wine in whom moisture
brings on a cough; it's thus reckoned best for asthmatics.
When mixed with Pepper and powerful wine, it gives aid
by working on those weakened or affected by excessive cold.

6.2.18 Gum Tragacanth, *Astragalus gummifer* Labill.

Gum Tragacanth is often placed in proven antidotes,
for a gentle drink of it soothes pains of a hardening
and it moistens in the first and cools in the second degree.
It is excellent for the eyes, and fitting for a cough and the lungs,
for hoarse voices, the bladder, and the kidneys.
Very gentle itself, it soothes a roughness of the tongue.

6.2.16 SQVILLA / **Sea-Onion** *Constantine, 'Scilla', 362*

6.2.17 SILER / **Sermountain** *Constantine, 'Seseleon', 364*

6.2.18 DRAGAGANTVS / **Gum Tragacanth** *Constantine, 'Dragagantum', 360–61*

6.2.19 DIAGRIDIVM

Ecce diagridium quantum eminet antidotorum
Celsius excelsis et acucius omnibus unum!
Hoc ex lacte feri desiccatur titimalli,
Res preclara nimis, uis et decus antidotorum:
Ista iuuant cunctos, iuuat ista iuuancia cunctos.

6.2.20 AMONIACVM

Tercius in calido gradus, in siccando secundus
Est amoniaco, quod uiscida flecmata purgans,
Mollit, dissoluit sciasim, rapit atque podagram
Arteticosque iuuat; splen adiuuat oximel illi
Iunctum; sanat epar cataplasmatum per acetum,
Siccat apostema melli nitroque iugatum.

6.2.21 BDELLIVM

Sunt humecta gradu primo feruentque secundo
Bdellia, quapropter dissintericis medicantur.
Soluit apostema durum species superuncta,
Hec lapidi ualet et tussi, sed morsibus obstat.
Acri cum uino superuncta iuuat crepituram,
Hec quoque si sapa commixta sit atque cerusa
Lenificat testes, Galieno teste, tumentes.

6.2.19 DIAGRIDIVM *P* 46r: Dyagridium
1 quantum] *scripsi*, quos *P*

6.2.20 AMONIACVM *D* 192v: De Amoniaco | *P* 46v: Amoniacum
1 secundus *om. P* 2 flegma *D* 4 artericosque *D*

6.2.21 BDELLIVM *D* 192v: De Bdelliis (*lines 1–4*) | *P* 46v: Bdelium
4 thussi *D* 6 hoc *P*

6.2.19 Scammony, *Convulvulus scammonia* L.

See how much higher stands Scammony than the noblest
of antidotes, how much sharper it is alone than all the rest!
It is dried from the juice of wild spurge,
a very famous thing, the virtue and grace of antidotes—
they help everyone and this helps all those helping everyone.

6.2.20 Gum Ammoniac, *Dorema ammoniacum* D. Don.

The degree is third in heat and second in drying
for Gum Ammoniac, and by purging viscous phlegm,
it softens and releases sciatica, takes away gout,
and helps the arthritic; vinegar-honey added to it
aids the spleen; as a plaster with vinegar it cleans the liver
and dries an abscess when mixed with honey and Soda.

6.2.21 Bdellium, *Commiphora africana* A. Rich.

Bdellia are moist in the first and hot in the second degree,
for which reason they cure those with dysentery.
In an ointment this spice dissolves a hard abscess,
is good for the stone and a cough, and works against bites.
In an ointment with vinegar it helps cracking
and if this is mixed with wine must and white lead
it soothes swollen testicles, so testifies Galen.

6.2.19 DIAGRIDIVM / **Scammony** *Source unknown*

6.2.20 AMONIACVM / **Gum Ammoniac** *Constantine, 'Amoniacum', 375*

6.2.21 BDELLIVM / **Bdellium** *Constantine, 'Bdellium', 359*
1 *Cf.* Gen. 2: 12–13, Num. 11: 7

6.2.22 ACORVS

Est acorus feruens gradu siccansque secundo.
Huius munda facit preclaraque lumina succus.
Splen, stomachum uino sumptum confortat eparque,
Pectoribus laterique simul fractisque lacertis
Et spleni prodest achori decoccio sumpta,
Pro quo reu semis ponunt equeue cimini.

6.2.23 CAMPHORA

Arboris est gumma quam profert India diues
Camfora, digna deis et in omni nobilis euo.
Dulce sapit, dulce fraglat, res grata puellis,
Si non olfactu uel potu. Frigida ualde,
Rite tuos premeret, Venus infitiabilis, ignes
Et quia sicca gradu perstat uel frigida quarto,
Cephalicum premit olfactu narisque cruorem.
Caniciem properam nimis assuefacta ministrat
Et iam, grata prius, fit res ingrata puellis.

6.2.24 NVX MVSCATA

Nux muscata gradu calet exsiccatque secundo.
Os fetens curat, uentrem constipat eparque
Roborat et stomachum, uentum depellit et auget
Vim digestiuam. Galienus predicat illam
Condecorare cutem, splen curat eparque tumescens.

6.2.22 ACORVS *P* 46v: Accorus
3 stomachum] *scripsi*, stomacho *P* 4 laterique] que *add. P*

6.2.23 CAMPHORA *D* 192v: De Camphora | *P* 46v: Camphora
1 gumma] *scripsi*, gummi *DP et P add.* et in omni *et. canc. P* 2 euo] *scripsi*, ewo *P* 3 flagrat *D* 5 promeret *P* 7 cephalicum] *scripsi*, cephalicam *DP* 8 aswefacta *P*

6.2.24 NVX MVSCATA *D* 192v: De Nuce muscata | *P* 46v–47r: Nux muscata
1 exiccatque *D* secundo] 20 *P* 4 Galyenus *P*

6.2.22 Yellow Flag, *Iris pseudoacorus* L.

Yellow Flag is hot and dry in the second degree.
Its juice can make the eyes both clean and very bright.
Taken with wine, it strengthens the spleen, the stomach, and liver,
and taking a decoction of Yellow Flag is good for the chest and side,
as well as for broken arms and the spleen. In place of this
they give half as much Rhubarb or an equal amount of Cumin.

6.2.23 Camphor, *Cinnamomum camphora* T. Nees & Eberm.

Camphor is the gum of a tree that wealthy India gives,
worthy of the gods and noble in every age.
Sweet is the taste, sweet the smell, a pleasing thing for girls,
but not by smell or in a drink. It's very cold, so it should
rightly quench your fires, unspeakable Venus,
and because it's dry and cold in the fourth degree,
by its odour it brings out blood of the head and the nose.
Taken too habitually it hastily supplies gray hair
and, once a pleasing thing, it becomes unpleasant for the girls.

6.2.24 Nutmeg, *Myristica fragrans* Houtt.

Nutmeg is hot and dries in the second degree.
It cures a stinking mouth, stops up the belly
and strengthens the liver and esophagus, forces out wind,
and increases digestive power. Galen claims it beautifies
the skin, cures the spleen and a swollen liver.

6.2.22 ACORVS / **Yellow Flag** *Constantine, 'Acorus,' 355*

6.2.23 CAMPHORA / **Camphor** *Constantine, 'Camphora,' 370*

2 *Cf.* Juvenal, *Satires* 12. 114 5 *Cf.* Ovid, *Ars amatoria* 2. 414 8–9 *Cf.* Godfrey of Winchester, *Epigrammata* 134, 1

6.2.24 NVX MVSCATA / **Nutmeg** *Constantine, 'Nux muscata,' 355*

6.2.25 NITRVM

Dicit Aristotiles quod mundet flecmata nitrum.
Hoc oculos albos oleo iungens, sed aceto
Aures sanabit; ualet interius in aceto,
Sed neruis stomachi nocet intestinaque ledit.
Hoc tamen adiuncto festinat pocio fluxum
Cumque oleo corpus febre cassabit superunctum.
Fungos expugnat uulue, nimis humida siccat.

6.2.26 THIMVS

At thimus feruetque gradu siccatque secundo.
Thimus res grauis est: dum pessima flecmata purgat,
Ledit epar, facit ut stomachus non appetat escas,
Quapropter ueteres huic dant selinon <et> anisum.
Iunxerunt et amigdaleon; Hiis morphea cedit
Et morbi ueteres necnon angustia feruens.

6.2.27 ANACARDVS

Quarto uero gradu siccans, feruens anacardus
Nil nisi magna potest: hinc antidotum preciosum
Conficitur quod uim, quod nomen traxit ab illo.
Morbos qui ueniunt frigdore uel humiditate
Antidoto curat: sanat letargum acerbum,
Vim memorem seruat, fit mollibus utile neruis.
Hec dat coniunctum, sed mortis acumina solus.

6.2.25 NITRVM *D* 192v: De Nitro | *P* 47r: Nitrum
1 flegmata *D* 7 expungnat *P*

6.2.26 THIMVS *D* 192v: De Thimo | *P* 47r: Thimus
1 at] et *P* 2 flegmata *D* 4 quapropter] et *add. P* dant] daucum *D* et] *scripsi*, *om. DP* 5 his morfea *D*

6.2.27 ANACARDVS *P* 47r: Anacardus
2 hinc] *scripsi*, lhi*n*c (?) *P* 5 curat] *scripsi*, curant *P* 7 solus] *scripsi*, soluit *P*

6.2.25 Soda/Natron (sodium carbonate, Na_2CO_3)

Aristotle says that Soda will purge phlegm,
Mixing this with oil will repair cloudy eyes, but ears
with vinegar; it is good for the insides with vinegar,
but it harms the stomach muscles and injures the intestines.
Yet a potion, with this mixed in, hastens the flux
and it will free a body from fever if applied with oil.
It conquers vaginal yeasts and dries the excessively moist.

6.2.26 Garden Thyme, *Thymus vulgaris* L.

But Garden Thyme heats and dries in the second degree.
Thyme is a heavy thing, for while it purges the worst of phlegm,
it injures the liver, and prevents the stomach from digesting foods,
for which reason the elders add Celery and Anise to it.
They also add almond paste: a scurf departs from these,
as do old diseases, as well as a burning constriction.

6.2.27 Marking Nut, *Anacardium orientale* L.

But the Marking Nut, drying and heating in the fourth degree,
can do nothing but great things: from this a precious antidote
is made, which took its power and took its name from it.
In an antidote it cures diseases that come
from cold or humidity: it repairs a sharp lethargy,
preserves the memory, and is useful for weak tendons.
As a mixture, it gives these things, but alone, the pricks of death.

6.2.25 NITRVM / **Soda** *Constantine, 'Nitrum', 384*

6.2.26 THIMVS / **Garden Thyme** *Source unknown*
5–6 *Cf.* Constantine, 'Epithymum' (*sic*), 368

6.2.27 ANACARDVS / **Marking Nut**
Constantine, 'Anacardi', 382

6.2.28 CALAMVS AROMATICVS

Cum calamus sit aromaticus uirtute coruscus
Et nil utilius stet odoribus in speciebus,
† Plerus * * * * * * ob idem † speciem dicemus opimam,
Augentes meritam (quod possunt carmina) famam.
Subtilis, frangi facilis, citreique coloris
Ex Yndis uenit et Persis sed fit pocioris
hic precii calamus quem mittit odorifer Yndus.
Temperie multa nature conuenit omni
Temperiesque loco feruet siccatque secundo.
In uino si detur epar pectusque iuuabit;
Si suffumigium fiat tussim releuabit—
Delicie regum cum solo fiant odore!
Sed quid condignum merito retinemus honore
Cum sic multa parans incepisset peregrinus?
Vesperus aduenit simul auditorque recessit.

6 <EPILOGVS>

Floriger eoas species, herbas philogeas
Centum sex decies claudens concluditur ortus.
Quis, cuias, cui uel, ipsum plantauerit auctor
Si queris, 'cuias' tibi baldemonia dicet;
Si 'cui,' carpe rosas oleumque require rosarum.
In primo primi titulum deprendito libri.

6.2.28 CALAMVS AROMATICVS *P* 47r–47v: Calamus aromaticus

2 stet] *scripsi*, extet *P* 3 plerus . . . ob idem] *There is no space in* P, *but a word or two is necessary here for metre and sense.* 14 sic] *scripsi*, sit *P*

---

6 <EPILOGVS> *P* 47v: [no title] | *Sternberg*: [no title] *First edited by Kaspar Sternberg,* Abhandlung über die Pflanzenkunde in Böhmen *(Prague 1817–18), 1. 64, and then by Rigg, 287–8.*

2 concludit *Sternberg* 3 plantavit *Sternberg* 4 tibi] *P*, *om. Rigg*

6.2.28 Sweet Sedge, *Acorus calamus* L.

Since Sweet Sedge is gleaming with virtue
and nothing can be more useful among spices for its odours,
[. . . . .] for the same reason, we will call it a splendid spice,
increasing its deserved fame, a thing which songs can do.
Slender, easily broken, and of a lemony colour,
it comes from Indians and Persians, but this Sedge
which fragrant India delivers has a greater value.
By a great moderation it agrees with every nature
and this moderation heats and dries in the second place.
If it is given in wine it will help the liver and chest.
If a fumigation is made, it will relieve a cough—
royal delights may happen with the odour alone!
But why do we detain him, worthy of proper honour,
since the pilgrim had thus begun, preparing many things?
Evening has come and, at once, the hearer has departed.

6 Epilogue

The flowering garden, enclosing one hundred and sixty
eastern spices and herbs that love the earth, is done.
If you ask what author planted it, from where,
or if you ask for whom, Baldmoney will tell you 'where';
and if 'for whom,' go pluck some Roses and ask for oil-of-Rose.
Find the title of this work in the first entry of the first book.

6.2.28 CALAMVS AROMATICVS / **Sweet Sedge** *Constantine, 'Calamus aromaticus,'* 357
4 *Cf.* Ovid, *Met.* 7. 167

---

6 <EPILOGVS> / **Epilogue** *Original*

Commentary

<PROLOGVS> / Prose Prologue

This Prose Prologue appears to be incomplete or was culled from a longer prologue by a careless scribe. Rigg calls it 'incoherent and probably textually deficient' (248). While that assessment is true for portions of the Prologue, the whole is generally clear and serves the purpose of setting the herbal poems in a wider context. There is a time, Henry says, for religious matters and for secular matters. This brief Prologue fulfils his obligation to speak religiously, and he seems eager in the last paragraph to turn to the secular matters (*secularibus*) of herbs, flowers, medicines, and spices. The comparison between righteous and wicked men seems like it should be related to the theme of health and sickness, though the connection is not made explicitly. As described in the Introduction above (15–17), the last paragraph of the Prologue introduces the pattern of the square garden with a theatre in a lake at its centre, which will serve as the guiding metaphor for the entire herbal (though the lake is not mentioned again). References are to line numbers of the Latin; the English line numbers are different.

1–2 *Cf. HA*, Prologue, lines 3–4: 'Principium rerum, uegetatio, finis earum, / Hoc opus aspira, deduc finique precamur.' The failure of the poet to elide *terminum* makes this line suspect, for Henry usually followed the classical rule of eliding a terminal *-m* before a vowel. Rigg suggests (248) that the couplet could be a version of the couplet in the *Historia* 'garbled' by a scribe or compiler.

3 *religiosis et secularibus*] *Cf.* Henry's poem 'Satira communis' (*HA* 780–84), where he writes successively for *clero*, *monachis*, and *laicis* (lines 1, 43, 61).

3 *diuersissimis*] *Cf.* Henry's introduction to *De contemptu mundi*, in *HA* 584–5: 'ut pateat pluribus (id est minus doctis).'

4 *et . . . differunt*] There is no easy emendation for this confused passage. A lacuna seems likely after *et est*.

7 *Quod ut elucescat*] *Cf.* 2 Pet. 19: 'donec dies elucescat, et lucifer oriatur in cordibus uestris.'

7–8 *Quod . . . hoc modo*] As the sentence stands, *uespera* must be the subject, but it would make more sense if it were something like *unusquisque* ('each man'), to match *cuiusque*. If that is the case, then *uespera* is ablative ('in the evening').

8–9 *Septies . . . Domino*] Ps. 118: 164; *Regula Sancti Benedicti* c. 16.

10 *suus*] Understand *seruus* or even emend to *seruus*, as Rigg suggests (248).

12–13 *Aurum . . . michi*] Eccles. 2: 8, 'coacervavi mihi argentum et aurum et substantias regum.'

29 *Vbi est quod agisti?*] A common trope, but compare Henry's *De contemptu mundi* c. 18: 'Ubi est quod heri fecit? . . . Ad nichilum deuenerunt' (*HA* 616).

29–30 Zeph. 1: 15, but perhaps better known to a cathedral canon like Henry from the responsory *Libera me*.

36–37 *Inepta ... asserit*] Another garbled phrase, from which something is clearly missing. It would make sense if we omit *ut frigidum*, but that is too drastic an emendation when we have only one manuscript.

40 *omnia cooperantur in malum*] An inversion of Rom. 8: 28, 'diligentibus Deum omnia cooperantur in bonum.'

49 *theatrum*] Henry will return to this vine-covered theatre in 4 Epilogue 1 (258–61).

1 <PROLOGVS LIBRI PRIMI> / Prologue of the First Book

The complete poem is found only in *S*, but John Leland, *De uiris illustribus* (ed. Carley, 336) reproduced lines 11–14 and I have included the key variants in the apparatus. This poem was discussed in 1997, even before Ruppel and Rigg's identification of the herbal, by Thomas Haye in *Das lateinische Lehrgedicht im Mittelalter. Analyse einer Gattung*, Mittellateinische Studien und Texte 22 (Leiden 1997), 97 n224 and 150–51 nn81–3. He briefly treats the herbal of the 'hochmittelalterlichen englischen Dichters Henricus' together with those of Macer Floridus and Walahfrid Strabo. Haye considers that the herbal collection in *S* is a '*Summa*' and 'für die Zeit nicht untypische' (151). Presumably following John Harvey ('The square garden of Henry the Poet,' *Garden History* 15 [1987], 1–11), Haye states that this 'Henricus' is not Henry of Huntingdon, and he provides a poor transcription of this poem in note 81. The sentiment of this poem echoes the opening of Henry's letter *De contemptu mundi*, which he wrote for his friend Walter of Leicester (on his identity see *HA* cxiii–cxiv, 584–5 n2):

> Walter, once the flower of youth and the darling of your age, now, alas! you are being wasted by a lingering illness and consumed by grievous pain. In the joyful prime of our lives, I wrote for you a book of epigrammatic verse, and I also composed a poem on Love, which was worthy of your acceptance. As a young man, I dedicated to you, also young, the writings of my youth; as an old one, I send you, now also old, the work of my old age. (*HA* 585, trans. Greenway)

This passage from the *Historia* provides a possible context for the poem above. The *iuuenis* in line 2 could be any youths who might read Henry's youthful lyrics, but he could specifically mean Walter, for whom Henry composed many of his verses. In fact, the *Anglicanus ortus* may have been intended for Walter as well, if we can take Henry's epitaph for Walter literally: 'I, Henry, who bear garlands to you, first brought epigrams, next the contests of love, and then medicinal herbs' (*De contemptu mundi*, c. 19, trans. Greenway, in *HA* 619). So in both the *De contemptu mundi* and this verse prologue he remarks on their passage together from youth to old age and refers to his earlier epigrams. Walter was clearly an important part of Henry's life and an inspiration for much of his poetry.

1 The opening of the poem is reminiscent of Boethius, *De cons. phil.* 1 met. 1.

1 *epigramata*] Henry may be using 'epigrams' to mean any poem, or he could be referring specifically to his many short, witty poems dependent on Martial.

2 *seria*] The scribe's *serta* does not scan. *Seria* plays nicely off *ludens* (line 1), and was first conjectured (or misread, as he does not give the original reading) by Haye, *Das lateinische Lehrgedicht*, 150–51 n81 (and cited by Ruppel, 'Ein verschollenes Gedicht,' 204, who does acknowledge the manuscript reading). It most likely refers to the two books of *epigrammata seria* appended to later redactions of *HA* (see the Introduction above, 8).

4 *senibus*] Rigg (251) emends *seminibus*, the reading in *S*, to *satis*, but given that Henry wrote epigrams for boys (line 1) and serious writings for a young man (line 2), it makes sense that this third work is for *senibus*, old men. Lines 5–6 repeat the formula of three stages of life.

11 *Cf.* Ovid, *Remedia amoris* 76: 'carminis et medicae Phoebe repertor opis.'

12 The vale of Tempe in Thessaly was known in Greek mythology as a favourite haunt of the muses. *Tempe* is neuter plural and thus the subject of *resonant*.

13 *prius*] Perhaps referring to the composition of the *Historia Anglorum*, another time when Apollo (*Phebe*) crowned Henry with 'flowering ivy' (*edera florente*). In classical verse the *-us* should be shortened before a vowel, but lengthening is common at the caesura in medieval Latin.

14 *parate*] Ruppel ('Ein verschollenes Gedicht,' 204), following Haye, says that *parare*, found in *S*, is the correct reading. The reading *parate*, however, was witnessed by John Leland, *De uiris illustribus* (ed. Carley), 336.

1.1 ARTHEMISIA / Mugwort, *Artemisia vulgaris* L.

Based partly on Macer, 'Artemisia,' lines 1–30. Henry's lines 1–4, 15–18, 20–21, 23, and 25 are original or from another source. Henry is particularly didactic in this poem, glossing the difficult medical words (*menstrua*, *steras*, *hicterici*, *opium*) as if he were speaking to a student. He uses this technique in later poems (*cf.* 1.10, 4; 1.19, 7–8; 3.8, 24–5), though hardly to the extent he does here, where he provides four glosses in response to questions posed either by himself or his student.

2 *Nature racio*] The 'law of Nature,' a Stoic concept known to Henry perhaps from Cicero, *De officiis* 3. 23: 'Atque hoc multo magis efficit ipsa naturae ratio, quae est lex divina et humana.'

2 *pretulimus*] It is odd to find the spelling *preferrimus* in both manuscripts, and it may be a case of shared error. *Preferimus* with one 'r' does not scan, and it may have been a gloss at one point for *pretulimus*.

3–4 These three varieties are not in Macer, nor do they appear in the Latin Dioscorides under 'Artemisia' (10. 428–9). The Latin Alphabetical Dioscorides (fol. 31v), however, does give the names *monoglonos*, *tegenes*, and *leptafilos* in the entry on *Artemisia*, and Pseudo-Apuleius provides three separate entries for 'Herba artemisia monoclonos,' 'Herba artemisia tagantes,' and 'Herba artemisia leptofillos' (nos. 10–12, pp. 42–5).

3 *Diascorides*] Pedanius Dioscorides (*ca* 40–90 CE) was the author of *De materia medica*, the ancestor of most medieval herbals and pharmacopoeias, and thus is not surprisingly one of the most often cited authorities in this work. Most of Henry's references to Dioscorides come by way of Macer or Constantine the African.

9 *deducere menstrua*] One of the most common effects of medicines in this and Macer's herbal is emmenagogic, forcing menstruation to begin. While this might seem, to a cynical, modern reader, no more than a veil for an abortifacient, medieval emmenagogues may often have had a 'pronatal' effect, according to Monica Green, supposedly cleaning out the uterus to prepare it for more effective conception. See Monica H. Green, 'Flowers, poisons and men: Menstruation in Medieval Western Europe,' in *Menstruation: A Cultural History*, ed. Andrew Shail and Gillian Howie (Basingstoke 2005), 51–64, at 53.

13 *Fouere* can simply mean 'to warm' but here it probably means more specifically 'to apply as a poultice' (*fomentum*).

16 *Phebeque*] Diana, here in her role as goddess of the moon.

20–21 A description of *stera* similar to this is found in the Macer cited by the late thirteenth-century herbalist Rufinus, where Macer's line 13 is glossed: 'Duritias stericas—*sterica passio est duritia circa matricem*—solvit pellitque tumorem' (Rufinus, 43).

23 *Hicterici* (more properly *icterici*) are people with jaundice, so *galuicies* apparently is equivalent to *galbities*, 'yellowness,' from *galbus*, 'yellow.' However, I have not found this word in any other source, and it is not surprising that the scribe of *P* supplied *calviciem*, 'baldness.'

26 *Plinius*] Perhaps Pliny 26. 24, where a variety of plants including *artemisia* are prescribed for *struma* (scrofulous sores), though he does not specify how the *artemisia* is prepared. This is the first of many mentions of Pliny the Elder (23–79 CE), author of the *Natural History*, a major source for medieval herbalism. Some references to Pliny, such as this one, come by way of Macer's poems, while others appear to come from Henry's own research in the *Natural History* or derivations thereof.

1.2 OZYMA / Basil, *Ocymum basilium* L. [starts 346!!!!!]

Most of the poem is based on Henry's personal experience, and I have found no direct source for the medical information. Basil appears twice in manuscript *S*, under the titles *Basilica* and *Ozoma*. This poem forms a pair with the following, *Crocus*, in which the two plants fight for supremacy and crocus itself criticizes basil's powers. The Trinity Compiler used Henry's lines 2–3, 12 and 14 within his new poem on 'gariofilatum,' one of two types of basil named by Constantine (349): 'Est enim gariophyllatum et citreum.'

1 *matrem*] That is, *mater herbarum*, artemisia in poem 1.1.

4–5 *decus et dolor*] *Cf.* Martial, *Ep.* 11. 13. 5, 'Romani decus et dolor theatri,' and Henry's epitaph on Henry I, 'Rex Henricus obit, decus olim, nunc dolor orbis' (*HA* 492). The epitaph (*funereum . . . carmen*) on Matilda is not found in Henry's surviving epigrams, but in *HA*, 462–3.

6 *inter*] A poetic postpositive preposition.

11 *redolens*] A non-classical usage. The subject is Matilda and she is, of course, smelling the basil, and not being redolent herself.

13–15 The claim in these lines that basil can dissolve poisons is challenged by the crocus in the following poem 1.3, at line 19, where it implies, speaking in the first person, that its ability to conquer poison is greater.

1.3 CROCVS / Saffron Crocus, *Crocus sativus* L.

Much of this poem, describing the battle of crocus and basil, is original to Henry. Lines 20–22 are based on Macer 2025–6. The explicitly medical lines seem to come from diverse passages in Pliny. The Trinity Compiler includes lines 14–22 in his longer poem 'Galbo,' changing crocus's self-references into impersonal statements, and the Digby Excerptor does the same. EMA translates this poem ('Safron,' 194) and Daniel Arundel (fol. 60r) translates lines 14–17 under 'Cartamus.'

4 The pun on blades (*comas*) works well in Latin and English.

7 Pliny 21. 34: 'uiret bruma et colligitur.' Perhaps influenced by Lucan, *De bello civili*, 1. 17: 'Et qua bruma rigens ac nescia vere remitti.' Lucan was a major source for Henry's *Historia Anglorum*.

14–18 Pliny employs saffron for eye problems (20. 187, 21. 131, 25. 169) and specifically praises saffron's efficacy for them (21. 137–9). None of these passages, however, seem to be the immediate source for Henry's poem.

19 This is an attack on the claim in the previous poem, 1.2, 13–15, that basil can counteract poisons.

20–22 *Admisce . . . eque*] This information comes from Macer's poem 'Lolium' (ll. 2015–28), which was also called *nigella*, where the plant is mixed with *thus* (ll. 2025–6): 'Mulsa decoctum commixto thure crocoque / Apponas coxae, sciasis quam vexat iniqua.' These lines are also imitated in Henry's poem on *Lolium*, below at 5.1.10, 7–8.

21 The scribes and editor of EMA show confusion concerning *coxa*. Frisk's edition of EMA at this point reads 'ley hem alle to-gyder to þe ȝye þat is greued with sciatica passio' (194), and notes that one manuscript reads 'thye' for 'ȝye.' Even though most manuscripts read 'ȝye,' 'thye' is an acceptable translation for *coxa*, which can refer to the thigh as well as the hip.

1.4 LAVREOLA / Laureole (= Spurge Laurel), *Daphne cnidium* L.

The name *laureola* could apply to several kinds of spurge (*Euphorbia* spp.) or laurel (*Daphne* spp.). I have not identified Henry's immediate source. Dioscorides treats the similar plants δαφνοέιδης (4. 146, spurge laurel, *Daphne laureola* L.) and θυμελαία (4. 172, spurge flax, *Daphne cnidium* L.), but it is the latter that produces the 'Cnidian grain' (called *coccus cnidius* in the Latin Dioscorides, 11. 83). The Latin Dioscorides does not use the name *laureola*, but *Circa instans* gives separate entries to *laurus* and *laureola* (fols. 201r and 201v, respectively) and Rufinus classifies *laureola* under 'Alipiados. id est, laureola et semen eius dicitur cocognidum,' also providing the synonym 'Mezerion' (Rufinus, 16). This poem is translated in EMA as 'Laureole,' 191–2, and is abbreviated by the Digby Excerptor. As Henry clearly distinguishes between *laurus* and *laureola*, I have treated *laureola* as different from the several occurrences of *laurus* in other poems below.

2 An echo of Ovid, *Amores* 1. 8. 3, 'Ex re nomen habet.' The passage would make more sense, however, linguistically and botanically, if the line were reversed, *i.e.* laureoles take their name from the matter of laurels. *Cf.* Marbode of Rennes, *De lapidibus* (*Marbode of Rennes' [1035–1123] 'De lapidibus' Considered as a Medical Treatise*, ed. John M. Riddle [Wiesbaden 1977]), line 420 (*De eliotropia*): 'Ex re nomen habens est eliotropia gemma.'

4 The subjunctive *uideatur* seems unnecessary, and may be used only to preserve the correct metre.

7 *Animosi . . . oris*] *Cf.* Ovid, *Amores* 1. 15. 19, where the epithet applied to the playwright Accius.

7 *Persius*] There is no mention of *cocognidon* in the extant satires of the Roman poet Persius (34–62 CE), nor was he known for medical or botanical knowledge. Henry cites Persius at 6.1.9, 16, though incorrectly calls him Ovid. Henry could mean another author entirely (though 'animosi . . . oris' is an apt description of Persius) or *Persius* could also refer to 'the Persian,' but it is not clear who this would be. The EMA translator gives this name as *Prosius* (191), and the editor Gösta Frisk suggests that this is an error for the late antique physician Theodorus Priscianus, whose work was included in the eleventh-century *Passionarius* of Gariopontus, and who mentions *coccum cnidium* in one medical work (EMA, 329). Regardless, *Priscianus* would not scan here.

8 *cocognidon*] = *Coccum Cnidium*, or the 'Cnidian grain.' Pliny 27. 70 ('Coccum Cnidium'), Robert Cricklade (*Roberti Crikeladensis Defloratio Naturalis historiae Plinii Secundi*, ed. Bodo Näf [Berlin 2002], 334, 'De cocognido'), and Constantine ('Cocognidium,' 364) all treat this seed. The *Laud Herbal*, no. 349, is clear about its source: 'Coconidium .i. semen lauriole.' The *coccum cnidium* is similar to a peppercorn and was used to counteract hemlock poisoning and to loosen the bowels. It is the seed either of *Daphne gnidium* or of widow-wail (also spurge olive, *Cneorum tricoccum*), Pliny 21. 53–5.

11 The efficacy of *laureola* for all things internal echoes Dioscorides' description of *Daphne laureola*, 4. 146, where it induces vomiting and menstruation, purges phlegm, and causes sneezing.

1.5 BALDEMONIA / Baldmoney (also Spignel), *Meum athamanticum* Jacq.

Source unknown. The first two lines were printed from *P* by Kaspar Sternberg in *Abhandlung über die Pflanzenkunde in Böhmen*, 2 vols (Prague 1817–18), 1. 65. Partially translated (lines 10 and 14–15) by EMA as 'Baldemoyne' (190), and abbreviated twice by the Digby Excerptor. The same plant, or a variety of it, is treated under the name 'Meu' in poem 4.19. I have found no source for the medical information in this poem. The description could come from personal experience, as Henry was a native of the English fens (*paludes*) where *baldemonia* grows. Henry speaks fondly of the *paludes* several times in his *Historia* (*HA*, xl–xli, 320–21, 354–5, 692–3). My thanks to Diana Greenway for pointing out this connection.

4 *ude . . . paludes*] Reminiscent of Ovid, *Met.* 1. 418: 'caenumque udaeque paludes.'

7–11 It is rare for Henry to advocate carrying an herb or spice as a protective amulet. Usually he is dismissive, or at least wary, of amulets and urges proper ingestion or direct application for a cure to be effected (*cf.* lines 1.7, 44, and 2.1, 35–6).

9 *lacescat* = *lacessat*

1.6 AMBROSIA / Ragweed, *Ambrosia artemisiifolia* L.

Henry's poem on *ambrosia* is based primarily on Strabo's poem 'De Ambrosia,' lines 369–74, though the first line is based on one from Strabo's 'De Agrimonia.' Henry has embellished the poem with references to Virgil (*i.e.* Maro), Homer, and the Muses. The Trinity Compiler used only the last two lines within a new poem of a purely medical nature, EMA translates lines 7–9 under 'Ambrosiana' (200), and the Digby Excerptor used the poem in two separate entries. Henry, like Strabo, is more concerned with the ambrosia of the gods than the medicinal properties of the real plant. Apart from the single cure, all we have for identification is the name. Dioscorides uses the name αμβροσια for sweet wormwood (*Artemisia maritima*, 3. 114), though today 'ambrosia' is used primarily for the ragweed family (Ambrosiae). Pliny (27. 28) admits that the name is applied to many plants: 'Ambrosia vagi nominis et circa alias herbas fluctuati'.

1 Strabo 361: 'ordinibus facile est discernere pulchris.'

5 *Pyerides*] The Muses, daughters of Pierus. See Jan M. Ziolkowski, 'Classical influences on medieval Latin views of poetic inspiration,' in *Latin Poetry and the Classical Tradition: Essays in Medieval and Renaissance Literature*, ed. Peter Godman and Oswyn Murray (Oxford 1990), 15–38.

7–9 *Cf.* Strabo 372–4: 'Medici tamen arte suapte / hanc utcumque colunt, tantum quae sanguinis hausta / absumit, quantum potus ingesserit almi.' The sense is that *ambrosia*, when drunk in a potion, presses out of bodies the same measure of blood as was ingested of the original drink. I was aided in the translation of this difficult passage by the EMA: 'Ambrosiana wole dryve out of þe body þat blediþ inward also mikel blode as the pacient drinkeþ iuus of þis herbe' (200). The translator has interpreted Henry's remedy as applying to internal bleeding, which is not obvious in the original Latin.

9 *Vergit* was a difficult word for the scribes, but is probably the correct reading albeit not exactly equivalent to Strabo's *ingesserit*. It can mean 'poured in' as in Ovid, *Ex Ponto* 1. 9. 52: 'in gelidos versit amoma sinus.'

1.7 ORIGANVM / Oregano, *Origanum heracleoticum* L.

Based closely on Macer's 'Origanum,' lines 1285–1324. The only notable differences from Macer's poem are the astrological reference in line 40 (see below), and the wry dismissal in line 44 of Macer's amulet against dangerous animals.

1–2 *Exigui* and *eximii* play nicely off each other in Latin, but the alliteration is difficult to recreate in English.

7–8 A rather awkward adaptation of Macer 1304–05: 'Naribus infusus irino mixtus olivo / Invisum capiti coget manare cruorem.'

14 *haustum*] The subject has switched from *succus* to *origanum*.

16–17 Macer's cure (lines 1323–4) is for the hip, rather than the leg.

21 An *oxifalum* (thus in *P*, *S*, and Macer 1294) is a fluid measure of fifteen drams, originally called an *oxybaphus* (literally, 'vinegar-cup'). The classical name is hinted at by *oxifabi*, used by the Digby Excerptor, a spelling also used by the Latin Alphabetical Dioscorides in the passage on *Anchusa* (fol. 13va).

29 *acoras* = *achores*

37 A liberal paraphrase of Macer 1289, 'Cum mulsa sumptum prodest aconita bibenti.' *Infrendens* ('gnashing angrily') is an odd, perhaps suspicious, word to describe *aconitum* (wolfsbane, monkshood, or poison in general). Perhaps a more serious problem is that, while *aconitum* is the proper singular, it always appears in the plural *aconita* in Henry's favourite texts (Virgil, *Georgica* 2.152; Ovid, *Met.* 1.147, 7.419; Ovid, *Ars amatoria* 3.465; Isidore of Seville, *Etym.* 17.9.25), and that is the reading given by *P*. In that case, *infrendens* needs to be in the plural. The only singular I have found in a common text is the Graecized *aconiton* in Ovid, *Met.* 7.407. As nothing found in Macer's poem is missing here, I feel confident in leaving the line as found in *S*.

38 *rosiriaco* = *rhus syriacus*, ground sumac berries (*Rhus coriaria* L.), still a popular condiment in the Middle East.

40 *Cf.* Martial, *Ep.* 1.2.1: 'Quid nunc saeua fugis placidi, lepus, ora leonis?' or 6.93.3: 'Non ab amore recens hircus, non ora leonis.' But also compare Ovid, *Met.* 2.81: 'Haemoniosque arcus violentique ora Leonis.' Henry displays a rare reinterpretation of Macer here, giving the time by the place of the sun in relation to Leo, instead of Macer's 'quando Sirius ardet' (line 1308). While Henry may have seized this opportunity to borrow from Martial, one of his favourite poets, the passage now refers to a different time than Macer's original. Sirius is at its height around the summer solstice, but the sun is within Leo (that is, it 'holds the mouth of Leo,' *tenet ora Leonis*) from 23 July to 22 August. In either case, high summer is indicated, but this lack of astrological precision suggests that Henry cares more for the quality of his verse than of his recipes. See poem 6.2.1, line 26, for a similar astrological expression of time.

1.8 LAVANDVLA / English Lavender, *Lavandula vera* D.C.

Lavender is not found in Pliny, Pseudo-Apuleius, Strabo, or Macer, nor does Henry's poem bear any relation to Dioscorides 3.26, στοιχάς (French lavender, *Lavendula stoechas* L.), or Pseudo-Dioscorides, cap. 13, 'Sticas' ('Pseudo-Dioscoridis *De herbis femininis*,' ed. Heinrich F. Kästner, *Hermes* 31 [1896], 578–636, at 598). Thus this poem appears to be a rare and pleasant example of Henry's application of his own knowledge and observation. The Digby Excerptor condensed Henry's poem to only one line, no doubt because of the lack of medical information.

3 Lavender oil is still used as a natural insect and rodent repellent.

7–10 Henry explains why lavender has little or no medicinal use. She is a haughty (*superba*) plant, proud of her powerful odour. If she had medicinal powers, they would surely match the strength of that odour, and would apparently be too strong a medicine. The force of *uix* is unclear. It may essentially mean *non*, but it could also indicate that lavender has some small medicinal value, not worth mentioning in a discussion of its excellent odour.

1.9 SALVIA / Sage, *Salvia officinalis* L.

The middle of this poem (lines 12–22) is a reworking of Macer's much shorter poem 'Salvia,' lines 870–81. Henry begins the poem (lines 1–11) with a discussion of the herbalists who came before him, Macer and Walahfrid Strabo (*Stabus*). Henry, like many in the Middle Ages, believed that the herbalist Macer was the classical poet Aemilius Macer (d. 16 BCE), and therefore that the medieval Strabo (d. 849 CE, and not the geographer, 64/63 BCE–23 CE) would follow in Macer's footsteps (*sequens Macri uestigia*) rather than the reverse. Henry did not seem to notice that Macer cites Strabo (lines 900, 906). In the final section (lines 23–35) Henry provides a recipe for an antidote called the 'Ten-Herb Medicine,' not found in Macer. The Digby Excerptor used only this section for his entry on *Saluia*. Daniel Arundel translates lines 9–10 and 23–35 in his discussion of 'Elifagus,' noting that the rest of his poem is the same as Macer's.

3 This line is problematic. *P* has omitted it entirely and the line in *S* hardly makes sense without creative punctuation. We should probably understand an *est*: 'whose happy gift [is] sure health.' The reading in *S* of *predacio* ('pillaging' or 'plundering') makes little sense in the mood of these lines, even ironically. *Prestacio* makes better sense, yet is still difficult to fit syntactically: 'whose happy gift (a guarantee) is sure health.'

6 *Cura orti* seems personified—perhaps the goddess of horticulture (*i.e. cura orti*)?

10 This line is not in Macer as Henry claims. It is actually found, with slight variation, in the medical poem called the *Regimen sanitatis salernitanum* or the *Flos medicinae*: 'Cur moriatur homo cui salvia crescit in horto?' (*Collectio Salernitana* 5. 31, line 1102). Most or all of the *Regimen* was written after Henry's poem, so the author(s) of the *Regimen* either borrowed the line from Henry or, what is more likely, the line was a common adage. If the latter is true, the misreading in *S* (*infirmatur* for *cur moriatur*) is surprising. Another variant of the line appears in the herbal of Rufinus, attributing it to the *Tabula Salernitana* (another name for the *Regimen sanitatis Salernitanum*): 'Cur moritur homo, quia salvia crecit in orto' (Rufinus, 285). Henry Daniel notes correctly that 'Henry Anglicus' is wrong in his attribution of this line to Macer: 'And þerefore þis is þe vers þat Macer hymsilf made of sauge: *Cur infirmatur homo cum salgia credit in orto?* Þus he. But in þe text of Macer fynde Y

nozt þis vers' (Daniel Arundel, *Elifagus*). For more on the history of this famous verse, see Jonathan Usher, 'Simona and Pasquino: "Cur moriatur homo cui salvia crescit in horto?"', *MLN* 106 (1991), 1–14.

11 *Arguat* ('prove,' 'argue,' 'blame') is a curious verb to use here. Perhaps Henry wanted to suggest a tone of moral superiority or the feeling of a legal proceeding.

18 It is not entirely clear what *frequenti* modifies: the process could be done 'with frequent care' or done 'under the frequent sun,' maybe over several days or when the sun is clear and at its height.

19 The replacement of *quod si* in *S* with *nunquam* in *P* is curious. Both scan properly, but the use of the subjunctive *poscas* demands a word like *si* rather than *nunquam*.

20 *abortum*] There are many cases in this and other medieval herbals in which a herb effects or forces *abortum*, a word which can apply variously to a miscarriage, a premature birth, a dead foetus, or an abortion of a live foetus. John Riddle has argued that *abortum* should mean 'abortion' in most cases (*Eve's Herbs: A History of Contraception and Abortion in the West* [Cambridge, MA 1997], 23, 148, 223). Furthermore, the German translators of Macer Floridus always use *Leibesfrucht* ('embryo') to translate *abortum* or *abortivum* (*e.g.* Macer, lines 846, 872, 1722, in *Höhepunkte der Klostermedizin. Der 'Macer Floridus' und das Herbarium des Vitus Auslasser,* trans. Johannes Gottfried Mayer and Konrad Goehl [Holzminden 2001]), indicating that they understand the foetus still to be alive. However, I translate *depellit abortum* and similar phrases as 'expels a foetus,' based on Henry's adaptation in his poem on gentian, 6.2.7, line 10, of a passage from Constantine the African, *Liber graduum* (367). Constantine says that gentian 'mortuum foetum expellit,' which Henry adapted into verse as 'pellit abortum.' While it may have been the case that Macer intended *pellit abortum* to mean 'cause an abortion,' Henry's reading of Constantine shows that he understood *abortum*, at least in that one case, to mean a miscarried foetus and I have carried that interpretation to the other instances of *abortum*. Nonetheless, it is likely that readers of medical works like this interpreted such phrases as they wished depending on the circumstances.

21 Identical to Macer 878. This may be laziness on Henry's part, or an error by an earlier scribe who was too familiar with Macer's version.

25 Henry introduces here the kitchen which, with its cook, will play a dramatic role in Book 5, where Henry has created an often spiteful dialogue between himself (in his role as poet/herbalist) and the 'Cook,' probably meant to represent the poet Martial, nicknamed the 'Cook' (see Rigg, 218–19 and Wolfgang Maaz, *Lateinische Epigrammatik im hohen Mittelalter* [Hildesheim 1992], 262–7). The *cocus* is always eager to chatter and argue (*certans garrire*).

28 This line witnesses a rare instance in which the copy of the *Exceptiones* in *O* has a better reading than the primary manuscripts. I have used *tanetico* in *O* as the basis for the emendation to *taneticumque*, since *tanetumque* in *P* and *S* does not scan.

33 *cifulum* = *scyphulum*, a small bowl or cup (RMLWL, *s.v.* 'scyphus').

1.10 RVTA / Rue, *Ruta graveolens* L.

Based on Macer, 'Ruta,' lines 267–331. Daniel Additional (fol. 60r–60v) cites this poem in his passage on 'Bisara.'

1 *Ruta decens*] Possibly inspired by Ovid, *Amores* 3.1.9: 'Forma decens ….'

1 *decimo*] Referring to the tenth place in the garden bed and the tenth poem in this book.

1–2 These lines would work as they appear, transposed, in *P*, but Henry more often points out the location of a plant in the very first line (see poems 1.11, 1.21, 2.21, 3.21, 4.2, and 4.21).

4 *illis*] The plural in *S* seems to work better than *illi* in *P*, since it refers to the herb's hot and dry *uires*, and not to the plant itself.

7–8 'Naso' is Ovid, *Remedia amoris* 801–802: 'You would rather usefully gather rue, which sharpens the eyes, as well as whatever keeps our bodies from Venus' ('Utilius sumas acuentis lumina rutas / et quidquid Veneri corpora nostra negat').

10 *Cytharea*] Classically *Cytherea*, for Venus.

11 This line does not follow logically. The first part makes sense if we understand *horum* to apply to all of the other herbs: 'none of these [other plants] is better.' There is no indication what *neutrum* in the second part signifies. Perhaps the absence of this line in *S* is an indication that it is a later addition by an inferior poet.

19–22 King Mithridates of Pontus (135–63 BCE) was particularly wary of poison, and had an antidote developed particularly for him, *mithridatium*. See Gilbert Watson, *Theriac and Mithridatium: A Study in Therapeutics* (London 1966). This was one of the most popular antidotes of medieval and early modern medicine. It is described by Quintus Serenus, 1061–8. The *Antidotarium Nicolai* calls it 'mater omnium antidotorum' (89).

32 *lyeum*] Lyaeus (λυαιος, 'the relaxer'), an epithet for Bacchus. Henry uses it so often to mean 'wine' that I do not capitalize it. *Acre lyeum* is vinegar.

33 Either reading, *compescis* or *compescit*, will work. I have opted for the third person, following *rapit* and *compescit* in lines 29–30.

34 *sumptum*] *Sumpta* would be expected but does not scan. We need to understand 'this thing, taken.'

42, 48, 51 *unguen*] The scribe of *S* does not seem to have known the difference between *unguen* (ointment) and *unguem* (accusative of *unguis*, a claw or talon), which could lead to serious confusion for a reader. Classically, *unguen* meant simply grease, but Henry clearly is using it as a synonym for *unguentum*, and both mean 'ointment.' However, in line 42, *unguen* can not strictly mean 'ointment' which implies topical, exterior application. If rue is to be injected with a clyster, then *unguen* here means something like 'a grease-based mixture.'

45 *curare*] The reading in *P*, *iuuare*, will not scan, and *curare tumentes* also appears at 2.5, 15; 5.1.3, 20; 5.2.3, 29; and 6.1.9, 18, whereas *iuuare tumentes* appears nowhere else.

47 *Quidem* does not serve any purpose here other than to complete the metre.

49–50 *Cerusa* is a chemical compound of lead, called burnt lead, white lead, or Venetian ceruse, which was a common base for white paint until the modern era.

51 *Sacer ignis* is usually understood to apply to erysipelas or St Anthony's fire, though it could be used for any number of red skin inflammations.

52 A *derta* is a type of itching, probably scabies. See Choulant's note on *derta* at Macer, line 299.

52 *Herpeta* is not modern herpes, but any spreading, itching skin eruption.

58 Either reading, *conficitur* of *P* or *conficiunt* of *S*, is possible. While one could take *Greci* or *medici* as the implied subject of *conficiunt*, I have retained the passive tense used in line 57.

58 Spelled *diapiganon* in Macer 320. This is the first of several antidotes in the herbal with the Greek prefix *dia-* or *dya-* ('across'), all compound medicines in which the primary ingredient is the substance after the prefix. Hence *diapaganon* is a compound antidote based on *paganon*, or rue.

59 *Ciminum* was the classical spelling for cumin. While the scribe of *S* usually spells it *cuminum*, I have followed *ciminum* from poem 6.1.9 for the sake of consistency.

63 The reading of *P* would also work, though it seems somewhat forced: *Roborat hoc stomachum quod forte dirigat escas* ('This [antidote] strengthens the stomach so that it forcefully directs food'). I have emended to *digerat* following Henry's use of *digerat escas* at 2.14, 29; 6.1.5, 9; and 6.1.9, 15, and *digerit escas* at 6.1.7, line 8, and 6.2.17, line 2.

65–66 These lines hardly make sense. Part of the difficulty comes from the fact that scribes used the same abbreviation ($\overline{qm}$) for different words: *quam* and *quoniam*. It appears the scribe of *P*, reading *quam*, added another *ualet* to help the line scan. Rigg suggested the drastic emendation of *Quam* to *O*, but *quoniam* preserves the sense better with the least modification. Apart from those difficulties, the rest of the line (*hoc ... hoc est*) may be grammatical, but is essentially meaningless. The manuscripts are identical for line 66, and I cannot propose an alternative without drastic emendation. My translation is only a literal attempt at the supplied line.

1.11 YSOPVM / Hyssop, *Hyssopus officinalis* L.

After the first nine lines on Solomon's praise of hyssop, the remainder of Henry's poem is a close adaptation of Macer's 'Ysopum,' lines 1503–31. Since the neuter *ysopum* is used in line 30, I have read the title *De Ysopo* in *S* also as neuter and the title *Isopus* in *P* as an error.

1–9 These lines refer to the book that Solomon is said to have written on 'plant life, from the cedar of Lebanon to the hyssop that grows out of walls' (1 Kgs. 4: 33).

1 *undenum*] A reference to the poem's position, eleventh in Book 1.

7 This line is identical to line 29 of Henry's epigram 12. 1, 'Laus Dei summi' (*HA* 806–807), in which he devotes a stanza (lines 28–31) to David and his song of thanksgiving (1 Chr. 16: 7–36).

9 *iactancia*] Used substantively as 'a boasting' or 'ostentatious show.'

10–11 Henry's explanation of *antidotum* is incorrect. An antidote is any cure that is 'given against' (ἀντίδοτον) something, and is not specifically for interior complaints. Most *antidota* in the *Anglicanus ortus* are compounds of numerous ingredients. Hyssop is unique here as a simple antidote (that is, a cure with one ingredient). I have not found the source for this remedy.

13 An awkward passage, only a little clearer in Macer 1504–05: 'Eius decoctio facta / Sic ut cocta simul sint mel, ficus quoque sicca.' Apparently the method of cooking figs in honey was common enough that Macer, and Henry in turn, could apply it to the preparation of herbal remedies.

15 *ptysimque*] *Ptysis* (classically, *phthisis*) is consumption of the lungs which involves much spitting (the usual meaning of *ptysis*). The spelling is supplied from Macer 1511 (*phthisimque*) and Henry's own spelling at lines 4.3, 41 and 4.18, 12. The scribe of *S* did not know this word and interpreted it as 'thirst' (*sitim*).

18 *clarissima clarum*] A common pun in Latin, but difficult to reproduce in English, since we use different words for 'famous' and 'clear.' Literally, it says '[Since it is] very clear, when drunk first, it makes a sore [throat] clear.'

23 *cardama*] Not cardamom, but rather *cardomum*, a type of garden or water cress, described below in poem 4.7, 'Nasturcium.'

27 *sonitus . . . auris*] Apparently some form of tinnitus.

31 For *calor*, both manuscripts read *color*, an understandable reading when discussing a plant described as *uirens*. Yet, as its power to heat is stressed, I have emended to *calor*.

1.12 CAMEDREOS / Wall Germander, *Teucrium chamaedrys* L.

The poem, apart from lines 4–7 and 19–23, is based closely on Macer, 'Chamaedrys,' lines 1903–17.

4 *bis genito*] An epithet of Bacchus (Ovid, *Met.* 3. 317).

5–6 *Lauduni . . . Anselmi*] These lines make clear that Henry spent time studying under Anselm of Laon (d. 1117). His presence at Laon should not be surprising, as several of his fellow ecclesiastics, all nephews of Bishop Roger of Salisbury, also studied there: Alexander 'the Magnificent,' archdeacon of Salisbury then bishop of Lincoln, and dedicatee of Henry's *Historia Anglorum*; Alexander's brother David, archdeacon of Buckingham; and his other brother Nigel, archdeacon of Salisbury and bishop of Ely. We do not know the exact dates when Henry was there, but he may have found himself in the august company of Adelard of Bath, Gilbert de la Porée and Peter Abelard. *Cf.* Edward J. Kealey, *Roger of Salisbury, Viceroy of England* (Berkeley 1972), 47–9. This line is discussed by Diana Greenway in 'Henry of Huntingdon as poet: The *De herbis* rediscovered,' *Medium Ævum* 74 (2005), 329–32.

6 *Fontibus . . . manancia*] A popular metaphor, but perhaps known to Henry from St Jerome, *Ep.* 49. 13 (*Sancti Eusebii Hieronymi Epistulae*, editio altera, ed. Isidorus Hilberg and Margit Kamptner): 'legimus, o eruditissimi viri, in scolis pariter et Aristotelia illa vel de Gorgiae fontibus manantia simul didicimus.' *Cf.* Pseudo-Virgil, *Culex* 78 (in *Virgil*, vol. 2: *Aeneid Books 7–12, Appendix Vergiliana*, ed. and trans. H. Rushton Fairclough, rev. G. P. Goold, Loeb Classical Library [Cambridge, MA 2000]): 'semper opaca novis manantia fontibus antra.'

7 *solebatis . . . ciues*] Henry is addressing the citizens of Laon, from whom he learned the recipe for mixing germander with wine. This makes this already difficult passage more confusing, for he addresses both germander and the people of Laon in the second person.

8 *depellis abortum*] See note to poem 1.9, line 20.

9 *Conquassata* is an odd word to use substantively, but it comes directly from Macer 1907. It is translated into German as 'Prellungen' (bruises), which is plausible, but I have found no precedent. It could also mean broken bones, whiplash, or any sort of damaging shaking.

19–23 This recipe is not in Macer or *S*. It could be a later addition by Henry or another poet-scribe. Conversely, it could be another passage where the scribe of *S* may have been unduly influenced by the fact that he had copied Macer elsewhere in the same manuscript, and thus cut or overlooked this recipe.

20 *bracteos*] Derived from βϱαθύ, a name for juniper (*sauina*) described below in poem 4.25, where it is called *brateon*.

1.13 CAMOMILLA / Chamomile, *Chamaemelum nobile* (L.) All.

Based closely on Macer, 'Chamomilla,' lines 549–91. Five kinds of chamomile are discussed in the poem. Apart from true chamomile (*camomilla*), there is *amaruscus*, which is stinking chamomile or mayweed (*Anthemis cotula* L.); *leucantemon*, the ox-eye daisy (*Chrysanthemum leucanthemum* L.); *crisantemon*, one of the many members of the *Chrysanthemum* genus; and *anthemis*, which can be applied to all chamomiles (line 37) but is also given specifically to wild chamomile (*Matricaria chamomilla* L.).

5–9 The difference between sweet-smelling chamomile and stinking chamomile (*amaruscus*) was a common subject in medieval herbals and medical verse. Rufinus (99) records the verse, 'Fetet amarissa; redolens olet camomilla' ('*Amarissa* stinks; chamomile smells sweet'), and a later herbal glossary gives a similar line emphasizing their similarity: 'Fetet amarusca, redolet similis camomila' ('*Amarusca* stinks; chamomille, similar, is fragrant,' in San Marino, Huntington Library, MS HM 64, fol. 186ra, discussed by Jerry Stannard, 'A fifteenth-century botanical glossary,' *Isis* 55 [1964], 353–67, at 366).

11 *colubrinis*] Most likely referring to *colubrina*, or dragon arum, treated below in poem 2.7. It could also be an adjective used substantively: 'serpentine things.'

18 *depellit abortum*] EMA (144) translates Macer 574 (*pellere . . . abortum*) as 'delyuere a woman of here deed childe.' See the note to poem 1.9, line 20.

20 *egilopas* = *aegilopes*, a tumour in the tear duct.

21 *feda*] Macer's original *hypochondria turgida* (swollen), line 577, makes more sense.

24 *exantumata* = *exanthemata* (singular *exanthema*), skin eruptions occasioned by a variety of diseases such as measles and scarlet fever.

26 I cannot find this exact recipe in Pliny. Henry learned it from Macer 580–83. Pliny does relate a cure using capers (20. 166) which must be used for thirty-five days and also purges spleen.

33 *nigellis*] Since chrysanthemums come in many colours, but not true black, I think *purpureus* and *nigellus* need to be understood as red and purple, respectively.

1.14 BVGLOSSA / Ox-Tongue (Bugloss), *Anchusa arvensis* L.

Based on Macer, 'Buglossa,' lines 1127–38. Henry's lines 2–4 are original.

5 *tepide*] I am following Macer 1133 ('Mixtus aquae tepidae'), but *tepidus* in *P* could be what Henry intended and thus applies to *succus*.

13 Pliny does say this about *buglossos*: 'quod in vinum deiecta animi voluptates auget.' He also says that it is called 'euphrosynum, the plant that cheers' (25. 81). The language, though, is closer to that of Pseudo-Dioscorides, *De herbis femininis*, cap. 2, 'Buglossos': 'haec in vino missa hilaritatem convivio faciunt' ('Pseudo-Dioscoridis *De herbis femininis*,' ed. Heinrich F. Kästner, *Hermes* 31 [1896], 578–636, at 591).

1.15 SANICLA / Wood Sanicle, *Sanicula europaea* L.

The EMA translates this poem as 'Sanicle' (189). Sanicle is not found in Macer, Strabo, Pliny, or Dioscorides. Hildegard of Bingen, writing after Henry, does include an entry on *sanicula* in her *Physica* (Strasbourg 1533), 2. 42, which is rather different except for the last line: 'Qui autem ferro uulneratus est: succum saniculae exprimat, et eam in aquam fundat, et pransus bibat, et uulnera eius interius purgat, et bene sanat.' Sanicle's healing properties, particularly for sword blows, must have been well known, or else Henry and Hildegard share a source. The fourteenth-century *Sinonoma Bartholomei* (ed. J. L. G. Mowat [Oxford 1882]) contains *sanicula*, and gives 'wodemerche' as a synonym (38), as does *Agnus Castus* (202), where the brief description is seemingly based on personal observation and not taken from Henry. Hunt notes numerous other glosses of *sanicula* as 'wodemerche' or 'wodewort' (228). In the Old English herbal tradition, Bald's *Leechbook* includes 'wudu merche' (wood parsley) in an eye salve (Stephen Pollington, *Leechcraft. Early English Charms, Plant Lore, and Healing* [Norfolk 2000], 382–3), and the *Lacnunga*, an Anglo-Saxon medical collection (London, British Library, MS Harley 585), names it for use on a neck tumour (Pollington, *Leechcraft*, 186–7, and see the editor's note on 167). The only cure in any way similar to Henry's is in the *Lacnunga*: *wudumerces sed* ('wood parsley's seed') is one of many ingredients in a healing potion concocted for a certain King Arestolobius which is good 'against all infirmities which stir up a man's body.' One of the cures given is for the 'seondre exe,' or seeping cerebrum (Pollington, *Leechcraft*, 240–41). The figure of Arestolobius is probably based on one of the four real kings of Judea in the first century BCE, all named Aristobulus. See Debby Banham, 'Arestolobius, the Patriarch of Jerusalem and bark that comes from Paradise: What did the Orient mean to compilers of Old English medical collections?,' in *Proceedings of the Thirty-Eighth International Congress on the History of Medicine*, ed. Nil Sari *et al.* (Ankara 2005), 459–68.

1 *Huic ... subest*] *Huic* refers to the previous plant *buglossa*, which is paired with *sanicla* because of the similar wound-healing properties, and it is sanicle that *subest*. Compare *subit* at 1.17, 1.

2 The name *sanicla* comes supposedly from *sanare*, to heal. *Cf.* EMA 189: 'Sanicle hauyþ her name for-þi þat she helyþ woundes.'

5 *stomachi penetralia*] Either *stomachi* in *P* or *stomacum* in *S* could work, but the choice changes the meaning of *penetralia*: 'inner parts of the stomach' for the former, and 'the stomach and the innards' for the latter. Since I have found no precedent for *penetralia* on its own meaning 'innards,' I have opted to use *stomachi*.

7 *Talem conspicies qualem potauerat eger*] Apparently the potion of sanicle was believed to appear in the open wound, not having been digested or otherwise modified by the stomach. So says the EMA: 'This herbe wole seke boþe bon and wounde, and in þe wounde she wole shewyn her al such as þe pacient drinkyth here' (189).

8 *Dum proprius uigor huic superato corpore restat*] A difficult line to interpret, especially since *S* gives a markedly different reading (which does not scan). If the Latin of *P* is not corrupt, Henry seems to mean that the potion of sanicle will travel past the stomach, through the body, and come out in a wound, provided it still has its original power (*proprius uigor*) and the patient survives (*superato corpore*). That is, however, a generous reading and the passage may be corrupt.

12 The *pellicula seruatrix* is one of the protective skins (*meninges*) covering the brain, either the *dura mater* or the *pia mater*. *Cf.* William of Conches, *De philosophia mundi* 4.24, De cerebro: 'Sub craneo duae pelliculae sunt, miningae dictae, quarum exterior, durior est; duraque mater dicitur: propinquior vero cerebro, ne laedat ipsum, tenuior, diciturque pia mater' (PL 172: 95). The translator of EMA understood what *pellicula* denoted (189): 'she assendiþ in-to þe hed and in-to þe brayn and brekeþ þe skyn of þe brayn þat is clepid pia mater, and so she sleþ þe pacient.' See also Ynez Violé O'Neill, 'William of Conches and the cerebral membranes,' *Clio Medica* 2 (1967), 13–21.

1.16 COSTVS / Cost (Costus Root), *Costus speciosus* J. König

This poem bears no relation to 'Costus' in Macer, lines 2165–81, which is the only poem from Macer's herbal that Henry did not use. Some of Henry's poem (lines 1 and 7–9) comes from Strabo's poem on clary sage, 'De Sclarega' (lines 275–83); *costus* is described in that poem's last three lines as growing near the clary sage. Macer's *costus* is an aromatic ingredient found in unguents and perfumes, described by Pliny (13. 15–18), and identified as *Costus speciosus* (crape ginger) by the recent translators of Macer (*Höhepunkte der Klostermedizin*, trans. Mayer and Goehl, xlvii), but *Saussurea Lappa* (costusroot or the Himalayan snow lotus) by the editor of Pliny (see the index to the Loeb edition of Pliny, *Natural History*, vol. 7).

2–3 *species ... herba*] Henry distinguishes the herb *costus* from the spice or aromatic *costum*, which in classical Latin is neuter rather than masculine.

1, 7–9 *Cf.* Strabo, 'De Sclarega,' 281–3: 'eam iuxta hortensis non extima costi / silua latet, stomachique moras uentremque salubri / prouocat auxilio radicis munere coctae.'

12 *finxisse putent*] Perhaps echoing Ovid, *Fasti* 6. 3–4: 'sed erunt qui me finxisse loquantur, / nullaque mortali numina visa putent.'

12 *uerbum non amplius addam*] Horace, *Satires* 1. 1, 121.

1.17 ANGLICA COSTVS / English Cost or Costmary, *Tanacetum balsamita* L.

Translated in Daniel Additional (fols. 69r–69v) and Daniel Arundel (fol. 72v) under 'Costus.' I have found no source for this poem. It seems more original than most in the herbal, and provides an interesting example of anti-Scottish sentiment in Anglo-Norman England (line 3).

2 *costus*] Three genders are used to distinguish three species: this type of *costus* is a feminine, fourth-declension noun, as compared to the masculine *costus* and neuter *costum* described in the previous poem 1.16, lines 2–3.

10 *empicos* = *empyicos*

10 *iuuato*] *iuuaret* in *P* would also work, but we would lose the rhyme with *grato*.

1.18 BETA MAIOR / Burdock, *Arctium lappa* L.

Lines 1–6 and 8–13 are based on Pseudo-Apuleius no. 36, 'Herba Personacia' (pp. 81–2). I have not found the source for line 7. The final four lines are original to Henry. Henry misread his copy of Pseudo-Apuleius or had an alternate version, for in the standard edition the root and *spina* (lines 8–9) are used for *uulnera uetera* rather than for dog bites (line 10). Likewise, where Henry calls for *beta* with honey to cure only old ulcers, Pseudo-Apuleius uses that combination twice: for curing intestinal pains and burns. *Beta maior* and *beta minor* (see the following poem 1.19) are both some form of burdock, rather than of the modern beet. Lines 5–12 are translated in Daniel Additional (fol. 30v) under 'Bleta.' The name *personatia* or *personancia* was applied to many large-leaved plants like beet or burdock (Hunt, 202).

7 This line presents several problems. The placement of *sed* makes little sense without the forced punctuation. Moreover, the line is also the only one in the poem which does not come from Pseudo-Apuleius, which suggests that it may be an interpolation by a later scribe.

8 *spina*] There is no indication here or in Pseudo-Apuleius as to what this *spina* might be. The term can apply to any number of spiny bushes, like the blackthorn (*cf.* 'Spina alba' for hawthorn or barberry in Hunt).

10 *superatum*] Latin use of a passive participle in place of the finite verb *superabis*. Strictly, the line reads 'Thus you will escape the overcome bite of the rabid dog.' The remedy makes sense in English only if the bite is overcome afterwards: 'you will overcome . . . the bite.'

11 *ciatum* = *cyathum*

13–14 As he usually does, Henry expresses doubts about cures that could be construed as amulets or, in this case, a crown made of the herb.

14 *uetiti non credere*] A distinctly unclassical construction, but Henry is having fun creating the paradox of 'certain people forbidden to disbelieve anything,' *i.e.* they believe everything. As this reading is in both manuscripts, scans, and makes some sense, I think it best to keep it, however awkward.

15–17 This is the only passage in the herbal in which Henry advocates any sort of scientific method, but compare *HA* 9. 1 (ed. and trans. Greenway, 622–3): 'However, if miracles are narrated to me in this way I do not openly contradict them unless they are obviously frivolous, nor give them constant affirmation unless I observe them to be fully corroborated by well-known proofs and trustworthy persons' ('Michi autem si narrentur huiusmodi miracula, nec aperte contradixero, nisi aperte friuola sint, nec constanter affirmauero, nisi notissimis indiciis et probatissimis personis ad plenum roborari perspexero').

1.19 BETA MINOR / Lesser Burdock, *Arctium minus* Bernh.

Translated by EMA as 'Beta the lesse' (190). I have found no direct source for this poem. As with *beta maior* in poem 1.18, this is probably not our modern beet, but some kind of burdock.

1 *lecto . . . equo*] *Beta minor*, while lesser in many ways than the *beta* of poem 1. 18, is still in the same bed, or in a bed at the same height.

7 *Galienus*] Galen of Pergamum (129–200/216 CE) was considered, along with Hippocrates, as one of the fathers of rational medicine. Henry does not seem to have read any of Galen's works (many would not be widely available to Latin scholars until the thirteenth century) but instead gathered his information indirectly from sources such as Macer and Constantine the African.

7–8 *Theodoricon* (also spelled *theodoriton*) is a name given to some important antidotes. There are at least two varieties: *theodoricon hipericon* and *theodoricon anacardinum* (Constantine the African, *Tratado médico de Constantino el Africano. Constantini Liber de Elephancia*, ed. Ana Isabel Martín Ferreira [Valladolid 1996], 122). The latter is alluded to below at 6.2.27, 2. Two variations on *theodoriton* given by Constantine do not include *beta* (203, 206). There are also two versions of *theodoriton* given in the *Antidotarium Nicolai* (155–7), both of which are beneficial for head pains and injuries, though neither features beets or burdock. *Theodoricon* is glossed as 'given by God' in a copy of *Alphita* in our manuscript *D* (Oxford, Bodleian Library, MS Digby 69), fol. 94r: 'Theos. Deus. Hinc

Theodoricon a deo datum.' The recipe closest in name to *theodoricon* found in Galen's genuine works is called *Theodotion*, but it bears no relation and does not mention *beta* (*Claudii Galeni Opera Omnia*, ed. Karl Gottlob Kühn, 20 vols in 22 [Leipzig 1821–33], 12. 754). Galen's discussion of the burdocks ('Arctium maior et minor,' *Opera Omnia* 11. 837) does not mention *theodoricon* or any use for head injuries. It is difficult to tell what case Henry intended *theodoricon* to be. If we read it as accusative, it becomes an ingredient (parallel with *hanc*) added to medicines rather than the antidote itself. The following lines, however, show that Henry knows it is an antidote, so I am inclinded to take it as indeclinable noun, and thus parallel with *medicaminibus*.

1.20 APIVM / Celery (Smallage), *Apium graveolens* L.

Based on Macer, 'Apium,' lines 332–65, less 336–7, which reports that the word *apium* is derived from *apis* (bee), an insect that loves celery's white flowers. Perhaps Henry ignored those lines in preference to the etymology used in line 1, whereby *apium* comes from *apex*, the 'summit' of the victory helmet crowned with celery. While the etymology in the first two lines comes from Macer 332–3 (and ultimately from Isidore, *Etym.* 17. 11. 1), Henry anthropomorphizes the celery, which steps forward as the 'triumphal herb' (line 3), replacing the hero whose helmet bore the celery in the first place. Henry may also have had in mind the triumphal arch, which *apium* imitates in its height and strength.

1 *Sic*] The reading of *hic* in *S* would work as well, but *P* is generally less prone to contamination.

4 Henry puns on *procedit*, with the double meaning of a plant springing forth and a soldier marching.

5 *minantem*] There is another double meaning here, since *minans* can mean 'projecting up' (like a plant) or 'threatening' (like a soldier). *Cf.* Silius, *Punica* 4. 2: 'saxa minantia caelo,' and Virgil, *Aeneid* 2. 240: 'minans inlabitur urbi.'

6 *Althydes* = *Alcides*, an epithet for Hercules.

6 *cuncta*] The neuter plural probably refers to Hercules' tasks, rather than enemies as one might assume.

7 *subter . . . coronam*] Exod. 25: 27.

11 *sanxitur* = *sancitur* (probably by analogy with the perfect form *sanxi*).

13 In classical Latin the first syllable of *porus* is short, which Henry knows, but it is lengthened in Henry's source, Macer 347: 'Desiccans poris assumpta repellit apertis.'

31 The *lacrimum* of the egg is part of the white (*albumen*), either the germinal disc or the chalazae, the transparent cords that hold the yolk in place.

On *lacrimum* instead of *lacrima*, see Macer 212 and Choulant's note, as well as Macer 364, 2205, and 2220.

35 *P*'s reading of *uiridem* could work as well as *crudam*, but the latter preserves a weak rhyme, towards which Henry was often inclined. *Viridem* is most likely an intruded gloss.

1.21 PETROSELINVM / Parsley (no. 1), *Petroselinum crispum* (Mill.) Nyman

I have found no direct sources for this poem. The Digby Excerptor dramatically condenses the entire poem, while the Trinity Compiler uses Henry's lines 1–4 and 21–31 within his own, longer poem 'Petrosilinus' (*T* 102v–103r). This poem introduces the characters of Apollo (lines 14–15) and the Cook (lines 16–17), a humorously abusive figure who will take over the narration from Henry in Book 5, Part 2. The Cook is probably meant to represent Henry's favourite poet, Martial, who was nicknamed 'the Cook' (Rigg, 218–19, 256). Parsley is the only herb to receive two separate poems. Poem 5.2.5 also treats parsley, but in the voice of the Cook. Henry the Herbalist and the Cook exchange positions: Henry gives culinary recipes here and the Cook gives medical cures in 5.2.5.

1 *Viginti uisis*] The twenty plants already examined in the garden and described in Book 1. He will repeat this formula in the following books at poems 2.21, 3.21, and 4.21.

2 *Danai*] Danaans, a synonym here for all Greeks, also used below in poem 3.24, line 1. The term is used frequently by Virgil, Ovid and Statius, all favourites of Henry.

2 *triannem*] I have found this name only in the *Laud Herbal*, no. 1148: 'petrosilinum id est perresil. triannem.' The *Glossary* is part of an early-twelfth-century medical collection in Oxford, Bodleian Library, MS Laud Misc. 567. See also Willem F. Daems, *Nomina simplicium medicinarum ex synonymariis medii aevi collecta* (Leiden 1993), 373. It is tempting to imagine this collection on Henry's shelf, but I have found no evidence.

3 *Cf.* Rabanus Maurus, *De rerum naturis* 19. 9, *De oleribus*: 'Petrosilenon uocatum quod sit similis apio.' *Apium*, smallage or celery, is discussed in the previous poem 1.20.

7 Rigg's emendation to *qua* works only if *ea* is made ablative and scanned long, which does not fit the metre. Since *que* is in both manuscripts and makes sense ('doing those things which that one can do') I see no reason to emend.

11–12 *Petroselinum* gets its name from the stones (*petra*) it breaks up and removes from the body.

13 Henry's plan to relate antidotes which employ parsley is interrupted by Apollo. It is only in the second poem on parsley, 5.2.5, that he is able to give these antidotes, but there in the voice of the Cook.

15 *Talia*] Thalia is the muse of comedy and light verse. She is also named in Henry's poem 3.5 on *Nimphea*, at line 4. *Cf.* Martial, *Ep.* 7. 17. 4, 'lasciuae fuerit locus Thaliae.' Strabo also refers to Thalia in his poem on pennyroyal (324–5): 'Quod nisi me currens deponere uela Thalia / cogeret et tandem portus intrare moneret.'

17 The second syllable of *uatis* must be lengthened for this verse to scan.

21–32 Both of the recipes given by Henry are good examples of the thin green sauces popular in medieval cuisine which are now mostly lost to the modern cook, outside of the Argentinian *chimichurri*.

22, 29 *ius danna*] I do not know what this 'juice' could be. It is clearly a spicy flavouring similar to cress (*nasturcium*), but better.

30 *ciminum*] Preferred to *cuminum*. On this spelling see the note to poem 1.10, line 59, and poem 6.1.9, 'Ciminum.'

1.22 SOLSEQVIVM / Calendula (Pot Marigold), *Calendula officinalis* L.

Based partly (lines 5–9, 16–21) on Pseudo-Apuleius no. 49, 'Herba Heliotropia' (pp. 99–100), and possibly on Pliny's desciption of 'heliotropium' (22. 57–61), though it is stated there that it possesses blue flowers, and hence is most likely turnsole (*Chrozophora tinctoria* L.). The poem also owes much to Ovid's tale of Clytie transformed into a sunflower or heliotrope, *Metamorphoses* 4. 256–73. The name of the plant is *solsequia*, apparently singular in line 2, but it changes to *solsequium* in line 18, which agrees with the title in *P*. Henry's golden flower (line 3) would suggest something like the calendula or pot marigold (and not the standard marigold, or the sunflower, both of which are native to the Americas). EMA translates this as 'Rodewort' (190–91) and Daniel Arundel (fol. 66v) as 'Cicoria, Rode,' common English names for the pot marigold (Hunt, 242). The *Agnus Castus* says it more clearly: 'Solsequium ys an erbe that me clapyth Roddys or marigoldys' (203). The Trinity Compiler used most of this poem (lines 9–14, 16–18, 21) within a longer poem; most of the changes are too drastic to report in the apparatus.

1–8 Pseudo-Apuleius no. 49: 'Huius herbae diuinae ad solis cursum floscelli se uertunt, et cum sol occidit, floscelli se cludunt [*sic*]; rursum cum sol oritur, floscelli se aperiunt.' Henry's introduction is similar to Dioscorides' account of 'Eliotropium' as cited by Rufinus (119): 'nomen accepit quod primo solstitio estivo floreat vel quod foliis maturibus circumacta conveniat, unde et a Latinis solsequia nuncupatur. Nam et sole oriente flores suos apperit. Item recludit cum sol occubuerit.' Also compare Aldhelm's riddle 'Eliotropus' (*The Riddles of Aldhelm*, ed. James Hall Pitman [New Haven 1925], 28), which refers, as Henry does, to the plant's yellow flower:

> Sponte mea nascor fecundo cespite vernans;
> Fulgida de croceo flavescunt culmina flore.
> Occiduo claudor, sic orto sole patesco:
> Unde prudentes posuerunt nomina Graeci.

3 The subject of *nutrit* is not given, but it must be the sun, a point not worth mentioning when discussing a plant called 'sun-follower.' *Cf.* Ovid, *Met.* 1.496: 'sperando nutrit amorem.'

5 *ille* = *flos*

7 *Vergit et ad solem*] *Cf.* Ovid, *Met.* 4.270: 'vertitur ad Solem.'

11 *febris acuta*] *Cf.* Pliny 22.61, who says the 'Magi' advise tying either three or four pieces of heliotropium against the tertian or quartan ague, respectively. Henry's cure based on merely seeing the plant is only slightly more ridiculous.

12 *Gysta* is a variant of *gutta*, a common Anglo-Latin word for gout or any number of other ailments (DMLBS, *s.v.* 'gutta'). It is not unworthily (*indigne*) called *gutta* ('drop of liquid') since the various conditions called 'gout' in the Middle Ages were said to come about by the flow of liquid into one part of the body, usually a lower extremity.

12 *illam*] It is tempting to use *istam* from *T* for the sake of the rhyme, but that manuscript cannot be used as a faithful witness to Henry's original poem.

15 *Bis genito*] An epithet for Bacchus, so the herb is cooked with wine. See note to poem 1.12, line 4. The scribe of *S* has curiously left a large blank where *bis genito* should be, most likely because he could not read his example but perhaps because it offended his Christian sensibilities.

17 *luxus*] Dislocation of a joint. *Cf.* Pseudo-Apuleius no. 49: 'Ad luxum. Herba heliotropia contusa et adposita efficaciter sanare dicitur.' The EMA translator did not know or misread *luxus* and changed this cure to 'For the flux' (191).

1.23 PARVENCA / Periwinkle, *Vinca minor* L.

The entire poem seems original to Henry and the descriptions come probably from personal experience. As the poem is primarily about love and its vagaries, it may give us some insight into Henry's lost collection of poems *De amore* (see the Introduction above, 7–8). It is abbreviated twice by the Digby Excerptor, who relates only the few, brief medicinal uses of the herb.

1 *umbrosum*] The shady bed of *paruenca* is placed in contrast to the sun-loving *solsequium* of the previous poem 1.22. *Cf.* Ovid, *Met.* 7.75: 'quas nemus umbrosum secretaque silva tegebat.'

4 *amanti*] The reading of *amare* in *S* would also work ('she loves and always strives to love the earth'), but that seems needlessly repetitive and *S* is more apt to be corrupt.

5–6 Henry is describing climbing plants which seem to hate the earth and love the air, which is the opposite of periwinkle's behavior.

7 The second *hec* refers to the *aera* which periwinkle flees.

7–10 These stories of flight and escape come from Ovid, *Met.* 1.452–567 and 5.379–424.

14 The observation that periwinkle blooms even in the snow appears to be original to Henry. It is not found in any other herbal, most of which are primarily Mediterranean in origin.

20, 23 *uenerem*] In most instances where *uenus* is a direct object, it means 'sexual intercourse,' 'sexual appetite,' or even 'semen,' and in those locations I have not capitalized the word.

24–27 There are several problems in these lines. Rigg could not make sense of line 24, which is confused in each manuscript. Michael Winterbottom has suggested the emendation to *ultro quaeque* in line 24, which helps but is drastic, and posited a lacuna in line 26 or 27, which seems likely. *S* has not recorded lines 25–26, no doubt due to eyeskip from one *uelitis* to the other (lines 24, 26). With only *S*, it is difficult to tell if Henry intended *dabitis* in line 25. Strictly speaking, its last syllable must be short, but as Rigg notes (259), Henry is known to lengthen a final *-is* at the caesura. See Henry's Epigram 1.2, lines 37, 55 (*HA* 782).

24 *quaeque* = *quaecumque*

25 The final syllable of *dabitis* must be lengthened for this line to scan properly, which is common at the caesura in medieval Latin verse.

28 *uictoriolam*] Another name for periwinkle. See 3.13, 25, below for another example. The Digby Excerptor makes this passage clearer in his second excerpt of the poem: 'Victoriola etiam uocatur quia guttam uincit' (*O* fol. 91v).

29–30 *uincere . . . uincire*] Henry is playing on *peruinca*, another common name for periwinkle. I could not recreate the alliteration on *u* in English.

1.24 STRVCION / Masterwort, *Peucedanum ostruthium* L.

Based on Macer's 'Ostrutium,' lines 907–27. Only the last two lines (21–22), giving the plant's English name, are original to Henry. This is a difficult plant to identify. The EMA calls the plant 'Bysshoppeswort' (191, and note on 222).

Numerous English herbs were called 'bishopsweed' or 'bishopswort,' most commonly wood betony, *Betonica officinalis* L. (Grieve, 'Betony, Wood'), however betony and bishopswort are listed as separate plants in the late Anglo-Saxon medical text known as Bald's *Leechbook* (translated and discussed by Karen Louise Jolly, *Popular Religion in Late Saxon England: Elf Charms in Context* [Chapel Hill, NC 1996], 154–5, 207 n55). 'Byschopeworte' and similar spellings are given occasionally as glosses to *ostrutium* and *strutium* (Hunt, 194, 247). Another option is soapwort (*Saponaria officinalis* L.), given by Hunt as a possible identification for *strutium* (247).

5 *elleboro*] Hellebore, treated below in poems 2.2 (*elleborum album*) and 2.3 (*elleborum nigrum*). This line is probably referring to one of the virtues of white hellebore, described at 2.2, 31: 'Sternutamentum contractum nare mouebit.'

5 *Replicatur*, which usually applies to folding and unfolding, is an odd word choice here, where the forcing out of phlegm by sneezing is clearly meant. Macer 924 is clearer, as is often the case: 'Sternutamentum per se pulvis movet eius.' Macer also specifies white hellebore (*veratro ... albo*, line 925).

7 *sclirosim*] Without this line in *S* for comparison, it seems wise to follow Macer 911 ('Durum, quem Graeci sclirosim dixere, repellit') for this difficult word, which could easily have lost the macron over the terminal *-i*.

9 *ortopnoicis*] Those suffering from orthopnoea, difficulty breathing when lying down (DMLBS, *s.v.* 'orthopnoea').

17 I have translated *lepra* throughout as 'leprosy,' but *lepra* could apply to any number of scaly or degenerative skin conditions and even cancers in antiquity and the Middle Ages, as well as to the chronic disease now known as Hansen's disease.

21 *pontificalem*] This name is not in the list of Latin names in Tony Hunt's *Plant Names of Medieval England*. Perhaps Henry is actually translating the English name 'bishopswort' into Latin (*pontificalis* = 'episcopal').

1.25 MIRTVS / Myrtle, *Myrtus communis* L.

It is fitting that a plant sacred to one of the deities often named in the herbal, Venus, should round out the first book. The Trinity Compiler uses Henry's lines 2–3, 13–14, and 16 in his twenty-eight-line poem on myrtle. The discovery of *T* justifies much of Rigg's emendation to line 3. The Digby Excerptor used lines 8–19. Lines 1, 8–9, and 13–18 are translated by EMA ('Mirtus,' 193–4). I have found no source for this poem; it bears little similarity to Pliny's lengthy passage on myrtles (15. 118–26) or to the several sources cited by Rufinus (192–3).

1 *ultima*] The last, twenty-fifth, plant in this bed and book of the herbal.

1 *partis . . . borealis*] That is, of the northern quadrant of the garden. The EMA translator misunderstood the purpose of this line and translated it, 'Mirtus is habundaunt in þe fer north' (193). Not satisfied with this statement, EMA adds 'She growiþ in þe colde mery, and ȝit she is hote in kynde' (193), in an attempt to explain the apparently cold habitat and hot virtue of the plant.

2 Virgil, *Ecloga* 7. 62, 'formosa myrtus Veneri, sua laurea Phoebo,' and Pliny 12. 3, 'Apollini laurus . . . Veneri myrtus.'

3 *terre . . . equo*] A troublesome phrase, as should be clear from the *apparatus criticus*. Rigg's emendation works well, but I think it is prudent to keep the subjunctive *amet* found in both *S* and *T* and treat the *quod* like an *ut*.

4–7 These lines are problematic in all of the manuscripts. Michael Winterbottom has suggested that there is a lacuna of one or two lines after *labor* in line 6. As sense can be made from *P* and *T* taken together, I see no need to posit missing lines.

5 *odores*] In this case, *odorare* must be taken as a transitive verb meaning 'to sniff' or 'to smell.' This is rare, but not unknown; see *The Later Letters of Peter of Blois*, no. 30, ed. Elizabeth Revell (Oxford 1993), 163, line 86.

7 *hinc*] 'From this height,' namely, from the bed at ground level rather than from the usual knee-level.

16 *ciliacos* = *coeliacos*. The term applies not specifically to those with modern coeliac disease, but to anyone suffering a wide range of abdominal and bowel disorders.

2 PROLOGVS SECVNDI LIBRI / Prologue of the Second Book

The poem is addressed to Clio, the muse of history, perhaps a favourite of Henry's because of his *Historia Anglorum* (though she is not mentioned in that work). The poem is written in couplets which rhyme on the last two syllables, except for lines 11–12. The first three lines were transcribed from *S* by Haye, *Das lateinische Lehrgedicht*, 150 n81.

1–2 Clio celebrates gods and heroes in Horace, *Odes* 1. 12, 1–6. These lines are also reminiscent of Horace, *Ars poetica* 83–5: 'Musa dedit fidibus diuos puerosque deorum / et pugilem uictorem t equom certamine primum / et iuuenem curas et libera uina referre.'

4 *nec qui moritur morte*] A common religious sentiment, but perhaps echoing Ambrose, *De benedictionibus patriarcharum* c. 9: 'qui autem accipit, non morietur peccatoris morte' (PL 14: 686D).

5 *serta*] These garlands, once given to Henry by Clio, probably recall his writing of the *Historia Anglorum*.

7–8 The theme of magnifying little things will be repeated in poem 2.10 on roses (lines 1–2).

12 *leuem . . . leuemque*] Henry is showing off his metrical skill, using both meanings of *leuis*, which scan differently. An emendation of *leuemque* to *leuisque* is desirable for the sake of the rhyme, but it would make little sense grammatically.

2.1 MANDRAGORA / Mandrake, *Mandragora officinarum* L.

After an original introduction (lines 1–10), the rest of the poem is based on Pseudo-Apuleius no. 131, 'Effectus herbae mandragorae' (pp. 222–5), for the subject but much indebted to Ovid's *Metamorphoses* for the language (see the commentary below). The Trinity Compiler uses most of Henry's poem (with some lines changed drastically but lines 4–5, 11, 19–31, 35–36 copied directly) and adds sixteen lines of his own for his entry on 'Mandragora.' This poem is discussed by Anne Van Arsdall, 'Exploring what was understood by "mandragora" in Anglo-Saxon England,' in *Old Names—New Growth. Proceedings of the 2nd ASPNS Conference, University of Graz, Austria, 6–10 June 2007, and Related Essays*, ed. Peter Bierbaumer and Helmut W. Klug (Frankfurt am Main, 2009), 57–74, and in Anne Van Arsdall, Helmut W. Klug, and Paul Blanz, 'The mandrake plant and its legend: A new perspective,' in the same volume, 285–346. I am grateful to Dr Van Arsdall for supplying me with copies of these essays in advance of publication.

1 *excelso . . . lecto*] Portions of Henry's imaginary garden are composed of raised beds, perhaps because the plants in them need more sun or simply for the enjoyment and edification of the viewer.

2–3 These lines provide the best evidence that the author of this work resided in England.

3 *diuiciis*] Most likely referring to the many medical attributes of mandrake.

5 *corpore corpus*] *Cf.* Ovid, *Met.* 15. 89, 'pinguescere corpore corpus,' and Martial, *Liber Spectaculorum* 9. 6 (ed. and trans. Kathleen M. Coleman [Oxford 2006], 82 and notes on 93), 'corpore corpus erat.'

9 *radice tenentur*] *Cf.* Ovid, *Met.* 4. 269, 'quamvis radice tenetur,' and 14. 292: 'moly vocant superi, nigra radice tenetur.'

10 Ovid uses *frondescere* at the same point in a hexameter (*Met.* 4. 395: 'pendens frondescere vestis').

12–14 Rigg (263) has suggested that a line might be missing here. I doubt that, since we do have all the necessary information about collecting mandrakes. Nonetheless, the repeated *si . . . si* in line 13 and the use of the present participle *uellens*, instead of the subjunctive verb *uellerit*, are awkward.

12 *non . . . firme*] Once again, Henry has doubts about the stories that circulate about certain plants, such as the fatal power of a screaming mandrake root.

13 *gremio genitricis*] A common phrase in Marian literature, possibly learned from Juvencus, *Evangeliorum libri quattuor* 1. 198 (ed. J. Huemer, CSEL 24 [Vienna and Leipzig 1891]), 'Ecce simul parvum gremio genitricis Iesum.'

26 *sanare*] The verb *curare* in *P* would work equally well, but since the prose redaction of the poem in *Exceptiones*, by far the oldest exemplar of the herbal, uses the verb *sanat*, I will assume that was what Henry intended and *curare* is a synonym supplied by a later scribe. The same verb replacement is found below in poem 2.7, line 30, with *sanat* in *S* and *curat* in *P*.

35 *sarticulum*] Presumably from *sartus*, a mending or a patch, therefore a little patch or strip of the plant. The source passage in Pseudo-Apuleius no. 131 does not use this word, and also specifies that the cure is for children: 'Ad filacteria infantium propter fascinum aut indicium. Infantibus in collo suspendis in linteolo mundo et de tela ligabis, ita ut ad tempus non nomines.'

36 *philactorium* = *phylacterium* (*filacteria* in Pseudo-Apuleius), specifically a Jewish phylactery, but here probably any magical amulet with protective writing.

2.2 ELLEBORVM ALBVM / White Hellebore, *Veratrum album* L.

Based closely on Macer, 'Elleborus albus,' lines 1774–1832. In *P* a later hand has incorrectly added *niger* after the title *Eleborus*.

3 *Ypocras*] A common medieval spelling of Hippocrates of Cos (*ca* 460–*ca* 370 BCE), who was usually paired with Galen as the fathers of medicine. The reference to his *Aphorisms*, one of the best known works of the Hippocratic corpus in the Middle Ages, comes from Macer 1814. Hellebore is discussed in *Aphorisms* 4. 13–16 and 5. 1. *Ypocras*, scanned with three long syllables in Macer, is scanned short-short-long by Henry. This scansion is repeated every time the name is used (4 Epilogue 2, 11; 5.2.2, 1; 5.2.6, 5; 5.2.6, 18; 6.2.7, 4).

4 *Philo*] Perhaps Philo of Tarsus, a first-century CE physician and pharmacologist, but possibly Philo of Alexandria (*ca* 20 BCE–50 CE) who did occasionally write on medicine. However, there were numerous noteworthy Philos in the Greco-Roman world (*cf.* David T. Runia, *Philo and the Church Fathers* [Leiden 1995], 26–8).

5 *Themeson*] Themison of Laodicea, a first-century BCE physician and founder of the Methodist school of medicine. He appears in Macer lines 265 and 1825.

5 *Plinius*] Pliny devotes a lengthy passage to the hellebores (25. 48–61) and mentions them throughout his *Natural History*.

9 *sero*] To prepare his insides better for hellebore's purgative action, the patient may not eat late the night before (just as we still prepare for modern colonoscopies and similar procedures).

18 *scrupulos*] A *scrupulus* or *scrupulum* (also *scripulum*) is 1/24 of an ounce, but can also mean any tiny amount in general, such as a 'pinch.'

22 *in principio tamen*] Apparently dropsy is best cured only at its onset.

25 *limphaticus*] Frenzied or insane, either due to fear of water or possession by a water nymph (both called *lympha*).

29 *Temptans testabitur eque*] An awkward little sentence. Henry seems to suggest that one can test the effects of hellebore rather than simply believe a book, but both will provide the same answer.

2.3 ELLEBORVM NIGRVM / Black Hellebore, *Helleborus niger* L.

Based on Macer, 'Elleborus niger,' lines 1833–58, on lines 1774–8 of his 'Elleborus albus,' and perhaps with reference to Pliny 25. 48–61.

1 *subit . . . subit*] With the sense of 'is next to' in the garden.

3 A euphemistic manner of saying that white hellebore purges by causing vomiting and black hellebore by diarrhoea.

4–5 These lines do not seem to have come from Macer, and may be based loosely on Pliny's description of the two hellebores, 25. 48–61.

12 *flecma* = *phlegma*. While *flegma* in *S* is closer to the classical *phlegma*, the spellings in *S* vary dramatically, while *P* consistently uses *flecma* through all of books 1–6.

16 A *syringium* is a fistula or sore, particularly one cured by the use of a syringe (*syrinx*). Macer employs this word at lines 219, 1481, 1759 and 1844. The copy of Macer used by Rufinus (39) includes a gloss: 'Syringia, id est fistula.' Henry also has a cure for *syringia* using iris root (3.8, 30). He presumably derived this passage from Macer, who found it in Pliny (25. 53). Pliny's original cure, though, mentions nothing about necks (*collo*), providing instead a detailed description of how ancient physicians stripped the thin shoots from black hellebore roots with the heaviest skin (*gravissimi corticis*). It appears that some derivative of Pliny, or Macer himself, described the thick skin of the root as *callo*, which most scribes read as *collo*. Choulant, in his edition of Macer, has emended to *callo* to agree with Pliny, though he notes that most manuscripts and older editions read *collo* (Macer, note to line 1844). I am assuming that Henry also read and understood *collo*, and that the misunderstanding occurred earlier in the herbal tradition. Of the source passage in Pliny the editor notes, 'The whole sentence, however, is in any case very clumsy, with a loose, almost formless, structure' (Pliny 25. 53, note *e*). In this case I am not going to presume extensive medical knowledge on Henry's part. Had this been the case, he might have understood *syringia* as a synonym for fistulae, as it is used in Macer. Fistulae can be used to describe a variety of abscesses, but are generally around the anus in medieval texts. So if Henry did understand Pliny or Macer's original meaning of the passage, and used *callo*, we should read this passage as, 'Let a strip from the hard skin of the root be applied and removed after two days; it removes fistulae.'

24 Pliny 25. 54: 'datur ad leniter molliendam alvum plurimum drachma una.'

26 *quid rides*] A nod to Horace, *Satires* 1.1, 69–70 (ed. Fairclough): 'quid rides? mutato nomine de te / fabula narratur.' However, whereas Horace implies that the story of Tantalus could be applied to his audience, Henry seems to suggest that his auditor is a cow.

26–27 These lines give a strong indication that Henry had access to a copy of Pliny or an abbreviation or commentary on his work. The *rusticus* in question could be Melampus, a shepherd discussed by Pliny at the start of his section on the hellebores: 'Melampodis fama divinationis artibus nota est. ab hoc appellatur unum hellebori genus melampodion. aliqui pastorem eodem nomine invenisse tradunt, capras purgari pasto illo animadvertentem, datoque lacte earum sanasse Proetidas furentes' (Pliny 25. 47). Melampus, however, cured his she-goats, whereas the healing of cattle is mentioned later (25. 55).

2.4 AZIMVM / ? Ragwort, *Senecio jacobaea* L.

Source unknown. Ragwort should not be confused with ragweed, *Ambrosia artemisiifolia* L., described above in poem 1.6, or with its close relative groundsel, *Senecio vulgaris* L., in poem 5.1.6. A common name for ragwort was cankerwort, which seems to be the source of *cancrum* in line 2. It is also called Stinking Nanny in Britain (Grieve, 'Ragwort') and Stinking Willie in North America, both of which fit well with the overall unpleasantness of *azimum*. The final line further emphasizes this plant's unique lack of beauty. The Digby Excerptor incorrectly calls it *acinum* (raspberry), which obviously does not fit the description.

Ragwort is only the most likely identification after an exhaustive search for any other appearance of a plant called *azimum*. Since the poem seems to be entirely original, we cannot resort to finding a source which could provide a positive identification. Moreover, Henry's description is too vague to help, so we must depend on similarly-named plants in other herbals and herbal lists. In the first place, we can assume that *azimum* refers neither to unleavened bread nor to an actual azyme. The scribe of *S* may have thought the plant bore some relation to an azyme, hence the title *Herba azimi*. *Azimum* does not appear in Macer, Pliny, Strabo, Pseudo-Apuleius, or any other major herbal, nor does it appear in any herbal list examined by Tony Hunt. The herbal of Marcellus Empiricus (*ca* 400), possibly known to Henry, does mention a porridge made of *azomum*, though the few manuscripts are confused and the editors are at a loss for an identification (*cf. Marcelli de medicamentis liber*, ed. Max Niedermann and Eduard Liechtenhan [Berlin 1968], 336, line 3). Otherwise, the name is most similar to *ocimum* or *ozimum*, basil, but Henry has already treated basil (poem 1.2, above) and the description here of an ugly, foul-tasting plant can hardly describe that. The *Sinonoma Bartholomei* gives the name *ozimum* not to basil, but to basil seed (33). This poem, though, does seem to describe a plant rather than a seed. The *Laud Herbal Glossary* of the early twelfth century provides several similar names. Closest is *azimon*, no. 159, but that is an alternate spelling of *aeizon*, the houseleek ('Azimon .i. iouis barba. et semper uiua'). Henry treats *iouis barba* and *semperuiua* as synonymous in poem 3.25 and seems to know it well. Also similar in the *Laud Herbal* are *eucimo* (nos. 540 and 593) and *euzimum* (no. 554), both glosses for *eruca*, rocket or white mustard, which Henry describes in poem 4.4, below.

2 *cancrum*] The alternate name given in this line is troubling. Where *P* and *O* read *Cancrum*, *S* reads *Canor*. Moreover, a table of contents found in *S* gives the name of this herb as *Ozinum i. cauernum* (see Rigg, 229, 290). I have opted for the reading in *P* since *Canor* is more apt to be a misreading of *Cancrum* than the opposite, *cauernum* appears to be a variation of *cancrum*, *cancrum* also appears in the *Exceptiones* (*O* 92r), and because a number of medieval herbal lists include a *Herba cancri* or *Herba cancrosa* (which Hunt could not identify, 134). The *Laud Herbal*, nos. 411 and 428, glosses *cencron* as millet ('Cencron .i. milium') and *cacrius* as the rosemary seed ('Cacrius .i. semen roris marini'), neither of which makes sense in this context.

6 *Splendida uesano*] Another *fit* must be understood here, parallel to the previous lines.

7 *discretus*] Possibly with the double meaning of both 'distinguished' and 'able to distinguish,' that is, use reason.

2.5 PASTINACA / Parsnip:

1) Parsnip, *Pastinaca sativa* L.
2) Skirret (*Sium sisarum* L.), or Caraway root (*Carum carvi* L.)
3) Wild Carrot, *Daucus carota* L.

The recipes in lines 6–17 come from Macer's 'Pastinaca,' lines 1264–84. The distinction of three types of *pastinacae* (lines 1–5) is original to Henry. *Circa instans* has an entry for *daucus* rather than *pastinaca*, differentiating *daucus creticus* and *daucus asininus* (fol. 196v), but this does not seem to have influenced Henry. Until the modern period, carrots and parsnips came in a wide variety of sizes and colours, more often white and purple than orange. They were not always seen as distinct plants, but simply as varieties of the long, sweet root vegetable *pastinaca.*

2 *sceruuisam*] Most likely the skirret (Middle English *skirwhite*), the name given to the edible roots of several plants of the family Apiaceae. It is probably to be identified with the Roman *siser*, grouped by Pliny with the parsnips and named by the modern translator as a skirret (Pliny 19. 90). The name is now more often applied to *Sium sisarum*, though this appeared in England only in the fifteenth century (John H. Harvey, 'Vegetables in the Middle Ages,' *Garden History* 12 [1984], 89–99, at 93). *Sceruuisa* could also be the root of caraway (described in the following poem, 2.6), which Dioscorides notes can be 'edible as Pastinaca' (3. 66). The *Oxford English Dictionary* traces *skirwhit* to the Old French *eschervis*, which is from the Latin *carui*, or caraway. I would suggest that *sceruuisa* could apply to any number of long, white root vegetables and is here more likely parsnip or parsley root rather than caraway. In the Middle English herbal *Agnus Castus*, 'eruca' is called 'skyrwyt' (152). If Henry had wanted to discuss caraway root, he would have found his opportunity in the very next poem. In any case, the various white relatives of the parsnip all look and taste rather alike.

6 It is called *pastinaca* because it is good 'to eat' (*pastu*). The pun works only in Latin.

9 The *tumor uentris muliebris* is probably a large uterine fibroid.

14–15 Henry received this recipe from Macer, but his addition of *ut dicunt* ('as they say') reveals his typical skepticism about using herbs as amulets.

2.6 CARVI / Caraway, *Carum carui* L.

Caraway is not in Macer, and I have not found its source. Henry's poem is translated in EMA as 'Carui' (194). The Trinity Compiler provides a much longer poem on caraway (fols. 93v–94r), made up of original material, Henry's lines 2–3 and 9–10, and Henry's poem 6.2.10 on cardamom. In Constantine's *Liber graduum*, *cardamomum* is another name for wild caraway ('Cardamomum syluestre carui est,' 372). The presence in EMA's 'Carui' of the shape and appearance of chervil is possibly responsible for the lack of such description in 'Cerfoile' (EMA, 129–30).

1 *sexto*] That is, the sixth poem in the second book and the sixth plot in the second quadrant of the garden.

1 Caraway's nominal poverty (*paupercula nomine*) is a pun on 'careo, carui' ('I lack, I lacked').

3–4 The line 'uis acris et ignea ualde,' used twice here, is in the first line of

Macer's poem on chervil ('Cerefolium,' line 928), and Henry repeats the theme in his own poem on chervil, at 5.1.4, 1.

5–6 *Ceruleus* can be used to indicate any one of several deep colours, be it of the sky, sea, or leaves. Here it is probably a deep green, and the Middle English Macer takes time to explain cerule as 'yelowe as is wex or grene and blak to-gidere' (EMA, 194).

10 Caraway and cumin have often been confused, most likely because their seeds are almost identical in appereance, though quite different in flavour. The Germans called it *Kimmel*, the Italians *comino tedesco* (German cumin), and the French *cumin de près*. The English word 'caraway' probably comes from the Arabic *al-karawiya*, rather than from the Latin (*cf.* 'Caraway' in the online Spice Pages of Gernot Katzer through the University of Graz, <http://www.uni-graz.at/~katzer/engl/>). It is clear from this line, though, that Henry knew the difference between the two spices and valued cumin more highly.

2.7 DRAGANTEA / Dragon Arum, *Dracunculus vulgaris* Schott

Closely based on Macer, 'Colubrina,' lines 1728–65. Henry's own voice comes through in line 9 and in the asides in lines 3, 18, and 25. Dragon arum exudes a terrible odour (line 1), similar to rotting flesh, in order to attract pollinating flies. It is named for its similarity to snake skin (line 4), which provides one of the best examples in the herbal of the medieval adage *similia similibus curantur*: since it looks like a snake, it cures snake bites.

1 Henry, in directly addressing the plants in his garden, is following the tradition of Strabo, who arranged his *Hortulus* in the manner of a walk through his garden. He spoke to the Iris directly, 'Te neque transierim, Latiae cui libera linguae' (Strabo 217), which is clearly the inspiration for this line.

3 It is not clear why Henry urges against using the name *colubrina*. Both it and *dragantea* are given by Macer, lines 1728–9, without comment.

8 Either *harum* or *horum* will work, since *serpens* can be either gender. I have kept the feminine to correlate with the feminine *colubrina* and Macer's use of *illarum* (line 1735).

13 *granis*] Either the dragonwort seeds or a very small measurement, 'a grain.'

19 *emoptoicos* = *haemoptoicos*, those who suffer from *haemoptysis*, the spitting of blood. A gloss to Macer's poem on Arnoglossa, included in the thirteenth-century herbal of Rufinus (39), says 'Emoptoici dicuntur qui sanguinem spuunt vel vomunt.'

22–23 *pernio*] Chilblains (still called 'perniosis'). The name, according to Henry, comes from *pernicies*. The *plebs* called it *mula*, from the Old French *mule* (DMLBS, *s.v.* 'mula' no. 4). Macer also says this (line 1763).

29 *brionia*] Probably white bryony, *Bryonia dioica* Jacq., which does not otherwise appear in the herbal. *Cf.* Grieve, 'Bryony, White.' Henry has not made clear that bryony should be mixed with the dragon arum. Macer says, 'Si sit ei tritae cum melle bryonia iuncta' (line 1758).

30 *fagedenica* = *phagadaenica*, a variety of rodent ulcers, gaping wounds, or even bulimia (*cf.* Pliny 26. 111).

33 *matrix*] The direct address of the womb, or any body part, is unique but is clearly necessary to preserve the rhyme and metre.

2.8 SAXIFRAGA / Great Burnet Saxifrage, *Pimpinella major* L.

Great burnet saxifrage is only one of several possible identifications for the name *saxifraga*, which was given to many plants which could (or supposedly could) break apart rocks. In typical medieval fashion, the plant's ability to break apart rocks in nature was applied to stones in the human body. Saxifrage is not in Macer, but is found in Pseudo-Apuleius, no. 98 (p. 177). While Pseudo-Apuleius does describe how *saxifraga* cures stones (*cauculos*), the recipe is different and also mentions fevers. Rufinus cites four other herbalists on the subject of *saxifraga* (278–9). None are closely related to Henry's poem, though they all note that it breaks stones outside and within the human body. Marcellus also emphasizes the power of saxifrage against stones (*Marcelli de medicamentis liber*, 26. 93): 'Herba saxifraga, si ex oleo et liquamine manducetur, intra triduum calculos soluet.' EMA translates this as 'Saxifrage' (195) and Daniel Arundel (fols. 71v–72r) translates lines 1–5 and 9–10 as 'Colopendrya.'

1 For *petrosilinum*, see poems 1.21 and 5.2.5. The EMA translator misunderstood the comparison to *petrosilinum*, and took it to be the same plant: 'Saxifrage hauyþ his name for-þi þat it brekiþ þe stoon. Some men clepen hit petroselinum' (EMA, 195).

2 One of the clearest etymologies in the herbal: *saxifraga* is named from *frangit saxa*, which is most likely true.

3 An excellent example of the medieval doctrine of *similia similibus*, curing like with like. Very hard cherry pits are ground up in a cure for breaking up kidney stones.

6–8 These lines are difficult. *P* is lacking line 6, and we cannot refer to the translation of Henry Daniel, who did not have these lines available or decided not to use them. The scribe of *S* was clearly confused by the word after *teneram* in line 6. My emendation to *tantum* seems necessary to help lines 7–8 make sense and reflects the translation in EMA, which provides some guidance: 'Men seyn þat þer is no medicyne more profitable for þe stoon þan is þis. But þis takeþ nat a-wey but þe tendre stoon. And if þe stoon be of long tyme gadred, þan it must be distroyed with a strengre medecyne' (EMA, 195).

2.9 VIOLA / Sweet Violet, *Viola odorata* L.

Based on Macer, 'Violae,' lines 1342–94. Henry's lines 1–2, 9, 31, and 47–51 are original. The poem is presented in an explicitly religious context, beginning with a liturgical sequence in honour of the Assumption, as described below. This is a rare example of Christian language in the herbal, for Henry usually prefers to describe pagan Greco-Roman deities. Daniel Additional translates the cure in the last five lines in his entry 'Diana' (fols. 74v–75r). The first two lines of the poem introduce this poem and the following two (2.9–2.11, 'Violet,' 'Rose,' and 'Lily'), all of which form a botanical prayer of sorts to the Virgin, whose emblems include these three flowers. These emblems are repeated in the Book 5 Prologue, lines 4–5.

1–5 These lines show an impressive expansion of Macer 1342–3: 'Nec roseus superare decor, nec lilia possunt / Fragrantes Violas specie, nec vi, nec odore.' The comparison of the lily to the Virgin Mary would be well known to Henry outside of the herbal, but lines 1–2 are almost identical to part of a liturgical sequence of the eleventh or twelfth century for the Assumption, 'Purpurea et viola, roscida ut rosa, candens ut lilia' (printed by Gall Morel with the title 'Sanctae Mariae assumtio, sequentia' from a twelfth-century manuscript of Einsiedeln, in *Lateinische Hymnen des Mittelalters* [Einsiedeln 1868], no. 162, p. 99; discussed by Margot Fassler, 'Mary's Nativity, Fulbert of Chartres, and the *Stirps Jesse*: Liturgical innovation circa 1000 and its afterlife,' *Speculum* 75 [2000], 389–434, at 421). Line 2 may also be influenced by Strabo, 'De Rosa' (lines 392–428), where he also describes the lily as the emblem of Mary, faith and chastity: 'O mater uirgo, faecundo germine mater, / uirgo fide intacta, sponsi de nomine sponsa . . .' (lines 419–20).

3–4 These lines, with their repetition on *n* and *u*, show clearly how Henry liked to indulge in alliteration.

5 *formosaque lilia*] Vocative. Henry apostrophizes the lilies, ennobled as the Virgin's emblem.

10 *Iustus*] Perhaps Curtius Justus, an ancient physician cited several times by Gargilius (*Gargilii Martialis quae extant*, vol. 1: *Fragmenta ad holera arboresque pomiferas pertinentia*, ed. Sebastian Condorelli, Biblioteca di Helikon, Testi e studi 11 [Rome 1977]). See also the note to Macer 1389. Possibly to be identified by Actius Justus, author of *De muliebria*, also known as *Gynaecia* (Augusto Beccaria, *I codici di medicina del periodo presalernitano* [Rome 1956], *s.v. Accio Giusto, Gynaecia*).

12 *Cf.* Ovid, *Remedia amoris* 803: 'praecipiam de Bacchi munere'

21 *Herba* in this case refers not to the whole plant but specifically to the leaves.

28 *cerotis*] From *ceratum*, a wax plaster.

29 *ragadias*] *Cf.* Isidore, *Etym.* 4.7.39: 'Ragadiae dicuntur, eo quod fissurae sint rugis collectae circa orificium.'

34 The cure for *angina* in Macer 1352 calls only for water. Henry has added *angina* to the problems cured by violets with honey and water found in Macer 1364–6. *Angina* covers a variety of swellings in the throat, probably tonsillitis (*cf.* Constantine, *Liber de morborum cognitione et curatione* [= *Viaticum*], in *Constantini Africani* . . . *Opera* [Basel 1536–9], 2. 43–5).

35 *collectio*] A tumour or a boil, any sort of 'gathering.' The scribe of *P* probably did not know this sense of *collectio* and supplied the more familiar word *decoccio* in its place, regardless of the fact that it does not make sense.

41 *gliquiricie* = *glycyrrhizae*, a variant of *liquiritiae*. I cannot find this passage in Pliny's accounts of violets or liquorice. The citation comes directly from Macer.

47–51 This recipe is not found in Macer. It was commonly known as *mellicratum* if made without the violets. An English manuscript dating from the mid-twelfth century (Bethesda, MD, National Library of Medicine, MS E 8, fol. 17v) contains a recipe for *mellicratum* without the violets in the margin of a commentary on the *Aphorisms* of Hippocrates attributed to Alexander (*i.e.* of Tralles). The commentator describes *mellicratum*: 'Et ut scias qualis est uirtus mellicrati, superflua purgat et naturalia conseruat. Philosophi refert (*sic*) quia ad odorem mellis quadraginta dies uixit quidam.' ('And so you know what sort of virtue *mellicratum* has, it purges superfluities and preserves the natural states. The philosophers relate that a certain person lived forty days on the smell of honey.') In the margin a contemporary hand gives the recipe: 'unam partem mellis et duas aque celestis diu mixte ad solem diutius pone' ('place one part honey and two of heavenly dew, mixed well, in the sun for a long time'). Violets were renowned for their cooling power, and the violet syrup described here is a general cure for all *calores*. Nicholas Culpeper still voiced, in the seventeenth century, the common medieval opinion: '[Violet] is used to cool any heat or distemperature of the body, either inwardly or outwardly' (*Culpeper's Complete Herbal* [London 1880], 380).

48 *fialas* = *phialas*

2.10 ROSA / Rose, family *Rosaceae* L.

Based loosely on Macer, 'Rosa,' lines 776–807, but most of the poem is original to Henry. This poem ranks among Henry's most creative entries in the herbal. It takes the form of a conference between Henry, Erato (the muse of lyric and erotic poetry), Macer, and Walahfrid Strabo (called *Stabus*). Henry plays the role of inquiring student while Erato encourages the ancient herbalists to share their wisdom about roses. This poem forms a trilogy with the preceding Violet (2.9) and succeeding Lily (2.11), the three flowers of the Virgin.

5–6 The muse Erato is referring apparently to Henry's lost poem *De amore*. It would seem, according to these lines, that he wrote briefly in that work on the subject of plants, undoubtedly in imitation of Ovid.

10 *Tempe*] See note to line 12 of the Prologue to Book 1.

12–13 A paraphrase of Macer 776–7: 'Dici flos florum nobis Rosa iure videtur, / Quod specie unctos praecedat odoreque flores.'

12, 18 *florum flos*] Peter Dronke has traced the popular themes of *flos florum* and *rosa rosarum* in ancient and medieval Latin and Greek lyrics (*Medieval Latin and the Rise of European Love-Lyric*, 2nd ed., 2 vols [Oxford 1968], 181–92), and notes that they were 'common currency' by the twelfth century (*Medieval Latin*, 186).

15 The *fera incola* could be Pegasus itself, perhaps its tamer Bellerophon or, in later legends, Perseus. See John M. Steadman, 'Perseus upon Pegasus and *Ovid Moralized*,' *Review of English Studies*, New Series, 9 (1958), 407–10.

15 *incola fontis*] Parallel construction with Ovid, *Met.* 1. 512: 'incola montis.'

16 Rigg noted (265) that it is strange for Henry to say that *Stabus* (Walahfrid Strabo) is following in the footsteps of Macer, since not only did Macer write centuries after Strabo but Henry should have known that for Macer cites Strabo in his own herbal (lines 900, 906).

17–18 A paraphrase of Strabo, 'De Rosa,' 400–401: 'herbarum uicisse comas uirtute et odore / dicitur, ut merito florum flos esse feratur.'

29 *Anglia felix*] *Cf. HA* 9. 53 (ed. Greenway, 694): 'Felix Anglia tantorum patrum tantis insignita splendoribus!'

31 *pro!, cedat*] I owe this creative punctuation of *procedat*, as it appears in both manuscripts, to Rigg (266) who acknowledges that 'The punctuation, interpretation and separation of "pro! cedat" are all uncertain.'

33 *Cf.* below, poem 4.1–2, line 24: 'dolor equus utrimque.'

45 The emendation to *solum* is based on Macer 806: 'Sub Phoebo tantum septem suspende diebus.'

46 *Palladii*] Rutilus Taurus Aemilianus Palladius, a fourth-century CE writer on agriculture. His work *De re rustica* was well known in the Middle Ages. The name comes from Macer 802.

50 *Parnasus . . . Aganippe*] Fountains sacred to the Muses. Virgil, *Ecloga* 10. 11–12: 'nam neque Parnasi uobis iuga, nam neque Pindi / ulla moram fecere, neque Aonie Aganippe.'

2.11 LILIVM / Lily, family *Liliaceae* L., probably *Lilium candidum* L.

Based on Macer, 'Lilium,' lines 808–42, without Macer's lines 816, 818, 828–9, and 839–40. Henry's lines 5–8 and 33 are original. Henry differentiates between two types of lily, red (*sanguineus*) and white (*niueus*), in line 8.

14 The sense here is that the poultice of lily bulbs and wine should be removed from the foot corns (*clauis*) only after three days have passed. Macer 823 is much clearer: 'nec solvas nisi cum lux tertia transit.'

15 *maturat turgida pusque*] The juice softens, or ripens, swellings and pus-filled boils. The use of *maturat* with *pus* is uncommon or simply incorrect; it is the swelling that contains the pus which 'matures' and not the pus inside. Macer 842 is clearer: 'Turgida maturat, pus concoquit et cito purgat.'

31 *uenando uenena*] The reading in *P* of *uirus uenando* would also work, but as in many other cases I have opted for the reading in *S*, all other things being equal. Henry's source, Macer 821, reads 'Sic quoque fungorum vetat ille venena nocere.' While Henry often likes to provide a synonym for words in Macer (such as *uirus* for *uenena*), he also likes to show off his own vocabulary, so it seems more likely that he would use both *uenena* and *uirus* in this passage.

2.12 CELIDONIA / Celandine, *Chelidonium majus* L.

A condensed version of Macer, 'Chelidonia,' lines 1690–1708. Henry has omitted Macer's lines 1690–92, where it is explained that there are two kinds of celandine, a greater (*Chelidonium majus* L.) and a lesser (*Ranunculus ficaria* L.), both good for the eyes. Henry's line 1 is original, in which he indicates the poem's location within the garden and book.

1 *duodeno*] That is, the twelfth poem in Book 2 and the twelfth plant in this bed.

2–3 The passage from Pliny is 15. 89–90, but Henry is paraphrasing Macer 1693–4.

4 *illa*] The *mater yrundo*, mother swallow.

5 The name *celidonia* comes from *chelydon* (χελιδών), the Greek name for the swallow.

2.13 PIGMENTVM / ? Meadowsweet, *Spiraea ulmaria* L.

Most of the poem is original to Henry, but line 6 is apparently based on Macer's 'Barrocus,' lines 1645–6, all of which poem Henry uses below for his poem 4.22, 'Boragum.' Little is provided to identify *pigmentum*. Countless flowers could be described as pleasing to bees (lines 5–6). This herb could be associated with the Old English *beowyrt*, identified either as sweet flag (*Acorus calamus*) or lemon balm (*Melissa officinalis*). See Pollington, *Leechcraft*, 100, for a discussion of these possibilities. Henry's own poem 4.22, 'Boragum,' is based on Macer's 'Barrocus,' and probably describes lemon balm. If we assume that

Henry has not made a duplicate entry and that this is a distinct species (according to modern taxonomy), it could be bastard balm (*Melittis melissophyllum*) or meadowsweet (*Spiraea ulmaria*). The glossary *Alphita* defines 'herba pigmentaria' as 'melissa.'

The name Henry uses for this herb is also troubling but can help in identification. *Pigmentum*, or the Old French *piment*, is the name given to a variety of spiced wines featuring honey. This is probably the *pigmentum* mentioned by Henry in his epigram 12. 8, 23 (*HA* 818), where a girl addresses her lover as a *stillula pigmenti* (which should be understood as a 'sip of *piment*' rather than 'a little drop of paint,' the translation given). *Pigmentum*, however, often bears the general meaning of a dye, and later any spice. Henry could be referring to the wine itself, but he does call it a 'herba.' The situation is complicated by the fact that most European vernaculars took *piment* or *pimento* to refer to some variety of hot pepper or to almost any spice. A British manuscript of *ca* 1300 (London, British Library, MS Additional 15236, cited by Hunt, xix, 84, 174) contains five different lists of herbs and their synonyms, two of which include the English name 'piment' or the French 'pigmentarie.' These are given as synonyms for 'citrago' or 'melissa,' both Latin names for balm. The fourteenth-century *Sinonoma Bartholomei* (29) tellingly provides definitions for two different *Melissae*: 1) 'Melissa herba est quae a quibusdam dicitur baume'; 2) 'Melissa, herba pigmentaria idem, an medewort secundum quosdam.' The first *melissa* is clearly the standard balm, but the second is probably meadowsweet, called 'meadwort' in medieval England, used in spiced wines and beers, and a favourite with bees (Grieve, 'Meadowsweet'). If we take *herba pigmentaria* in the *Sinonoma* to mean an herb for spicing a drink, the identification of *medewort* with Henry's *pigmentum* should be settled.

Pigmentum was prized by ecclesiastics other than Henry. In the thirteenth and fourteenth centuries priories in the western part of the diocese of Paris were required to supply the cathedral chapter of Notre-Dame-de-Paris with the herb called *pigmentum*. Every year, at least from 1280 to 1315, a different priory was obliged to gather and deliver a full cartload of the herb to be scattered on the floor of the cathedral on the Feast of the Assumption (Auguste Longnon, *Pouillés de la Province de Sens* [Paris 1904], xlv–xlvi, 369).

1 The use of *subintrat* here is curious. Nothing about the plant suggests the sneaking or silent movement meant by this verb. Perhaps Henry simply means that it 'enters next' or 'enters lower down' in comparison with celandine in the previous bed.

2 *uocant*] The collective singular *uulgus* has changed to the plural.

6 *Cf.* Macer 1645–6 (which Henry also uses for the opening lines of poem 4.22): 'Contritis foliis apium si vasa perungas / Non fugient, meliusque facis, si lac sibi iungas.'

2.14 VETONICA / Betony, *Betonica officinalis* L.

A close adaptation of Macer, 'Betonica,' lines 429–91. Henry's lines 2–4 are original. I have retained the spelling *uetonica*, as it appears consistently through *S*, the older manuscript. Daniel Additional mentions this poem under 'Betonica,' though does not describe it since 'Henricus Englisch seith but the same' as Macer.

2 *Quot uires*] Betony was credited with more potential cures than almost any other herb or spice. It alone was the subject of a treatise, *De herba vettonica*, credited to the first-century imperial physician Antonius Musa (published by Ernst Howald and Henry E. Sigerist, *Antonii Musae De herba vettonica liber, Pseudoapulei Herbarius, Anonymi De taxone liber, Sexti Placiti Liber medicinae ex animalibus* [Leipzig 1927], 3–11).

2 *Natura creatrix*] Echoes of Lucretius, *De rerum natura* 1.629, though the phrase could have been idiomatic by Henry's day. I can find no clear Lucretian influence elsewhere in the herbal.

2–4 There are several difficulties in these lines. The sense (that betony has so many medicinal virtues that they cannot be described) is clear, but the grammatical subject is not, and I have treated the entire phrase as an exclamation. *Mea mens* is part of a relative clause, therefore the best option for a subject is *omnis* in line 4; however, that seems to be part of an aside starting with *nec*. Moreover, each *sufficit* (with the subjects *mens* and *omnis*) needs to lead to the single infinitive *tradere*. Beyond that, in line 2, *quantasque* must be elided awkwardly in order to scan, while a long syllable is missing after *tibi*.

7 *preest*] The first syllable must be shortened for the line to scan properly.

11 *per subteriora*] This is most likely what Henry inteded, as it is found in most manuscripts of Macer, and he used the same phrase above at 1.4, line 11, but Choulant opted for the rarer reading *per subtiliora* (Macer 451 and apparatus). It is not clear what either would mean in a medical context. The German translators understand Macer's 'per subtiliora / Dicitur expelli' (451–2) as 'soll . . . in Brodem und Dünste verdünnt' (*Höhepunkte der Klostermedizin*, trans. Mayer and Goehl, 47*). It appears that Henry understood the harmful blood to be flushed out through the 'lower parts,' *i.e.* in the urine, rather than through the airy exhalations suggested by *subtiliora*.

22 *bis bina*] The reading in *S*, *quaterna*, does not scan and is probably an intruded gloss.

23 *uiginti quatuor*] Macer 458 gives *viginti septem* which, as it will not scan at this point, seems to have been changed by Henry for the sake of metre without regard for the efficacy of the recipe. It also could have resulted from a misreading of *xxuii* as *xxiiii*.

25 Henry indulges in a pun on two meanings of *potes*.

28 *necne*] A poetic form of *necnon*, since a negative is not intended here. Macer 480 reads 'Pondere vero fabae pulvis cum melle voratus.'

38 *punctus . . . frigoris*] Apparently the first, violent onset of chills during a fever. This line is almost identical to 2.23, 16 below.

41 Pliny 26. 40: 'faciles praestat vomitiones radix vettonicae, hellebori modo quattuor drachmis in passo aut mulso.'

44 Pliny 25. 101: 'moribus inponitur vettonica praecipue, cui vis tanta perhibetur ut inclusae circulo eius serpentes ipsae sese interimant flagellando.'

46 *proprio morsu*] The transposed reading in *P* will also work. Macer 485 reads *morsu proprio*, and Henry usually tries to rewrite his source lines, even if using the same words.

47–48 In Macer 490–91 this cure is attributed to an unnamed 'they' (*dicunt*), rather than to Pliny. I cannot find this cure in Pliny.

50 *carmen*] An addition not found in Macer, nor can I find it in Pliny. Perhaps it comes by way of Pliny 25. 84, discussing betony: 'tantumque gloriae habet ut domus in qua sata sit tuta existimetur a periculis omnibus.'

51 *Menetamus*] Menemachus, a Greek physician working in Aphrodisias in the second century CE, a member of the Methodist sect who is quoted by Caelius Aurelianus, Galen and Oribasius (*Dictionary of Greek and Roman Biography and Mythology*, ed. William Smith, 3 vols [Boston 1870], *s.v.* 'Menemachus'). He appears in the herbal of Macer Floridus at lines 486 and 1166 as 'Menemachus,' though that is over-correction on Choulant's part, since the name is spelled differently in nearly every manuscript.

2.15 FRAGA / Strawberry, *Fragaria vesca* L.

Source unknown. Strawberries are not found in Macer, Strabo or Dioscorides, and this poem bears no relation to Pseudo-Apuleius no. 37, 'Fraga' (p. 83). The Digby Excerptor condenses the poem to one line, while the Trinity Compiler used only lines 2 and 5 in his longer poem 'Fra.'

1 *sequitur*] That is, which follows betony (poem 2.14).

6 *liuor*] Envy is a theme to which Henry returns frequently in the herbal, especially during his arguments with the drunken cook, *e.g.* at 5.2.5, 1, and 5.2.6, 1.

7 The tree in question is the arbutus, or strawberry tree (*Arbutus unedo* L.), a native of southern Europe whose fruits look like those of the ground strawberry, and are edible but tasteless (hence the *unedo* of its botanical name). Henry probably knew Ovid's description of the arbutus and strawberries, food of the first men (*Metamorphoses* 1. 103–104): 'contentique cibis nullo cogente creates / arbuteos fetus montanaque fraga legebant.'

9 *figmenta . . . parantes*] This rhyme and alliteration also appear below in poem 4.24, 'Palma Christi,' 9–10.

2.16 PVLEGIVM / Pennyroyal, *Mentha pulegium* L.

Based on Macer, 'Pulegium,' lines 626–77, though highly abbreviated. Henry's introduction, lines 1–4, is based on Strabo's 'De Puleio,' lines 300–326. Henry does not use Macer's lengthy explanation of afterbirth (*secundas*) in lines 631–41 (which has been transferred to poem 3.8 below on *Iris*), nor Macer's lines 629, 650, 665, 668–71, and 673–7. Choulant remarks (note to 668) that many manuscripts of Macer are lacking lines 668–77. It would seem that Henry had a manuscript from this family, but for the fact that his last line is based on Macer's line 672. Among the poems based directly on Macer, this one is remarkable for how thoroughly Henry has rearranged the material. For example, Henry's lines 10–13 are drawn from Macer's lines 666 (*tussim*), 647–9 (*nausea, morsus*), 662 (*spleni*) and 629 (*menstrua*). *Pulegium* and *Puleium* are both common classical spellings and are interchangeable here.

1–2 Strabo 302–304: 'Hoc aput Indorum tanti constare peritos / fertur, aput Gallos quanti ualet Indica nigri / congeries piperis . . .'.

2–4 *Tonans* was a common classical epithet for *Jupiter* or *Jovis*. Henry borrowed this usage from Strabo. These lines are based loosely on Strabo 308–16:

> . . . O magni laudanda Tonantis
> uirtus et ratio, nullis quae munera terris
> larga suae non pandit opis; quae rara sub isto
> axe uidere soles, aliis in partibus horum
> copia tanta iacet, quantam uilissima tecum
> efficiunt; rursus quaedam quae spreta uidentur
> forte tibi, magno mercantur ditia regna,
> altera ut alterius potiatur foenore tellus,
> orbis et in toto per partes una domus sit.

Henry expands on this sentiment—that God has dispersed healing plants in varying quantities across the world for different peoples—in poem 2.20, *Conferba*.

10 *tepido*] Wine (*uino*) must be understood, which we find in Henry's source Macer 666: 'Tussim compescit cum vino sumpta tepenti.'

11 *sumpta*] Henry switches to an implied feminine subject, most likely *herba*.

16 *aut lente*] The addition of this ingredient is curious. It is not found in Henry's source Macer 659–60: 'Et quosvis alios solet emendare tumores, / Si superadditur tepidae permixta polentae.' Moreover, we would expect the dative *lenti* to match the *tepide polenta*, rather than the ablative. But since it is found in both manuscripts and can be made to work (with some forcing), I have not emended.

18 *hec et multa*] Assume a verb like *facit* here.

24 *malfacio* = *malefactio*, a fainting or swooning. Rufinus adds a gloss to this word in his quotation of Macer: 'Malfactio est defectus totius corporis ex nimio fluxu sanguinis' (257).

2.17 SERPILLVM / Wild Thyme, *Thymus serpyllum* L.

A close adaptation of Macer's 'Serpillum,' lines 1325–41, less only 1341, concerning *menstrua*.

1 *Serpillum* supposedly derives its name from *serpere*, since it twists like a *serpens* along the ground. The *poeta* in question is most likely Virgil (see note to lines 16–17 below).

2 The comparison to pennyroyal (*pulegium*), treated in the previous poem, is Henry's addition to Macer's lines 1325–6.

6 *S* reads *linito* (which does not scan) for *mulceto*, probably an intrusion based on Macer's *perline* (line 1328).

15 *tutus liberque quiescat*] Perhaps borrowed from the anonymous eleventh-century *Psalmi Turonenses*: 'Sicque regente Deo tutus liberque quiesco' ('Psalmus David,' xxii. 32), in 'Die Psalmenparaphrase eines Anonymus aus Marmoutier,' ed. Peter Orth (26 November 2007), MGH Poetae Latini medii aevi 6, Nachträge zu den Poetae aevi Carolini, Ergänzende Texte, <http://www.mgh.de/~Poetae/Texte/Psalmi-Turonenses.pdf>.

16–17 Virgil, *Ecloga* 2. 10–11, where the subject is Thestylis: 'Thestylis et rapido fessis messoribus aestu / alia serpyllumque herbas contundit olentis.' Virgil also discusses *serpyllum* in *Georgica* 4. 30–32: 'Haec circum casiae virides et olentia late / serpylla et graviter spirantis copia thymbrae / floreat inriguumque bibant violaria fontem.'

2.18 PIPERA / Lesser Burnet, *Pimpinella saxifraga* L.

Based in part on Strabo's 'De Agrimonia' (lines 359–68), though Henry's poem is on a different plant. The description of its shape and flowers, lines 5–6, is not in Strabo's poem. *Pipera* has nothing to do with *piper* (black pepper) and is probably a variation of *pimpinella*. The EMA translator thought as much, translating this as 'Pympernolle' (190). The *Sinonoma Bartholomei* glosses *pimpinella* as 'assimilatur minori saxifragiae' (34). For the true saxifrage (great burnet) see poem 2.8 above. The name pimpernel now applies to a small blue or red flower (*Anagallis arvensis*) which is unrelated to the medieval pimpernels, members of the saxifrage family (Pimpinellae). Moreover, the white flowers and many branches described by Henry (lines 5–7) are more indicative of the flower-packed umbels of a saxifrage or burnet than of a pimpernel. The Trinity Compiler reproduces lines 1–2 and 5–8, but has rewritten line 1.

1–2 Strabo 359–61: 'Hic quoque sarcocolam, campos quae plurima passim / uestit et effetis siluarum inuenta sub umbris / nascitur, ordinibus facile est discernere pulchris.'

8 This line provides one of the few cases of shared error (*uulnera* in *S* and *T* instead of *mundaque* in *P*), pointing to the unsurprising conclusion that the English manuscripts are related. *Mundaque* must be correct, given Henry's love of rhetorical devices like the *climax* here, also employed in the next poem (2.19, 6–7).

2.19 BENEDICTA / Avens (Herb Bennet, Hare's Ear), *Geum urbanum* L.

Avens is placed together with burnet because of their shared ability to clean and close wounds. The first half of this poem seems original to Henry, but I have not found a source for the cures in the second half, except line 8, which seems to be borrowed from Strabo's poem 'De Abrotano,' 91–8. There is no similarity to Pseudo-Apuleius no. 61, 'Herba leporis pes' (p. 115). Rufinus includes this plant under 'Gariofilata,' since it smells like cloves (*gariofili*). He notes that it is also called 'pes leporis, sana munda, avancia et herba benedicta' (146). EMA translates lines 2 and 6–7 under 'Benet' (195).

1–2 The name *benedicta* reflects the plant's 'blessed' qualities, while *auricula leporina* describes its appearance.

6–7 These lines offer another fine example of rhetorical *climax* like that in the previous poem at 2.18, line 8.

8 *Cf.* Strabo 97: 'quos incerta premit furtiuae iniuria guttae.' But this may have come from Macer's poem on southernwood ('Abrotanum,' lines 31–51; Henry's version is poem 2.23 below). This line does not appear in Choulant's text, but he does note its presence in some manuscripts (Macer, note to line 51).

8 *preest*] The *prodest* in both *P* and *S*, which is clearly wrong, may point to a shared exemplar.

2.20 CONFERBA / Comfrey, *Symphytum officinale* L.

Comfrey is not found in Macer. Most of lines 17–24 come from Pseudo-Apuleius no. 59, 'Herba Confirma' (pp. 112–13), but for most of the poem

Henry has indulged in a novel commentary on herbs in general and their confusing array of powers, as well as on the balance of four qualities and four humours. Rufinus (24) includes it under the name 'Anagallis,' where he notes that it is the same as 'symphytum et consolida maior.'

1 *qui dedit omne bonum*] God, or perhaps Mother Nature.

8 *mors improuisa*] This phrase adds a touch of spiritual dread to this otherwise philosophical passage. A sudden and 'unexpected death' was one of the greatest fears of the medieval Christian, and it is implied here that a proper knowledge of the four humours and the medicines to keep them in balance is useful for avoiding such a *mors improuisa*.

1–15 This is a fascinating and unique passage in the herbal. This is the only instance in which Henry explains some of the medical theories underlying his poem, outlining (but not clearly) how every body possesses a unique complexion of the four humours. His main concern seems to be with doubt about divine providence with relation to herbal medicine. The very fact that God, or his representative Nature, has placed different plants with the same Galenic qualities around the world is a testament to His concern for human bodily health. Henry's description of the four qualities and the four humours is primitive in comparison to the elaborate medical philosophy already being taught at the same time in Chartres and Salerno, but for him it is a rare attempt at rationalizing the medicinal effects of herbs upon bodies. The conjunction of Galenic humoral theory with Aristotelian natural philosophy based on the four qualities is typical of the new medical theory taught from the later eleventh or early twelfth century. *Cf.* Nancy G. Siraisi, *Medieval & Early Renaissance Medicine: An Introduction to Knowledge and Practice* (Chicago 1990), 4, 13–16.

17–19 A difficult passage made more so by the verse. The *hec* in line 18 refers to the original pieces (*frusta*) of meat, which will break into even more pieces under normal circumstances when boiled. Comfrey's marvellous ability to knit wounds is demonstrated by the fact that the many pieces of meat are bound into one lump (*unum*, line 18) when boiled with comfrey. The source is Pseudo-Apuleius no. 59: 'Haec herba hoc argumento intelligitur: carne bubula concisa et in caccabo missa, si eius radicem miseris ad dragmas II, coctca bubula in unum cohaerebit.' This idea is clearer in Latin Dioscorides II. 14, 'De alio sinfitu': 'Carnes incisas frustis et in caccabo missa in se glutinare facit.'

22 *regem*] A trope of medieval medicine, though Henry's source might be Quintus Serenus 299–300, 'Qui stomachum regem totius corporis esse / contendunt, vera niti ratione videntur,' or possibly Strabo's 'De Apio,' line 334: 'Corporis hunc regem turbans si nausia uexet.'

23 *Oxigarum* is fermented fish sauce (*garum*) with vinegar. *Cf.* Robert I. Curtis, *Garum and Salsamenta: Production and Commerce in Materia Medica*

(Leiden 1991).

24 Pseudo-Apuleius no. 59 gives only a cure *ad tussim*. There is no mention of *splen*, *os*, or *intima*.

24 *os nodat*] A troubling phrase. Since *os* must a long syllable, it means 'mouth' and not 'bone.' *Nodat* literally means 'ties in knots,' so it is not clear what that means in the context of a mouth without a known source for this line. *Os* in a medical context can refer to the *os stomachi*, the bottom of the esophagus, and thus *nodat* is some sort of beneficial tightening of the *os* for the sake of digestion.

2.21 VIOLA <HYEMALIS> / Winter Violet, *Viola hiemalis* L.

Apparently original to Henry. The winter violet seems a likely choice based on the description, but it could be one of any number of cold-blooming flowers in the family Violaceae.

1 *Viginti . . . uisis*] That is, twenty plants in this bed (and twenty poems in Book 2) have now been examined and passed by.

4 *equant*] The reading of *equantur* in *P* makes as much sense but does not scan.

6 *ista . . . illa*] Sweet violet in poem 2.9 and this winter violet.

2.22 BASILISCA / Autumn Gentian or Felwort, *Gentiana amarella* L.

Basilisca is not found in Macer, nor is it translated by EMA or Daniel. Nor will it be found among the many plants with names based on 'draco'—these are generally bistorts/adderworts (see poem 2.7)—nor among the basils, usually called *ocimum*, though occasionally *basilica* or *basilicon* (see poem 1.2). Pseudo-Apuleius treats a *herba basilisca* (no. 130, pp. 218–9) which is known especially for its ability to protect against the dreaded basilisk. However, while Pseudo-Apuleius provides the classic description of the basilisk's deadly gaze, Henry attributes great powers to its breath. Several English herbal lists give *basilisca* as a name for felwort (Hunt, 48), now often called autumn gentian. Some manuscripts of Pseudo-Apuleius provide a dramatic illustration of *basilisca* with several serpents writhing about before the plant. The image of *basilisca* found in Oxford, Bodleian Library, MS Ashmole 1431, fol. 30r, looks quite similar to members of the family Gentiana. A manuscript of *ca* 1300 (London, British Library, MS Harley 2851) has a passage titled 'De herba Basilisca seu Gentiana' (Eleanour Sinclair Rohde, *The Old English Herbals* [London 1922], 192).

1 *proximus . . . locus*] That is, the next plot after *uiola hyemalis* in poem 2.21.

4 *uires ex nomine pensa*] That is, the name *basilisca* indicates its primary effect, defeating the poisonous breath of the basilisk.

5 *basiliscus*] The basilisk would have been well known to any educated person in the Middle Ages, but perhaps Henry's source is Isidore's description of the basilisk (*Etym.* 12. 4. 6–9).

2.23 ABROTANVS / Southernwood, *Artemisia abrotanum* L.

Closely based on Macer's 'Abrotanum,' lines 31–51, with a line from Strabo's 'De Abrotano,' 91–8. It is not clear whether Henry knew the plant in the neuter form *abrotanum* or if the masculine form *abrotanus* found in both manuscripts is correct. The allusions to Strabo and Pliny come from Macer. Daniel Arundel (fol. 4r) notes under 'Abrotanus' that 'Henricus seyth þe same, and but lytel more.'

1–2 Strabo 98, 'praeterea tot habet uires quot fila comarum.' Also see the note below to lines 24–25.

2 This line, as received from *P* and *S*, does not scan. I have added *illi* to complete the hexameter based on a similar reading above at 1.11, 11.

4 *coctana* = *cottana*, a Syrian fig. But at this point Macer calls for *cidonia*, or quinces (line 45), and *cotonia* or *cotonea* were classical variants for *cidonia*.

9 *disnoycos*] Those suffering from a type of eye disease (*cf.* Macer, *Der deutsche 'Macer.' Vulgatfassung mit einem Abdruck des lateinischen Macer Floridus 'De viribus herbarum'*, ed. Bernhard Schnell with William Crossgrove [Tübingen 2001], 156 n35).

12 *habunde* = *abunde*

16 *punctus . . . frigoris*] See note to 2.14, 38.

21–23 Based on Macer 50–51, from Pliny 21. 162: 'si subiciatur pulvino, venerem stimulari aiunt, efficacissimamque esse herbam contra omnia veneficia quibus coitus inhibeatur.' However, Henry used a copy of Macer attesting lines rejected by Choulant, whose edition of Macer reads: 'Haec etiam venerem pulvino subdita tantum / Incitat, et veneri nocuis potata resistit.' Choulant (note to line 50) notes that several manuscripts of Macer replace those two lines with the following three: 'Plinius ut scribit venerem movet illius herba / Si fuerit tantum pulvino subdita nocte / Et cunctis veneri nocuis potata resistit.' Henry was using this alternate version. The Trinity Compiler likewise uses these alternate lines in his own poem on *abrotanum* (*T* fol. 89r).

23 *ueneri*] Both manuscripts originally read *ueneri*, preserving the original sense in Pliny 21. 162 (see previous note), but the scribe of *S* added an 's' making the dative a genitive, which could reverse the sense of the line. If dative (*ueneri*), it 'hinders all things harmful to sex,' which reading is more in accord with the previous two lines. If genitive (*ueneris*), southernwood 'hinders all the harms of sex,' that is, it is an anti-aphrodisiac.

24–25 These lines are not in Choulant's edition of Macer. See the note above to 2.19, 8. Choulant notes that one manuscript adds two more lines at the end (Macer, note to line 51), which may be Henry's source: 'Quos incerta premit furtivae iniuria guttae / Adiuvat et tot habet vires quot fila comarum.' These lines are not original to Macer, but are from Strabo, 'De Abrotano,' lines 97–8: 'quos incerta premit furtiuae iniuria guttae; / praetera tot habet uires quot fila comarum.' Henry could have borrowed 2.23, line 1, directly from Strabo or second-hand from Macer. These lines are translated in EMA (60): 'and also it helpith agen the gowte; that is proue.' That both Henry and the EMA translator had a version of Macer that Choulant deemed inferior is indicative that there may be a specifically English tradition of Macer manuscripts.

2.24 TANETICVM / ? Tansy, *Chrysanthemum vulgare* (L.) Bernh.

Translated in EMA as 'Tansey' (191), and this is one of the few cases in which EMA translates the entire poem, including even Henry's non-medical commentary in lines 5–6. It is abbreviated by the Digby Excerptor in one line. The Trinity Compiler uses lines 1–4 of this poem in his much longer 34-line poem 'Taneticum,' but only the second half of line 3 and all of line 4 are copied closely. Here are the first five lines of that poem for comparison:

> Taneticum agreste talis medicaminis extat,
> Taneticum ortensem vulgo dicunt tanacetum.
> Acra sit illa licet lenem confert medicinam
> Namque iuuat pectus. Nec solum pectora purgat
> Set simul omne latens quod celant corpora curat.

4 *omne latens*] It is not clear what these 'secrets' or hidden ailments are. Perhaps Henry is echoing the common trope of the philosopher discovering the 'hidden' causes of nature. *Cf.* Alexander Neckham, *De laudibus divinae sapientiae* 9. 273–4, in *Alexandri Neckam De naturis rerum libri duo. With the Poem of the Same Author, De laudibus divinae sapientiae*, ed. Thomas Wright, Rerum Britannicarum Medii Aevi Scriptores 34 (London 1863), 492: 'Sed quis naturae vires causasque latentes, / Arcanas leges enucleare queat?'

2.25 LIGVSTICVM / Lovage, *Levisticum officinale* Koch

Based on Macer's 'Ligusticum,' lines 882–906, and Strabo's 'De Lybistico,' lines 229–35. The final lines expressing doubts about Walahfrid Strabo (*Stabus*) are from Macer. Henry has borrowed Macer's ideas and phrases, but quotes directly from Strabo's *Hortulus*.

1 *finis*] Namely, the end of the second book and of the second bed of the square garden.

3–4 *S* places these two lines at the end of the poem after line 25. As both Macer and Henry tend to place explanations of a plant's name at the start of their poems, I have followed *P*'s placement of the lines.

3 *Ligurum terra*] Liguria, a territory of an ancient people in northwest Italy. This etymology comes initially from Isidore, *Etym.* 17. 11. 5, but Henry takes it directly from Macer.

13 *dictis . . . omnibus*] Apparently a decoction of the root alone will help the same ailments listed above (lines 7–8). *Dulcis* will also work, but Henry is most likely rewriting Macer's *supradictis* (line 897). Either reading will also work for the last word of this line: *ista* as the subject *elixatura* or *istis* agreeing with *dictis . . . omnibus*.

16 *si nectas desuper*] That is to say, you can also tie (*nectas*) a plaster of lovage to a poisonous bite using part of the herb, and the rest in a potion.

17 *statuerunt*] The implied subject must now be something like *medici* or *ueteres*.

18 This line provides some striking variants. First, where Macer and *S* read *digestibilibus*, *P* provides *que uentrem soluunt*, which seems to be an intruded gloss. Second, I have used *stiptica*, the reading of *S*, though it seems neither scribe knew the word intended, *peptica*, *i.e.* 'digestive' (*cf.* Macer 899: 'quod inest sibi peptica virtus').

20–21 *gemellis . . . mereri*: Henry is borrowing directly from Strabo 231–4 here, as Macer does not use this wording:

> Hoc germen suco quamuis et odore gemellis
> orbibus officere et tenebras inferre putetur,
> semina saepe tamen quaesitis addere curis
> parua solet, famamque aliena laude mereri.

22–25 The doubts expressed in these may sound like an original addition by Henry, but are actually in direct imitation of Macer 902–906.

24–25 The use of *reperio* in *S* for each instance of *inuenio* is one of the more curious readings in the herbal. It does not scan, and if we assume Henry is well trained in metrics, it is not clear why any scribe would replace either verb with the other, both being common verbs, in no way representing the sort of technical language that is more often replaced by scribes of the herbal.

3 PROLOGVS IN LIBRO TERTIO / Prologue of the Third Book

The first three lines present a tripartite approach to medicine, as taught by *Physica*, which is similar to the division of medicine found in the *Isagoge* of Johannitius (Ḥunayn ibn Isḥāq), first adapted in Latin in the later eleventh century by Constantine the African and perhaps available to Henry. Constantine explains that medicine is divided into practice and theory, while theory is divided again into naturals, unnaturals, and contra-naturals. *Cf.* 'Johannicius. Isagoge ad Techne Galieni,' ed. Gregor Maurach, *Sudhoffs Archiv* 62 (1978), 148–74, at 151. While Henry's division of medicine into health, sickness, and sex is different than Johannitius's into theory and practice, they both are clearly part of the same rational approach to medicine gaining popularity in the later eleventh and early twelfth centuries. This poem is hardly proof that Henry had studied academic medicine, but he does show familiarity with the new medical theory often associated with the physicians of Salerno.

4–5 This passage is compact. Judging from the context, *ista . . . ista . . . illa* must refer, respectively, to 1) the sick, 2) the healthy, 3) those engaged in sexual activity, even though lines 2–3 give those aspects of *Physica* in a different order.

10 *Editus Phebo*] Asclepius, the son of Apollo (Phoebus), who wanted to grant immortality to mankind but was stopped by Hades and Zeus with a deadly lightning bolt: Ovid, *Met.* 2. 642–8. Isidore also relates the tale in his *Etym.* 4. 3. 2.

14–15 Compare Henry's final poem of the *Historia Anglorum*, dedicated to King Henry II: 'Hec aurora tuos precessit, Phebe, nitores . . . His igitur radiis, dum sceptra decora decoras . . .' (*HA* 10. 40, pp. 776–7, lines 8, 13).

16 Rigg's emendation (269) of *hos* to *has* seems reasonable, though I believe that it refers to *causas* rather than *herbas*, as he suggests.

18 *perhennis* = *perennis*

3.1 DIPTANNVS / Dittany of Crete, *Origanum dictamnus* L.

This poem has to be one of the strangest in the *Anglicanus ortus*. We begin with the image of dittany leading a procession with a sceptre held aloft (lines 3–4). That personification is immediately abandoned to provide one of dittany's medical uses (extracting arrows and blades); this information does not come from Henry's usual medical sources, but from Virgil. There follows a bizarre tale about giants and a woman who gives birth to an ape, all of which is somehow related to dittany. The poem ends with a moral platitude about moderation. See the commentary below for more on these lines.

Most of this poem is original to Henry apart from the reference to the *Aeneid*. Partially translated by EMA ('Ditayne,' 195–6). As described in the Introduction above, 15–17, this is one of the poems which situates the reader clearly in a physical space: 'on the emerald cloister's southern side' (line 1). The word *claustrum* gives a good indication of the garden Henry had in mind. While it need not imply an actual monastic or cathedral cloister, it still implies an enclosed, perhaps walled, square space. To be sure, he may have chosen the word simply to rhyme with *austro*.

1 *austro*] That is, in the southern quadrant of the garden cloister. The EMA translator misunderstood this line, as he did with poem 1.25 on myrtle, and took this cardinal direction to mean a location in the world rather than in a garden: 'Ditayne is habondant in þe souþ' (195).

4 *prehit = praeit*

5–11 Virgil, *Aeneid* 12. 411–15, where Venus removes an arrow from Aeneas using dittany. This cure is also found in Pliny 26. 142.

9 *tenerorum mater Amorum*] Venus, Aeneas's mother (Ovid, *Amores* 3. 15. 1). *Cf.* Henry's epigram 'De amore' (*HA* 11. 25, p. 802): 'Qui tenerorum uulnus Amorum non reueretur, / Innumerorum tela dolorum perpetuetur.'

13–14 It is not clear what about dittany is *similis* to this strange woman. Whoever she is, she has doubts about the birth of the giants, who were produced directly from the earth (Ge or Terra) when Uranus's blood fell on the goddess. *Cf.* Ovid, *Met.* 1. 151–62, and *HA* 560–61, for the giants of England. The giants will reappear in the next poem at 3.2, line 3. The mood and tense of the verbs in this passage is also odd. Why the subjunctive mood of *fatear*? Why the repeated perfect infintive *peperisse*? There are many problems here yet to be resolved.

14 The source for the ape is obscure. Ernst Robert Curtius, in his excursus on 'The Ape as Metaphor,' remarks that *simia*, when used instead of *simius*, can refer to an ape aping man rather than simply being an ape (Curtius, *European Literature and the Latin Middle Ages*, trans. Willard R. Trask [New York 1953], 539). This exploration of *simia* and *simius*, while providing some interesting twelfth-century parallels, does not otherwise help explain this passage. Perhaps an incubus is meant by *simia*, as in later legends about Albina, founding mother of England. *Cf.* Lesley Johnson, 'Return to Albion,' *Arthurian Literature* 13 (1995), 19–40, and Julia Marvin, 'Albine and Isabelle: Regicidal queens and the historical imagination of the Anglo-Norman prose *Brut* chronicles,' *Arthurian Literature* 18 (2001), 143–91. I am grateful to Jocelyn Wogan-Browne for insight on this passage.

15 As with the previous lines, this last one is also unclear. The *Nam* leads us to make line 15 dependent on lines 13–14, but the story of the doubting woman and her ape-child does not seem to offer the sort of moral about moderation or modesty which the *Nam* suggests. This line seems more connected to line 12, where Henry draws back from adding anything more to dittany's powers, as if admitting that one impressive cure makes a better poem than the many smaller cures found in other entries.

3.2 FENICVLVM / Fennel, *Foeniculum vulgare* Gært.

Based on Macer, 'Feniculum,' lines 678–710. Henry's introduction, lines 1–7, is original; in it he praises the size and powers of fennel, recalling the giants who appear in the previous poem. Macer's lines 680 and 692, which touch on fennel's powers against all poisons, are not paraphrased directly, but are hinted at in the introduction. Daniel Arundel ('Fenellus,' fol. 85v) says that Henry gives the same information as Macer.

3 *terrigenas . . . Gigantes*] A pun on 'earth-born,' since fennel obviously grows from the earth, but the giants were born from Ge (Terra, Earth). See the note to poem 3.1, lines 13–14. *Terrigena* is also the epithet specifically of Typhoeus, one of the most powerful of the giants (Ovid, *Met.* 5. 325), although Henry may also have known this phrase from Isidore, *Etym.* 11. 3. 13.

4 *mediantes*] It is not clear if this is accusative and modifies *Gigantes*, in which case it means 'cutting in half,' or if it is nominative and Henry has converted the collective singular of *turba* into a plural, in which case it means 'being half the size.' The diminutive status of other plants next to fennel is clear.

5 *tanta*] The implicit subject has switched from the neuter *feniculum* to feminine *herba*, a change Henry often makes for the sake of the metre.

5 *renitescis*] Perhaps intentionally echoing *renitens . . . renitencius* in the previous poem 3.1, line 2, used to describe dittany.

7 This line is repeated (but for *habetur* in place of *haberis*) in the second line of Henry's poem on the stone jet (*De gagate*, no. 29) in Black, 84.

11 An expansion on Macer's statement 'atque experiendo probatum' (line 683). The subject of *putauerunt* is presumably *medici* from line 8.

18–20 This recipe is not in Choulant's edition of Macer. It may have been in Henry's copy of Macer, though, as Henry's original additions are rarely of a medicinal nature.

18 *felleque galli*] This can refer to the bile of a rooster, or the entire gall bladder.

27 *nefreticis*] Those with nephritis, a kidney disease.

36 This line is a standard addition for Henry, emphasizing an herb's powers to treat both whole bodies and individual parts. Here, though, the line is more compact than elsewhere.

40–41 These lines are rather more awkward than Macer's original (lines 709–10): 'Tradunt auctores eius iuvenescere gustu / Serpentes et ob hoc senibus prodesse putatur.' They also display a superstition that Henry generally avoids or comments upon.

3.3 ANETVM / Dill, *Peucedanum graveolens* Benth.

Henry starts this poem in lines 1–22 with a complex, perhaps confused, explanation of why some herbs, particularly dill and fennel (discussed in the previous poem), look alike. This is one of the few passages in the herbal where he gives a theoretical discussion of plants, their natures, and larger cosmological themes. His description of prime matter (*yle* = *hyle*) and the elements (lines 12–17) places him firmly in the *avant-garde* of twelfth-century natural philosophy, in good company with Adelard of Bath, William of Conches, and Bernardus Silvestris. The second half (lines 23–52) is based on Macer, 'Anethum,' lines 395–428.

1–22 This passage is unlike any other in the herbal. Most of it is original to Henry, though the language at the start seems indebted to both Orientius, 'De trinitate,' line 58 (ed. Robinson Ellis, in *Poetae christiani minores*, CSEL 16 [Vienna 1888], 246), 'sede sedens patria, super omne salutifer aeuom,' as well as Claudian, *De raptu Proserpinae* 1. 248–51 (*Claudii Claudiani Carmina*, ed. John Barrie Hall [Leipzig 1985], 300):

> hic elementorum seriem sedesque paternas
> insignibat acu, ueterem qua lege tumultum
> discreuit Natura parens et semina iustis
> discessere locis . . .

Also compare Boethius's Platonic hymn 'O qui perpetua' (*De cons. phil.* 3 met. 9), in which he explains the Creator's binding of the elements.

4 A verb is needed with *ficus* as the plural object, such as 'plants' or 'gives.' After Henry has explained how dill seed is annually renewed into dill plants, we are given an intentionally absurd example of how seeds do not work: only a fool would plant a fig in order to produce dill. I have seen similar statements in seed catalogues old and new, and it is probably a gardening adage of great antiquity.

6 *pende . . . pendere*] Perhaps the time when the flower heads are heavy with seeds, or when the herbalist hangs the plants up to dry.

12–13 *elementata*] A relatively new word in Henry's day. He may have learned it from William of Conches's *De philosophia mundi*, 22, 'De elementis': 'Si ergo illis velimus imponere digna nomina, particulas praedictas dicamus elementa, ista quatuor quae videntur elementata' (PL 172: 49, there ascribed incorrectly to Honorius Augustodunensis). The term also appears during the twelfth and thirteenth centuries in commentaries on the *Isagoge* of Johannitius and the *De natura hominis* (*Premon physicon*) of Nemesius of Emesa, translated by Archbishop Alphanus of Salerno (see Irene Caiazzo, 'Un inedito commento sulla *Isagoge Iohannitii* conservato a Parigi,' in *La Scuola Medica*

Salernitana. Gli autori e i testi, ed. Danielle Jacquart and Agostino Paravicini Bagliani [Florence 2007], 93–123).

Henry's passage is strikingly similar to Bernardus Silvestris, *Cosmographia*, Megacosmus 4. 7 (ed. Peter Dronke [Leiden 1978], 118): 'Precedit Yle, Natura subsequitur elementans; elementati Nature elementa, elementis elementata conveniunt. Sic principia principiis, sed a principe principio, coheserunt.' This is probably a coincidence of two intelligent clerics reading the same sort of works in the early twelfth century. See Theodore Silverstein, '*Elementatum*: Its appearance among the twelfth-century cosmogonists,' *Mediaeval Studies* 16 (1954), 156–62, with additional information by the same author in 'Guillaume de Conches and Nemesius of Emessa: On the sources of the "new science" of the twelfth century,' in *Harry Austryn Wolfson: Jubilee Volume on the Occasion of His Seventy-Fifth Birthday* (Jerusalem 1965) 2. 719–34; Peter Dronke, 'New approaches to the School of Chartres,' *Anuario de estudios medievales* 6 (1969), 117–40, *elementatum* discussed at 128–9; and Winthrop Wetherbee's commentary on this passage in *The* Cosmographia *of Bernardus Silvestris* (New York 1973), 153 n128. Silverstein posits that William of Conches wrote the *De philosophia mundi* in the late 1120s. This does little to help date Henry's herbal, though it does say something about the circulation of new philosophical works in his day. I am grateful to Father Édouard Jeauneau for his assistance with this passage.

13 After this line *S* has added the line 'Frumenti granum fieri locum (*recte* lolium) doluerunt,' repeated in its proper place at line 21.

13–15 These lines reverse the Neoplatonic tone of lines 12–13, in which creation proceeds from the one to the many. Here the language has Aristotelian elements, in which 'you see' (*uides*) both that a *genus* is composed of separate *species* and that a group of *species* create a *genus*. Cf. Boethius, *De cons. phil.* 3 met. 9, line 21: 'Ad te conuersas reduci facis igne reuerti,' and Bernardus Silvestris, *Cosmographia*, Megacosmus, 3. 203–204 (ed. Dronke, 109): 'Distrahitur genus in species, naturaque simplex / Unaque non uno particulata modo.'

16 *cognita uis lippis*] That is, known to all the world. An allusion to Horace, *Satires* 1. 7. 3: 'omnibus et lippis notum et tonsoribus esse.' Also employed by Adelard of Bath, whose teachings and works Henry may have known, in *Quaestiones naturales*: 'patet enim hoc et lippis tonsoribus' (Adelard of Bath, *Conversations with His Nephew*, ed. and trans. Charles Burnett [Cambridge 1998], 98).

17 *puluis erunt*] A common theme, but Henry may have had in mind his lengthy Epigram 11. 23, 'De contemptu uisibilium,' lines 39–40 (*HA* 800): 'Sperma prius, modo uas ceni, post uermibus esca; / Ordine cernis homo quid fuit, est, et erit.'

17 *esse*] The 'essence' of a thing, used here as a direct object. Henry employs this use of *esse* elsewhere; see Epigram 12. 4–5 (*HA* 812).

18–19 The connection between deer's horn and smallage is perhaps based on their similar shape (suggested to me by Susan Crane), though it is not clear if Henry actually believes this, is relating a folk legend, or is giving an intentional absurdity. This passage is perhaps dependent on Dioscorides' description of asparagus, which he claims can grow from broken ram's horn: 'alii uero dicunt cornu hircinu, si contusu spargatur, sparagos nasci facit' (*cf.* Latin Dioscorides, 'De sparagu,' 10. 221). John Riddle discusses this curious passage in 'Byzantine commentaries on Dioscorides,' *Dumbarton Oaks Papers* 38, Symposium on Byzantine Medicine (1984), 95–102.

19 *equo*] Since this lacks a noun, I have translated it in the idiomatic, substantive sense of 'propriety' or 'what is proper,' but it could also be taken as referring to the ground: 'growing rather thickly on the level ground.'

21 *lolium*] Cockle (*Agrostemma githago* L.), a flowering weed, treated by Henry in poem 5.1.10, which is commonly found in fields of wheat and other cereals. Its appearance was explained as a spontaneous transformation of wheat.

27–28 *genitale . . . iter*] Probably the prostate and urethra, or their proper use. The sense of *tollit* is not clear. Apparently the *iter* is the successful transfer of semen, and that is what is damaged or 'taken away' by too much dill.

31 *tollit*] The alternate reading of *pellit* in *P* would also work, and this is what Macer uses (line 428).

32–33 The sense is that a powder of burnt dill seed relieves (*suspendit*) a swollen uvula. *Cf.* Macer 411–12: 'Uvaque si nimio turgens humore gravetur, / Suspendit pulvis combusti seminis eius.'

34 *acrior*] It is difficult to tell if this is a good thing or not, for *acrior* could mean the cure with ashes of the root is 'harsher' or 'more bitter,' but it could also mean 'more effective.'

35 *habundanter* = *abundanter*

39 *os stomachi*] The base of the esophagus, where it meets the stomach.

48 *infusus*] This word, as used by Macer and Henry, usually is close in meaning to our modern 'infusion,' but here it has to have the literal sense of 'poured on.'

50 *condilomata*] From *condyloma*, pimples or boils, or specifically the swellings of haemorrhoids (Macer Floridus, *Höhepunkte der Klostermedizin*, trans. Mayer and Goehl, 156 n33).

3.4 FEBRIFVGA / Feverfew, *Chrysanthemum parthenium* Bernh.

Lines 1–3 are translated by EMA as 'Fetherfoy' (196) and abbreviated by the Digby Excerptor. The Trinity Compiler uses lines 1–11 of this poem in his poem 'Febrifuga,' but seriously rewrites some of the lines, so I have supplied only the relevant variants in the apparatus. Henry repeats Horace's 'sub iudice lis est' (*Ars poetica*, line 78) in lines 7, 9, and 11. He quotes it more fully, 'et adhuc sub iudice lis est,' in the final line 13. The case in question asks whether feverfew is a type of centaury (line 6) or artemisia (line 8). The irony of this poem would not be lost on readers familiar with Horace's work, in which the dispute is over the history of elegiac verse, used for much loftier occasions than identifying varieties of centaury and artemisia.

The Trinity Compiler usually borrows lines from other herbalists to create his poems, but in a few instances he has written new material. In the poem 'Febrifuga,' in particular, the Compiler used Henry's poem but decided to resolve the dispute over the identity of *febrifuga* once and for all. After repeating, with some modification, Henry's lines 1–11, the Compiler adds the following:

> Nos igitur paci temptantes reddere lites,
> Dicimus entallos septemfoliumque latine
> Esse febrifugam, que centaurea uocata
> Est, ergo aut species eiusue sub altera tantum.
> De centaureis diuisim denique dicam:
> At arthemesie species si dicitur esse
> Tercia tunc erit a consolida pene remota
> Et minus intense quam prima ualet facit ista.
> Ergo participet cuiuscumque speciei
> Hec tamen a cunctis manet altera sola, sed ipsa
> Colliriis faciet et plagis, multis quoque causis.
> Set quia constat eis sentencia verior esse
> Qui centauream dicunt hanc esse minorem,
> Nunc taceo, sed tunc ex hiis que nouero dicam.

This fascinating passage deserves translation, although the inferiority of the grammar, prosody, and scribe make this difficult:

> So, in an attempt to bring the disputes to a peaceful settlement, we say that *entallos* (= *eptaphilos*) and *septemfolium* is feverfew in Latin, which is called centaury (therefore either a species of it or only under the second). To sum up, I will speak separately about the centauries, but if it is said to be a type of artemisia, then the third will be quite different from comfrey and accomplish those things less intensely than the first is able. So let it partake of any species, yet the second remains apart from all others, and it will be effective for eye salves and blows and many complaints. But because the judgment of those who say that it is *centaurea minor* is understood to be more valid, I'll now be quiet but then speak about those things which I understand.

Rather than settling the dispute, the Trinity Compiler has managed to hopelessly confuse the case by bringing in different plants like comfrey (*consolida*) into the court, as well as new names (*septemfolium*) which Henry did not mention.

1–3 The name *febrifuga* comes from *febres fugat* ('it fights fevers').

6–7 Daniel Arundel (fol. 61r) espouses this opinion in the passage on 'Centaurea': 'The grete Centorie is febrifuga, febrefu.' Rufinus takes the other view, however, citing a work called the *Synonima*, and says that 'Centaurea minor febrifuga vel fel terre idem est et tota herba utimur' (79). Henry treats centaury in poem 3.19, below.

9 *eptaphilos*] A variety of artemisia, called *eptapolos* above in poem 1.1, line 4.

10 *horum*] Apparently the other plants, *centaurea* and *eptaphilos*. One would expect *harum*, but both manuscripts have *horum*.

3.5 NIMPHEA / Figwort, *Scrophularia nodosa* Pursh.

Henry offers several names for the plant. *Nimphea* is usually the name given to the water-lily (*Nymphaea alba* L.), yet that plant does not seem intended here. *Millemorbia* is generally applied to the figwort, a common medieval remedy for all sorts of ailments, especially scrofula, hence the botanical name (Grieve, 'Figwort'; André, 'millemorbia' and 'nymphaea'). I have not found a source for this poem. It has the tone of personal knowledge to it, since it is dedicated to alternate names and comparisons to other plants rather than to the sort of recipes Henry learned from Macer or Constantine. Translated by EMA, 'Mille-morbia,' 196–7. See also Gösta Frisk's discussion of the name, EMA, 229–30, 282.

3–4 *millemorbia*] This word cannot scan in hexameters, and thus it is 'dreaded' by poetry.

4 *nostra Talia*] 'Our Thalia,' the muse of comedy. See note to poem 1.21, line 15.

6 *fyalam*] I have opted for this spelling since it is *fiala* in the edition of EMA and *phiala* in one of its manuscripts (196). Frisk suggests that if *millemorbia* is the water-lily instead of figwort, *fiala* ('shallow bowl') could be a descriptive nickname for the plant, which has a bowl-like flower (EMA, 230). It is spelled *fiola* in *S* and in one of the herb lists found in that manuscript (Rigg, 291).

7 *conferba*] Comfrey's powers are discussed in poem 2.20, above.

8 *rute ... acute*] This line echoes line 8 in Henry's poem 1.10 on rue, where he quotes Ovid, *Remedia amoris*, 801–802: 'Utilius sumas acuentis lumina rutas / et quidquid Veneri corpora nostra negat.'

9 *fera gutta*] It is not clear if this is a specific disease or if *fera* is added simply for effect. EMA translates this as 'wode gowte' (197).

9 *leporinam*] Henry is recalling his poem on avens (*Benedicta*, 2.19), also called herb bennet or hare's ear (*auricula leporina*), which is used against gout and is also called *diuinam* (2.19, 8–9).

11–12 Between these two lines *P* has added 'quod querat dubitans et adhuc et cetera non soluit.' This is probably not part of this poem, but rather a gloss on the previous poem, or a mutilated version of line 13 from the previous poem 3.4 ('quod querat dubitans et adhuc sub iudice lis est').

3.6 ASARVM / Hazelwort or Asarabacca, *Asarum europaeum* L.

Loosely based on Macer, 'Asarum,' lines 1532–68, less lines 1541–2. Henry's lines 1–2 are original. The reorganization of information in the poem is more creative than most, as Henry has thoroughly rearranged Macer's lines 1543–68 for his lines 5–31.

4 Where Henry attributes the name *asarum* to the *medicis*, Macer 1532 says the name occurs *graece*, which may tell us something about Henry's views about Greeks and his sources, namely that if he heard that something was said in Greek, it was implictly said by or for physicians.

5 Macer 1535 gives only *Provocat urinam* and does not mention *flecma grossum*.

12–19 This passage, which reads like a medical checklist, works grammatically if we supply the verb *circumspice* from line 10 for each of the terms in lines 12, 14, 16, and 18.

21 *quamlibet herbam*] The plural *quaslibet herbas* in *P* is probably borrowed from Macer 1554, which also has the plural.

22 *Communiter omnibus ista*] A highly truncated phrase, to which I have supplied 'rules' in the translation to make sense of *ista*, and we must assume a verb like *dixi*, as found in Macer 1556–7: 'Sed quia de cunctis dixi communiter herbis, / Quo sit danda modo proprie Vulgago docebo.'

25–26 *P* reads *uino* in place of each instance of *mero* in these lines. This is most likely an intruded gloss.

3.7 MACEDONIA / Alexanders or Black Lovage, *Smyrnium olusatrum* L.

Based on a conflation of Strabo's 'De Lybistico' (lines 229–34) and 'De Cerfolio' (235–47), the latter of which mentions *Macedonia* explicitly, but not *Cerfolium*. Henry may have received it without a title and assumed it treated only *Macedonia*. Henry's lines 3–6 are original. Alexanders is a common plant (line 3) which was often used as a leafy vegetable (line 4) like common lovage. The

Laud Herbal, no. 852, gives *macidonea* as a synonym for a type of iris: 'Iris illirica .i. macidonea, que fuerit grauissimi ponderis.'

1 Strabo, 229: 'Inter odoratam memorare lybistica silvam.'

2 *infirmis . . . aristis*] Alexanders produces numerous tiny pods and flowers on each of its flower heads (umbels). *Cf.* Strabo, 239–41: 'Infirmis diuisa licet Macedonia ramis / spargitur et crebris ignobile semen aristis / sufficit . . .'.

4 *facilis*] Best understood as 'easy to cultivate' in this context.

5 *per se crescit*] It 'grows on its own,' which is why it *spernit laborem* (line 4).

8 The prescription of an *uncia* is Henry's invention. Strabo 244 reads *solet obuia gustu* at this point.

3.8 YRIS / Iris, *Iris pseudacorus* L.

Closely based on Macer, 'Iris,' lines 1456–88 and partly on Strabo's 'De Gladiola,' lines 217–28. Lines 25–9 are mostly new, and show Henry's more didactic side; in these lines he gives a clear explanation of *secundae*, afterbirth.

1–2 *Yris* is the goddess of the rainbow, or a rainbow itself, and thus her name is given to a flower found in many colours.

3 The etymology, while immediately from Macer, comes originally from Isidore, *Etym.* 17. 9. 9–10.

4–5 Henry is referring to the iris's other name, gladiola, meaning 'little sword,' from *gladius*, a gladiator's short sword. This etymology is given by Isidore, *Etym.* 17. 9. 83, and by Strabo 217–18: 'Te neque transierim Latiae cui libera linguae / nomine de gladii nomen facundia finxit.'

25–29 This description of afterbirth (*secundae*) is not found in Macer's 'Iris,' but there is a long description in his poem on pennyroyal, Macer 631–41, on which Henry seems to base his version. In Henry's poem 2.16 on pennyroyal he omits the description of *secundae*, apparently saving it for this point.

30 *curat*] *Purgat* in *P* will also work.

3.9 YREOS / Yreos (fictional plant) or *Iris florentina* L.

'Yreos' was known to some in the Middle Ages as a distinct variety of iris, bearing a white, rather than purple, flower. A mnemonic couplet explained the difference between the flowers (*Agnus Castus*, 99): 'Irus [*sic*] purpurium florem gerit, yrios album, / Gladiolus roseum, sed spatula fetida nullum.' Rufinus quotes five authors on the plant (156–7), noting it is larger than the normal iris or gladiola. The *Laud Herbal* no. 819, however, says 'Ireos .i. gladioli ortensis radix,' in which case it is a part (the root) of the usual iris (here, the gladiola) rather than a different variety. *Yreos* is, in fact, no more than a grammatical confusion. Medieval writers did not recognize a late genitive form of the Greek ιρις (Jerry Stannard, 'Medieval reception of classical plant names,' in Jerry Stannard, *Herbs and Herbalism in the Middle Ages and Renaissance*, ed. Katherine E. Stannard and Richard Kay [Aldershot 1999], 153–62, at 158). *Yreos* is not the *Irio* of Pliny (18. 49, 58, 96; 22. 158), identified by the editors as the seed of winter cress.

2 *Tyma* and *tyme* (singular *tymum* and *tyma*) appear to be names of different varieties of thyme, possibly used to distinguish the bushy garden thyme from the creeping wild thyme (called *serpillum* in poem 2.17). Garden thyme is treated below in poem 6.2.26.

3.10 MENTA / Mint, genus *Mentha* L.

Based primarily on Macer, 'Mentha,' lines 1569–84, with one line from Strabo's 'De Menta,' lines 284–99.

1 *quoque*] Henry is referring to the similar powers of iris in poem 3.8, line 6.

4 *Cf.* Strabo 287: 'raucisonam claro rursus redhibere canori.'

4 *rehibere* = *redhibere*

12 *sanat*] The reading of *purgat* in *P* will also scan.

13 The dramatically different reading in *S* (*festinat anelum* for *solet accelerare*) suggests either the censoring of feminine cures or that a line is missing.

15 *P* includes a useful gloss above *paritura*: 'id est non.' Based on this, I have emended *hanc*, found in both manuscripts, to *haud*. For a discussion of mint's contraceptive properties see Riddle, *Eve's Herbs*, 61–3.

16 The scribe of *P*, or a contemporary reader, has marked the words of this line with numbers for ease of reading: 5, 1, 3, 4, 2, respectively, appear above the words. Perhaps this is an indication of the low level of Latinity in one of *P*'s readers.

3.11 ABSINTHIVM / Wormwood, *Artemisia absinthium* L.

Based on Macer, 'Absinthium,' lines 52–114. Henry has rearranged the content of Macer in a much more thorough fashion than in most of his poems. The interjections of lines 28, 43, and 55 are original to Henry.

3–9 A clever reworking of Macer 107–14. The passage from Pliny is 27. 7.

5 *solitos*] The reading of *solito* could be forced to work ('by custom'), but it

seems more likely that Henry closely followed Macer 110 ('Absinthii succum solitos donare bibendum') and that the final *–s* was dropped by a scribe.

9 *Precio* in *P* and *preciis* in *S* will both work here, though offering slightly different meanings. *Precio preciosior* is also used in poem 1.9, line 1, concerning sage.

20 *anginam*] See note to poem 2.9, line 34.

22 *epar*] Henry uses this word as synonym for *iecur*, 'liver,' though they can apply to different organs. See Charles Burnett's discussion of livers and gizzards in Adelard of Bath, *Conversations with His Nephew*, 229 n18.

24–28 This cure is from Macer 53–9, but the language is pure Henry.

25 *aerio*] If we follow *P* and read *aereo*, this could mean 'in an open copper pot,' which may have been what both scribes understood. But the structure of the line comes probably from Strabo, line 323, on pennyroyal, 'in aerio si te perflarit aperto,' where air is intended rather than a pot.

25 *frigidata*] The first syllable must be short for the line to scan.

35 *Mollit* in *S* or *lenit* in *P* will work. Macer 100 reads *resolvit.*

45 The odd *sius iungas* in *S* is due most likely to a misreading of the abbreviation '9' for *con–* as the similar abbreviation for the terminal *–us*, since *sius* is written *si9*. The scribe of *S* never uses a '9' for *con–*. I owe this observation to Diana Greenway.

54 *P* placed this line after line 56 and marked its proper place.

54 Here *tinea* must have the usual meaning of a worm or moth which destroys clothing and books; however, in all other cases below (4.10, line 4; 5.1.4, line 11; 5.2.6, line 11), *tineae* are found inside the human body and are most likely tapeworms. *Tinea* also appears as a superficial condition in other works, and in such cases is almost definitely ringworm, *e.g.* Bartholomaeus Anglicus, *De genuinis rerum coelestium, terrestrium, et inferarum proprietatibus* 7.2 (Frankfurt 1601; repr. Frankfurt 1964), p. 278: 'Item patitur caput quandam in pueris familiarem passionem, quam Constantinus vocat squamam, nos autem dicimus tineam, quia ad modum tineae superiorem cutis capitis substantiam corrodit, et quasi inseparabiliter tenet eam.'

56 *incaustum* = *encaustum*

3.12 BALSAMA / Horsemint, *Mentha longifolia* (L.) Huds.

Henry and other authors perhaps confused *balsamita* (horsemint, *Mentha longifolia* Huds. [Hunt, 44–5], or water mint, *Mentha aquatica* L. [Hunt, 241]) with *balsamum* (the balsam tree, Balm of Gilead, *Commiphora opobalsamum* Engl.), which receives its own poem at 6.2.1, 'Balsamum.' While lines 5–8 are based on Pseudo-Apuleius no. 106, 'Herba Sisimbrium' (p. 189), lines 1–3 are apparently original to Henry and sound more like they are describing the famous balms of the Orient. Translated by EMA as 'Bawme' (196). The Trinity

Compiler has used all of this poem in his 'De Balsama,' but has rewritten it extensively and added 28 more lines (*T* 91r–91v). I have provided only the relevant alternate readings.

4 *terralis*] I have found no source for this name. It is not in Pseudo-Apuleius, nor is it recorded by Hunt in *Plant Names of Medieval England*.. EMA gives it as *ciralis* (196).

4 *sisimbria*] 'Sisimbrium' is usually glossed as horsemint or water mint (Hunt, 241).

5–8 Pseudo-Apuleius no. 106, 'Herba Sisimbrium': 'Ad uesicae dolorem stranguiriam. Herbam sisimbrium contritum excepto suco scripulos II, febricitanti ex aqua calida, non febricitanti ex uino potui dabis, remediabis mire.' EMA offers further explanation to *stranguria*: '. . . euel that is clepid stranguria, the whiche streyneth the meates and weyes of the vryne, so that a man hauyth ofte-sithes difficulte for to pisse . . .' (196). This could be a translation of a line lost from Henry, or more likely a gloss added by the EMA translator.

3.13 RAPHANVS / Horseradish, *Armoracia rusticana* Gaertn. Mey & Scherb.

Source unknown. This poem bears little relation to Strabo's 'De Rafano,' lines 387–91. I have found two copies of another poem on *Raphanus* by another, unknown author (Oxford, Bodleian Library, MS Digby 13, fol. 90r; Cambridge, Trinity College, MS O. 9. 10, fol. 104r), but it is quite different. The identification is made based on the description of *Radix* in the following poem as being similar to *Raphanus*, but lesser in virtue and, by implication, smaller in size. An entry in the *Laud Herbal*, no. 1254, may complicate matters ('Rafanus .i. radix'), but it simply confirms that the two herbs are similar. Only in lines 1–10 and 40–41 does Henry treat *raphanus* directly. Lines 11–39 address broader issues of binding wounds and the creation of an impressive remedy called the 'Medicine of Twenty Herbs,' which does not include *raphanus*. The first six lines are translated in EMA, 'Nepe,' 197.

1–3 I have found no source for applying a frog (*rana*) to a wound. The EMA translator also understood *ranam* as frog: 'first bynd to þe cancre al a froissh' (197). Several cures employing frogs are found in Quintus Serenus, *Liber Medicinalis*, lines 114, 668, 782, 912. Cures using burnt frog ashes and frog skins are also given in the Latin translation of the *Cyranides* (*Textes latins et vieux français relatifs aux Cyranides*, ed. Louis Delatte [Liège 1942], 101–102), though that work has been firmly dated to 1169. Rigg suggested to me that 'frog' may have already been used in twelfth-century English to refer to a toadstool, so perhaps some sort of fungus is intended, though the emphasis on the skin (*pellem*) of the *rana* seems to require an animal. In the end, however, it is not clear how the frog helps cure the *cancer*, when all that seems to have been effected is the horrible death of a frog.

3 *uix pellem*] An awkward phrase, and one with which the scribe of *S* clearly had trouble. A large space was left in the middle of this line before an extraneous *est*.

5 *siligineus*] Usually means 'of wheat,' though EMA translates it as 'flour of rye' (197).

7 *griasque rubescens*] Madder (*Rubia tinctorum* L.) is a prime source of red dye (hence *rubescens*) and was sometimes called *grias* (Hunt, 130).

8 *uarenca*] A variant of *warencia*, another name for madder (Hunt, 266). Charlemagne called for *warentiam* in the 'Capitulare de villis' (*Kapitularien*, ed. Reinhard Schneider [Göttingen 1968], 27).

8, 26 *canabum = cannabis/cannabum* (Hemp, *Cannabis sativa* L.)

9 *yrigeron*] Groundsel, which has its own poem below, 'Senecion,' 5.1.6.

11 *multas*] I have translated this as 'many herbs,' but *medicinas* could also be understood.

18 *Herbarum matrem*] Artemisia, or mugwort, treated in poem 1.1.

18 *agrimoniam*] Agrimony, *Agrimonia eupatoria* L., which does not have a poem in this herbal.

20 *sinula*] A type of mallow, treated below in poem 3.17.

21 *Plantago* and *lanceolata* are the two main varieties of plantain discussed in poem 5.1.1, the greater plantain and ribwort plantain.

22 *fabiculam*] I am not sure what the 'little bean' is. Perhaps lupin (described in poem 4.11), since most other peas and beans are not regularly included in herbals.

22 *ruuetam*] Apparently a variant of *rubetam*, a rare word which Henry probably learned from Ovid, *Met.* 1.105: 'haerentia mora rubetis.' It is not clear if *ruueta* is another ingredient in this potion, or if it is a place where the *fabicula* is to be found.

24 *acidula*] Sorrel, *Rumex acetosa* L., the subject of poem 5.1.5.

25 *uictoriolam*] If the emendation is correct (both scribes seem confused by this word), *uictoriola* is periwinkle, also called the *Herba Victorialis* (Hunt, 142). This name is also given in Henry's poem on periwinkle (1.23, 28).

27 *reginam*] Meadowsweet, described above in poem 2.13, where it is called *pigmentum*. The *Agnus Castus* says that 'Regina prati is an herbe that men cleputh medsowte or medwort or brydwort' (202).

27 *melandram*] Beebalm, *Melissa officinalis* L. (Hunt, 173), described below in poem 4.22, 'Boragum,' or simply another name for meadowsweet.

28 *duo ... contraria*] The two things are apparently the concoctions mixed in lines 18–22 and 23–7, respectively. They are contrary because the herbs of the first mixture are typically purgative while those in the second are of a binding virtue. The total mixture, however, is used for binding wounds while the amount of comfrey added dictates how quickly the wound will knit. Presumably the physician should dictate the speed of healing in order not to upset the humoral balance.

30 *consolide*] A synonym for *conferba* from line 23.

30, 34 *done*] I have not found what a *dona* could be. It could be a measurement, a synonym for horseradish (which would explain the presence of this recipe within the poem), or a different plant entirely.

34 *iunctas*] Agreeing with an assumed *herbas*?

36 *religes*] Henry seems to have taken this as the future indicative, which would be expected with *sanabitur*.

39 *uiginti . . . herbarum*] It is difficult to calculate just which twenty herbs Henry means. If we count *mater herbarum* (*i.e.*, artemisia), *agrimonia*, *buglossa*, *sanicla*, *sinula*, *terrestre piretrum*, *elna*, *plantago*, *lanceolata*, *fabicula*, *conferba*, *portulaca*, *acidula*, *pipera*, *uictoriola*, *canabum*, *regina/melandra*, and *consolida* we have eighteen ingredients. That suggests that *ruueta* in line 22 and *dona* in lines 30 and 34 are also ingredients to be added, whatever they might be. See the notes to those lines.

3.14 RADIX / Radish, *Raphanus sativus* L.

I have not found a direct source for this poem, but it could share a source with *Circa instans*, 'Radix' (fol. 207v), which also follows an entry on 'Raffanus': 'Radix calida est et sicca in secundo gradu. Herba est cuius radix simili nomine appellatur que cum inuenitur in passionario. Semper poni debet radix raffani. Virtutem similem habet raffano et contra easdem causas et eodem modo, sed non est adeo efficax.' Translated by EMA as 'Radissh' (197–8), and abbreviated by the Digby Excerptor.

3 This description seems to confirm the identification of poems 3.13 and 3.14 as horseradish and radish, respectively. Radishes are smaller and weaker in flavour than horseradish, but are otherwise similar.

6 *tempore Martis*] The time when Mars reigns in the sky, or simply the month of March. *Cf.* Claudian, *In Eutropium* 2. 567 (*Claudii Claudiani Carmina*, ed. Hall, 188): 'ei mihi, quas urbes et quanto tempore Martis.'

7 *aminiculis* = *amminiculis*

7 *producunt tempora mortis*] Literally, 'draws out the time of death,' *i.e.*, lengthens life.

3.15 ENVLA / Elecampane, *Inula helenium* L.

Based on Macer, 'Enula,' 1489–1502, though Henry has turned it into a dialogue with the plant. The Trinity Compiler's poem 'Enula campana' (*T* fol. 95v) is primarily a copy of Macer's 'Enula.' The first line, though, indicates that the Compiler knew Henry's version as well. Macer 1489 reads 'Enula, quam Graecus Elnam vocat Eleniumque,' whereas *T* has 'Enula, quam uulgus elnam uocat elenumque.' *T* probably made the change from *graecus* to *uulgus* based on Henry's first line.

6 *ortomicis*] Those with *ortomia* (modern orthopnoea; see poem 1.24, line 9 and poem 6.2.1, line 17) are usually called *orthopnoici*.

13 *turpe*] She is presumably being scolded for dwelling on feminine problems and cures, though this does not bother our narrator in any other poem.

13 *Vates odere loquaces*] Reminiscent of Horace, *Satires* 1.9, 33–4: 'Garrulus hunc quando consumet cumque: loquaces, / si sapiat, vitet, simul atque adolaverit aetas.'

3.16 ALTEA / Marsh Mallow, *Althaea officinalis* L.

Based on Macer, 'Althaea,' lines 366–94. Only Henry's line 4 appears to be original.

1–2 In each line, *alta est* must be elided for the line to scan properly. This reinforces the pun on *altea*.

3 *euiscum . . . uisco*] The etymology of naming sticky hybiscus from birdlime (*viscum*) is from Macer 368, and though it sounds like it would come from Isidore's *Etymologiae*, it is not found there.

4 The name *ybiscus* is not in Macer. The hibiscus is not part of the same genus as the marsh mallow, but both are now considered to be members of the larger family Malvaceae.

11 *fotu*] A warm compress, as opposed to an internal medicine, which is prescribed in lines 9–10.

18 *apostemata*] Plural of *apostema*. For sake of convenience, I have always translated *apostema* as 'ulcer' or 'abscess' (rather than the antiquated 'aposteme'), and Henry likely did not think too deeply about the meaning of the term. However, in the course of the high and later Middle Ages, the pathology and definition of *apostemata* became a serious concern for professional surgeons. See Michael R. McVaugh, 'Surface meanings: The identification of apostemes in medieval surgery,' in *Medical Latin from the Late Middle Ages to the Eighteenth Century*, ed. Wouter Bracke and Herwig Deumens (Brussels 2000), 13–29.

3.17 SINVLA / Mallow:
1) Curled Mallow, *Malva verticillata* L.
2) High Mallow, *Malva sylvestris* L.

Based on Macer, 'Malva,' lines 1962–92, less lines 1984 and 1974–7, probably since they provide an aphrodisiac and a cure for breast diseases. Henry's introduction, in lines 1–7, and line 32 are original. The primary plant discussed is the common, or high, mallow, as based on Macer's poem. Macer, however, does not mention the variety of mallow which Henry calls *sinula*, probably the 'crisped' or 'curled' mallow, which spreads widely over the ground instead of growing tall, like high mallow or like hollyhock (*Althaea rosea* L.). Pseudo-Apuleius uses the name *malva erratica* (no. 40, pp. 87–8), though Henry took no cures from that source. The name *sinula* supposedly comes from *sinuo*, because the plant twists and wanders. This poem confirms Hunt's tentative identification of 'Sinnula,' found in a fourteenth-century herbal glossary (London, British Library, MS Sloane 420, fols. 115r–121r), as a variety of *Malvaceae* L. (239).

4 *subiecti . . . signa*] Signs of death, specifically, or of any type of corruption. I am taking *subiecti* to refer to the patient, but it could also be understood with *corruptio* in the previous line, so that it could be translated as 'so that no corruption of the patient occurs.' That would not change the meaning seriously.

5 I have used the common English name curled mallow, but the Latin name is literally 'wandering mallow.'

7–8 The explanation of the mallow's name (*maluam* = *molliat aluum*) comes from Macer (line 1962), but originally from Isidore's *Etym.* 17. 10. 5. As with most Isidorean etymologies, this is not reproduceable in English. There is no reason for *molliat* to be in the subjunctive except to preserve the metre.

12 *cacostomacham*] Literally, 'stomach-spoiling.'

12 *Sextus Niger*] Sextius (as he was originally known) wrote a *De Materia Medica* between 10 and 40 A.D., now lost. It was a major source for both Pliny and Dioscorides (*cf.* John M. Riddle, *Dioscorides on Pharmacy and Medicine* [Austin 1985], 13–16). Henry probably knew of Sextius only through Macer's poem 'Malva.' See also M. Wellmann, 'Sextius Niger, eine Quellenuntersuchung zu Dioscorides,' *Hermes* 24 (1889), 530–69.

20 *Thebanus Olimpius*] A misreading of the female doctor Olympias of Thebes (*Thebana Olympias*) at Macer 1978 and Pliny 20. 226. Her identity is otherwise unknown; perhaps she was thought to be Olympias, mother of Alexander the Great. Given that both manuscripts of Henry clearly read 'Thebanus Olimpius,' the error was probably on Henry's part. Several manuscripts of Macer, though, do provide the masculine *Thebanus* (Macer, note to line

1978). Bruce P. Flood, Jr. suggests that one of two philosophers named Olympiodorus is intended ('Macer Floridus: A medieval herbalism,' PhD diss. [University of Colorado, 1968], 344).

23–25 I am positing that an earlier scribe, from whose manuscript both *P* and *S* are descended, fell prey to *homoioteleuton*, skipping from *oliuo* (line 23) to *oliuum* (line 24). Line 24, in its original form, was most likely a variation on Macer's line 1987. In lines 22–6 Henry adapts Macer's lines 1981–9, from which it will be clear that a line is missing in Henry's poem describing the use of olives in a mallow plaster:

> Contritis foliis illius cum sale pauco
> Egilopas pelles, succoque medeberis eius
> Puncturis apium; cui si coniungis olivum,
> Corpus et inde linas, apium te nulla nocebit.
> Decoctam lotio capiti superaddito malvam,
> Sic turpes achoras pelles furfurque nocivum;
> Decoctis eius foliis si iungis olivum,
> Extingues ignem sacrum cataplasmate tali.
> Et combusturis illo bene subvenis ignis.

The use of *oliuo* in line 23 without a governing verb or participle is odd, but Henry uses *oliuo* the same way below in poem 6.1.1 at line 16: 'utraque uim iecori digestiuam dat oliuo.'

27 This is the only appearance in the herbal of *salix*, the willow, a popular ingredient in medieval *materia medica*, although Henry avoids trees for the most part in his garden.

3.18 PIRETRVM / Pellitory:
1) Pellitory, *Anacyclus pyrethrum* D.C.
2) Pellitory-of-the-Wall, *Parietaria officinalis* L.

Based on Macer, 'Pyrethrum,' lines 2086–2108, with a nod to Strabo's 'De Lilio,' lines 248–61. The title in *S*, 'De piretro terestri,' indicates only one variety of pellitory, in differentiation from pellitory-of-the-wall (*Parietaria officinalis* L.). Henry mentions this poem below in 'Aloe,' 6.1.12, lines 37–38. Henry's introduction to pellitory (lines 1–4), the commentary on its name (lines 5, 7–9) and lines 24 and 27 are original. He makes a distinction, not found in Macer, between pellitory the herb and pellitory the spice. The two effect all the same cures. The Digby herbalist condenses the entire poem to one terse line.

1 *sinula*] Curled mallow, discussed in the previous poem (3.17), which provides a splendid pun with *si nulla*, not reproducible in English.

3 It is not clear what the *problema* is; this word does not possess in Latin our sense of 'problem,' as in a difficulty to be removed, but rather means a puzzle or riddle. The puzzle could be whether *sinula* or *piretrum* is more useful, or what is the relationship between *piretrum terrestre* and true *piretrum*.

4 *Cf.* Strabo 248–9: 'Lilia quo uersu candentia, carmine quoue / ieiunae macies satis efferat arida Musae?'

7 *speciosa . . . speciei*] A common pun in the herbal ('beautiful . . . spice'), which cannot be easily imitated in English.

22 Not our modern tetanus, but a painful cramp in the neck or upper back. *Cf.* Isidore, *Etym.* 4. 6. 12: 'Tetanus maior est contractio nervorum a cervice ad dorsum.'

26 *soluit*] The reading of *ducit* in *S* would also make sense, but it is more likely that Henry would prefer the echo with *resoluit* at the end of the line.

26 *resoluit*] This is usually a positive verb in the herbal, used for the soothing and loosening of various conditions, but here it is clearly some sort of pathological effect on the limbs, such as enervation or loss of control.

3.19 CENTAVREA / Centaury, *Centaurium erythraea* Rafn.

Based on Macer, 'Centaurea,' lines 1709–27, less line 1716, which gives a cure for bringing old wounds to scab. It is odd that this sort of cure would be omitted by Henry, since it would be expected after his line 10. It may have been missing from his own copy of Macer, or it may be an indication that *P* and *S* share the loss of the same line. Henry's statement that centaury heats and dries in the second degree (lines 3–4) is not in Macer, and may come from Constantine's 'Centaurea' (362–3). Macer 1714 is briefer on the subject: 'Desiccativae virtutis dicitur esse.' Daniel Arundel translates this under 'Centaurea' (fol. 61r) but attributes it to Macer. His translation is preceded by 'Henry Anglicus seeth þat þer is mykel dowte and strif bytwene manye of þe mykel centorie and of þe litle, and he determyneth neyþer but passeþ.' This is in reference to the dispute over the types of centaury mentioned in Henry's poem 3.4, 'Febrifuga.'

1–2 *minor . . . maior*] There are many species in the genus *Centaurium*, so it is impossible to know which ones Macer and Henry considered the 'smaller' and 'larger' varieties.

3 *tibi nota canam*] A poetic trope, but perhaps reminiscent of Ovid, *Ex Ponto* 4. 19, 'teque canam quacumque nota, tibi carmina mittam.'

3.20 MARRVBIVM / Horehound, *Marrubium vulgare* L.

Lines 1–15 are based on Macer, 'Marrubium,' lines 1437–55, and the last ten lines, not found in *S*, supply an antidote from Constantine the African (or his companion Johannes Afflacius). These last verses are so inferior metrically (particularly lines 19–20) that I am tempted to see them as a later addition by a scribal 'Pseudo-Henry.' However, until another manuscript appears without these lines to agree with *S*, I will follow *P* and include them with the genuine Henry. For the spelling of the title I have used *marrubium* from the poem itself rather than the titles given in *P* or *S*.

4 *caligine*] This term usually does not appear on its own, but is often used to describe eyes. Here it could take the accustomed meaning of 'cloudiness of the eyes' but on its own it could mean 'dizziness' or a 'fogginess' of the head.

7 *ptysicos*] Those suffering form *ptysis* (see note to poem 1.11, line 15 above).

15 *renibus*] *Naribus* in *P* would also work, but *S* agrees with Macer 1455, 'His, qui vesicae morbo renumque laborant.'

16–25 The antidote *dyaprassion* is from Johannes Afflacius (usually attributed to Constantine), *Liber Aureus de Remediorum et Aegritudinum Cognitione*, in *Constantini Africani ... Opera*, 1.205: 'Diaprassium nostrum: Rec. ireos, unc. 4. prassii, pulegii, calamenthi, ficus, ana, unc. 3. liquiriciae, unc. 4. scyllae, hyssopi, nucleorum, unc. 2. foenugraeci, drach. 1. infusi in aqua, die ac nocte. Haec cocta sufficienter, et colata, iterum colatura coquatur, cum tantundem mellis, da cochlearium unum ter in die.' The recipe is essentially for horehound drops, which are still available from some candy stores and were a popular remedy for coughs and sore throats well into the twentieth century.

18 This line scans only with much forcing. *Prassii* must be scanned differently (short-short-long, the classical scansion) from *prassion* in line 1 (long-short-short). This use of *prassii* matches Afflacius's recipe for 'diaprassium' noted above. Both *prasion* and *prasium* appear in classical Latin. The spelling *calmenti* in *P* is not otherwise attested and scans much better as *calamenti*. *Puleium*, though, is an acceptable variant of *pulegium*, or pennyroyal, treated in poem 2.16 above.

18 *calmenti* = *calamenti*, another name for catnip (*nepta, nepeta*). See the commentary on poem 3.23 below.

19 *gemine*] The final syllable must scan long, so this should be read as the dative, agreeing with *uncie* or *unceole*, *i.e.* 'with two ounces' (literally, 'to a twin ounce').

20 The *octo* refers to the number of ingredients in lines 17–19, but *unam* refers to ounces.

3.21 SCLAREGA / Wild English Clary, *Salvia verbenaca* L.

Based partly on Strabo's poem 'De Sclarega,' 275–83. Translated by EMA ('Sclarye,' 198) and abbreviated by the Digby Excerptor. The identification is made based on Henry's description of the larger *sclarega maior* in the following poem. The true clary is about twice the size of wild clary (Grieve, 'Clary').

2 *calde*] For *calide*, used as a substantive with the implicit meaning *aqua calida*. *Cf.* Strabo 279, 'dulci tamen indita caldae,' and the editor's note on this line. EMA, however, understood *calde* to mean some sort of condition like *gutta calida* and says 'Sclarye, as leches seyne, is gode for þe hote gowte' (198).

3 *fermenta*] Here, not yeast, but fermented beverages made with yeast. Clary sage has commonly been used to flavour beers and wines for centuries. *Cf.* Strabo 280–81: 'et vires et odorati fermenta saporis / prestat.'

5 It is not clear how *S* came to provide *refragatur* for *fit inepta*. Their meanings are similar, though *fit inepta* is certainly a more subdued reading. Regardless, *refragatur* does not scan and may be an intrusive gloss or an attempt by a later scribe at a more dramatic verb.

3.22 SCLAREGA MAIOR / True Clary, *Salvia sclarea* L.

Source unknown. For the identification, see the commentary on poem 3.21 above.

3 *cum lacte capelle*] Goat's milk does not appear anywhere else in Henry's herbal, and not at all in Macer's. It seems Henry knew this ingredient from Quintus Serenus, line 197 or 312, both of which end *cum lacte capellae*. Neither of these cures, though, includes clary or is for chest pains. Serenus does not specify a white (*niuee*) goat, though this may be a poetic embellishment on Henry's part.

3.23 NEPTA / Catnip, *Nepeta cataria* L.

Based on Macer, 'Nepeta,' lines 592–625, less lines 614 and 618, the former of which provides an abortifacient. Here, 'calamint' appears to be another name for catnip (stated more explicitly in Macer 592–3), rather than modern calamint (*Calamintha* genus) which is a different, albeit closely related, type of plant. The last eight lines, not found in *S*, come from Pseudo-Oribasius. Daniel Arundel translates the entire poem for his entry 'Balsamyta.'

1 Henry gives a clever pun on *nepta* and *inepta*, not found in Macer. *Cf.* Henry's epigram 'De Philiro' (*HA* 792) in which he similarly compares *ineptum* and *aptus*.

25 A clever rendition of Macer 625: 'Hocque modo venerem prohibet potata frequenter.'

26–33 Pseudo-Oribasius 1. 129, 'Antidotum Diacalamentum': 'Hoc antidotum, dicit Galenus tam esse salubre, ut plurimis annis homo possit sanus seruari. Recipe nepitae unc. vi. petroselini unc. vi. siseleos unc. vi. pulegii unc. vi. piperis nigri unc. vi. libistici unc. ii. thymi unc. v. apii sem. unc. i. mel quod sufficit' (printed as part of *Physica S. Hildegardis* [Strasbourg 1533], 139). The antidote *dyacalamentum*, like *dyaprassion* above (poem 3.20), is described by Rufinus (65–6, 120, 342). Rufinus's recipes and cures, though, are different. The recipe given in the *Antidotarium Nicolai* ('Diacalamentum', 55) is similar, but more complex. This was a popular remedy. A Belgian abbot, writing in 1147, urges a friend to take *diacalamentis* for a cold instead of the more expensive *diamargariton* made of pearls (discussed by Carmélia Opsomer-Halleux in 'The medieval garden and its role in medicine', in *Medieval Gardens*, ed. Elisabeth B. MacDougall, Dumbarton Oaks Colloquium on the History of Landscape Architecture 9 [Washington, DC 1986], 93–114, at 105). Henry discusses *dyamargariton* below in poem 5.2.5, line 9, and in his lapidary *De gemmis preciosis* no. 14, 'De Margarita', line 7: 'conficiunt medici "diamargariton" ab illa' (Black, 77).

28 *sisileos*] *Circa instans* equates *siseleos* with sermountain (*Laserpitium siler* L.), treated below in poem 6.2.17: 'Siseleos sive siler montanum' (fol. 209r). This could also be its close relative laserwort, *Laserpitium latifolium* L., a powerful and popular purgative.

29 *ligusticos*] Apparently a Latin transliteration of the undeclined Greek nominative. We should expect the Latin genitive *ligustici*.

3.24 PORTVLACA / Purslane, *Portulaca oleracea* L.

An abbreviation of Macer, 'Portulaca', lines 748–64. Henry has not included Macer's lines 751 (on purslane's grades), 759 (a cure for the eyes) and 763–4 (a comparison to sorrel, 'Acidula', treated in Macer, lines 711–43, and Henry's next poem, 3.25). *T* uses only Henry's line 4 with most of Macer's poem in the entry 'Portulaca'.

1 *andraginis*] A common variant of *andrachne*, also called *andrago* in some herbals, under the assumption *andraginis* is genitive. *Cf. Sinonoma Bartholomei*, 149: 'Portulaca uel portacla, andrago, uel andragnis, pes pulli idem.'

1 *Danais*] See note above to poem 1.21, line 2.

3 *Causon* (*s.v.* RMLWL) is discussed by Constantine in his *Liber de morborum cognitione et curatione* (= *Viaticum*), in *Constantini Africani . . . Opera*, 2. 142–4.

9 Choulant's edition of Macer does not include Henry's source for this line ('Est haemoptoicis haec saepe comesta salubris') in the body of his edition, but he does note its presence in most manuscripts (note to line 762). However, it is curious that this line does not appear in *P*, and it may have been inserted by the scribe of *S* from his copy of Macer.

3.25 SEMPERVIVA / Houseleek, *Sempervivum tectorum* L.

An abbreviation of Macer, 'Acidula,' lines 711–42, without lines 711–12, 714–15, 730, and 739. While *acidula* usually refers to some form of sorrel (*Rumex acetosa* L.), Henry applies it to the wide variety of succulents in the *Sempervivum* (houseleek), *Sedum* (stonecrop), or *Jovibarba* (hens and chicks) genera, all in the family Crassulaceae. Henry does not use Macer's description of *semperviva* (*acidula minor*), lines 743–7, which is omitted in many manuscripts of Macer (*cf.* note to Macer line 744). It is curious that Henry also omits Macer line 711, 'Dicimus Acidulam, quam Graecus dicit Aizon,' since Henry usually delights in giving as many alternate names as possible for his plants, particularly those of Greek origin. Henry treats *barba Iouis* as a plant distinct from *semperviva* in lines 22–3, though in Macer 741 it is merely a synonym. Henry addresses the plant directly in lines 1–3 and 22–3.

3 *Plinius*] Henry learned this idea from Macer 742, but I have not been able to find it in Pliny. It may be related to Pliny 25. 162, where he compares houseleek (*aizoum*) to *andrachle*, which is used for several eye complaints and headaches.

8 *cephalargia* = *cephalalgia*, which simply means 'headache' in Greek.

13 *Lumbrici rotundi* are probably our modern parasitic roundworms (phylum Nematoda), particularly of the genus *Ascaris*. See note to poem 6.1.2, line 17 below.

4 LIBER QVARTVS / The Fourth Book

Inspired by Boethius, *De cons. phil.* 1 met. 7, also in adonics. Neither *P* nor *S* has reproduced the poem in this format. Each scribe, either misunderstanding the metre or employing a space-saving measure, wrote the poem in 18 lines rather than 36. However, each also paired the lines in a different way, producing different and mostly nonsensical lines. See Rigg, 271, for the reconstruction of this poem from the corrupt exemplars. Michael Winterbottom suggested a change in punctuation to lines 18–19 from Rigg's edition, which I have followed.

1–6 While the entire poem is clearly indebted in its metre to Boethius, *De cons. phil.* 1 met. 7, this passage is also reminiscent in its content of lines 1–4 of that poem: 'Nubibus atris / condita nullum / fundere possunt / sidera lumen.'

11–12, 31–32 *Physica* and *Ethica*, along with *Logica* were traditionally the three branches of philosophy, according to Augustine, *De Civitate Dei* 8. 4, and Isidore, *Etym.* 2. 24, 1–16.

15 *Sidera fulgent*] Boethius, *De cons. phil.* 2. met. 2, 4. Also compare Horace, *Carmina* 2. 16. 3–4: 'neque certa fulgent / sidera nautis.'

4.1–2 <IACINCTVS ET NARCISSVS> / Hyacinth, *Hyacinth orientalis* L. and Narcissus (Daffodil), *Narcissus pseudonarcissus* L.

Henry drew on a wider variety of sources for this poem than for most others: Ovid, the book of Proverbs, Statius, and perhaps Pliny. Isidore also groups these two flowers together (17. 9. 15–16). For the myths about Hyacinth and Narcissus Henry is dependent primarily on Ovid, *Met.* 10. 163–219 and 3. 339–510. The medicinal attributes of narcissus may come from Pliny 21. 128–9 but Pliny's description of hyacinth (21. 66) does not give any remedies. This poem and the Epilogue 1 to Book 4 are the only instances in the herbal where Henry included two distinct plants (as opposed to two species of the same genus) in a single poem. The two flowers must be counted separately in order to reach the total of one hundred plants for books 1–4 (see the Introduction above, 12–13). The Digby Excerptor has condensed this poem to a few brief phrases. Most hyacinths are *Hyacinthus orientalis* L. (Grieve, 'Grape Hyacinth'; André, 'hyacinthus'). The name *Narcissus* could apply to any of the leaning, trumpet-flowered members of the daffodil family, but it could be the true narcissus, *Narcissus tazetta* L. Identification is complicated, however, for Henry says the *narcissus* is red (*roseum*); see the note to line 23.

The Trinity Compiler used lines 25–9 in his own poem 'Narcisus' and I employ only those in the apparatus. 'Narcisus' is the only poem in the Trinity compilation where the author seems to comment on Henry's poem, and it is worth reproducing it in its entirety here:

> Narcisum fabula iuuenem sophistica florem
> Narrat; Iacincto necnon deconuenit (?) idem.
> Vulnere Narcisus periit, nunc uulnera curat;
> Feruores aliis reprimit feruore peremptus.
> Contusus contusa iuuat luxataque sanat,
> Ast hic quem Veneris feruens extinxit acumen,
> Si caput inde laues, febres extinguit acutas,
> Sicque dedit pueri candorem fabula flori
> Sicut et alterius Iacinctum purpura tinxit.
> Narciso gelida magis autem sicca potestas

Hinc magnas plagas curat magisque iacentes (*sic*).
Serpentis morsus sanat superaddita trita.
Si iungas eque, coniuncta lilia potes,
Extenuatur eo nimia processio potu.

While the Compiler has reproduced only five lines, and those not exactly, it is clear from his lines 1–2 and 8–11 that he knew all of Henry's poem. The information in his lines 13–15 comes from another source. The Compiler may have been insulting by calling the story or Henry's poem a 'sophistic fable' (*fabula . . . sophistica*, line 1).

1 This line and line 11 are discussed by Thomas Haye in the context of the relation of author to reader within didactic poems (*Das lateinische Lehrgedicht*, 151). He compares this line to similar ones in Virgil (*Georgica* 3. 290: 'angustis hunc addere rebus honorem') and Strabo (*Hortulus* l. 75: 'ut ingenti res paruae ornentur honore'), both of whom also endeavoured to increase honour by means of little things.

7–8 *cures . . . curet . . . curantem*] The double meaning of *curare* as 'to cure' and 'to care/to be anxious/to be concerned' cannot be reproduced in English.

9 *res homini labor est*] *Cf.* Eccles. 6: 7

9–10 *natura . . . testante*] *Cf.* Prov. 30: 18–20 or Wisd. 5: 11.

15–16 *tu . . . hic*] Hyacinth . . . Narcissus.

17 *leuis*] Rigg, 273, notes that *lenis* can also be read here and make sense, though *leuis* is preferable because of Narcissus's 'smooth' reflection in the water.

20 Ovid, *Met.* 3. 466, 'inopem me copia fecit.'

23 *roseum*] A fine example of ancient authority trumping observation: no variety of narcissus or daffodil is red, but Henry is working from Ovid, *Met.* 3. 482, 'pectora traxerunt roseum pecussa ruborem.' Pliny (21. 128) says 'Narcissi duo genera . . . purpureo flore,' but the editor notes that 'The adjective *purpureus* probably refers here to the red nectary of the flower, but it is always a difficult word both to interpret and to translate' (note to 21. 128). Such is also the case with *roseum*. If Henry actually means that the petals of the flower are red, he may have had in mind the amaryllis, a relative of the narcissus, though it is more likely he was simply imitating his source.

24 *Cf.* poem 2.10, line 33 above: 'uigor equus utrique.'

25–31 I have not found a source for this medical information. It could perhaps be a simple application of the legendary boys' attributes to their respective plants: the hot one can cure fevers, they are both beautiful so they both clear the skin, and so on. However, Pliny's passage on narcissus (21. 128–9) has some similarities, though not enough that I feel comfortable including it among Henry's sources (see Table 2 in the Introduction above, 30–34):

> Narcissi duo genera in usum medici recipiunt, purpureo flore et alterum herbaceum, hunc stomacho inutilem et ideo vomitorium alvosque solventem, nervis inimicum, caput gravantem et a narce narcissum dictum, non a fabuloso puero. Utriusque radix mulsei saporis est. Ambustis prodest exiguo e melle, sic et vulneribus et luxatis, panis vero cum melle et aerina farina. Sic et infixa corpori extrahit. In polenta tritus oleoque contusis medetur et lapide percussis. Purgat vulnera permixtus farinae, nigras vitiligines emaculat.

Pliny's narcissus is effective against burns, wounds, and dislocations. It appears that Henry intends hyacinth, and not narcissus, to heal *contusa* and *luxata* (line 27), but the language is close enough to suggest possible influence.

32 *gloria fame*] *Cf.* Martial, *Liber Spectaculorum* 15. 1, 'Summa tuae, Meleagre, fuit quae gloria famae . . .'.

35 Henry is referring to the *Thebaid* of Statius and the *Aeneid* of Virgil.

36 Nisus and Euryalus are young warriors in Virgil's *Aeneid* (9. 176–223) famous for their close bond and, in some readings, their homosexual love. Dymas and Opleus (= Hopleus) are similar characters in Statius's *Thebaid* (10. 347–448). Statius himself compares them to Nisus and Euryalus (10. 447–8): 'forsitan et comites non aspernabitur umbras / Euryalus Phrygiique admittet gloria Nisi.' The close bonds shared by these two pairs of warriors are thus, by implication, shared by the personified hyacinth and narcissus.

4.3 SINAPIS / Mustard, *Brassica alba* L. or *Sinapis alba* L.

Based on Macer, 'Sinapi,' lines 1139–1200, without lines 1143, 1155–6 and 1159–60. It is odd that Henry did not include material from these lines, which treat mustard's extreme heat. Henry may have had a defective copy of Macer for this poem.

1 *Tercia*] Third poem in the fourth book, and third plant in the fourth bed of the garden.

2 *Pitagoras*] Pythagoras of Samos (*ca* 580–500 BCE) appears numerous times in Pliny's *Natural History* as a medical authority, judging mustard at 20. 236 and several other plants at 24. 156–60.

5 Pliny 20. 240: 'semen ac radix, cum inmaduere musto, conteruntur manusque plenae mensura sorbentur ad confirmandas fauces, stomachum, oculos, caput sensusque omnes.'

7–8 *Salubre* and *potatum* agree with *mustum* in line 5.

9–11 This recipe for a mustard bath is still a common home remedy.

12–13 This strange passage, whatever it may mean, is based on Macer 1147–8: 'Si tritum iungas tepidae versesque palate / Ad solem capitis purgabit flegma nocivum.' The cure seems to ask that the patient suffering 'harmful phlegm' look at the sun and turn mustard paste in his mouth, though it may simply be a poetic way of saying the patient should hold it on the roof of his mouth.

14 Translated literally, this means 'The wise men mix this into their sneezes,' but the sense is clearly that powdered mustard can be taken like snuff to force out nasal blockages.

31 *Mansa*] The switch to the feminine probably reflects a switch from *oleum* or *semen* to an implicit feminine *herba* or *sinapis*.

32 *Menemacus*] See note to poem 2.14, line 51.

36 *sinapismus*] A mustard-based antidote. Henry learned it from Macer 1773.

37 *habundat* = *abundat*

38 *Lenior* gives a different sense to the passage (more soothing, gentle) than Macer's original *debilior* (line 1174).

4.4 ERVCA / Rocket, *Eruca sativa* Mill.

Eruca is paired with *sinapis* (poem 4.3), since both are forms of mustard (line 1). Based on Macer's 'Eruca,' lines 1016–36. Daniel Arundel ('Eruca,' fols. 81r–81v) notes that Henry says the same things as Macer. The name *eruca* applied to a wide variety of plants (Hunt, 110) and is the source of both the modern names 'rocket' and 'arugula.' Nearly any plant in the family Brassicaceae (mustards and cabbages) could be intended here. The best candidates are rocket (*Eruca sativa* Mill.) or charlock (*Sinapis arvensis* L.). My choice of the former is based on line 16, since rocket has long been used as a leafy vegetable. The scribe of *S* includes after the last line of 'Eruca' the first line of 'Lactuca' (poem 4.5), an indication that he had on hand a continuous version of the herbal, like that in *P*.

1 Perhaps a parody of Virgil, *Aeneid* 1. 565: 'Quis genus Aeneadum, quis Troiae nesciat urbem.'

2–3 Choulant's edition of Macer gives the hot and dry properties of *eruca*, though without the grades (lines 1016–17). Some manuscripts of Macer add a line after 1017, 'Tertius erucae fertur gradus esse caloris,' which version Henry most likely was using (Macer, note to line 1017).

3 *digerit*] Most instances of *escas* in the *Anglicanus ortus* appear with *digerit* or *digerat*, and never with *egerit*. While *egerit* is shared by both manuscripts, it does not make much sense in this context and the change may have been influenced by the *egerit* in the next line, which does make sense. *Egerit* would make sense in this line only if *eruca* were a purgative, which is unlikely given that it is popular in sauces (lines 16–17).

7–11 Henry, using the first person, seems to be speaking as a knowledgeable physician. For some reason the scribe or a reader of *P* has dramatically cancelled the word *lino* in line 7 although it is necessary.

12 *uatum*] It is not clear who these 'poets' are. The idea comes from Macer 1034: 'Confirmant pariter medici pluresque poëtae.'

13 Henry's direct address of Venus is a novelty not in Macer 1033–4. The scribe of *S* omitted *Venus* from this line, which may simply have been oversight but could be an intentional case of Christian censorship, as a similar case occurs at poem 1.22, line 15, where *S* omits *bis genito*, an epithet for *Bacchus*.

14 *mira canam*] Ovid, *Fasti* 4. 267.

16–17 A brief restatement of Macer 1029–32. Macer notes that the seed is called *euzomon* by the Greeks, a point oddly not included by Henry.

4.5 LACTVCA / Lettuce, *Lactuca sativa* L.

An abbreviated version of Macer, 'Lactuca,' lines 765–75. The compiler of *S*, in the process of putting the herbal into alphabetical order, split up this poem. The first line ended up on fol. 61v at the end of *Eruca*, poem 4.4, while the rest begins on fol. 65r. Lettuce is related to mustard and rocket (poems 4.3 and 4.4) and is similar in appearance when flowering, hence its placement here. The brevity of this poem should be striking to the modern reader, for whom lettuce is very common. In the Middle Ages many other greens were available which could provide more flavour and, probably by extension, more medicinal uses.

1 *Hanc*] Henry is referring to the hot and dry *eruca* of the previous poem 4.4.

6 *Sompnia uana*] Echoes of Ovid, *Met.* 11. 614.

8 After this line in *P*, a contemporary hand has added an explanation: 'Nocet oculis quia caligines inducit diu comesta.'

4.6 SATVREIA / Savory, *Satureia hortensis* L.

Based on Macer, 'Satureia,' lines 843–69. *P* includes at the top of fol. 26v, above line 17, two extra lines related to savory, taken from Macer, lines 868–9: 'Si desit thimus pro thimo ponere tymbram / Precipiunt medici quia vis est una (*Choulant ed.* aequa) duabus.' Henry knew its other name, *timbra*, from Virgil, *Georgica* 4. 30–32: 'Haec circum casiae virides et olentia late / serpylla et graviter spirantis copia thymbrae / floreat inriguumque bibant violaria fontem.'

1 Macer does not provide the degrees for savory, but does differentiate its hot and dry powers: 'Illi sicca minus vis est, sed fervida valde' (line 844). Perhaps Henry interpreted *valde* as the strongest degree, fourth. Constantine (379) places savory in the third degree: 'Satirion calidus est et siccus in tertio gradu.'

2 *Argi*] The reading *Argiui* in *S* is tempting to use as the *lectio difficilior*, but the sentence needs the *hanc* in *P* and so also the reading *Argi*.

12 *hec . . . hic* = *frenesis . . . letargus*

13 *distendat*] Macer uses *commiscens* at this point, so the sense of *distendere* here must be 'to soften/expand an ingredient with a liquid,' in this case, vinegar.

19 *satiris*] Savory (*satureia*) is supposedly named after satyrs, who are exceptionally lascivious (hence the *nimis* in line 18). Henry received this statement from Macer, who apparently misread Isidore, *Etym.* 17.9.42–3: 'Satureia calida et prope ignita. Vnde illi [et] nomen inditum credunt, quod pronos facit in Venerem. Satyrion dicta a Satyris propter incendium libidinis, quam vulgus stincum vocant; Venerem enim suscitat. Idem et orchis . . .'. Both plants discussed are aphrodisiacs, but only *satyrion* (orchid) is said to be named after the lascivious nature of satyrs, since the roots of some orchids resemble testicles. See also Grieve, 'Orchids.'

4.7 NASTVRCIVM / Cress, *Nasturtium officinale* L.

Medieval *nasturcium* is cress and not the modern nasturtium (genus *Tropaeolum*), a native of South America, so named for the similarity between the shape and taste of its leaves and those of European cress. Based on Macer, 'Nasturtium,' lines 988–1015, though thoroughly rearranged. The indication that it is dry in the fourth degree (lines 1–2) is apparently from Constantine's 'Nasturtium,' 384, although there is no other indication that Henry had Constantine's work available to him when he was writing books 1–4. Daniel Additional (fols. 114r–114v), after outlining Macer's *nasturtium*, says in his passage 'Nasturcius,' 'Henricus þe same.'

1 *septima*] Seventh poem in this book and seventh plant in this quadrant of the garden.

3 *ruta*] Henry treats rue above in poem 1.10, though that poem does not mention its anti-aphrodisiacal properties.

11 *Linchenas* = *lichenas*, impetigo or some other skin disease. Pliny discusses this condition at length (26.2–4).

19 Almost identical to poem 4.25, line 13, on juniper ('Sauina'). *Antraca* is usually a synonym for *carbunculi*, and the explanation of the name comes from Macer 496. For a discussion of these names, see Léon Rippinger, 'À propos de quelques noms de maladies chez Celse et Scribonius Largus,' in *Études de linguistique générale et de linguistique latine offertes en hommage à Guy Serbat* (Paris 1987), 207–18, at 212–17. Curiously, in two passages cited by Rippinger from the Latin Oribasius, *antracas* are said to be called *malas pustellas* by rustics. Perhaps Macer, in calling them *bona ulcera*, was making fun or was confused.

20 *furunculus*] Literally, a 'little thief.' Pliny uses it to mean a burning sore or boil (20. 130).

22–23 *sumpta . . . posite*] The implicit subject here has switched from the neuter *nasturcium* to the feminine *herba*. Macer uses the neuter at the end of his poem.

4.8 AMEOS / Giant Hogweed, *Heracleum mantegazzianum* L.

Ameos is a name applied variously to numerous umbellifers, such as cow parsley, hemlock, and goutweed (Hunt, 20–21). The editor of Constantine's *Liber de Elephancia* identifies *ameos* as *Ammi maius* L., called 'bishop's weed' in England (*Tratado médico de Constantino el Africano*, ed. Ana Isabel Martín Ferreira [Valladolid 1996], 104), but that plant rarely grows over four feet. The same is the case for small bullwort, *Ammoides pusilla* (Brot.), the identification given to *ameos* by Giovanni Cristofolini and Umberto Mossetti in the medical works of Guilielmus de Saliceto (*ca* 1290): 'Interpretation of plant names in a late medieval medical treatise,' *Taxon* 47 (1998), 305–19, at 308. Giant hogweed is the most likely candidate in this case because of size and habitat; it is a native of Britain and can reach a height of fifteen feet. Henry emphasizes the plant's great size (line 1). I have not found the source to this poem. It bears no relation to the 'Ameos' described by Latin Dioscorides (10. 404–405) or Constantine (369).

8–9 Henry returns here to his favourite metaphors of battles and war.

13 The *sed* should be understood as 'and also' rather than 'but.'

13 *singula*] Henry employs here the literary topos of impatience. The listener is assumed to be growing impatient, but in the following poem (4.9, line 13) he loses his own patience.

4.9 PSILLIVM / Fleaseed (Psyllium Plantain), *Plantago psyllium* L.

The ability of *ameos* in the previous poem to fight all types of cold leads naturally to *psillium*, which is considered colder (in a Galenic sense) than any other herb. Source unknown. Henry's *psillium* bears no relation to Constantine's 'Psyllium,' 363, nor to Latin Dioscorides's 'De Psillion' except that the latter also says 'Virtus est semini eius frigida' (11. 37). The end of this poem shows Henry becoming either playful or irritable, refusing to answer another question from his student about a Greek medical term. The Trinity Compiler used this poem in his entry 'Spillia,' but only lines 8–12 are copied closely.

3 *trociscum*] A medicinal pill. As this word does not appear in the standard herbals, Henry may have learned it from the *Antidotarium Nicolai*, where it is common (especially at 157–63).

5 *lampade Phebi*] A common classical epithet for the sun (*e.g.* Silius Italicus, *Punica* 1. 193), also used by Henry in his Epigram 12. 8, line 48 (*HA* 818), 'Lampade Phebea.'

10 *alia … luce*] That is, returning every third day, if counting inclusively in the medieval fashion, *e.g.* the tertian fever. The change made by *T* in this line (*ternas* for *alia*) reflects this meaning, but also destroys the sense of *alia … luce*. Compare *alterna febris* in poem 4.10, line 8.

12 *cephalargia*] See note to poem 3.25, line 8.

13 *per singula curram*] Sedulius, *Carmen paschale* 3. 358. See note to poem 4.8, line 13, on this theme.

4.10 CORIANDRVM / Coriander or Cilantro, *Coriandrum sativum* L.

Closely based on Macer, 'Coriandrum,' lines 957–87, less lines 986–7, where Macer says that some believe too much coriander can bring about death! Henry's opening (line 1) and the final recipe (lines 26–8) are original. These lines suggest that coriander featured prominently in Henry's dishes, and also are a witness to the relative cost of various spices in the twelfth century.

1 *subit*] That is, it follows *psillia* in poem 4.9, and in the previous plot. The two are paired because of their notable cooling tendencies.

1 *et superest*] The alternate reading of *frigidum* in *P* is surprising. It does make sense, given how cold coriander is paired with cold psyllium in the previous poem, but it does not scan. Perhaps the scribe of *P* felt the cold nature of coriander needed to be emphasized further.

8 *alterna febre*] A fever coming to crisis every other day, usually called a tertian fever in medieval medicine.

14 *fabe* = *seminis* (since coriander seeds are so large).

24 *Xenocrates*] Xenocrates of Chalcedon (396–314 BCE), a student of Plato and his successor as head of the Academy. This statement attributed to him is found at Macer 984–5 and Pliny 20. 218.

26–28 The Trinity Compiler's poem 'Coriandrum' is primarily a copy of Macer, but the last two lines seem based on Henry's version (*T* fol. 92v): 'Qui uesci pipere formidat propter aceume (*sic*) / Pro condimento gelidum iungat coriandrum.' It is not clear what *aceume* means. In Henry's version, *pauperies* takes pepper away, but here *aceume* seems to indicate taste rather than cost.

Perhaps it is an error for *aciem* (*i.e.* the sharp flavour of pepper), although that would not scan.

4.11 LVPINVM / Lupin, probably *Lupinus albus* L.

Translated by EMA, 'Lupinus,' 199–200, and condensed by the Digby Excerptor. EMA adds an original description of the plant, something he generally does not do in other passages taken from the *Anglicanus ortus*: 'Lupinus is an herbe þat groweþ a-bowte in þe felde. It beriþ large and sharp prikkes . . .' (199). Masculine *lupinus* and neuter *lupinum* both exist in classical Latin. I have followed the neuter form used in line 1 in both manuscripts rather than the masculine used in the title of *P*. Henry's main theme is lupin's ability to combat drunkenness and he was therefore able to turn to several classical texts on the subject of wine and inebriation. I have found no direct source for the medical material in lines 8–10 (but see note to line 10).

1 *concutit arma*] Ovid, *Met.* 1. 143.

2 *Thebeum . . . deum*] In some traditions, Bacchus is the god of Thebes, especially in Statius's *Thebaid*, which Henry knew (see poem 4.1–2 above). Hercules could also play this role, but since the lupin is an effective cure against drunkenness it has, as it were, declared war on Bacchus.

2–3 *granaria . . . ampla*] The seedpods of the mature lupin.

4 *legumen*] Apparently the scribe of *P* misread this word and supplied *lyea*, an attempt at *lyeo*, a common word in this herbal.

5–6 These lines form a reply of sorts to Horace, *Epistulae* 1. 5. 19–20: 'Fecundi calices quem non fecere disertum, / contracta quem non in paupertate solutum.'

7 *cornua*] Horns = strength or bravery. *Cf.* Ovid, *Ars amatoria* 1. 239, 'Tunc veniunt risus, tunc pauper cornua sumit,' and Ps. 68: 32–3.

10 *lumbrici*] The efficacy of lupins against stomach worms is found in numerous sources and is thus difficult to trace: Pliny (22. 155), Latin Dioscorides (as cited by Rufinus, 175–6), Pseudo-Apuleius's 'Herba lupinum montanum' (no. 111, p. 196), *Circa instans* (fol. 201r), Pseudo-Pliny's *Medicina Plinii* 86. 1–3 (*Plinii Secundi Iunioris Qui feruntur De medicina libri tres*, ed. Alf Önnerfors, Corpus Medicorum Latinorum 3 [Berlin 1964]). Pseudo-Apuleius and *Circa instans* share Henry's prescription of lupins with wormwood (*absinthium*). Isidore, following a line from Virgil's *Georgica*, says only that lupins cause sadness (*Etym.* 17. 4. 7). See also Pseudo-Galen's *Alfabetum Galieni* no. 149 ('Lupinus'): 'Farina vero eorum cum marrubio pari pondere in vmbilico imposita lumbricos expellit' (*Galeni Opera Omnia. Galeno ascripti libri* [Venice 1562], fols. 88–101). I owe this last reference to Dr Nicholas Everett of the University of Toronto.

4.12 FENVGRECVM / Fenugreek, *Trigonella foenum-graecum* L.

Perhaps based on passages from Pliny, especially 24. 184–8, though direct imitation is difficult to prove. Henry continues the battle imagery from the previous poem. Fenugreek is named for *faenum Graecum*, 'Greek hay.' It is still used as animal fodder and as an edible green or seasoning. Translated by EMA, 'Femygrek' (198) and by Daniel Arundel, 'Fenugrecus' (fol. 86r). The Trinity Compiler uses most of Henry's poem (lines 2–3 and 5–9) in his thirty-six-line poem 'Fenigrecus.'

1 *in cetum*] A phrase used frequently in the *Ilias Latina*. Perhaps the fact that this herb is called 'Greek' reminded Henry of the Trojan legend.

1, 7 *Fenugrecum* needs to be scanned differently in each of these lines to preserve the metre.

2 *Cf.* Pliny 24. 184: 'vis eius siccare, mollire, dissolvere.'

3 The Trinity Compiler modified this line to include another species of mallow, presumably Henry's *sinula*: 'Si tres maluarum species tamen iunxeris illi' (*T* 96r). Henry treats these three types of mallow in poems 3.16 and 3.17 above.

4 *quas*] The antecedent is *duricias* ... *collecturasque*.

5–6 The ingredients for this cure are in Pliny 20. 251, but his recipe is for simple stomach pains. I have translated *cum polline* simply as 'with flour,' but Pliny 24. 186, possibly Henry's source for this passage, calls for not just flour but 'fenugreek meal': 'Farinam feni cum hordeo aut lini semine decoctam aqua mulsa.' Henry may have misunderstood this passage, taking *pollen* as a synonym for *farina* and as a separate ingredient from the fenugreek, not merely a description of its preparation.

6 *encathisma*] Apparently an error, since an *encathisma* is a hot bath for soothing stomach problems or a compress, and the rest of the line would make no sense if that sense were intended. Here the word is used as some sort of medical condition which fenugreek cures. Perhaps Henry intended *encathis* (swelling of the eyelid)? EMA does not seem to have known what it was: 'A plastre ... wole destruye þe euel þat is clepid encaresma' (198).

7–9 This cure could be dependent on one of Pliny's discussions of cabbage (20. 88): 'vel aqua ipsa cum hordeacia farina, sucum ex aceto vel cum feno Graeco. sic aliqui et articulis podagrisque inponunt.'

4.13 PAPAVER / Poppy, *Papaver somniferum* L.

Based on Macer, 'Papaver,' lines 1037–86, less lines 1040 (naming a separate 'field poppy'), 1052 (describing the black seeds of the red poppy), 1060–61 (warning against deadly overdose of poppy), and 1085 (suppository to bring on sleep). It is not clear why Henry would cut any of these lines, particularly the warning against overdose, since he usually adapts the entirety of each of Macer's poems.

1 *tredecimus*] Thirteenth plant in this book and in this bed of the garden.

3 *ille est* must elide to scan properly.

10 *Huic*] That is, to the second type of poppy.

17 *subactis*] Literally 'conquered' or 'subdued', but in the case of medicinal leaves, 'pounded' or 'ground up' seems to be intended.

19 *cantu*] Excessive singing which brings on a sore throat.

21 *iunctum*] This word refers to the plaster (*cataplasma*), but it is not clear what the plaster is to be joined with, unless we are to read the word simply as 'when mixed together.'

24, 28 These questions address information taken from Macer, but their format is original to Henry and typical of how he tried to make the material more entertaining and accessible.

28 *nominis extat*] Ovid, *Ars amatoria* 2. 637.

29 *fame ingentis*] Henry uses the same phrase in his epigram 'De Zoilo' (*HA* 11. 22, p. 796).

4.14 GIT / Git or Nigella, *Nigella sativa* L.

Git, also called nigella or fennel flower, is best known today in Indian cuisine, but it has a long history in Europe as well. *Git* appears several times in Pliny's *Natural History* (10. 167–8; 20. 182–4; 27. 121; see the Introduction above, 46–8) and Charlemagne called for it to be grown on royal estates in his 'Capitulare de villis' (*Kapitularien*, ed. Schneider, 27). Henry apparently derived his information from Pliny, though he has omitted the herb's many medicinal qualities given at 20. 182–4. This poem is translated by EMA, 'Git', 199, and condensed by the Digby Excerptor. After the final line the scribe of *S* attempted to rewrite the first line: 'Git cornute tuos prouisit musa triumphos.'

1 *cornute*] The seeds of git grow in four conjoined pods which curve up towards each other like little horns (Pliny 27. 121).

5–6 These lines may come from Henry's personal experience, but are more likely derived from Pliny's account of git (19. 167–8). Pliny says that it is used in baking festive breads, whose tops are seasoned with poppy seeds and bottoms with celery seed and git. Indian naan or papadums are the closest modern equivalents.

4.15 GAZARA / Knotweed, family *Polygonaceae* L.

Source unknown. Translated by EMA as 'Azara' (199), and in both versions of Henry Daniel under 'Gazarus.' Hunt (125) identifies the medieval *Gazarus* as knotgrass or knapweed (*Centaurea scabiosa* L.), which can grow rather tall, but has nothing tree-like about it. If *gazara* is a type of knotgrass or knotweed, it is clearly not the most common variety, prostrate knotgrass (*Polygonum aviculare* L.), which grows close to the ground. Some members of the knotweed family, especially the rapacious Japanese knotweed (*Polygonum cuspidatum* Siebold & Zucc.) or giant knotweed (*Polygonum sachalinense* F. Schmidt), are hardy and grow quite tall. The latter two species did not reach Europe until the nineteenth century, so some other tall variety must be intended, as Henry stresses that it can look like a tree. Pliny describes four types of knotweed under the name *Polygonum* (27. 113–17), but gives no name similar to *gazara*. The fourth variety is most similar to Henry's description, in that it seems more like a tree (*paene arboris modo frutex*) and because herbalists employ it more than almost any other plant. However, Pliny's recipes bear little relation to Henry's, so the immediate source of this poem must be sought elsewhere. See the Introduction above, 47, for more on this passage. The Trinity Compiler rewrote line 6, and added a half line at the end: 'Virtutis calide est.'

4.16 PIONIA / Peony, *Paeonia officinalis* L.

Closely based on Macer, 'Paeonia,' lines 1605–40, which also provides the allusions to Galen and Dioscorides.

8 *scotosim*] Henry's definition of this word is not found in Macer. Choulant notes (on Macer 1612) that some manuscripts read *sclerosim* or *sclerosin*. If *scotosis* is not a misreading of *sclerosis*, it is likely related to *scotoma*, a condition either of dimming eyesight or of flickering lights on the periphery of the vision associated with a migraine, but Henry understands *scotosis* simply as a headache. I have found *scotosis* defined only in Charles du Fresne Du Cange, *Glossarium latino-germanicum mediae et infimae aetatis*, ed. Lorenz Diefenbach (Frankfurt 1857), 520c: 'dass ist dar abe der man mit schonen augen nicht gesicht.' No source is given for this definition, and it may have come from Macer, which does not help in its definition.

21 *suspensa*] Worn as an amulet from the neck, as is made clear in the following lines.

4.17 AQVILEIA / Columbine, *Aquilegia vulgaris* L.

The whole of this poem is most likely original to Henry, and it seems intentionally placed near poems 4.14 and 4.15, which are also dedicated primarily to the appearance of their plants. Henry gives no medicinal recipes, merely describing three of the plant's names: *aquileia*, *argentilla* and *herba puellaris*. The name *aquileia* applied to several plants in the Middle Ages: balm, meadowsweet, houseleek and columbine (Hunt, 31). *Argentilla* applied to even more plants (Hunt, 32), though Henry obviously considered them the same plant. I have based the identification with columbine on Henry's description of the flowers, as columbines do indeed look like inverted raptor's talons. None of these names appear in Pliny, yet Pliny does group together the magical plants *coracesia et calicia*, which the editor translates as 'girls' plant' and 'beauty plant' (24. 156 and note *a*). The similarity is striking to the *herba puellaris* of Henry's line 5. The Digby Excerptor copied the first four lines more closely than he did for most other poems, for which reason I have included variants from those lines in the critical apparatus.

1 *quatuor . . . aquilis*] Because columbine's inverted flowers, with sharp petals, look like talons.

2 *pulcrior argento*] Marbode of Rennes, *Liber decem capitulorum* c. 4, 'De matrona,' line 35 (ed. Rosario Leotta and Carmelo Crimi [Florence 1998], 42).

3–4 This passage gives one of the few detailed descriptions of a plant's appearance in the entire *Anglicanus ortus*, and suggests direct observation on Henry's part. While columbines come in many colours, the common European columbine usually wears a purple or mauve shade (*purpura cedit ei*).

7 *gustata*] The reading of *P*, *gestata*, will also work here, but Henry seems to avoid cures which call simply for carrying the plant as an amulet, relying more on ingested and applied cures.

4.18 VERBENA / Vervain, *Verbena officinalis* L.

Based on Macer, 'Verbena,' lines 1859–1902. This poem seems unfinished. Problems in scansion and grammar occur in lines 4–5 and 13–15.

1 *statillina*] I have not found a source for this name. It does not appear in Macer, though the other names come from Macer 1859–60.

2 *perysterion*] The name means 'dovecote' in Greek.

2 *yerabotanum*] For *hierobotanum* (ἱεροβότανον), which means 'holy herb' in Greek. The holy nature of *verbena* is emphasized by Pliny 22. 5.

4–5 In *P* these lines are given as one line, which is identical to Macer 1885. This is probably a coincidence, rather than influence of Macer on the scribe of *P*. Unfortunately, for line 4 to scan, the *aptari aptam* must be elided, which is not typical of Henry's verse.

9–12 Pliny 26. 37–8: 'verbenaca vero omnibus visceribus medetur, lateribus, pulmonibus, iocineribus, thoraci; peculiariter autem pulmonibus et quos ab his phthisis temptet radix herbae consiliginis . . .'. Macer (1887–91) misread Pliny, who within a passage on vervain explains that *consiligo* is good for the lungs and *phthisis*.

13–15 This sentence is incomplete. A verb like *iungatur* would help 13–14 and in 15 we need to understand *illis* before *quos*.

13 *foliis de mille*] = *millefolia*, yarrow (*Achillea millefolium* L.). This line is similar to two lines by Quintus Serenus: 'herbaque cum seuo foliis de mille vocata' (line 693), and 'herbaque quae nomen foliis de mille recepit' (line 813).

15 *anxius angit*] Virgil, *Aeneid* 10. 89: 'nunc sollicitam timor anxius angit.'

19 *dolores*] It is not clear where this word belongs. The cures for jaundice and poisonous bites come from Macer 1862–5, but *dolores* are not mentioned there. *Hictericus* is usually substantive, referring to a jaundiced person, but if we take it as an adjective here, it will work.

26 *Cf.* poem 1.14, line 14.

28–30 Most of this semi-magical explanation comes from Macer 1881–3, but the final comment (*nam mortis signa patescunt*) is original to Henry.

31–34 Pliny 25. 106, speaking of *hiera botane* which is also called *verbenaca*: 'sed Magi utique circa hanc insaniunt; hac perunctos inpetrare quae velint, febres abigere, amicitias conciliare nullique non morbo mederi.'

34 *quodcumque petas pocieris*] Echoes of Ovid, *Met.* 7. 683: 'consequitur, quodcumque petit, fortunaeque missum . . .'.

35–36 Henry has changed the focus of Macer 1902, which refers to these recipes as 'old wives' tales' (*vana . . . anilia*). Henry emphasizes proof by experimental testing (*nisi temptarim quod celem*) rather than dismissing old superstitions.

35 *Natura potens*] *Cf.* Horace, *Satires* 2. 1. 51: 'imperet hoc natura potens, sic collige mecum . . .' and Boethius, *De cons. phil.* 3 met. 2, 1–2: 'Quantas rerum flectat habenas / Natura potens . . .'

36 *non . . . possim*] *Cf.* Ovid, *Ex Ponto* 2. 4. 5: 'Non ita di mihi sint tristes ut credere possim.'

4.19 MEV / Spignel, *Meum athamanticum* Jacq.

The herb *meu* seems to be the same plant as baldmoney, described in poem 1.5, above. Perhaps Henry differentiated two varieties where we now have the single species *Meum athamanticum*. The direct source is unknown. *Meu* is not in Constantine and Henry's poem bears little relation to the entry for *Meu* in the Latin Alphabetical Dioscorides (Cambridge, Jesus College, Q. D. 2, fol. 93v).

1 *diureticum*] Pliny emphasizes the diuretic powers of spignel (20. 253, 'urinam ciet in aqua pota radice trita vel decocta'), but does not give any of the other cures and does not use the word *diureticus*, a technical term Henry is eager to use. Henry has placed *meu* (4.19) and *ciperus* (4.20) together because of their diuretic virtue.

4 *pauper nomine*] Poor, since *meu* is such a short name.

5–7 *Alexander*] Probably the sixth-century Byzantine physician Alexander Trallianus (Tralles), several of whose works were available in Latin redactions from an early date (seventh century) and to whom was attributed a popular *De pulsibus et urinis*. See D. R. Langslow, *The Latin Alexander Trallianus: The Text and Transmission of a Late Latin Medical Book* (London 2006), 4–5, and Langslow, *Medical Latin in the Roman Empire* (Oxford 2000), 70. Less likely candidates are Pope Alexander, to whom were credited magical powers, or Alexander the Great, to whom several Hermetic works were attributed, especially the *Liber de septem herbis*, in which seven magical herbs are aligned with the seven planets. The same work is sometimes described as written for Alexander by Hermes: *De septem herbis ad Alexandrum* (to appear in *Hermes Latinus* IV.2. *Textus Medici*, ed. Paolo Lucentini, CCCM 144A). That Alexander also appears in Henry's poem 3.7, 'Macedonia.'

5–7 *Galienus*] Again, it is not known to what work Henry is referring. If he does have a specific work in mind, it could well be pseudonymous, but in this case, it seems Henry is being coy, referring the reader to authorities when he does not actually know any more virtues for *meu*.

4.20 CIPERVS / Cyperus, *Cyperus longus* L.

Based on Macer, 'Cyperus,' lines 1585–1604, which Daniel Arundel translates, yet attributes to Henry ('Ciparus,' fol. 68v). Cyperus, also known as sweet galingale, is a marsh grass related to papyrus, and is not to be confused with galangal, which has its own poem below ('Galanga,' 6.1.7). The scribe of *S* understood *ciperus* as a fourth declension noun, changing *ciperum* to *ciperu* in line 1 and writing *ciperui* in line 8. In all other sources it is second declension.

1 *diureticum*] *Ciperus* is known for its diuretic powers and Henry has thus paired this poem with poem 4.19, in which *diureticus* is defined.

6 *Apollodorus*] There are numerous classical authors of this name, but Apollodorus the Epicurean of Athens (3rd or 2nd century BCE), known for his biological writings, was probably intended.

6 *lienem*] A case of synecdoche where 'spleen' refers to a diseased or enlarged spleen, or to an excess of humours in the spleen.

8 The dramatically different reading of *S* seems due to the scribe's confusion of Macer 1588–93:

> Dicit Apollodorus, quod pellere possit abortum,
> Si mulier foveatur aqua, qua coxerit illum;
> Asserit hic idem consumere posse lienem

Illius fumus, si saepius ore trahatur;
Si se sanus homo fumo subfumiget illo,
Dicit eum fieri firmum magis et leviorem.

15 Understand the verb *dixit*.

4.21 VALERIANA / Valerian, *Valeriana officinalis* L.

Source unknown. Henry's description is closest to that of 'Alexander' (Trallianus?) cited by Rufinus, 319, but there are not enough similarities to prove any connection. Lines 1–7 are paraphrased by EMA, 'Valerian,' 199. The Digby Excerptor abbreviates this and the Trinity Compiler uses lines 2–11 within a much longer poem.

1 *Viginti uisis*] Twenty plants have been seen in this bed of the garden, and twenty described in this book of the herbal.

1–5 The impressive alliteration in these lines cannot be reproduced in translation. *Valeriana* supposedly derives its name from being so beneficial (*multa ualet*, 'it is good for many things').

10–13 These lines are essentially the same in *P* and *S* and present difficulties. Why are *morbus* and *hostis* in the nominative? Does the sentence in lines 10–11 relate to the final one? The enemy (*hostis*) could be the disease or 'envy' (*liuor*) in line 12, who denies that valerian does anything beneficial. We may have here an important case of shared error.

12 *Ergo neget liuor te*] Perhaps echoing Marbode, *De ornamentis verborum* III. 'Complexio,' l. 4 (ed. Leotta and Crimi, 4): 'Egregios igitur livor neget Andegavenses.'

4.22 BORAGVM / Balm, *Melissa officinalis* L.

Based on Macer, 'Barrocus,' lines 1641–63, less line 1647. *Boragum* is not borage, but rather Henry or a scribe's attempt at *Barrocum*.

1 *quam*] Antecedent is an implied *herba*.

1 *Mellisophilos* is Greek for 'honey-loving.'

1 *Achiui* are the Achaeans, standing for Greeks in general.

3 *lac . . . perungas*] See note to poem 2.13, line 6.

5 *Plinius*] In reference to Pliny 21. 150.

8 *cyliacos = coeliacos*

9 The addition of *antiquos* at the end of this line in both manuscripts is one of the strongest pieces of evidence for shared error. For *ortobnoicos* see the note to poem 1.24, line 9.

10 Either reading (*fedis* or *sedis*) could work. Choulant opted for *sedis* in the comparable line of Macer, so the recent translators have therefore understood *vitiis . . . sedis* as 'Haemmorrhoiden.' However, Choulant notes that most manuscripts read *foedis*, so I am assuming that was the reading in Henry's copy of Macer. Regardless, *uiciis fedis* ('foul vices') is so vague as to be meaningless.

15 It is not clear what *hec inflacio* is or if it is related to the dog bite in the previous line. Macer 1654 reads 'Tali discutitur inflatio noxia potu.' The whole of line 15 seems unfinished or corrupt. It is unlike Henry to repeat a word at the caesura and end of a line unless as a pun. I am tempted to emend the second *potu* to *fotu*, but the manuscripts do not support such a change.

17 *ictibus*] The reading of *morsibus* in *P* is probably an intruded gloss.

4.23 ARISTOLOGIA / Birthwort or Dutchman's Pipe, genus *Aristolochiaceae* L.

Based on Macer, 'Aristolochia,' lines 1395–1436, less lines 1406 and 1430–32, giving feminine cures, and lines 1409–10, a recipe for cleaning wounds. Three varieties are identified: *rotunda*, *longa* and the Greek *clematis*, probably to be identified with the modern *Aristolochia rotunda* L., *Aristolochia sempervivens* L., and *Aristolochia clematitis* L., respectively. Macer's poem is organized in three sections according to the abilities of these three types. Henry, however, thoroughly rearranged Macer's poem in order to separate the cures 'in aqua' (lines 11–16) from those 'cum uino' (lines 17–20). The reference to Pliny (line 27) is taken from Macer.

1 *Rotunda est* must elide for the line to scan.

3 *clematis*] Not the flowering vine clematis, but *Aristolochia clematitis* L., the European birthwort.

7–8 These lines exhibit bizarre shifts in mood not typical of Henry: there is no need for the subjunctive verbs *ungas* or *mundas*.

10 *frigida*] Refers to *aqua* in the previous line.

16 *leuior*] Lighter, perhaps meaning relieved of excess humour, or simply that the suffering or rigour of paralysis is eased. It is not clear, though, how a paralytic is *arens*, 'dry' or 'thirsty.' Macer 1420 reads simply, 'Et sic fit sumpta levior paralyticus illa,' which I have followed in emending *sit agit* shared by *P* and *S*.

17–18 The scribe of *S* realized he had made a mistake here and inserted the correct line 17 ('cum uino morsus curat potata malignos') after line 31, with an arrow indicating its proper position.

18 *opungnare* = *oppugnare*

22 *sancte*] This is an odd adjective for Henry to use, and it is not in Macer.

Perhaps its supposed ability to scare off demons (lines 32–3) lends it an air of holiness. There is very little in the herbal that could be called 'holy,' apart from St Mary's seal, described in the following poem 4.24.

24 *pisces*] This does indeed say that this herb will kill fish (thus also in Macer 1435–6). The source of this dubious fishing technique is Pliny 25. 98: 'Piscatores Campaniae radicem eam quae rotunda est venenum terrae vocant, coramque nobis contusam mixta calce in mare sparsere. Advolant pisces cupiditate mira statimque exanimati fluitant.'

26–27 This reference to Pliny comes from the same section, 25. 97–8.

32 *laudabilis*] Genitive, *i.e.* 'of the praiseworthy herb.'

4.24 PALMA CHRISTI / St Mary's Seal (Solomon's Seal), *Polygonatum multiflorum* L.

The Trinity Compiler uses lines 1–3 and 8 in his own poem on 'Palma Christi.' The Digby Excerptor calls it 'Herba fera uel palma' and adds an extra comment at the end: 'Venerem eciam cohercet.' Lines 4–10 are translated by Daniel Additional (fol. 118r) under 'Palma Dei.' The plant called *palma Christi* or *palma Dei* was also called St Mary's seal, now usually known as Solomon's seal (Hunt, 238), although *palma Christi* has also been identified as motherwort, *Leonurus cardiaca* L. (Hunt, 196–7; Stannard, 'A fifteenth-century botanical glossary,' 360–61). Whether this poem is dedicated to St Mary's seal or motherwort, it was a suitable place for a meditation on, even a hymn to, the Virgin Mary. The *Alphita* is of little help for identification, simply saying 'Sigillum Sancte Marie herba est.' The editor of the *Agnus Castus* identifies *Palma Christi* as dead-nettle (284), even though the author states that 'Palma Christi is an herbe that me cleputh mannes moderwort' (197). Motherwort would make sense here based on its name, but it has no fruit to speak of, as mentioned in lines 6–7. Solomon's seal thus seems the best option, though I have found no evidence of its use in food or painting (lines 8–10).

8–10 This passage echoes a phrase in Henry's poem on strawberry (*fraga*), 2.15, line 9: 'ni populo figmenta ferant pigmenta parantes.' By analogy with that line, I have supplied *ferant* in line 9, where a word is needed. Henry clearly enjoyed the alliteration and rhyme of *figmenta ferant—pigmenta parant*. This time he added a twist: those who prepare pigments might be telling lies to 'those seeking that skill' (*artem querentibus illam*), possibly in order to protect the secrets of a trade guild.

10 *Eius*] Of her, that is, the Virgin Mary.

11–16 Henry abandons here the herbal's classical pagan themes and indulges in a rare passage of Christian devotion, similar in content to portions of the Athanasian Creed. He treats the Trinitarian paradox of the son without a father, who is his own father nonetheless. While this theme was a common one to educated ecclesiastics of the twelfth century, Henry may be thinking of Augustine, Sermon 217, c. 1: 'sed generans fons et genitus fons unus est fons: quemadmodum generans Deus et genitus Deus unus est Deus, de Patre scilicet natus Filius. Pater non est Filius, Filius non est Pater; Pater non est de Filio, Filius de Patre est; sed tamen Pater et Filius unum sunt propter unam substantiam, et unus est Deus propter inseparabilem divinitatem' (*Sermones*, ed. Miguel Fuertes Lanero, Obras Completas de San Agustín 7, 10, 23–26 [Madrid 1981–5]).

13 *mater . . . filia*] Several motets and masses from the later Middle Ages are titled 'Mater patris et filia,' and it was likely a common trope by Henry's time.

15 *Virgo parens*] *Cf.* Sedulius, *Carmen paschale* 1. 323: 'Virgo parens, aliaeque simul cum munere matres.'

17–18 The final two lines hardly seem to follow from the contemplation of the Virgin Mary, especially since the *cuius* must refer to the plant and not Mary. It almost seems that these lines are meant to come immediately after line 7, and all the intervening lines are parenthetical.

4.25 SAVINA / Juniper, *Juniperus sabina* L.

An extended version of Macer, 'Sabina,' lines 492–506. Lines 1 and 4–9 are original to Henry. The reference to Oribasius (line 22) comes by way of Macer 506, though the description of him 'balancing the known with the unknown' is original to Henry.

1 *ultima*] That is, the last poem in Book 4 and in the four-book herbal *De herbis*.

3 *brateon*] Also called *bracteos*. See note to poem 1.12, line 20.

6 Juniper is also known as *Sabina cacumina* since the tender tops (*cacumina*) were the source of a volatile oil for use in medicine. *Cf.* Ovid, *Met.* 1. 552: 'ora cacumen habet.'

13 Almost identical to poem 4.7, line 19. See the note to that line concerning *antracas*.

17–20 For juniper's powers as an emmenagogue and abortifacient see Riddle, *Eve's Herbs*, 54–5.

20 The emendation from *leuiter pota* in *P* is based on Macer 498: 'si cum vino sit sumpta frequenter.'

22 *Cf.* Book 4, Epilogue 2, line 20: 'nota quod ignotis iubet Oribasius equans.'

22 *Oribasius*] The first mention of Oribasius, already an important source for Henry. He was a Greek physician, *ca* 325–400 CE, who worked for the

Roman emperor Julian the Apostate. Portions of his massive medical encyclopedia *Collectiones Medicae* were translated into Latin in the early Middle Ages.

4 <EPILOGVS 1. PALMES ET LACTERIDIS> / Epilogue 1
1) Vine, *Vitis vinifera* L.
2) Squirting Cucumber, *Ecballium elaterium* A. Rich.

This epilogue brings us back to the theatre and lake in the middle of the garden which Henry introduced in his Prose Prologue above: 'in medio uero laci sedes est quasi theatrum, palmitibus conductis Phebo resistens' (lines 49–50). The bucolic and peaceful nature of the final lines will be interrupted, at times rudely, by Apollo and his audience of medical experts in the following books. This poem is found only in *P* and is particularly corrupt; Rigg (275–6), Winterbottom, and I have all made emendations. See the Introduction above, 12 and 14, for the importance of this poem in determining the arrangement of the *Anglicanus ortus*. Though no recipes are given for the vines (*palmes*), both they and *lacteridis* must be included among the 160 ingredients mentioned in the final Epilogue after Book 6 (340–41).

The Digby Excerptor used only lines 10–11 for his entry on 'Lacteridis.' *Lacterida* is listed in Charlemagne's 'Capitulare de villis' and *lacterides* is in Constantine, 380, but they bear no resemblance to Henry's poem. *Lacterides* is a name given to several members of the spurge genus possessing milky resin (Hunt, 153). The juice of the caper spurge is a violent purgative (Grieve, 'Spurges'), which is in agreement with Henry's line 12. However, the plant here is more likely the squirting cucumber, which was called *elacterium* (Hunt, 104), and the milky juice of which *Circa instans* uses in many recipes (fol. 197v). Latin Dioscorides says that 'Elateriu sucus est cucumeris agrestis' (11.67). The wild cucumber known as manroot, *Echinocystis lobata*, is a native of North America.

1 *centum*] The one hundred herbs are those treated in Books 1–4.

5 *frondea tecta*] *Cf.* Virgil, *Georgica* 4.61–2: 'aquas dulces et frondea semper / tecta petunt.'

6–8 It seems that lines 7–8 (*uernus . . . flores*) are an explanation of Henry's poetic fancies in lines 6–7, hence the drastic emendation from *que* to *nam*. If the *que* in *P* is correct we may be missing an entire line for the relative clause. As Rigg has noted, these lines are flawed, particularly because *eos* has no clear referent. I would suggest that *eos* are those figures who are in the garden: our narrator, his interlocutor, the Cook, and those characters we will meet in Books 5 and 6, Apollo and the Old Man (see the Introduction above, 17–19).

6 *zaphirea* = *sapphirea*

10 Rigg admits that *aeno* is a 'wild conjecture', but one with which I am apt to agree.

13 *gelidos ... ortus*] Ovid, *Ibis* 11: 'Ille relegatum gelidos aquilonis ad ortus.'

14 *fessos ... artus*] *Cf.* Pseudo-Virgil, *Culex* 204–205 (in *Virgil*, vol. 2, ed. Fairclough, rev. Goold): 'cum grege compulso pastor duplicantibus umbris / vadit et in fessos requiem dare comparat artus.' This perhaps also echoes Strabo, *Hortulus*, line 392: 'Iam nisi me fessum via longior indupediret ...'.

4 <EPILOGVS 2> / Epilogue 2

This curious poem juxtaposes two incongruous themes: King Henry I's military endeavours, and Henry the poet's supposed sources for the poem. It has a tone of finality to it which suggests that it may originally have served as the conclusion to the original herbal of four books and one hundred plants. After this poem, at the base of fol. 32r, the scribe of *P* has added 'Sequitur quintus liber Anglicani orti' which provides the title for this work. See the Introduction above, 11–12.

1 *Hec*] Poems, presumably.

2–6 These lines seem to refer to Henry I's return from Normandy, suppressing rebellions in 1123–4 (Rigg, 277), and we can assume this poem was written relatively soon after that. They seem dedicatory in nature, but they are not at the head of the work, as one would expect, and nowhere else does the work seem to have a dedicatee.

9–20 These lines resemble an early medieval poem (ninth century at latest) attributed variously to Marcellus Empiricus and Dioscorides which begins 'Quod natum Phoebus docuit, quod Chiro Achillem', edited in Marcellus (ed. Niedermann and Liechtenhan, 2. 624–7); see also Riddle, 'Dioscorides', *Catalogus translationum et commentariorum: Mediaeval and Renaissance Latin Translations and Commentaries* 4 (1980), 141–2. Most of these authorities' names come from Macer's herbal, apart from the *sorores*, Prodymus, Justus, Stephanus and Philo. Verbs must be supplied throughout this passage for it to make sense, such as *cecinere* (line 10), *memorat* and *diuinat* (line 13), and *asseruere* (line 15).

9 *Phebus*] Apollo, the original god of medicine.

9 *Pheboque satus*] Asclepius, Apollo's son, and also god of medicine, named explicitly in line 17. He was possibly conflated with Asclepius of Bithynia (born 124 BCE), a Greek physician of the Methodist school in Rome.

9 *Olympius*] See note to poem 3.17, line 20.

10 *Themeson*] See note to poem 2.2, line 5.

10 *Apollodorus*] See note to poem 4.20, line 6.

10 *Sorores*] Probably the Muses, but they are in odd company, and not typically associated as a group with medicine.

11 *Ypocras*] See note to poem 2.2, line 3. 'Divinely sick' is a curious way to describe Hippocrates and his medical knowledge.

12 *Prodymus*] Identification unknown. Perhaps we should read not a name, but the verb ('we say'). It would not be unlike Henry to include himself in a list of authorities.

12 *Crisipus*] Chrysippus of Soli (*ca* 280–207 BCE), Stoic logician. The scansion and spelling of *Crisipus* differs from his other appearances as *Crisippus* in poem 5.2.3, line 22, and 6 Interlude, line 8. Chrysippus also appears in the prologue of Henry's *Historia Anglorum*, by way of a quote from Horace (*HA* 2).

12 *Plinius*] See note to poem 1.1, line 26.

13 *Iustus*] See note to poem 2.9, line 10, for a discussion of Justus.

13 *Galienus*] See note to poem 1.19, line 7.

14 *Xenocrates*] See note to poem 4.10, line 24.

15 *Catho*] Cato the Elder (234–149 BCE). His only complete surviving work is *De agri cultura*, and he is cited by Macer at lines 1205 and 1219.

15 *Pittagoras*] Pythagoras of Samos (sixth century BCE).

15 *Palladius*] See note to poem 2.10, line 46.

16 *Stephanus*] Not mentioned elsewhere in the herbal. Possibly Stephanus of Athens (or of Alexandria, *ca* 550–630 CE), an Alexandrian author of commentaries on Hippocrates and Galen. See Wanda Wolska-Conus, 'Stéphanos d'Athènes et Stéphanos d'Alexandrie: Essai d'identification et de biographie,' *Revue des études byzantines* 47 (1989), 5–89.

16 *Mellicius*] Possibly the Greek physician Meletos of the early first century CE. His remedy books served as a source for Pliny's *Natural History*. This name appears again below at poem 5.2.3, line 44, and is cited by Macer at line 1262. He is not likely to be the fourth-century pope Melecius or the third archbishop of Canterbury, Mellitus (d. 624).

17 *Asclepiusque*] See note to line 9 of this poem.

18 *Dyascorides*] See note to poem 1.1, line 3.

18 *Philo*] See note to poem 2.2, line 4.

18 *Menetamus*] Menemachus. See note to poem 2.14, line 51.

19 *Macer . . . Stabus*] See the Introduction above, 25–6 and 30–41.

20 Almost identical to poem 4.25, line 22 on *Sauina*. See the note to that line for *Oribasius*.

21–22 *Cf.* Ovid, *Met.* 2. 27, 'cinctum florente corona,' and Virgil, *Aeneid* 9. 808, 'cava tempora circum.' Henry will return to the theme of 'girding temples' in the Prologue to Book 5, line 14.

5 <PROLOGVS LIBRI QVINTI> / Prologue of the Fifth Book

This poem is the only verse prologue in hexameters, and presents one of the few cases of Christian language in the herbal, with its powerful descriptions of paradise, martyrdom and virginity. Henry, however, quickly abandons the religious tone and returns to his pagan deities (Venus and Apollo). Overall, it is one of the most original and artful poems in the entire work, as Henry brings together his themes of herbs and spices, authority and performance, Christianity and paganism, and considers the place of Books 1–4 and 5–6 in his lifetime of poetic composition. See the Introduction above, 10–11 and 17–20, for a fuller discussion of the importance of this poem for understanding the structure of the *Anglicanus ortus*.

1–2 The opening lines of this poem might be inspired by the opening lines of the Pseudo-Ovidian poem *De medicamine aurium* that begins: 'Ne tibi displiceat quod sum corpore paruus. / Ortulus iste breuis mitia poma gerit.' The twenty-one-line poem is edited by F. W. Lenz, 'Das pseudo-ovidische Gedicht *De medicamine aurium*', in *Ovidiana: Recherches sur Ovide*, publiée à l'occasion du bimillénaire du poète par Niculae I. Herescu avec le concours de D. Adamesteanu, Vasile Cristea, E. Lozovan (Paris 1958), 526–40, with the text and apparatus at 536–9. The poem is discussed by Klaus-Dietrich Fischer, 'A mirror for deaf ears? A medieval mystery', *Electronic British Library Journal* (2008), Article 9, <http://www.bl.uk/eblj/2008articles/article9.html>. The earliest copy known to Fischer (p. 3) comes from the mid-twelfth-century manuscript Oxford, Bodleian Library, MS Rawlinson C 235, which could mean it was available to Henry. For Middle English versions of the poem, see George R. Keiser, 'Verse introductions to Middle English medical treatises', *English Studies* 84 (2003), 301–17.

2 *plasmator eorum*] *Cf.* Bernardus Claravallensis, *Tractatus de gradibus humilitatis et superbiae* 3. 12: 'Sed plasmator eorum Deus requirens quod perierat . . .' (PL 182. 948).

4–5 The rose, lily, and violet are addressed above (poem 2.9, lines 1–2) as emblems of the Virgin Mary. They were also grouped together by pagan authors: *cf.* Ovid, *Ars amatoria* 2. 115–16: 'Nec violae semper nec hiantia lilia florent, / Et riget amissa spina relicta rosa.' Isidore treats the three flowers together in the same order: rose, lily, violet (*Etym.* 17. 9. 17–19).

4 *rosa martirii . . . lilia uirginitatis*] A common religious trope, but among Henry's notable contemporaries are Bernard of Cluny, *De contemptu mundi* 1. 177 ('Tunc rosa sanguine, lilia virgine mente micabunt') and 1. 317–18 ('Sunt tibi lilia pura cubilia virginitatis, / Est rosa sanguine, purpura lumine sobrietatis'), in *Scorn for the World: Bernard of Cluny's* De Contemptu Mundi, ed. and trans. Ronald Pepin [East Lansing, MI 1991], 22 and 30. *Cf.* Alexander Neckham, *De laudibus divinae sapientiae* 5. 105–106 (ed. Thomas Wright

[London 1863], 442): 'Quos rosa martyrii, flos campi, donat honore, / Tanto purpureas dicimus esse rosas.' The popular eleventh-century poem 'O Roma nobilis' also contains the flowers of martyrdom and virginity:

> O Roma nobilis, orbis et domina,
> Cunctarum urbium excellentissima,
> Roseo martyrum sanguine rubea,
> Albis et virginum liliis candida.

7 This line appears in Henry's *Historia Anglorum*, prologue, line 3 (ed. Greenway, 6): 'Principium rerum, uegetatio, finis earum,' and is varied in the first line of the *Anglicanus ortus* at the start of the Prose Prologue, line 1: 'Principium rerum, generacio, finis earum.' See the Introduction above, 10–12 and 17.

9 *Ter*] Henry 'shone three times' in his past poems, which is reflected in line 8: *ludens* (probably referring to his epigrams), *Veneremque fugans* (apparently in the lost work *De amore*), and *gramina plantans* (writing books 1–4 on herbs of the *Anglicanus ortus*). In the fourth place he has 'woven a book in square' (*quadratum texo libellum*), in which he intends to treat twelve more herbs, twelve spices, twelve gems and twelve stones. This plan will not succeed, as is explained in the Introduction above, 17–19. These lines echo the first lines of the concluding poem in *De contemptu mundi* written for his fellow archdeacon Walter (*HA* 618): 'Henricus tibi serta gerens, epigramata primum, Prelia mox / Veneris, gramina deinde tuli.'

9 *texo*] See Henry's letter to King Henry I, c. 1: 'Henrice compulsus epistolam contexui' (*HA* 502–503), and his *De contemptu mundi*, c. 1: 'Carmen etiam in amorem acceptabile contexui' (*HA* 584–5). See note 64 in the Introduction above on the theme of weaving and composing.

12 *postrema duo*] Referring to gems and stones in line 11, which were also believed to have medicinal uses (and not to poems 5.1.11–12 on hemlock and cocklebur, according to Rigg, 279).

14 *cinxit tympora sertis*] A common classical image, but perhaps drawn from Statius, *Achilleid* 1. 611, 'cinxit purpureis flaventia tempora vittis.'

15–17 These lines refer to Henry's lapidary *De gemmis* which was intended to make up books 7 and 8 of the *Anglicanus ortus*. See the Introduction above, 9–10 and 62.

16 *interpellabo*] This verb usually has the sense of 'interrupt' in the context of a conversation, but in the case of inserting gems into a garland, 'intersperse' seems to be the sense. It is a curious verb to use here, especially with its generally negative connotation of disturbing or molesting.

18 *Cf. HA* 10. 40, lines 13–14 (p. 776): 'His igitur radiis, dum sceptra decora decoras, / Tu diadema magis quam te diadema perornat.'

20 *Orientis aromata*] In reference to the eastern spices of Book 6.

5.1.1 PLANTAGO / Plantain:
1) Greater Plantain, *Plantago major* L.
2) Ribwort Plantain, *Plantago lanceolata* L.

Based on Macer, 'Plantago,' lines 196–266, though thoroughly reorganized. Macer differentiates *plantago maior* (lines 203–204) and *minor* (lines 242–3), a distinction which Henry has not used, attributing all the cures to either variety. Henry's final lines, 57–64, provide an antidote not found in Macer, and this is the only section reproduced by *D*. Henry's introduction in lines 1–4 is also original, as is his gloss to *emoptoicis* at line 22. Daniel Additional mentions in 'Butalmon' (fols. 38v–39r) that Henry wrote more about plantain than Macer. He translates Henry's introduction (lines 1–6) and the recipe for *dyarnoglossa*.

2 *plantauit*] Supply the object *te*, implied in *tibi*.

4 *occurrit*] Henry switches to the third person to describe plantain after the direct address in lines 1–3.

6 *lanceolata*] Macer 201 adds that this type of plantain received its name because it looks like a lance (*lancea*).

9 *Arnoglossa* means 'lamb's tongue' in Greek, hence *lingua agni* in Latin.

22 An odd use of *rite*, which cannot have the usual positive association, but must express simply a sense of regularity.

28 The first letter of *ciliacos* is badly smudged by what appears to be a later correction. I have retained the original spelling of *ciliacos* as that is what appears in the poem on myrtle (1.25, line 16).

34 *sperma*] Glossed with 'id est semen' in *P*.

44 *cyatos*] A later hand has added a footnote to this line: 'Sciathus est uncia et semis.'

46 *febris ... tercia*] A circumlocution for the tertian ague, *febris tertiana*.

51 On the use of *lacrimum* over *lacrima*, see the note to poem 1.20, line 31.

53 Pliny 25. 80: 'mira vis in siccando densandoque corpore, cauterii vicem optinens.'

54 *cauteria*] The sense here is that the drying power of plantain is so great that it works on the body like a branding iron, a drastic form of humoral therapy which was used to pull out or destroy excess humours. *Cauteria*, however, is glossed with *incisa*, indicating that the scribe or contemporary reader apparently understood it to mean a form of bloodletting or perhaps scarification rather than branding.

55 *Themeson*] See note to poem 2.2, line 5. This work on the virtues of plantain has not been identified.

57–64 *Dyarnoglossa* is a compound medicine made primarily of *arnoglossa*. This passage may not be by Henry, but rather the addition of a later scribe. I have not found a similar source; it is not in the *Antidotarium Nicolai*.

58 *guttam . . . caducam*] The 'falling gout', probably epilepsy, where *gutta* refers to any sort of disease.

59 *castoreum*] Strongly scented secretions of a male beaver's genital castor sac, a favourite ingredient in medieval and early modern medicine.

59 *lasar*] For *laser*, juice of asafoetida, *laserpitium*, or a similar plant.

59 *opoponacem*] Opoponax, an aromatic gum (*Opoponax chironium* Koch.).

60 *dentes equi*] A plant of some sort. The name is given to numerous species (Hunt, 99), and no indication is given here what might be intended. The *Alphita* glossary defines it as 'Dens equinus. Sulfuratura herba', which does not help in identification.

61 *quod sufficit*] However much honey is needed to form the ingredients into a pill.

62–63 The sequence of events is not entirely clear. Since a single pill cannot be given when the moon is waxing and waning (*crescente . . . descrescente*), either more than one dose is assumed or the *decrescente* applies to the period afterwards when the patient is supposed to avoid *uenerem uinumque*.

64 This line, as received in both manuscripts, seems corrupt. The first word in both is either *pons* or *pous*, but it is not legible in the gutter of *D*. Rigg has suggested that Henry wrote *pous*, the Old French word for 'pulse' (*cf.* Latin *pulsus*, and 'pous' in Tobler-Lommatzsch, *Altfranzösisches Wörterbuch* [Wiesbaden 1955–2008]). While Henry does use Latin words of French origin (*e.g.* 'mula' at poem 2.7, line 23), this would be the only instance of an actual French word in the text (or rather, Anglo-Norman: *Anglo-Norman Dictionary*, ed. William Rothwell et al. [London 1977–92], *s.v.* 'puls'). The same spelling is used in Middle English, as found in a lyric about the founders of medicine: 'Phebus fonde first the craft of medecine / By touche of pous and urine inspections' (No. 113, ll. 1–2, in *Middle English Lyrics: Authoritative Texts, Critical and Historical Backgrounds, Perspectives on Six Poems*, ed. Maxwell S. Luria and Richard L. Hoffman [New York 1974], 111).

Daniel Additional's translation provides some clues to another possible reading: 'Thereof is mad a medecyn þat is cald *diarnoglossa*, and it is cald *gutta caduca*; also ageyn *lunatica passio*' (fol. 39r). While Daniel seems to have misunderstood the fact that *gutta* is the disease, and not the medicine, the second technical term, *lunatica passio*, seems to come from Henry's line 64. An emendation of *Pous* to *Passio*, using *et* from *O* for the metre, is tempting, but then we would also have to change *tremulus* and *lunaticus* to feminine adjectives. Given these difficulties, I think it best to retain *Pous* and accept that Henry Daniel may have read *pous* as an error or abbreviation for *passio* (which can be abbreviated as *pas°*). A final possibility is that Henry was transliterating from the Greek *pous*, for 'foot', but that is properly two syllables, not one, nor does Henry show any genuine knowledge of Greek. Finally, it is also not clear to what *istum* refers. Perhaps the *antidotum* is meant, in which case taking the pulse could prove whether or not the antidote had been given or was working.

5.1.2 VRTICA / Nettle, *Urtica urens* L.

Based on Macer, 'Urtica,' lines 115–60. Henry's line 26 is original, and line 37 is a clever variation on Macer 159–60. *D* reproduces only lines 22–5, 27–30 and 36–7. There are over 500 species of nettle (family Urticaceae) but the most common, and surely the one intended, is the stinging nettle, *Urtica urens* (*cf.* Grieve, 'Nettles'). The final two lines provide rare instructions, for this work, on the collection and preservation of the medicine; in this case, nettle seeds should be gathered in August.

2 *acalife*] According to Hunt (3), *acalephe* (also *acalifa*) is a name given to some nettles; see also André, 'acelephe.'

3 The *-cal-* in *acalife* is indicative of nettle's great heat (*calor*).

8 *defluuium capitis*] Literally, 'a flowing over of the head,' but Pliny uses this phrase as a synonym for *alopecia*, or hair loss (11. 230; 22. 34).

34 *Veneris motus*] *Cf.* Ovid, *Amores* 2. 10. 36: 'at mihi contingat Veneris languescere motu.'

34–35 This is one of the few veterinary cures in the herbal. Classically, the first syllable of *quadrupes* is scanned long, but Henry treats it as short.

36 *Sextilis*] Sixth month of the old Roman calendar, later renamed August.

5.1.3 IVSQVIAMVM / Henbane, *Hyoscyamus niger* L.

Lines 9–30 are based on Macer, 'Iusquiamus,' lines 1933–61. I have found no source for the opening recipe in lines 1–8. Daniel Arundel mentions Henry's poem under 'Caniculata' (fol. 58v) and partially translates lines 1–7, though he leaves out all the ingredients.

1 The postpositive *nam* is unlike Henry and might indicate an unfinished revision.

1 *Iusquiamon* is apparently an antidote featuring *iusquiamum*. This name is closer to the Greek name for the herb *hyoscyamon*.

2 *confire*] Comfrey. This name seems drawn from early English or French rather than from the classical Latin *conferba* (treated in poem 2.20). *Confiria* also appears at a very early date (*Oxford English Dictionary*, 'comfrey').

3 See note to poem 3.23, line 28, on the plant *sisileos*.

5 I have found no other reference to a plant called *soffroacus*.

10 *reum* = *rheuma*

15 *obolus*] A small weight, based on the coin of the same name, essentially a halfpenny-weight, or one-sixth of a dram. We should expect the neuter *obolum*, but Henry might not have known the classical spelling.

16 *Myconis* here is based on *mycon* (classically *mecon*), a different name for poppy from *miconius* at poem 4.13, line 1.

17 The equivalent lines in Macer (1954–5) read: 'Et dicunt haemoptoicis sic posse mederi, / Vel quocunque modo sanguis iactetur ob ore.' The gloss given by Henry may come from his own knowledge, but more likely from Macer's poem on leeks ('Porrum'), lines 510–11, where he orders their juice be given: 'Aegrotis, qui reiiciunt sputantve cruorem, / Quos haemoptoicos soliti sunt dicere Graeci.' The version of Macer used by Rufinus adds a gloss to the word *emoptoicis* in the poem on plantain: 'Emoptoici dicuntur qui sanguinem spuunt vel vomunt' (39).

25 *caniculatam*] Elsewhere, henbane is called *canicularis* (Hunt, 65).

5.1.4 CERIFOLIVM / Chervil, *Anthriscus cerefolium* (L.) Hoffm.

Based on Macer, 'Cerefolium,' lines 928–46, less line 932 ('Cum mulsa bibitum pituitae noxia solvit'), perhaps because Henry did not know the meaning of *pituita*. This appears to have been a problem for other scribes, since Choulant says (note to Macer line 932) that one group of Macer manuscripts adds a gloss after the line in question: 'Humor viscosus pituita est conglomeratus.' The information in Henry's lines 16–17 is not found in Macer, but given their purely medicinal nature, these lines are likely not original to Henry.

3 The *tamen* is unnecessary since lines 3–5 simply provide cures for the *uertigo* in line 2, and in no way modify or correct the previous statement.

11 *repellit*] *P* reads *superabit* which does not scan. I have emended to *repellit* based on *pota repellit* at poem 1.10, line 39, and poem 1.14, line 7, as well as *pota repellis* at poem 5.1.9, line 6. *Repellit* was probably replaced by its gloss *superabit* in an earlier manuscript.

12 *uirgine*] *Virgo* is used here as an adjective in place of *uirginea*, *i.e.* virgin (white or unused) wax. The phrase comes directly from Macer 937: 'Virgine cum cera vetus huic axungia mixta.'

14 *cancris* = *canceres*

5.1.5 LAPAPHVM / Dock or Sorrel, family *Rumex* L.

Lapatium, given as the title of this poem in the margin of *P*, was a more common spelling than *lapaphum*. However, since *lapaphum* is used in the poem itself I have retained that spelling for the title. This poem is an abbreviation of Macer, 'Paratella,' lines 1993–2014. Henry has not included Macer's lines 1994–5 (an explanation of dock's four varieties) or part of 2012 (a remedy for restraining *menstrua*). There are numerous kinds of dock; the species intended is probably common dock (*Rumex obtusifolius* L.) or sorrel (*Rumex acetosella* L.).

2 *urtice spicula*] Nettles, discussed in poem 5.1.2. This remedy is not in Macer, and it sounds as if it comes from personal experience. 'Nettle in, dock out,' and its opposite, were popular proverbs in later medieval England. *Cf. Proverbs, Sentences, and Proverbial Phrases*, ed. Bartlett Jere Whiting and Helen Wescott Whiting (Cambridge, MA 1968), no. D288, 'In Dock out nettle.'

16–17 This passage is not found in Macer. Pliny, in his main passage on *lapathum* (20. 231–5), gives several applications of the root for various skin problems, though he does not name *pruritus* or *scabies*, nor does he mention sulphur.

5.1.6 SENECION / Groundsel, *Senecio vulgaris* L.

Based on Macer, 'Senecion,' lines 1664–89. The identification is helped by *Agnus Castus*: 'Senacion ys an erbe that me clepyth growndswthele' (203). *Senecion* is indeclinable (see line 3).

1 The etymology of *senecion* from *cano tincta colore* ('dyed with a grey colour') is a simplification or misreading of Macer 1664–5, where *senecion* is named from its similiarity to grey hair: 'Erigeron Graeci, nos Senecion vocitamus, / Quod canis similis videatur flore capillis . . .'. Macer's etymology is, in turn, a modification of that given by Isidore, *Etym.* 17. 9. 53, who says the name comes from *senescat* ('grows old'): 'Erigeron a Graecis dicitur, quod vere primo senescat: unde et eam Latini senicionem vocant.' The etymology is not reproducible in the English translation.

5–8 Originally from Pliny 25. 167, by way of Macer. Henry usually rejects or criticizes magical cures of this nature.

13 It is not clear who is the subject of *probarunt*. The unnamed *quidam* in line 9 consider *senecion* dangerous, and it seems more likely that Pliny, who favours it, would 'prove these things.' An emendation to *probauit* is tempting, but not justified by the one manuscript.

20 *capitelli*] In all other instances, Henry uses the neuter form, *capitella*.

22 *thabulatis* = *tabulatis*, 'floorboards.' *Tegulatis* (rooftiles) in Macer 1666. It is plausible that groundsel could grow up through the cracks in a poorly laid floor.

23 *facili medicamine*] Quintus Serenus 299.

5.1.7 MAVRELLA / Black Nightshade, *Solanum nigrum* L.

Based closely on Macer, 'Maurella,' lines 1918–32. Henry's poem is a close paraphrase of Macer's, yet he livens it up by addressing the reader directly in lines 9–10. Daniel Arundel notes that Henry says the same as Macer (in a section on nightshade incorrectly titled 'Faba lupina,' fols. 83v–84r).

1 *Mirmidone*] In the tongue of the Myrmidons, *i.e.* in Greek. Macer says only *Graeci*, line 1918. Daniel Arundel misunderstood the meaning of this line, taking *mirmidone* as referring to an alternate name for nightshade: 'mirmydon or mirmidona mirmidonius or mirmidonia maior' (fol. 84r). Perhaps Henry's knowledge of the Myrmidons came from Isidore's discussion of Greek peoples in *Etym.* 9. 2. 75.

12 This line is identical to Macer 1931.

5.1.8 YSATIS / Woad, *Isatis tinctoria* L.

Based closely on Macer, 'Gaisdo', lines 1766–73.

2 *tinctoribus*] Woad was the main source of blue dye in Europe until the early modern era, and is best known today as the blue paint supposedly applied by ancient British and Celtic warriors before battle.

4 This line, with the addition of *licet*, necessary for metre and sense, is identical to Macer 1769.

5 *decipit*] The sense seems to be more 'fail' than 'deceive'.

5.1.9 CYNOGLOSSA / Hound's-Tongue, *Cynoglossum officinale* L.

Henry addresses hound's-tongue directly. I have not found a source for this poem. It is not similar to Pseudo-Apuleius no. 97, 'Herba lingua canis' (pp. 175–6). Translated by Daniel Arundel as 'Cinoglossa' (fols. 67v–68r).

2 *certa salus*] Perhaps a sacrilegious play on Venantius Fortunatus's *Crux mihi certa salus*, but more likely recalling Martial, *Ep.* 2. 91. 1: 'Rerum certa salus, terrarum gloria, Caesar.'

2 *sic . . . sapientes*] Understand *uocant* for the subject *Greci sapientes*.

8 *dyacynoglossa*] A potion or electuary made out of *cynoglossa*. It is understandable that the scribe of *P* read *dyarnoglossa* at this point, having written it in its proper place just above in the poem on plantain (5.1.1, line 57). A recipe for 'Pilule cinoglosse' in the *Antidotarium Nicolai* (123), while probably composed after this herbal, is too similar to ignore as it includes most of Henry's ingredients: 'Recipe cinoglosse opii seminis iusquiami omnium trium an. ʒ .iiii. mirre trocliten ʒ .vi. olibani . ʒ .v. gariofilorum ʒ .ii. cinnamomi ʒ .ii. et cor. cubri ʒ .ii. temperentur cum rodostomate idest cum aqua rosarum.'

9 *Cf.* Ovid, *Met.* 4. 393: 'redolent murraeque crocique.'

11 *libani*] Variant of *olibanum* (*cf. Alphita*, 'libanum' and 'olibanum' and Hunt, 190–91), a name for the frankincense (*thus*) tree, *Boswellia thurifera* L. (poem 6.2.15).

11 Supply *uncias* or *unciolas* to *tres*.

12 See note to poem 5.1.1, line 59, about *lasar*.

13 *ana dimidiam*] *Ana* is a preposition meaning 'at the rate of' or 'in the amount of' (DMLBS, *s.v.* 'ana').

15–18 These four lines are preserved only in *D*. *P* is missing lines 15 and 17. It is more likely that the scribe of *P* or an earlier scribe skipped these lines than that the scribe of *D* added them.

5.1.10 LOLIVM / Cockle, *Agrostemma githago* L.

Based on Macer, 'Lolium,' lines 2015–28. Henry does not address the fact that cockle is harmful to food crops, as Macer does in line 2015: 'Frumentis nocuam Lolium Graecus vocat herbam.'

2 The remedy in this line is used for *cancros* and *pascentia vulnera* in Macer 2017–18, which ailments Henry has placed in his final line without any clear cure.

3 *zernas*] Acute impetigo (RMLWL, *s.v.* 'zerna').

5 The ingredient is 'quick sulphur' (*sulphure cum vivo*), or naturally occurring sulphur, in Macer 2020.

7–8 See poem 1.3, lines 20–22, above and the associated note.

8 *pariens*] An abbreviation of Macer's *parturiens mulier*, line 2027. It is not clear here or in Macer's version if this recipe is an abortifacient or an aid to live birth.

10 *ulcera . . . carnes*] Probably what are now called rodent ulcers.

5.1.11 CICVTA / Hemlock or Herb Bennet, *Conium maculatum* L.

An abbreviation of Macer, 'Cicuta,' lines 2029–55, less lines 2029–32 (stressing how deadly it is) and 2035–6 (lamenting Socrates' death). Translated by Daniel Additional as 'Benedicta' (fols. 26r–26v).

1–2 The first two lines are original to Henry and show that he was confused about hemlock or had a different plant in mind; no hemlock is safe to eat, even for strong English boys. (He may also be pulling the reader's leg, but his humour is usually more refined than that.) He may have understood one of many similar umbellifers like wild carrot or water parsnip, though the latter is also toxic.

3 *benedicta*] Henry adds that hemlock is also known as *herba benedicta*, or 'herb bennet' (Hunt, 81), which is not to be confused with avens, also called 'herb bennet' (treated above in poem 2.19).

4 The reading supplied by *P* is clearly wrong: 'Herba cicuta reos pre iure solebat Athenis.' Future manuscript discoveries may reveal how the scribe came up with *pre iure*. Perhaps it was a gloss to *pena*.

10 *epiforas* = *epiphoras*, an overflow of tears ususally caused by a blocked tear duct.

12–15 The Latin of this passage is awkward and possibly suspect. If the readings are correct, then Henry certainly slipped from his usual quality.

12 *Anasialus*] Anaxilaus (*cf.* Macer 2045 and Pliny 25.154), a Pythagorean physician and philosopher, banished from Rome in 28 BCE for practicing magic (EMA, 328). Choulant reveals in his note to line 2045 of Macer that none of his manuscripts actually read *Anaxilaus*, but rather gave names closer to Henry's *Anasialus*.

17 *amarus amor*] A common medieval pun, discussed by Jan M. Ziolkowski, '*Amaritudo mentis*: The Archpoet's interiorization and exteriorization of bitterness in its twelfth-century contexts,' in *Codierungen von Emotionen im Mittelalter*, ed. C. Stephen Jaeger and Ingrid Kasten (Berlin 2003), 98–111, at 107. *Cf.* Venantius Fortunatus, *Carmina* 3.23a, 12: 'nil cui subripuit carnis amarus amor' (*Venanti Honori Clementiani Fortunati Presbyteri Italici Opera Poetica*, ed. Friedrich Leo [Berlin 1881], 74), and Hans Walther, *Proverbia sententiaeque Latinitatis Medii Aevi. Lateinische Sprichwörter und Sentenzen des Mittelalters in alphabetischer Anordnung*, 6 vols (Göttingen 1963–9), nos. 2387 ('prodit amarus amor'), 10775 ('quam sit amarus amor'), 11058 ('amaro ... amori'), and 17235 ('si sit amarus amor').

21 *longis*] Assume *uerbis*. This line is identical to line 31 in the poem on periwinkle (1.23). While it may sound like a line original to Henry, it is a variation on Macer 2054, 'Singula cur memorem.'

22 *nocuos* ... *tumores*] Henry's source (Macer 2054) has *nocuum* ... *calorem* instead.

5.1.12 LAPPA / Cocklebur, *Xanthium spinosum* L.

Source unknown. While Hunt (154–5) identifies *lappa* as burdock (*Arctium lappa* L.) and lesser burdock (*Arctium minus* Bernh.), Henry seems to have treated both of those above in poems 1.18–19 under the names *beta maior* and *beta minor*. While it is certainly possible that one of those plants also fell under the name *lappa*, if we do assume that Henry intended a different plant, the clotbur or cocklebur seems most likely. This is supported by *Agnus Castus*, which says that 'Lappa is an herbe that men clepe burrus or clote' (173). The first two lines of Henry's poem are completely different in *D* and the third line is only in *D*. Could this be evidence of another redaction of the herbal, or merely of a scribe freely rewriting?

1–2 Calliope is the muse of epic poetry, and the idea that she should be singing about common herbs is probably intended to be humorous. Her presence ironically inspires the militant language in the following lines. While it is implied that she has sung or inspired the previous eleven poems, it is not clear in this instance why she would refuse to sing about *lappa*. These two lines are very different in *D*: 'Nunc igitur quoniam uulgares pandimus herbas / Lappa sit in medio, qua non uulgarior herba.' This is a paraphrase of Henry's lines (assuming those in *P* are the original), perhaps by a scribe who did not know who Calliope was or did not like the reference to her.

5 *porcinam . . . herbam*] One of the several plants called hogweed or pigweed. See the notes to poem 4.8, 'Ameos,' on giant hogweed.

7 *leuis*] I have translated this as 'trifling,' but perhaps Henry intended it to mean 'easy [to find]' or even 'cheap.'

5 <INTERLVDVM> / Interlude

This poem introduces us to the comic figure of the Cook, alluded to in poem 1.21, 'Petroselinum,' the first of two poems on parsley (the second is poem 5.2.5). Henry as Narrator gives up the narration of the following six poems (5.2.1–6) to the Cook, who is more knowledgeable about the medical uses of common kitchen vegetables. See the Introduction above, 12 and 14, for this poem's role in the herbal's structure.

1–2 The presence of Apollo, along with the metaphor of repaying a debt of one hundred things, has obvious echoes of Martial, *Ep.* 9. 102:

> Quadringentorum reddis mihi, Phoebe, tabellas:
>   centum da potius mutua, Phoebe, mihi.
> quaere alium cui te tam vano munere iactes
>   quod tibi non possum solvere, Phoebe meum est.

1 *monitu*] The admonition given in the Prologue to Book 5, lines 15–21.

1 *duodenas*] The twelve poems in Book 5, Part 1.

3 *prescriptis centum*] The one hundred herbs of books 1–4.

8 *inglorius*] A strange word in this context, and it is the best Rigg or I could make out of *inglōr*. *Cf.* Virgil, *Georgica* 4. 94: 'latam trahens inglorius alvum.'

12 *proth* = *proh* or *pro*. *Pro Iuppiter* was a common classical oath, and Henry probably learned it from Virgil, *Aeneid* 4. 590 ('flauentisque abscissa comas 'pro Iuppiter! ibit') or Ovid, *Met.* 13. 5 ('intendensque manus "agimus, pro Iuppiter!" inquit').

13–14 We have here a rare criticism of Henry's dependence on written authorities, which has prevented him from observing the common plants around him.

15–16 Possibly a parody of Job 34: 32–3: 'Si erravi, tu doce me; si iniquitatem locutus sum, ultra non addam. Numquid a te Deus expetit eam, quia displicuit tibi? Tu enim coepisti loqui, et non ego: quod si quid nosti melius, loquere.'

16 The *ecce* points not only to the following poems, but also, it seems, to a bed of vegetables in Henry's fictional garden, or even to a basket of vegetables in the theatre, since we have now left the garden proper and are sitting in its centre.

5.2.1 CEPA / Onion, *Allium cepa* L.

Based on Macer, 'Cepa,' lines 1087–1126, less 1097 (on the use of onions as a sleep aid) and 1123 (on their use for haemorrhoids). The cure for *glandes* in line 21 is not found in Macer.

3 *fellicis* = *fellitis*] Those with too much bile or gall (*fel*).

16 Using onions to cure stinking breath (*os fetens*) sounds like a bad joke, but this concept does come directly from Macer 1122: 'Oris foetori prosunt.'

17 *subito mutum*] Made mute by a disease, rather than since birth.

28 *Dyaschorides*] Latin Dioscorides, 'De cepulla' (10. 2, 229).

5.2.2 PORRVM / Leek, *Allium tricocum* L.

A condensed version of Macer's 'Porrum,' lines 507–48, less lines 515, 526–9 (a recipe for a potion made from leeks to aid the stomach) and 532–3 (a plaster of leeks and honey for wounds). *D* reproduces only lines 12–14.

4 Literally, this phrase says 'a head lamenting that it exists,' which is either a circuitous or intentionally humorous modification of Macer 542, who speaks merely of curing an 'immensum . . . dolorem' in the head.

6 Macer 538–9 adds mead (*mulsa*) to this remedy: 'Praestat idem pariter cum mulsa mixtus et auri / Infusus tepidus; fungis si manditur obstat.' Henry understood the mead to be included in the following remedy for *fungi*, which he has placed below in line 27.

7–11 Apart from the confusion in ingredients, this entire passage is awkwardly written and not of a quality typical of Henry's verses. For the passage to work grammatically, *porrum* and *unam* should be taken as the parallel objects of *iungas*, and *farine* and *dragmis* as those things in the dative to which they are respectively joined. Moreover, Macer's version (lines 512–14) does not call for all of these ingredients, but for only one of them: 'Cum galla dant hunc alii thurisve farina, / Aut geminis dragmis Porrorum seminis unam / Apponunt myrrhae, vino quoque trita resolvunt . . .'. Line 7, with the verb *iungas* on line 9, asks that leek be joined to 'incense flour' or 'powder of incense,' an odd ingredient, but it also appears in Macer 512: 'Cum galla dant hunc alii thurisve farina . . .'.

8 *ac*] Macer 513 has *aut* so that there are two separate, equivalent recipes rather than one, longer recipe.

10 *sistit*] Supply an infinitive verb such as *fluere* here.

11 *emoptoycis*] Henry did not think it necessary to define this word as Macer does in lines 510–11: 'Aegrotis, qui reiiciunt sputantve cruorem, / Quos haemoptoicos soliti sunt dicere Graeci . . .'.

22 *fracturas*] The reading in *P* of *iuncturas* could work ('it strengthens joints'), but Macer 545 reads 'fracturas solidat' and *iuncturas* seems more likely to be a scribal error than a change by Henry.

24 *nichilominus*] Henry adds this 'nevertheless' since he recognized leek's paradoxical and extraordinary ability (not remarked upon by Macer) both to close wounds and to keep them flowing, in order to clean out an ulcer.

5.2.3 CAVLIS / Cabbage, *Brassica oleracea* L.

This poem continues the Cook's recitation of medicinal vegetables. Based on Macer, 'Caulis,' lines 1201–63, less 1202–1203, 1207, and 1252. Henry, in the role of the Cook, adds lines 2, 4, 7, 26, and 34. *D* reproduces only sections of this poem (lines 12–13 and 31–4, then 35–40 and 45–54) within two separate poems titled 'De caule' (fol. 192r).

4 There seems no reason for Clio, the muse of history, to recall Cato's cabbage recipes, apart from the fact that we might see her as Henry's personal muse in his role as historian. The statements about Cato come from Macer's poem.

20 Macer 1219 specifies *tumores* rather than the more general *dolores*.

21 The appellation of *censor* to Cato is original to Henry, and is not found in Macer's herbal. Henry would not have known Cato's actual writings, but his position as imperial censor appears in several other works, such as the *De viris illustribus* of Pseudo-Aurelius Victor.

22 The statements about Chrysippus also come from Macer. See note above to Book 4, Epilogue 2, line 12, on Chrysippus.

24 Macer 1238 specifies *non scissum . . . alumen*.

34, 47 *probauit*] The Cook (or Henry) is concerned with providing suitable proof.

42 The *hec* is unnecessary and probably added just for the sake of metre.

44–54 Most of the recipes in this section which are attributed to *Mellicius* are still attributed to Chrysippus in Macer's version, except for the cabbage amulet in lines 46–7, which Macer 1262–3 does attribute to *Melicius*.

44 *Mellicius*] See note above to Book 4, Epilogue 2, line 16.

44 The final word (*oris*) is nearly illegible in *P*, the only exemplar for this line. The scribe knew he had made a mistake, and tried to fix it by crossing out the final letter and changing the penultimate letter. *Orsi* ('of the honeyed undertaking') is closest to what the manuscript has to offer, but *oris* seems more likely in this situation, and is also an echo of Book 4, Epilogue 2, line 16: 'quod melliti Mellicius oris.'

5.2.4 ATRIPLEX / Garden Orache, *Atriplex hortensis* L.

The first five lines are original to Henry. Lines 6–14 are based on Macer, 'Atriplex,' lines 947–56, though enlivened by their placement within the argument between Henry and the Cook. The arrangement of speakers in lines 1–5 is unclear. I have given most of the poem (lines 5–14) in the Cook's voice, but it could be Henry speaking, in an attempt to best the Cook on the subject of vegetables. In either case, the two characters are here reduced to playground name-calling.

1 *Ista* presumably refers to the information ('these things') in poems 5.2.1–3.

1–5 As should be expected, this passage is strongly reminiscent of passages from Martial's epigrams, particularly 8. 3, 11–12 ('Tune potes dulcis, ingrate, relinquere nugas? / Dic mihi, quid melius desidiosus ages?') and 13. 2, 4–5 ('non potes in nugas dicere plura meas / ipse ego quam dixi').

2 *latrasti*] The insult of barking like a dog is repeated below at 5.2.6, line 1.

7 The metre demands *aluum* instead of *uentrem*, the latter of which was probably an intruded gloss. See poem 5.1.2, line 19, for comparison.

5.2.5 PETROSILINVM / Parsley (no. 2), *Petroselinum crispum* (Mill.) Nyman

This is the second poem on parsley, the first appearing earlier at 1.21, and they are mirror images of each other. In the former, Henry was interrupted in his medical observations by Apollo, who summons the cooks (1.21, lines 15–16). This poem is started by the Cook, who includes parsley among his kitchen vegetables, but he provides medicinal antidotes, whereas Henry had given culinary recipes in the first poem on parsley (1.21, lines 18–32). The scribe of *P* has added a cross-referencing system to the poem: above each plant named in lines 17–20 is written the number of the folio on which that plant has its own poem. Portions of this poem, like in poem 5.2.4 above, could be repunctuated as a dialogue. It is difficult to tell who is speaking, particularly in lines 12–15. *D* reproduces lines 14–26.

1–2 As in the opening lines of the previous poem 5.2.4, this passage also echoes Martial, in this case, *Ep.* 11. 94, 1–2: 'Quod nimum lives nostris et ubique libellis / detrahis, ignosco.'

2 *nostre ... genti*] Perhaps the race of physicians or of poets, since Henry and the Cook, if he is indeed supposed to be Martial, are hardly of the same race or nation.

3 *apio*] Smallage or celery, treated above in poem 1.20, where it is paired with parsley's first poem at 1.21.

6 Perhaps Alexander Trallianus. See note to poem 4.19, line 5.

7 King Mithridates of Pontus was known for his fear of poisons and the antidote *Mithridatium* named after him. See the note to poem 1.10, lines 19–22.

8 The antidote *climax* (ladder), or 'Hermes' ladder,' is recorded by Lynn Thorndike, *A History of Magic and Experimental Science*, 8 vols (New York 1923–58), 2. 481, from the work of Gilbertus Anglicus (*ca* 1180–1250). With its sixty ingredients combined carefully in stages (*gradatim*), this antidote gives an indication of how much more complicated medieval recipes could be than the simples which make up most of this herbal.

9 *dyamargariton*] A compound made of pearls (*margaritae*), often ground into expensive wine. See also Constantine, *Liber de Remediorum et Aegritudinum Cognitione* (actually Johannes Afflacius, *Liber aureus*), in Constantine, *Constantini Africani ... Opera*, 1. 205, and Henry's poem on pearls in Black, 77–8.

10 This picks up the statement first made in poem 1.21, line 13: 'Hec solet antidotis, nec sepius ulla, reponi.'

11 *in solo selinon*] We must understand *uno* with *solo*: 'in one alone.' *Selinon* is given as the Greek name for celery/smallage (*apium*) in poem 1.20, line 9, though here it is a superior variety of parsley. Parsley and celery are closely related, so it may be that they were seen as the same plant in different strengths or exhibiting different qualities.

12 This line is especially problematic. I have followed Rigg's emendation of *inunctum* to *in uanum* and his reading of *g*[e] in *P* as *grece* seems logical, but this is a lot of conjecture. I would prefer *inunctum* ('the smeared/oily book'), but it does not scan. If *grece* is correct, we could read it as 'the little book in Greek' or 'gnaw Greekly/like a Greek.' The primary sense of the line is still clear: the Cook continues his abuse of Henry, who 'gnaws' on old books like a dog on a bone.

13 Most likely indebted to Ovid, *Ex Ponto* 1. 5. 15, 'Cum relego, scripsisse pudet,' and 4. 2. 3, 'nostros tacuisse libellos.'

14 *Dic michi*] A common phrase in classical verse, but here perhaps intentionally reminiscent of Horace, *Ars poetica* 141: 'Dic mihi, Musa, uirum ... .'

17–20 These twelve ingredients are all treated separately in their own poems: 1.21, 5.1.3, 4.23, 2.10, 3.9, 1.12, 1.20, 1.10, 2.16, 2.25, 3.20, and 3.2, respectively.

17 *aristologieque*] The scribe of *D* has glossed this word with 'plurale est,' presumably to indicate that it is not genitive.

24 I have opted for the reading in *D*, *nomina subicerem*, since it does not call for emendation, as does *uix subiunxissem* in *P* (see Rigg, 284).

26 *sidera gemmis*] An idea repeated below at poem 6.1.10, line 7.

5.2.6 ALLIVM / Garlic, *Allium sativum* L.

Based on Macer, 'Allium,' lines 161–95. Henry has curiously not included the qualities and degrees of garlic, found at Macer 162–3. Perhaps his character of the Cook is not expected to care about the more philosophical aspects of these vegetables. Henry may also have used Pliny, since the reference to him in line 21 is not from Macer but the information does appear in Pliny's primary discussion of garlic (20. 50–57). *D* reproduces only parts of the poem (lines 1–2, 5–6, 22–5, 30–31, and 33–7) and includes at the end two lines from poem 6.2.16, without any indication of a change. Most of the poem is in the voice of the 'Cook,' with whom Henry was arguing in the two previous poems. He insults Henry again (line 4) and turns the poem over to ancient authorities: Hippocrates in lines 5–17, Pythagoras in lines 18–23, Diocles in lines 24–9, and Macer in lines 30–36. Despite these attributions, all of this information is drawn directly from Macer who in turn was dependent on Pliny 20. 52–3 for the references to these Greek authors. The Cook ironically mocks Henry's habitual 'theft' of other authors' words (30–31) and finally gives his own thoughts on garlic's culinary uses (37–9). This poem and section of the book end in the voice of Henry as narrator as he teases the Cook but raises a forgiving glass to his efforts.

1 *latraui*] The Cook is echoing Henry's insult from 5.2.4, lines 2–3. If Henry is going to call him a dog, the Cook is willing to 'bark out' all he knows.

2–4 *allia*] Latin prefers the plural, while in English 'garlic' can be singular or plural, so I have translated *allia* . . . *allia* . . . *ista* in the singular.

7 Macer (lines 163–4) also includes scorpion stings in this cure.

17 *ipso*] Hippocrates (*Ypocras*) in line 5.

18–26 *Pittagoras*] This is most likely what Henry read and understood, but the equivalent line in Macer (180) reads Praxagoras, the name given in his source, Pliny 20. 52. Choulant notes that manuscripts of Macer provide many variants of each name, including *Praxagoras*.

21 Pliny 20. 53.

24–30 *Diocles*] Diocles of Carystus (*ca* 240–180 BCE), now known primarily as a geometer, though Pliny calls him a physician (21.61) and second only to Hippocrates in medical knowledge (26. 10).

27 *thenasmon* = *tenesmon*, a painful straining at bowel movement.

30 *Hec Diocles*] Written in *P* in a clear Gothic *textura* script and underlined, distinctly different from the usual *cursiva*.

41 This line contains mocking echoes of Psalm 64: 11 and Ezekiel 36: 30, in which *genimina* has positive connotations ('progeny'), as opposed to those verses with negative connotations (Matt. 23: 33, *genimina viperarum*).

6 <PROLOGVS LIBRI SEXTI> / Prologue of the Sixth Book

This poem is written in elegiac couplets, and serves as a medical gloss on Virgil's *Georgica* 2. 490, with which Henry begins the poem; he also begins the next poem (6.1.1, lines 1–2) with a modified quote from the *Georgica*. It is only here, towards the end of the herbal, that we get a glimpse of Henry's understanding of the value of medical learning. The happiest person is he who knows 'whatever will be the cause of health.' As noted in the Introduction above (55–6), Henry seems to be responding to contemporaries who disparage philosophy and the study of nature, or at least those who discourage the study of medicine as too worldly. Henry accepts that his skeptical audience might not want to heal others, but they have a duty to heal themselves (lines 3–4).

1 *Felix . . . causas*] Virgil, *Georgica* 2. 490.
2 *causa salutis erit*] Ovid, *Ex Ponto* 3. 9. 24.
5 *insanos*] A pun on 'unhealthy' and 'insane.'

6.1.1 PIPER / Pepper and Ginger:
1) Black Pepper, *Piper nigrum* L.
2) White Pepper, *Piper album* L.
3) Long Pepper, *Piper officinarum* L.
4) Ginger, *Zingiber officinale* Rosc.

Most of the poem is based on Macer, 'Piper,' lines 2056–85, less lines 2061–2 (a statement of pepper's qualities, *i.e.* dry and hot in the third degree) and 2083–5 (marvelling at how useful pepper is and how many recipes call for it). Macer also begins his poem with a statement that he is moving from herbs to spices, but most of Henry's lines 1–10 are original. The reader, he explains, is to study these spices all the more because they are so much more valuable than regular herbs (*graminibus*). Henry has also added an antidote not given by Macer, made from all three kinds of peppers (lines 28–35) and which he attributes to King Herod. Henry's lines 11–12 are based on Macer's shortest poem, 'Gingiber,' lines 2109–10, which therefore does not get its own poem in this herbal. Pepper also makes an appearance in Henry's Epigram 11.23, lines 43–4 (*HA* 796–802): 'Silua feras, Nereu pisces, piper India mitte: / His condita cibis uermibus esca placet.'

1–2 Imitation of Virgil, *Georgica* 4. 1–2: 'Protinus aerii mellis caelestia dona / exsequar: hanc etiam, Maecenas, adspice partem.' The reader of the herbal, therefore, has taken on the role of Maecenas, to whom Virgil addressed his *Georgica*.

4 *principio*] A normal word for beginning a new section, but it is probably again in imitation of Virgil, *Georgica* 4. 8: 'Principio sedes apibus statioque petenda . . .'.

8 Henry launches another attack on the Cook, despite the half-hearted apology at the end of poem 5.2.6, lines 40–41. Medicine and the kitchen are placed side by side in their praise of pepper, but the kitchen is clearly inferior as it is inhabited by the bibulous Cook. Henry undoubtedly has in mind Martial's passages on cooks and pepper: 'Sed cocus ingentem piperis consumet aceruum' (*Ep.* 7.27.7), 'o quam saepe petet vina piperque cocus' (13.13.2). The latter verse, from Martial's epigram on beets, seems to have influenced Henry's overall depiction of the Cook, who seeks out wine as often as he does savoury food.

16 *iecori*] Macer 2067 has *stomachi iecorisque*, which makes more sense, since in medieval medicine the liver does not digest food on its own; the stomach and liver work together.

18 *bachis*] From *baca*, a berry (thus, the bayberry) and not to be confused with Bacchus.

22 *periodica febris*] Probably the tertian or quartan ague.

26–27 An odd sentiment, suggesting that greater knowledge of the spice lessens its effectiveness. This statement recalls and perhaps pokes fun at the previous poem, in which the search for knowledge, particularly of medicine, is praised more highly than anywhere else in the herbal.

28–35 In his description of this antidote, Henry says that 'poetry abhors' it, *i.e.*, its name will not scan. However, he does give an alternate name, *confectio regis Herodis* (King Herod's Potion) in the final line. Henry was probably aware that the first syllable of *Herodes* scans long, but he was forced to scan it short to fit into his poem. It may also have been called *Herodium* or *Herodianum*, names difficult to put into verse.

6.1.2 MIRRA / Myrrh, *Balsamodendron myrrha* Nees

Based on Constantine's 'Myrrha' (359), from which also come the cures attributed to Flodius and Andromachus. The name of Dioscorides is not mentioned in Constantine's entry, but the cure attributed to him is. Latin Dioscorides mentions only *secunda* in 'De myris' (11. 55) and not *lumbrici* or *ascarides*. This could indicate that Henry believed he was reading Dioscorides, or that he merely added the name to lend authority to these cures. Lines 1–5 are original to Henry. At the base of fol. 39v of *P*, under line 3, a later hand has added: 'Mirra ita admodum auelani cum uino callido fetum mortuum expellit. Idem solet siccus perforare bibitus.' ('Myrrh, shaped like a hazelnut, with hot wine, thus expels a dead foetus. The same thing, when drunk dry [?], is apt to perforate [the stomach?].')

1 *Cf.* Matt. 2: 11, where the Magi give the Christ child myrrh, along with gold and frankincense.

3 See the previous poem 6.1.1, on pepper, for its inclusion in antidotes.

7 *Flodius*] This name is given as *Fledius* in Constantine's version. I have not discovered his identity.

8 Constantine indicates this plaster specifically for pains of the head.

12 *Andromachus*] Andromachus of Crete, a poet and imperial physician to Nero, 54–68 CE, and supposed inventor of the famous antidote *Theriaca Andromachi* (cf. Jerry Stannard and Peter Dilg, 'Camerarius' contributions to medicine and pharmacy: Observations on his *De Theriacis et Mithridateis Commentariolus*,' repr. in Jerry Stannard, *Pristina Medicamenta* [Aldershot 1999], Article 12, at 160–62).

17 *ascarides*] Parasitic worms of the intestine (possibly the giant intestinal roundworm, *Ascaris lumbricoides*), as opposed to *lumbrici*, which are found in the stomach.

22–23 Constantine specifies that these ingredients should be made into a pessary (*pessarium*).

6.1.3 SPICANARDVS / Spikenard, *Valeriana celtica* L.

Based mostly on Macer, 'Spica,' lines 2182–2203, less line 2184 (a cure for *iecur* and *dolor stomachi*). This poem is translated by Daniel Additional under 'Spiceceltica.' Line 3, extolling the odour of the spice, is original to Henry. The name *spicanardus* is given in the margin as the title, but is not used anywhere in the text. Henry has paired this aphrodisiacal spice (line 20) with the following aphrodisiac, cloves (poem 6.1.4, line 14), mentioning Venus in the last line of each poem. *Spica* can also refer to forms of lavender (*Lavandula* spp.), but the title in *P* indicates that spikenard itself was understood (at least by the scribe).

5 Henry adds this explanation of Celts and Gauls. Macer does not mention *Galli* or *gallica nardus*. *Cf.* Julius Caesar, *De bello Gallico* 1. 1: 'Gallia est omnis divisa in parte tres, quarum unam incolunt Belgae, aliam Aquitani, tertiam qui ipsorum lingua Celtae, nostra Galli appellantur.'

20 *infitiabilis* = *infitialis*] *Cf.* Ovid, *Ars amatoria* 2. 414: 'infitianda Venus.'

6.1.4 GARROFILVM / Cloves, *Syzygium aromaticum* (L.) Merrill & Perry

Based partly on Macer, 'Gariofilus,' lines 2141–6. Lines 1–2 and 9 are original to Henry. This poem is translated by EMA, 'Clowe gelofre.' Daniel Additional translates only the first two lines under 'Gariofilata.' He also mentions Henry in the much longer entry 'Gariofilus.' The same lines appear in Daniel Arundel under 'Garofilus.' The scansion of *garrofilum* is different from *gariofila* found at poem 1.5, line 12, above.

1 *gaudent reges*] *Cf.* Boethius, *De cons. phil.* 1 met. 5. 41: 'summos gaudet subdere reges.'

1–2 Versions of these lines are found in both manuscripts of Henry Daniel. As both suffer from confused Latin, I have not recorded their variants in the apparatus:

> Gariofilam gaudent reges imponere prel<is>.
> Gariofilum fauent summates ferre funeris.
> (Daniel Additional)

> Gayrofilam gaudent reges imponere prelis.
> Garofilum gaudent cines deferre crinu ouis.
> (Daniel Arundel)

In each manuscript the lines are also translated into English rhymes:

> It is plesaunt to kinges do gaurofle in her wyn.
> It is likyng to richemen bere garofle ther purses in.
> (Daniel Additional)

> Kyngys lovyn for to han gayrofle in here wyn,
> And other men lovyn for to bern clowys here bursys yn.
> (Daniel Arundel)

Henry Daniel's *prelis* seems more likely than *frenis* in *P*, which may have been a scribal emendation for the sake of a rhyme. Daniel's translation makes more sense than the Latin as he recorded it. The English verses may have existed independently.

5 *siccare, calere*] The original reading of *feruere calere* does not make sense, since they are synonyms, and because Macer 2141 gives *calidum siccumque*. In every other instance of *calere* in the herbal, it is paired with *siccare*, and I doubt this instance should be any different.

12 This line is drawn from a passage found in some manuscripts of Macer, but not included in Choulant's edition (*cf.* Macer, note to line 2143).

14 *Cincta Venus*] There is no way to make sense of *cuncta* in *P* except to read it as 'Venus entire', since it must be in the nominative of the feminine singular, or nominative or accusative of the neuter plural. Henry would be accustomed to his classical authors beginning a line of verse about Venus with a feminine adjective: Ovid, *Ars amatoria* 2. 397 (*laesa Venus*) and 3. 224 (*nuda Venus*); Virgil, *Aeneid* 10. 332 (*alma Venus*). Therefore, if we read it as *cincta*, then she could be seen as armed with *hac arte* (again echoing Ovid, *Ars amatoria* 1. 362 and 2. 480). If this is not what Henry intended, perhaps something describing the spice was intended. His source in Macer, lines 2144–5, reads: 'Accendit venerem si dragmae pondere tritum / Potatum fuerit cum vaccae lacte recenti . . .'. Something equivalent to *tritum* would give us an explicit subject for *bibatur*, but it is not like Henry to place only one word belonging to the preceding phrase on a new line.

6.1.5 CYNNAMA / Cinnamon, *Cinnamomum zeylanicum* Nees

Based on Macer, 'Cinnama', lines 2147–64. Lines 1–2 are original to Henry and rhyme. Since the scribe misinterpreted the name of the herb in the title and first line, I have used the spelling *cynnama* from line 13 in both places. *Timiama* or *tymiama*, as it appears in *P*, is a type of incense known from the Bible (*cf.* Exod. 30: 1). Henry has placed this poem and the following, 'Cassia', together, as these spices are almost identical in shape, taste and powers. In fact, most of today's cinnamon is actually the more common cassia bark. True cinnamon is much more expensive.

10 *tympana*] A type of dropsy called 'tambourine', in which the belly is stretched like the skin of a drum. It is described under the name *tympanites* by Constantine in his *Viaticum*, in *Constantini Africani . . . Opera*, 2. 100.

12 The disease in question is impetigo, which takes its name from *impetere* (see note to Macer line 2160), here given in the imperative 'attack!' *Cf.* Quintus Serenus, 155: 'Si uero uitium est quod ducit ab impete nomen'.

16 *P* provides only *Est preciosa magis* for this line, with a blank space following. This passage is based on the beginning and end of Macer's poem, lines 2147–9 and 2161:

> Cinnama tres species dicuntur habere, sed harum
> Est pretiosa magis, quae plus subtilis habetur
> Et quae plus mordet mixta dulcedine linguam . . . .
> . . . Grossa magis species fluxus haemorrhoidarum . . . .

If Henry ever finished writing this line, he probably rephrased elements from Macer's line 2149, producing something like: 'Est preciosa magis; linguam dulcedine mordet.' Otherwise, the phrase could be an intruded gloss on *subtilior* in the previous line.

19 *geminas . . . dragmas*] That is, of the spice cinnamon.

6.1.6 CASSIA / Cassia, *Cinnamomum cassia* Blume

Henry differentiates between *cassia* and *cassia fistula*, and throughout the poem he alternates between cures containing one or the other. The latter does not seem to be the modern *Cassia fistula*, the golden shower tree, but rather *fistula* is the fruit and *lignea* the branch of the one cassia plant. This poem is based on two entries in Constantine, 'Cassia fistula' (346–7) and 'Cassia lignea' (369), and is one of the more impressive examples of Henry reworking and rethinking his source. The reference to Galen comes from Constantine's 'Cassia fistula' and the citations of Cleopatra and Dioscorides come from his 'Cassia lignea.' The cure for cheek sores (*apostema bucce*) in line 17 is in neither of Constantine's entries. Though Constantine places *Cassia fistula* in the third grade of hot and dry, Henry places it in the second for those qualities (line 2). Lines 1–3 are translated by Daniel Additional in 'Cassia' (fols. 168r–168v). Daniel Arundel translates the whole poem under 'Cassia fistula' (fols. 60v–61r). See pages 45–6 of the Introduction for more on Henry's composition of this poem.

6 According to Constantine, Galen approved of *cassia fistula* because of its equal composition (*temperies*) of all four qualities: 'Vnde Galenus: Medicina temperata aequali compositioni uel complexioni similis, neque in calidum, neque in frigidum et humidum et siccum potest iudicari.' In this aspect of *temperies*, cassia is just like liquorice, described below in poem 6.1.11 as also possessing a level composition of qualities.

7 A large space is left between *confortat* and *sterasque* in *P*. Constantine reads: 'Stomachum, epar, uulnera, et omnia principalia membra confortat' (369). The *epar* has become *iecur*, and Henry may have supplied *steras* by reading *uulua* for *uulnera*, which leaves us lacking a cure for the stomach. Daniel Arundel (fol. 60v) translates Henry's lines 7–8, 'Cassia if it usid it conforteþ þe lyvere and þe stomac and þe matrice and alle þe principal menbris in man.' If Daniel's translation is trustworthy, the missing word is equivalent to 'stomac,' but *stomachum*, *aluum*, and *uentrem* will not scan unless the terminal *m* in either of the latter two is elided.

11 *apozimate*] From *apozima*, a salve made from an herb.

12 *sanguinis . . . uim . . . diram*] Perhaps Henry means that cassia will stop a wound from bleeding, or that it will assist an excessively sanguine person.

21 *stringni* = *strigni*, or nightshade, called *maurella* by Henry in poem 5.1.7. This spelling also appears in Constantine's 'Cassia fistula,' 347.

24–27 Most of our modern cinnamon is actually the more common cassia bark, a similarity not unnoticed in the past. *Cleopatra* here must be scanned long-short-short-long, a very different scansion from that of *Cleopatra* below at poem 6.2.5, line 17.

25 *Dyascoride*] Henry's immediate source was Constantine, but the Latin Dioscorides does say this: 'duplici pondere pro cinnamomum in antidotis intrat. est uero utilis in omnibus' (1. 62).

27 *summus*] The emendation is based on the translation of this line in Daniel Arundel (fol. 61r): 'Boþyn þey arn soveryn auctores; folwh whom þu wilt; þus He(nricus).'

6.1.7 GALANGA / Galangal, *Alpinia officinarum* Hance.

Based on Macer, 'Galanga,' lines 2125–30, less line 2127, which gives a remedy against trapped windiness. The absence of Galenic qualities in this poem is also found in Macer, who for some reason did not copy them (hot and dry in the third degree) from his source, Constantine, 'Galanga' (372). Henry's lines 1–4 are original. Galangal is an odoriferous root related to ginger. *Galanga* is a neuter noun, hence *sumptum* in line 7 and the emendation to *hoc* in line 8.

10 *indecorem*] Employed in the same metrical position by Virgil, *Aeneid* 11. 845: 'non tamen indecorem tua te regina reliquit.'

10 *stillando*] The meaning is unclear. Perhaps galangal, taken in liquid drops, was considered an aphrodisiac.

6.1.8 ZEDVAR / Zedoary, *Curcuma zedoaria* Roscoe

Closely based on Macer, 'Zedoar,' lines 2131–40. This poem, like the previous on *galanga*, is lacking a statement of the plant's qualities. Also like the previous poem, this lack is due to copying Macer who did not take the qualities (hot in the third degree and dry in the first) from his source Constantine, 'Zedoar' (374).

1 *at*] In response to the previous poem 6.1.7 in which *galanga* treats primarily an overly phlegmatic stomach.

6 *infectam . . . saliuam*] Saliva that has been thoroughly mixed with the juice of masticated *zeduar*.

6.1.9 CIMINVM / Cumin, *Cuminum cyminum* L.

Based on Macer, 'Cyminum,' lines 2111–24. Henry has added the introduction (lines 1–4), the information on pepper (lines 5 and 7), and the classical quotes (lines 21–3). Both *ciminum* and *cuminum* were acceptable spellings, but the former seems to have been more common in the Middle Ages.

5 *piper*] Henry does not actually give pepper's powers in its poem, 6.1.1.

9 *emoptoicos*] Macer's equivalent line (2118) gives the cure for *orthopnoicis*, but Choulant notes that several manucripts give *haemopticis*, which is the version Henry must have known.

19 *mulsa*] In Henry's source, Macer 2123, the recipe calls for *pusca*, vinegar-water.

22 Cumin was long believed to bring whiteness to the face, hence 'bloodless cumin.' *Cf.* Horace, *Epistulae* 1. 19. 17–18: 'Decipit exemplar vitiis imitabile; quod si / Pallerem casu, biberent exangue cuminum.' The idea that hot cumin could bring pallor to a face was a matter of debate for scholars of the High Middle Ages. The *Prose Salernitan Question* no. B 281 (*ca* 1200) brings up this problem: 'Quare ciminum cum sit calidum et humidum hominem eo utentem palidum reddat?' (*The Prose Salernitan Questions*, ed. Brian Lawn [London 1979], 135–6). Note, however, that the Salernitan *quaestio* says cumin is hot and moist, while Macer and Henry define it as hot and dry.

23 Not Ovid, but Persius, *Satira* 5. 55: 'rugosum piper et pallentis grana cimini.'

6.1.10 CEROTON / ? Carob, *Ceratonia siliqua* L.

Source unknown. This could be the carob seedpod (*Ceratonia siliqua* L.), a Mediterranean shrub. It was known in Greek as κεϱάτιον. If this identification is correct, perhaps the division into red and pale varieties refers to the dry and green forms of the seedpod, since it does not grow in the colours described. This identification can only be conjectural until Henry's source is found. It is clear Henry is not discussing *cerotum*, a wax plaster common in early medieval Latin medical works, particularly the *Medicina Plinii* (see note to poem 4.11, line 10) and the *Physica Plinii Bambergensis (Cod. Bamb. med. 2, fol. 93v–232r)*, ed. Önnerfors. *Ceroton* could otherwise be a variation on several other plant names: 1) *chironius*, for elecampane (*s.v.* DMLBS); 2) *carota*, for the carrot; or 3) *caryota*, the Syrian date, which appears in works familiar to Henry (Martial, *Ep.* 8. 33. 11 and 11. 31. 10; Statius, *Siluae* 1. 6. 20). None of these plants fit Henry's description, for here *ceroton* is some kind of plant which comes in a bitter, red variety of India (line 4) and a pale (*subalba*, line 5) variety grown in Arabian gardens. This description, with its separation into pale and red varieties, suggests the cherry and its sweeter pale and sour red varieties, so *ceroton* is a plausible misreading of *cerasus*, but it is clear that Henry knew the normal spelling (*cerasum* at poem 2.8, line 3). Rufinus quotes a 'Magister Salernus' in his entry on Cerasa: 'Hec cerasa non purgant sanguine sed pernecant lumbricos' (88). This agrees with Henry's line 19, but there were countless medieval cures for *lumbrici*. Given the fact that Henry discusses no other fruiting trees in his herbal, cherry seems less likely than carob.

1 *genus . . . diuersificatum*] In the context of a medieval medical work, this sort of language sounds positively Aristotelian, but it is unlikely Henry had read any of Aristotle's works, even of the Old Logic available in Latin translation. A more likely source for this sort of language is Boethius's translation of the *Isagoge* of Porphyry (in *Categoriarum supplementa: Porphyrii Isagoge translatio Boethii et anonymi fragmentum vulgo vocatum "Liber sex principiorum"*, ed. L. Minio-Paluello [Bruges 1966]), or possibly Isidore, *Etym.* 1. 37. 12: 'Eo enim et per speciem genus, et per genus species demonstratur.'

5 *nitentibus ortis*] *Cf.* Ovid, *Fasti* 5. 11. 543: 'Latona nitentibus astris.' The similarity of phrasing could be considered mere coincidence, if it were not for the fact that Diana and her stars appear in both poems.

7 *Latonia*] An epithet of Diana (adjectival form of Lato, mother of Apollo and Diana), personifying the moon.

7 *sidera gemmis*] An echo of poem 5.2.5, line 26, above.

8 *uiole rosulis*] To keep up the pattern of superiority, *rosulae uiolis* would be expected here.

8 *saliuncis*] The name *saliunca* was given to several plants (Hunt, 225–6). The translators of Pliny (21. 43) and Dioscorides (1. 8) identify it as Celtic nard (*Valeriana celtica* L.). Henry probably intended the wild nard mentioned by Virgil, *Ecloga* 5. 16–17: 'Lenta salix quantum pallenti cedit oliuae, / puniceis humilis quantum saliunca rosetis.' Both Virgil and Henry consider 'humble *saliunca*' of little worth when compared to stars, gems, roses and violets. However, in most of the bilingual plant lists recorded by Tony Hunt in *Teaching and Learning Latin in Thirteenth-Century England*, 3 vols (Cambridge 1991), 3. 142, *saliunca* is glossed with the Middle English *calketroppe* or its variants. This old spelling of 'caltrop' was used for a variety of thistle, which might make more sense in this case than a variety of nard, which could be valued as much as roses and violets.

15 *costo*] Used adjectivally with *oleo*. *Costino* would be expected.

16 *typum*] A medical term for the onset or appearance of the distinct character of a fever, *i.e.* tertian, quartan. Since Henry says *typum febris*, he cannot mean *typus* as a specific kind of fever, as used by Isidore, *Etym.* 4. 7. 10.

20 *amarus amor*] See note to poem 5.1.11, line 17.

6.1.11 LIQVIRICIA / Liquorice, *Glycyrrhiza glabra* L.

Based on Constantine's 'Liquiritia' (347). There are at least fourteen species in the liquorice family whose roots are used for food and medicine. Any one of them could be intended here. *Glycyrrhiza glabra* L. is the most common variety in western Europe (Grieve, 'Liquorice'). Henry allows liquorice to speak for herself in lines 7–20. This section is translated by EMA, 'Liquorice' (192–3), where the translator has taken the speech out of the first person, except for line 7: 'I am your helth, hastely come ȝe to me.'

3–6 Liquorice, like cassia above (poem 6.1.6), was remarkable to medieval physicians for its equal composition (*temperies*) of all four Galenic qualities. These lines seem to be an expansion of and even a challenge to Constantine's description of liquorice: 'Liquiritia temperati caloris est. Minus tamen quam calor naturalis. Humectat moderate, habet aliquantulum dulcedinis . . .'. Constantine places liquorice under the first grade, but Henry denies that it deserves even this: 'it cannot be even of the first degree.' Henry may have received this notion of *temperies* not from contemporary philosophical writings, but from Ovid, *Met.* 1. 51, where *temperies* is the balance between hot and cold in the habitable regions of the newly-formed earth: 'temperiemque dedit mixta cum frigore flamma.'

7 *Sum uestra salus*] *Cf.* Augustine, *Confessions* 1. 5: 'Dic animae meae: salus tua ego sum.'

7 *properate, uenite*] *Cf.* Isaiah 55: 1, 'O omnes sitientes venite ad aquas et qui non habetis argentum properate . . .'.

14 *chylum*] Classically, the juice of any plant, but Henry takes *chylum* specifically as liquorice juice. The Basel edition of Constantine appears to be in error at this point: 'Cocta in aqua cum recens fuerit, et succus extractus ab ea ac desiccatus, succus liquiritiae uocatur.' I believe that *succus liquiritiae* was originally a gloss to *chylum*, the word read by Henry, which word dropped out of the manuscripts of Constantine used in the edition.

17 *instrumentis*] *Instrumentum* (*s.v.* RMLWL) typically refers to a musical instrument, usually one with pipes, so the *instrumenta pulmonis et pectoris* are, by analogy, the trachea and bronchial tubes.

19 *costus eructans*] 'Belching cost.' The virtue of cost to cause belching (or vomiting) is transferred to the herb as an epithet. There is, however, no indication of this ability in Henry's poems on cost (1.16) and English cost (1.17).

19 *fremiscens*] A variant of *fremesco* ('to shudder,' *s.v.* DMLBS). Like cost in this same line, aloe is given an epithet according to its primary virtue or side effect: it causes shaking (*fremiscens*). It could be an error for *tremescens*. In either case, the effect of shuddering or shaking is not found in Henry's poem on aloe, 6.1.12, or his source, Macer 2233–69.

6.1.12 ALOE / Aloe, *Aloe vera* L.

Based closely on Macer, 'Aloë,' lines 2233–69. The first line and the last two are original to Henry. The last line provides the best evidence that the books 1–4 were composed independently of the second half of *Anglicanus ortus* and viewed at times as a separate work.

1–2 *corpore toto regnat*] The use of the *regnat* with the ablative is not classical, but this does seem to mean 'rules over the whole body' rather than 'rules with the whole body.'

8–10 These lines are problematic and seem unfinished. Henry's source, Macer 2244–6, reads: 'Si solvatur aqua, iuvat apostema labrorum / Et naris superappositum, nec non oculorum / Livoremque fugat, sic circa lumina factum.' Macer clearly outlines two effects of aloe as *iuvat apostema* and *fugat livorem*, but Henry has only the one verb *turpat*, which a scribe used to replace the more sensible *purgat*. More difficult to reconcile is *dolor*, which is clearly wrong: it is short in the first syllable and thus cannot scan in this position (Henry uses it properly everywhere else) and, moreover, it needs to be in the accusative. What is more, *dolor* is not in Macer, where *apostema* afflicts lips, nose and eyes. Everything suggests that *dolor* needs to be replaced, but I cannot say by what.

29 Macer (line 2265) is clearer: 'Vix unquam capitis vexabitur ille dolore.'

32 *uolunt*] The subject is not given, but is presumably *medici* or the *autores* named in line 34.

32 *geminans* = *geminatus*

33 *Dyagridium* is the juice of scammony, described below in poem 6.2.19.

35 Macer 2234–5 adds the information that the red variety looks like liver on the inside and is thus called 'liverish': 'Intus sicut hepar cum frangitur, haec epatite / Dicitur . . .'.

37 It is not clear why Henry makes this reference to his poem on pellitory, 3.18. The only similarity I can find is that pellitory comes in two varieties (an herb and a spice) which are equally efficacious, similar to aloe with its red and black varieties.

38 *ille liber*] Books 1–4 of this work. See the Introduction above, 12–13, on this passage.

6 <INTERLVDVM> / Interlude

This is the second interlude of the herbal, introducing the final section of the work (Book 6, Part 2) which is dedicated solely to exotic spices of the East. These poems are based primarily on the *Liber graduum* of Constantine the African. See the Introduction above, 18–19, for a discussion of this poem's function in the *Anglicanus ortus*. This poem also introduces an incongruous and satirical sexuality to the work. The language used to describe the old man, perhaps Apollo (Rigg, 286) or Constantine (Black, 66–7), seems intentionally sexual. He is described as *uerendus*, 'awesome'; *uerenda* was a euphemism for the sex organs. The poet immediately draws our eyes down the old man's beard to his genitals (*pubetenus*), reinforcing the *double entendre* on *uerendus*. Then we see him 'fondling' (*contrectans*) his beard, a word used for sexual groping or intercourse. It is not clear why Henry would portray his interlocutor in this manner. It certainly sets the scene in a comic tone, just as was done with the Cook in Book 5, though in an admittedly cruder fashion. The final two lines suggest that this new character is going to narrate the rest of the herbal (poems 6.2.1–28), though there is no clear evidence of conversation in the rest of the work as there was between Henry and the Cook in Book 5, Part 2.

1 *Finieram*] *Cf.* Martial, *Ep.* 8. 3. 9 ('Finieram, cum sic respondit') or Ovid, *Met.* 2. 103 ('Finierat monitus').

4 *signum . . . docendi*] Tugging one's beard might be expected of a venerable teacher.

5 *duodenas*] The twelve spices whose virtues Henry has just declaimed (poems 6.1.1–12).

8 *gente Crisippi*] Perhaps meaning all Greeks, philosophers in general, or specifically Chrysippus's students interested in medicine. See the note to Book 4, Epilogue 2, line 12, on Chrysippus.

11 *harum . . . aliarum*] Spices, namely the first twelve of Book 6, and the following twenty-eight (6.2.1–28), which are apparently related by the old man.

12 *Ille sub hec*] *Cf.* Virgil, *Aeneid* 5. 394, and Statius, *Thebaid* 3. 516.

12 *Arabs . . . Serus et Yndus*] It is not clear if Henry intends specific authors by these titles. They may simply be examples of eastern wise men, or foreign peoples known for medical knowledge. These lines may be indebted to Isidore, *Etym.* 17. 8. 1, 'aromata sunt quaeque fragrantis odoris India uel Arabia mittit.' The reference to three eastern peoples is very similar to those found in a pair of Isidore's poems (*Isidori Hispalensis Versus* xix and xx, ed. José María Sánchez Martín, Corpus Christianorum Series Latina 113A [Turnhout 2000], 229, 231):

> Quidquid Arabs aris, quidquid fert Indus odoris,
>   Quidquid et Ionii peruenit unda maris . . . (xix, 1–2)
>
> Hic odorata iacent hic spirant cinnama tura,
>   Quaeque serunt Seres quaeque Sabaea feret. (xx)

13 *eos*] Referring to plural Arabs. *Arabs* in line 12 is singular, but can refer to a single Arab or to all the people of Arabia.

6.2.1 BALSAMVM / Balm of Gilead, *Commiphora opobalsamum* L.

Based on Constantine's 'Balsamus,' 356–7. *Balsamum* is the gum of the balsam tree (Hunt, 45), which provides three separate ingredients: *carpobalsama* (line

16) is the seed, *xilobalsama* (line 22) is the branch and *balsamum* (lines 1–15) is the gum or juice. In Constantine's words: 'Cuius lignum, xylobalsamum, semen carpobalsamum, liquor balsamus dicitur.' Henry elaborates on this differentiation in the final lines (29–31). The corrections made in lines 22, 24 and 29–31 (*xilo* for *silo*) appear to be in a different, but contemporary, hand.

10 *Membri natiui*] The genitals. *Natiuus* here has the sense of 'natal,' concerned with reproduction.

11 A verb like *pellit* must be understood to govern *abortum siue secundas*.

12 *epitimatus*] A verbal form of *epithima*, a lotion. The word must be understood as a fourth-declension noun (*i.e.*, 'a lotioning') for the sake of the metre.

14 *peragorisat*] 'It soothes' (RMLWL, *s.v.* 'paregoricus').

15 *aquas*] Presumably water containing camphor or a distillation of it.

16 *carpobalsama*] Hunt (71) has identified this as wall germander (*Teucrium chamedrys* L.), which is clearly not correct.

17 *ortomia*] A variation on *orthopnoia*, modern orthopnoea. See note to poem 1.24, line 9 on *ortopnoicis*. Constantine uses *orthomia* in his entry 'Dactyli' (only in Isaac Israeli, *Opera omnia Ysaac* [Lyons 1515], 2. 79r), where it could refer to a different disease than orthopnoea.

21 If this line was written by Henry, and is not merely an intruded gloss, a typical conclusion might be '. . . nam multa ualet.'

26–28 This description of the abundance of gum is found in Constantine (and attributed to Dioscorides) but there is no mention of the time during which it should be done. 'When the sun holds burning Cancer and Leo' indicates high summer, middle or late July, when the sun is on the cusp between Cancer and Leo. *Cf.* Boethius, *De cons. phil.* 1 met. 6, 1–2: 'Cum Phoebi radiis graue / Cancri sidus inaestuat . . .'.

29–31 *Gutta* is not gout, as in most instances in the herbal, but a variant of *gumma*. The final lines are highly abbreviated, and it is necessary to supply verbs to understand the final line.

6.2.2 AGARICVM / Field Mushroom, *Agaricus campestris* L., or family *Agaricaceae* L.

Based on Constantine's 'Agaricus,' 346, though Dioscorides and Oribasius are not mentioned by him. The poem has similarities to one of the *spuria Macri*, 'Agaricus,' published by F. A. Reuss in *Walafridi Strabi hortulus Carmen ad cod. ms veterumque editionum fidem recensitum, lectionis varietate notisque instructum* . . . (Würzburg 1834), 91–105: no. 62 (repr. *Der deutsche 'Macer.' Vulgatfassung mit einem Abdruck des lateinischen Macer Floridus 'De viribus herbarum'*, ed. Bernhard Schnell with William Crossgrove [Tübingen 2003], 476). That poem is based on Constantine's account, rather than on Henry's poem. Daniel

Arundel says at the end of his passage on 'Agaric' (fols. 3v–4r) that 'Henricus Anglicus seyþ þe same' as Macer, but this is not true; he perhaps considered the spurious version to be genuine Macer. *Agaricum* could apply to any of the nearly five thousand gill-bearing fungi. We can probably narrow this down to the thousand or so of the well-known 'mushroom' type found in Britain, most of which are not poisonous. If we can assume one of the more common and edible varieties is discussed here, it is probably the field mushroom (*Agaricus campestris*) or the button mushroom (*Agaricus bisporus*).

3 *Hoc Dyaschorides*] Latin Dioscorides, 'De agaricu', 10. 375, is somewhat similar.

3 *Oribasius*] Referring to Oribasius, 'De Agarico', 4. 3.

8 *inquit magnus*] The transposition is necessary for the metre.

9 *opilata* = *oppilata*. This and its variant *opilatio* are consistently spelled with one *p* in the herbal.

10 *epilenticus*] A common medieval variant of *epilepticus* (*s.v.* DMLBS, 'epilepsia').

12 *philosophus*] Apparently the title given by Henry to Constantine, who ends his passage on 'Agaricus' with 'Curat etiam omnem dolorem qui est intra corpus.' Perhaps Henry thought he was reading Aristotle?

14 Henry is playing with the gender of the words here: though *agaricum* is neuter, one variety is masculine (*hic mas*) and the other feminine (*hec femina*).

15 The sense of *integer* is not clear. Constantine (346) says of the male variety only 'Masculus vero rotundus intrinsecus lenis.' Perhaps Henry misread *intrinsecus* or had another reading in his copy of Constantine.

15 *leuis*] Constantine gives *lenis* (346), though this could easily be the error of the early printed edition. Henry clearly understood *leuis* ('light'), as he compares it to the *grauis* female variety in the next line.

6.2.3 AMOMVM / Bastard Cardamom, *Amomum xanthoides* Wal.

Based on Constantine, 'Amomum', 376. Lines 1–4 and 10 are original. This *amomum* is not the *amomum* glossed as 'poppy' in a late English manuscript (Hunt, 21). Note the internal and end rhymes in the first four lines.

1 *mirabile*] The reading of *iocunde* in *P* does not scan and is probably an intruded gloss.

1 *fraglat* = *fragrat*

10 *que . . . referre*] It is tempting to add an *est* after *longum* ('and it is lengthy to relate these many things'), which could elide, but the phrase still makes sense without a finite verb.

6.2.4 STORAX / Gum Tree, *Liquidambar orientalis* Mill.

An abbreviation of Constantine's 'Styrax' (351). Although the marginal title is given as *storax*, both instances of *storace* in lines 1 and 9 are genitive, indicating that Henry may have believed that the nominative was *storaca*.

2 *Sigia* is the sap of the gum tree, also called *sagia* (Rufinus, 307).

2 *calamitam*] A synonym for *storax* (DMLBS, *s.v.* 'calamita' no. 2), not to be confused with *calaminta* or *calamenthum*, calamint (*Calamintha officinalis* Moench). Constantine calls this *calamenthum* which may be an error on his part, or that of a scribe or printer.

4 Henry has returned to the singular, perhaps for the sake of the metre, and because the two varieties can be treated as the one *storax*.

8 *pectus*] Constantine does not specify a cure for chests, but merely says that 'styrax calefacit.' But since most of the cures attributed to Dioscorides in this section treat conditions of the chest and throat, Henry probably assumed he meant the chest.

6.2.5 MASTIX / Mastic, *Pistacia lentiscus* L.

Based on Constantine's 'De Mastice' (354). Mastic is the dried resin of a shrubby member of the pistachio family (*Pistacia atlantica* L.). All of the authors cited by Henry appear in Constantine's entry except for Oribasius, to whom the cures in lines 1–9 are credited. Mastic, chewing gum's ancestor, is named from the fact that it can be masticated. The name refers only to the gum of the tree. The tree itself was called *Lentiscus* in the Middle Ages (*cf.* line 19 and Hunt, 158).

7 The emendation from *effectus* ('effects') to *affectus* ('moods') is based on Constantine's 'Malas quoque cogitationes aufert.'

7 *medicatus* = *medicina*

9 *bis*] Constantine does not ask for the ointment to be applied twice.

12 *Iohannes Damascenus*] Not St John of Damascus, but the medieval name for either Mesue the Elder (Abū Zakariyā Yūhannā ibn Māsawayh, d. 857), a Christian physician in Baghdad (or, more rarely, for Mesue the Younger, 924–1015, another Arab physician). Mesue the Elder was best known in the medieval West for a Latin translation of 132 medical aphorisms: Yūhannā ibn Māsawayh, *Le Livre des axiomes médicaux (Aphorismi)*, édition du texte arabe et des versions latines avec traduction française et lexique, Danielle Jacquart and Gérard Troupeau (Geneva; Paris 1980). It is doubtful that Henry knew Mesue's writings, but rather knew only the name from Constantine.

16 Henry's *tumidis* is probably from *tumentibus*, found only in Constantine, *Opera omnia Ysaac*, 2. 81r, not in *Constantini Africani . . . Opera*, 354.

17 The scansion of *Cleopatra* here is different from that in 'Cassia,' poem 6.1.6, line 24.

18 *gutta* = *gumma*. See note to poem 6.2.1, line 29.

19 *lenticii*] For *lentiscus* (mastic tree). Not to be confused with *lentitia*, 'stickiness.'

19 *pinee*] *Pinea* has replaced the classical *pinus*.

19 The words *eque aut* must elide for this line to scan properly.

19 *cipressi*] For *cupressus*, the cypress tree, *Cupressus* spp.

6.2.6 ANISVM / Anise, *Pimpinella anisum* L.

Based on Constantine, 'Anisum' (376), though with a creative twist on its aphrodisiacal properties (line 11). In the final line the 'winged boy' (Cupid) has given Love's darts (*spicula*) to anise, thus making it an aphrodisiac. Constantine simply says of it 'libidinem excitat.' Medieval *anisum* is most likely the same as today's anise (Grieve, 'Anise'). The marginal title is given as *Anisium*, but I have supplied the standard spelling here.

1 For the feminine *gratissima* and genitive *anisi* to make sense, we need to understand a feminine noun, most likely *species* with *anisi*. Classically, the second syllable of *anisum* was long, but Henry scans it short.

2 There seems to be an error here on Henry's part or the scribe's, since the manuscript reads *feruet dumque calescit*, both of which express heating. As *feruet* usually appears with *siccat* and Constantine reads 'Anisum calidum et siccum in tertio gradu,' I have emended to *siccat*.

5 It is awkward for all four objects to share the verb *confert*. Usually Henry says that a medication *dat lac* and *deducat* or *prouocat locium* and *menstrua*.

8 *reuma* = *rheuma*

11 *puer ales*] Cupid, the 'winged boy.' *Cf.* Horace, *Odes* 3. 12. 4.

11 *spicula*] This refers both to Cupid's darts and to the sharp little seeds of the anise plant.

6.2.7 GENCIANA / Gentian, family *Gentianaceae* L.

Based on Constantine, 'Gentiana' (367). This is also similar to the poem 'Gentiana,' another one of the *spuria Macri* (like 'Agaricus,' discussed in the commentary to poem 6.2.2 above) in *Walafridi Strabi hortulus*, ed. Reuss, 101–105: no. 62 (repr. in *Der deutsche 'Macer'*, ed. Schnell and Crossgrove, 476). Lines 1–4 are original to Henry, though it is not clear in what work Hippocrates (*Ypocras*) denies the efficacy of gentian. The gentian family has about 180 members (Grieve, 'Gentians'), so it is possible that this poem and 2.22, 'Basilisca,' both refer to some kind of gentian. *Circa instans*, as cited by Rufinus (147), notes that 'Gentiana dicitur etiam basilica' (this passage is not in the Venice 1497 edition used elsewhere in this work). *Basilisca* may have been intended.

1–2 Henry (as the Old Man) asks forgiveness for placing gentian in his verses, since *genciana* (scanned long-short-long in its first three syllables) cannot fit in hexameter verse.

1 *Da ueniam* is a common plea in classical texts, but Henry probably knew it best from Ovid, in *Heroides* 4. 156; *Ars amatoria* 2. 38; or *Met.* 11. 132.

3 *opes et opus*] A popular alliteration in classical verse, but Henry may have known this exact phrase from Hildebert of Lavardin, *Carmina Minora* (ed. Scott), *carm.* 46, line 9: 'in te fudit opes, et opus mirabile cernens.'

3 *sollers medicina*] *Cf.* Julius Firmicus Maternus, *Mathesis* 4. 19 (ed. Pierre Monat, 3 vols [Paris 1992–7], 2. 183): 'istas ualetudines uel praesidium dei alicuius uel sollers medicina curabit.'

4 *experiencia fallit*] A teasing reference to Hippocrates' *Aphorisms* which, in the new Latin translation of the twelfth century, begins, 'Vita brevis, ars vero longa, tempus autem acutum, experimentum vero fallax . . .'.

5 Constantine specifies *duobus scrupulis* of this potion.

10 *pellit abortum*] This is how Henry adapted Constantine's 'mortuum foetum expellit' and gives the best indication of how we should read the often vague and difficult word *abortum*. See the note above to poem 1.9, line 20.

6.2.8 EVFORBIVM / Spurge, probably *Euphorbia resinifera* Berg.

Based on Constantine's 'Euphorbium' (381). 'Euphorbia' could apply to any one of the more than three thousand species in the spurge family, Euphorbiaceae.

2 The pun on *species speciosis* is lost in English.

7 *bdellius*] Neuter, *bdellium*; described in its own poem 6.2.21, below.

9 *Hoc*] The reading of *hec* in *P* is possible, since Henry often switches his subject to an implied feminine singular *species*, but since *hoc* is used in the next line and clearly must be correct there (*mixtum*), the original reading in this line is probably an error.

12 As this line appears in the manuscript, it will not scan. The scribe may have rearranged it to fit *sciam*, a misreading of *sciasim* (a marginal note indicates that this cure is for *sciasi*). A serious rearrangement was necessary.

12 *aromaticis*] An abbreviation for *aromaticis potionibus* in Constantine, which alters the meaning somewhat. 'Aromatics' could refer to nearly any odoriferous ingredient and not just potions.

13–14 Henry may have misread his source, or had a faulty manuscript, for the passage in question does not mention the stomach (*uentrem*), but rather 'ueterem allopeciam curat' (Constantine, 381). Constantine also specifies 'oleo ueteri, aut laurino oleo,' rather than just *oleo*.

6.2.9 FOLIVM / Malabathrum, *Cinnamomum nitidum* Blume

Based on Constantine's 'De folio' (in *Opera omnia Ysaac*, 2. 81r, erroneously called 'Lolium' in the Basel edition, 361). Line 2 is original to Henry. *Folium* is short for *folium malabathri*, the aromatic leaf of a number of cinnamon varietals, probably *Cinnamomum nitidum*, also known as Japanese cinnamon. *Cf. Laud Herbal*, no. 1053: 'Malabatrum .i. folium de India.' Given its powerful scent (line 2), it could also be the patchouli plant (*Pogostemon patchouli* Pell.). The author of *Circa instans* also calls it 'folium paradisii' (fol. 203r). Daniel Additional names Henry in his passage on 'Mabatematicon' (fol. 197r) but claims incorrectly that Henry says 'it is ious of agnus castus.'

2 *inter odoriferas*] *Cf.* Venantius Fortunatus, 'Ad domnam Radigundem,' 7: 'Inter odoriferas tamen has quas misimus herbas . . .'.

3 *Hec*] Assume *species* rather than the neuter *folium*.

6 *Celtica nardus* is a type of spikenard, mentioned as *celtica spica* in Macer's poem on spikenard, line 2200. *Circa instans* also equates the two: 'Celticam dixit Galienus illius nature esse cuius est spica et illius actionis' (fol. 195v). Under 'Malabatrum' *Circa instans* gives this substitution: 'loco eius ponimus gariofil. vel spica nardi' (fol. 203r). The Latin Dioscorides notes that many mistake *folium* for *spicaenardi* (1. 61).

6.2.10 CARDAMOMVM / Cardamom, *Elettaria cardamomum* L.

Based on Constantine's 'Cardamomum' (347). There are two kinds of the sweet-smelling cardamom, one large and one small; the larger variety is not as effective for heating but has a stronger odour. Constantine has a second entry for a spice of this name (372), in which he says 'Cardamomum syluestre carui est.' This entry did not influence Henry's poem.

1 This line is a reply to line 2 of the previous poem 6.2.9, in which praises are also sung for *folium*.

3 *utraque*] Henry has made the common switch to an implied feminine *species* in order to preserve the metre.

5 *quoque* = *quantoque*

5 *calida*] Describing the feminine *species*, or perhaps *virtus*, rather than neuter *cardamomum*.

6 Constantine specifies *cholericum uomitum*.

7 *Aloes lignum* is not from the aloe plant, but is an incense derived from a

tropical Malayan tree, *Aquilaria agallocha* Roxb., still often called the lignum aloe or aloeswood (Grieve, 'Aloes'). It appears in many other medical texts (*e.g. Circa instans*, fol. 186v), so the absence of a poem dedicated to it in the *Anglicanus ortus* is surprising.

8 Constantine specifies *phlegmaticum uomitum*.

11 *ructura*] An adjectival form of *ructus*, belching. Cardamom was used primarily for digestive problems, as it was believed to bring out excess gas.

6.2.11 REV / Rhubarb, *Rheum rhaponticum* L.

Based on Constantine, 'Rheum' (354).

1 *Pontus*] In general, any sea, but often specifically the Black Sea (in full, *Pontus Euxinus*).

2 Henry has reversed Constantine's statement that 'Rheum tamen Indiae laudabilius.'

2 *primo*] This description differs from Constantine's classification of rhubarb, which is placed in the second degree for both hot and dry (354).

5 Constantine gives a remedy specifically for 'hypochondriorum extensionem.'

6 This line, as given in *P*, is clearly incomplete and corrupt: 'Hoc singultus hanelitus minatur.' Constantine's original passage reads: 'Anhelitum, singultum, uulnera intestinorum, diuturnam solutionem, et prolixam febrem amputat.' The cure for fever is given in line 7 and Constantine's *solutio* is probably interpreted as *dissinteria* in line 8. This leaves us with the *uulnera intestinorum* as the only missing cure. As Henry often simplifies the maladies and remedies from his source, it is plausible that he would shorten 'intestinal wounds' to 'wounds.' For example, Henry's cure for *ypocondria* comes from Constantine's 'hypochondriorum extensionem curat.' As for the loss of *inde*, the numerous minims found in the abbreviation of *inde* followed by *iuuantur* could be misconstrued as *minatur*. I am grateful to A. G. Rigg for the last suggestion.

6.2.12 EPITIMVM / Dodder of Thyme, *Cuscuta epithymum* L.

Based, incorrectly, on Constantine, 'Thymum' (368) and not on the previous entry 'Epithymum' (368). Translated by Daniel Arundel as 'Epithimus.'

1 *quarto*] Both *epithymum* and *thymum* are classified by Constantine as hot and dry in the third degree. If the degree was written in Roman numerals, it could easily have been misread or transcribed incorrectly.

2 A word or two is needed in the middle of this line to complete it metrically (scanning long-long or short-short-long). I am tempted to add *purgat*, which would lead into the following phrase, but no space is provided by the scribe and *Cum* is written with a majuscule C of the type usually given only at the start of the line by this scribe. Perhaps this indicates that this line was originally two separate lines and we are missing the second half of each, although there is nothing missing here from Constantine's entry 'Thymum,' unless there was further confusion between entries and Henry brought in information about another plant.

6.2.13 SAGAPINVM / Sagapenum, *Ferula persica* Willd.

Sagapenum is a resinous gum made from the root of *Ferula persica* (*s.v.* 'Sagapenum,' *The British Pharmaceutical Codex* [London 1907–73]). This poem is based on most of Constantine's 'Sagapinum,' 373 (it is not in the Lyons 1515 edition). Classically, the plant was known as *sacopenium* or *sagapenon*.

4 Henry has cleverly modified Constantine's statement that 'frigiditatem stomachi et uuluae extirpat,' essentially saying the same thing, but in reverse.

7 *exagium*] A weight or measure (DMLBS, *s.v.* 'exagium' no. 2) of unknown quantity. EMA, after translating a selection of Henry's poems, adds a brief paragraph on weights and measures, saying 'Exagius and solidus ben al one, but þe name is dyuerse' (200).

11 *Galbanum* and *opopanace* (= *opoponax*) are aromatic and medicinal gums similar to sagapenum. This line is also in Constantine's 'Sagapinum': 'Eodem modo ualet opopanax et galbanum.' On *opoponax*, see note to poem 5.1.1, line 59.

6.2.14 SQVINANTVM / Lemongrass, *Cymbopogon citratus* L.

Based on Constantine, 'Squinantum' (372).

7 A space has been left by the scribe between *uuluam* and *lapidesque*. Since Constantine says at this point 'epar et renes et uuluam mundificat, lapides frangit,' it is likely Henry also used the verb *frangit*.

6.2.15 THVS / Frankincense, *Boswellia thurifera* L.

This is the final poem in the *Anglicanus ortus* based on Macer's *De viribus herbarum*, in this case an abbreviation of his 'Thus,' lines 2204–32, without lines 2212 (a cure for an earache), 2213 (more ingredients for soothing breasts, mentioned by Henry in his line 7), 2224–6 (containing further comments on lines 2220–23, which Henry adapts in his lines 10–12), 2230 (for pain in the tongue), and 2232 (a plaster for burnt limbs). Medieval Europe would most likely know *thus* only as the odoriferous resin of the frankincense tree, which is native along the coast of the Red Sea (Grieve, 'Frankincense'). Poems 6.2.15–17 form a cohesive unit. In the following poem sea-onion (*squilla*) is defined in terms of frankincense (6.2.16, 1) and in the next, ser-mountain (*siler*) is compared to sea-onion (6.2.17, 2).

2 *odore beato*] While *thus* was almost synonymous with 'blessed odour,' Henry may have had in mind one of the many Biblical passages featuring it, *e.g.* Exod. 30: 34; Lev. 2: 1–2, 15–16; Eccles. 50: 8–9.

10 Macer 2220 calls not just for an egg, but 'lacrymumque albuminis ovi.'

15 *anate*] The use of *anata* in place of the usual *anas, -tis* is recorded in Anglo-Saxon glossaries (DMLBS, *s.v.* 'anata'). Henry may have been using the local Anglo-Latin for the sake of metre.

16 *panaria*] Not breadbaskets, but a truncation of *panaritia* in Macer 2210 (= *panaricium*), the condition of painful fingertips and extremities resulting from cold. One manuscript of Macer used by Choulant also reads *panaria* at this point (cf. Macer 2210 and note). Henry scans *panaria* with the first two syllables long, like *panarium* ('breadbasket'), whereas *panaricium* is properly scanned short in the first syllable.

6.2.16 SQVILLA / Sea-Onion, *Urginea scilla* Steinheil

Based on Constantine's 'Scilla' (362), though with some interesting variations: Henry's cure for cracked feet (line 6) calls for oil and reed (*oleo cannaque*), where Constantine calls for myrtle oil: 'Cataplasmatum cum oleo myrtino pedum fissuras curat.' Constantine also adds two sentences of warning against a deadly variety of *scilla* which grows in fields. *D* reproduces only the last two lines of this poem, including them at the end of 'De alliis' (fol. 192v).

1 *gradu quo thus manet*] Hot and dry in the second degree (from the previous poem 6.2.15, line 1).

1 *Humida spargit* ('scatters moisture') is an elusive way of saying that sea-onion dries (*siccat*) like *thus*. However, *humida spargit* seems to be synonymous with *aret* ('it is parched'), leaving us without sea-onion's second quality of heat, stated by Constantine (362), unless Henry understood *aret* to mean 'is hot.'

4 *uiscosa*] We probably should assume *flegmata*, which is often called *uiscosa* by Henry.

6 *canna*] Some manner of reed, of the genus *Calamus* L.

6.2.17 SILER / Sermountain, *Laserpitium siler* L.

The third poem on a series of three plants (poems 6.2.15–17) which are all hot and dry in the second degree, this is based on Constantine, 'Seseleon' (364), although without his remedies for menstruation and suffocation of the womb. *Siler* is not the brook willow given in classical dictionaries, but most likely sermountain (shortened from *siler montanum*). For identification of *siler* Hunt (238) cites *Circa instans*, 'Siseleos sive siler montanum,' and André identifies 'siler montanum' (*q.v.*) as *Seseli tortuosum* L., another umbellifer. Henry supplies *siler* above in other recipes, poem 3.11, line 50, and 6.1.1, line 33 (the first taken from Macer line 65). Sermountain is one of the rarer umbellifers, similar to parsley, producing a large seed with a sharp flavour. *Siler* is mentioned by Virgil (*Georgica* 2. 9. 12) and is identified by Holt Parker as staveacre or lousewort (*Delphinium staphisagria* L.), a member of the larkspur family: 'Vergil's mysterious *siler*: A possible identification from a lousy clue,' *The Classical Quarterly* 56 (2006), 623–9. While Parker may be correct about Virgil's use of *siler*, there is consensus about the medieval identification.

2 *Stat quo squilla gradu*] The sea-onion's grades are hot and dry in the second degree, so the sermountain's are as well. Henry is referring to the previous poem 6.2.16, line 1, which in turn refers back to poem 6.2.15, line 1.

5 *Pergendo*] A strangely vague word in this instance. Perhaps *purgando* was intended, but this still makes sense grammatically.

6.2.18 DRAGAGANTVS / Gum Tragacanth, *Astragalus gummifer* Labill.

Henry's poem is an abbreviation of Constantine, 'Dragagantum' (360–61), but not of the other 'Dragagantum' (383). 'Tragacanth' usually refers only to the gum produced by this small, thorny shrub (Grieve, 'Tragacanth'). This poem and the following three (6.2.19–21) all treat resinous gums.

1 *dragagantus*] I have retained the masculine declension of the spice, and changed the spelling of the title, since Henry uses masculine adjectives in lines 4–6.

2 *duri*] Understand *casus* or *morbi*, or it could be referring to any sort of hardened swelling.

6.2.19 DIAGRIDIVM / Scammony, *Convulvulus scammonia* L.

Source unknown. *Diagridium* is the juice extracted from the plant scammony. The *Alphita* says of it 'diagridium, scamonia idem; succus est cujusdam herbe in transmarinis paritbus nascentis' (50). Henry believes *diagridium* comes from *titimallus*, which seems to have been a comprehensive term for many succulent plants (Hunt, 252). Latin Dioscorides does say in 'De scamonia et diagridiu' that 'multi uero et sucu titimalli admiscunt [*recte* admiscent] ei' (11. 82), a passage which may have been confused in Henry's source. See also Rufinus, 'Scamonea' (288–9), who says that *diagridium* is only the juice of the herb. Constantine, however, does not say where it comes from ('Diagridium,' 369), and there is little similarity between his entry and this poem. Scammony is a variety of bindweed (family Convulvulaceae) long used in medicine (Grieve, 'Bindweeds'). The identification of *diagridium* with scammony is supported by Rufinus who, quoting Alexander (Trallianus?), says that 'Scamonea alio nomine dicitur diagridium, calidum et siccum' (288).

1 The second syllable of *quantum* must elide for this line to scan.

3 *feri . . . titimalli*] Any one of a number of succulent plants, usually spurge or houseleek (Hunt, 252). Henry has misunderstood the source of *diagridium*, saying that it comes from *titimallus*. This line seems to come from Latin Dioscorides, 'Multi uero et sucu titimalli admiscunt [*recte* admiscent] ei' (11. 82), where two separate plants are understood.

5 The first *ista* refers to the antidotes and the second to *res* (= scammony).

6.2.20 AMONIACVM / Gum Ammoniac, *Dorema ammoniacum* D. Don.

An abbreviation of Constantine, 'Amoniacum' (375). Ammoniacum, or gum ammoniac, is the resin gathered from the stem of the flowering ammoniacum plant (Grieve, 'Ammoniacum'). It is still considered a valuable expectorant, to which Henry attests (line 2). The scribe of *D* has added a note at the base of the page: 'Nota de amoniaco—Hic in presenti, non prius.' It is not clear to what this note refers.

4 Constantine specifies one dram of *amoniacum* in this recipe.

6 For Constantine, these *apostema* are specifically 'in neruis et articulis nascentia.'

6.2.21 BDELLIVM / Bdellium, *Commiphora africana* A. Rich.

Based on Constantine, 'Bdellium' (359). Galen is not mentioned in either printed version of Constantine. Henry may have added the reference to Galen (line 7) himself, or his copy of Constantine's *Liber graduum* included it. Bdellium is not the betel nut, but rather a resinous gum similar to myrrh. It is mentioned in the Bible (Gen. 2: 12–13, Num. 11: 7).

4, 6 Feminine *hec* refers to *species*, which is necessary to agree with *superuncta* in lines 3 and 5 and *commixta* in line 6.

4 *Sed* has the sense of *et* here.

5 *crepituram*] Constantine has *crepatura* ('fissure, crack') but *crepitura* could also be an alternative for *crepitus* ('creaking noise'), both from *crepo*. In the latter case, the word can mean 'farting,' but since the recipe calls for rubbing on an ointment, it seems more likely that Constantine and Henry both intended the word to mean some sort of cracking in the skin.

7 Note the bawdy pun on *testes* and *teste*.

6.2.22 ACORVS / Yellow Flag, *Iris pseudoacorus* L.

Based on Constantine, 'Acorus' (355). *Circa instans* says, 'Acorus radix est gladioli qui non tantum in humidis locis sed etiam in marinis et siccis crescit' (fol. 188v). Sweet flag (also known as sweet sedge) or yellow flag, marsh-dwelling members of the iris (gladiola) family, would fit this description. See also Hunt's entry on *acorus* (6). Assuming that Henry's poem 6.2.28, 'Calamus aromaticus,' treats sweet sedge, this is probably its close relative yellow flag.

6 Instead of rhubarb (*reu*) and cumin, Constantine suggests cloves and cumin: 'Pro eo uero poni potest, par pondus et dimidium fustium gariophyllorum aut cymini aequali pondere.'

6 *semis*] Henry has taken *semis* as an indeclinable noun.

6.2.23 CAMPHORA / Camphor, *Cinnamomum camphora* T. Nees & Eberm.

Based on Constantine, 'Camphora' (370). Its anti-aphrodisiacal powers are summed up in the popular Salernitan adage 'Camphora per nares castrat odore mares' (Rufinus, 63).

2 *digna deis*] *Cf.* Juvenal, *Satires* 12. 114: 'tantis digna deis.'

5 *Venus infitiabilis*] The same phrase is used above at poem 6.1.3, line 20. *Cf.* Ovid, *Ars amatoria* 2. 414: 'infitianda Venus.'

6 *quarto*] Constantine places camphor in the third grade, which could easily be misread if written in Roman numerals.

8–9 *caniciem properam*] *Cf.* Godfrey of Winchester, *Epigrammata* 134. 1: 'Praeproperam tibi canitiem, Tite, plangis adesse.' The tone of sad familiarity with grey hair suggests that Henry himself suffered from it and knew well that girls found it displeasing ('fit res ingrata puellis').

8 *assuefacta*] An odd word in this context which Henry must have learned from Constantine, who uses it twice in his entry on camphor: 'Eius tamen odor assuefactus libidinem extinguit: bibita uero melius operatur. Porro assuefacta caniciem uenire festinat . . .'.

6.2.24 NVX MVSCATA / Nutmeg, *Myristica fragrans* Houtt.

Based on Constantine, 'Nux muscata' (355). The reference to Galen comes from Constantine's entry. Henry does not include Constantine's explanation that mace (*macis*) is the rind found around a nutmeg nut. Translated by EMA as 'Notemuge' (193) and by Daniel Arundel in 'Careon' (fol. 59r). EMA adds a cure for gout not found in Henry: 'This wole ouer-come þe gowte maisterly, and, as it is seid, it wole close wondes faire.' The editor of EMA notes that this line is written in red ink (193 n18); it is most likely a later addition and not from Henry's herbal.

6.2.25 NITRVM / Soda or Natron (sodium carbonate, Na_2CO_3)

A dramatic abbreviation of Constantine, 'Nitrum,' 384, which runs fifteen sentences in the printed version. *Nitrum* (natron or soda) is not an herb, but a mineral, usually hydrated sodium carbonate, but also saltpetre (potassium nitrate). It was a standard ingredient in *materia medica*. Constantine does not provide qualities or degrees for *nitrum*, so neither does Henry.

2 *oculos albos*] Cataracts, apparently.

4 *Nerui* are usually tendons or sinews in a limb, but in the context of the *stomachum* (stomach or esophagus) they could be the surrounding muscles or ligaments.

6.2.26 THIMVS / Garden Thyme, *Thymus vulgaris* L.

This poem is not based on Constantine's 'Thymum' (368), which Henry used incorrectly as the basis for his poem on dodder of thyme, above at 6.2.12, 'Epitimum.' Unfortunately, there is little similarity between this poem and Constantine's entry 'Epithymum' (368), found immediately before 'Thymum.' However, it does appear that the two entries 'Thymum' and 'Epithymum' were somehow confused in Henry's manuscript of the *Liber graduum*, for most of Henry's lines 5–6 seem to be based on the last sentence of Constantine's 'Epithymum': 'Sed tamen quia epithymum angustiam generat et sitim, cum amygdaleo iungatur, neque subtiliter puluerizetur.' It is not clear where Henry found these degrees for *thimus*, since Constantine says that both *epithymum* and *thymum* are hot and dry in the third degree. Gargilius Martialis (no. 36, 'De thymo') says that thyme is hot and dry, but without giving the degree, and the rest of his passage is quite different. Henry's poem has little similarity to Latin Dioscorides, 'De tymo' (10. 394), but it is similar to several passages in Marcellus of Bordeaux, though that is probably not the direct source. Marcellus gives thyme alone as an excellent stomach remedy (17.7). He also provides a recipe for curing kidney and bladder pains (26. 94) which may come from the same tradition as Henry's poem, though the only common ingredients are *thymum* and *apium* which often appear together in Marcellus's work. Even closer is Marcellus's recipe for curing intestinal pains with the following ingredients: 'ex ruta et puleio, apio, origano, aneso, daucio, thymo, hysopo, panace, dictamno, anetho' (30. 42). Rufinus quotes one 'Alexander' (actually the *Antidotarium Nicolai*), saying that *thimum* is hot and dry, but in the third degree (315).

4 Classically *quapropter* is scanned short on the first syllable, but here and above at poem 6.2.21, line 2, Henry scans all three syllables as long.

4 *dant*] *D* gives *daucum* (carrot) here instead of the verb, which no longer scans, but does give an interesting modification to the recipe.

4 *selinon*] Another name for smallage (see poem 1.20, 'Apium'). In every other occurrence in this work *selinon* is scanned short-short-long, so another syllable is needed before *anisum*.

5 *amigdaleon*] A plaster made of ground almonds and vinegar.

5 *morphea*] Any of a variety of skin diseases (DMLBS, *s.v.* 'morphea' no. 2) characterized by discolored spots and moles; called 'morphew' in Middle English. Constantine mentions that ashwood cures *morphea* ('Fraxinus,' only in the Lyons 1515 edition, 2. 79r).

6.2.27 ANACARDVS / Marking Nut, *Anacardium orientale* L.

Based on Constantine, 'Anacardi' (382). The description of the antidote comes from another source. The better-known member of the Anacardiaceae family today is the eminently edible cashew (*Anacardium occidentale*), a native of Brazil. The *Anacardus* of medieval herbals is the marking nut, or anacard, whose poisonous nature most herbalists mention, though Henry does not.

2–3 The 'precious antidote' is *Theodoriton anacardinum* (in the *Antidotarium Nicolai*, 155, and Rufinus, 25). See the note on *theodoricon* above for poem 1.19, lines 7–8.

5 This line provides a rare instance of Henry not eliding from a terminal 'm' to a vowel: *letargum acerbum*.

5–6 *Cf.* Dioscorides: 'litargicos iuvant et mentem revocant et memoriam; frigus nervorum calefaciunt' (as cited by Rufinus, 25).

7 *solus*] An emendation from *soluit* in *P*, necessary to make sense of the *sed* and to reflect Henry's source better. Constantine says of *anacardi*, 'Soli tamen accepti, mortem aut lepram inferunt. Oportet ergo ut cum aliis odoriferis speciebus tribuantur.'

6.2.28 CALAMVS AROMATICVS / Sweet Sedge, *Acorus calamus* L.

Based on Constantine, 'Calamus aromaticus' (357), without several of his cures. Lines 1–4 and 12–15 are original to Henry. Daniel Additional says 'Henri þe same' in his passage on 'Calamus' (fol. 166v), though Henry's information is rather different from what Daniel provides. Daniel Arundel translates Henry's lines 6–12 under 'Calamus aromaticus.'

3 *plerus*] Another word or two is needed here to complete the metre and possibly help the sense. Something like *plerumque* is expected (though that does not scan): 'for the same reason, we will often call the spice splendid.' It is also tempting to provide a word ending in *-am* to replace *ob idem*, to complete a rhyme at the caesura and end of lines 3–4.

4 *possunt carmina*] *Cf.* Ovid, *Met.* 7. 167: 'quid enim non carmina possunt.'

8–9 The *temperies*, or the equal and temperate commingling of Aristotelian qualities, was a valuable attribute of certain plants (usually Eastern spices) which made them applicable for more remedies in more patients, and thus more valuable to the apothecary and physician.

13 *condignum*] It is not clear who the speaker is at this point or to what or whom *condignum* refers. Henry may have taken the narration back from the Old Man after line 12, in which case *condignum* refers to him. Conversely, the Old Man could still be speaking and thus *condignum* refers to Henry or to the plant.

6 <EPILOGVS> / Epilogue

The final poem of Book 6 is also the final poem of the entire herbal in six books. Books 7 and 8 apparently treated gems and stones (see the Introduction above, 9–10 and 19n61). Henry says that 160 herbs and spices have been surveyed and discussed, which provides the justification for including the squirting cucumber and vine mentioned in Book 4, Epilogue 1 among the counted herbs of the garden. This poem is placed after the scribe's colophon in *P*: 'Explicit hoc opus finitum per manus Martini de Tissnow scriptum in Humpolecz anno domini 1443° feria quinta ante festum Nicolai.'

1 *eoas species*] Although it is a later work, compare Johannes de Hauvilla, *Architrenius* 2. 245 (ed. Winthrop Wetherbee [Cambridge 1994], 44): 'Itur ad Eoas species . . .'.

4 *baldemonia dicet*] Poem 1.5, line 2, on baldmoney, explains that Henry comes from England: 'Anglia te speciem, me reddidit Anglia uatem.'

5 *carpe rosas*] Perhaps reminiscent of Strabo's poem on the rose, *Hortulus*, l. 422: 'Bello carpe rosas, laeta arripe lilia pace.' Henry's poem 2.10 on the rose

gives Henry's own name (2.10, line 41: 'Vis Henrice, tibi ius?'), but does not explicitly say for whom he wrote it, unless it is dedicated to Erato.

6 *titulum*] For a discussion of the possible candidates for a title, see the Introduction above, 11–12.

Appendix

Exceptiones de libro Henrici

Oxford, Bodleian Library, MS Digby 13, fols. 89v, 91r–92v (= *O*)

The *Exceptiones de libro Henrici*, or 'Excerpts from Henry's Book,' is a collection of short prose entries abbreviated from poems in books 1–4 of Henry of Huntingdon's *Anglicanus ortus*. The manuscript dates from the late twelfth century, making the *Exceptiones* the earliest witness to Henry's medical works. They are found in the manuscript immediately after a poor copy of the herbal of Macer Floridus on fols. 58v–89v. Given that the scribe of the manuscript shows no awareness of books 5–8 of the *Anglicanus ortus*, he may have used a manuscript similar to the one available to the scribe of *S*, Sloane 3468, which also witnesses only books 1–4. Some similarities in spellings between the Digby and Sloane herbals support this hypothesis. The *Exceptiones* are found in two separate sections of the manuscript. The first section is on fol. 89v and contains only three entries, drawn solely from Henry's Book 1. The second section is much longer, containing fifty separate entries from poems in books 1–4 of the *Anglicanus ortus*. The original three plants on fol. 89v are repeated, with longer entries, in the second section. Between these two sections are nine herbal poems, apparently intended by the scribe as companion pieces to the previous herbal of Macer. They belong neither to the herbal of Macer nor to that of Henry. Eight of these nine poems are also found in the later collection of herbal poems in manuscript *T* (Cambridge, Trinity College, MS O. 9. 10 [James no. 1422], fols. 89r–108r), which also includes poems by Macer and Henry.

In the diplomatic edition below, the italicized passages are those which are identical, or nearly so, to Henry's original. The notes indicate the lines of verse from which these excerpts were taken, along with occasional notes on grammar, spelling, and the transcription. I have made minor changes to the text where needed and indicated editorial suppressions and additions with square and angle brackets, respectively. Those lines used by the Digby Excerptor for his entries are given in the apparatus of the respective entries above.

{89vb}
...<P>aruinca est herba immo dicta quod alias uincat. Hec uincit guttam.[1]

Baldemonia est species sicce et frigide nature. Hec comesta cordis, pectoris, stomachi dolores curat. *Cor sanat, pectus releuat, stomachum refocillat.*[2]

Ambrosia herba que tantum cruoris potata tollit, quantum de ipsa bibitur.[3]

{91ra} Exceptiones de libro Henrici
Ozima uel basilea uel basilico est herba foliis rute similis, thuri odore, saluie flore, celidonie lacte. Contra letiferam potionem hausta ualet.[4]

Crocus messe surgit, uere cedit i<bi> hoc basilee contraria. Huius flores lacti muliebri commisce: qua mixta, diu seruata, oculos patientes superunge et multum proderit. Item contra letiferam potionem sicut basilea ualet. Item admisce ei thus et nigellam et hoc in mulsa coque et sciasim superponendo curabit. Picture etiam apta est ut medicine.[5]

Laureola est herba sic dicta quia lauro est similis, tamen in multis, tamen quia semper uiret. Cuius semen Persius coconidion dixit. Hinc optima fit potio que intima purgans per inferiora, et lenis est et non periculosa.[6]

Baldemonia feruida et sicca licet in palude oriatur que frigida est et humida. Cor sa{91rb}nat a dolore quolibet, pectus releuat, stomacum confortat. Solo morsu facit quod gingiber gariofilum piretrum cinnama, nam quod agunt empte facit hec inuenta palude, quodque datur pretiis, dat baldemonia gratis.[7]

Ambrosia pulcris ordinibus discernitur. Tantum demit cruoris quantum inde potatur.[8]

Origanum calidum et siccum in tertio gradu. Lacti coniunctum et in aures infusum dolorem extirpat. Naribus infusum cruorem prodire coget ṣi

---

1 1.23, 28–9
2 1.5, 6, 10
3 1.6, 8–9
4 1.2, 1–3, 15
5 1.3, 9–10, 14–15, 17–22, 24
6 1.4, 1–2, 8, 10–11
7 1.5, 14–15
8 1.6, 1, 8–9

iungitur iri. *Ore diu tentum plagis medicabitur oris, dente diu tritum denti medicabitur egro. Fauces et tumidas siccando comprimit uuas.* Puluis eius *cum melle tussim pellit. Cum calida morsus stomachi lenit, urine prodest,* lumbricos pellit. Omnibus interioribus ualet potata. Cum farris polline coxe appositum sciasim fugat uel opprimit. Fugat ydropisim et tumorem. Cum mulsa pondere oxifabi sumptum coleram nigram purgat. Deducit menstrua bibitum uel tritum uel coctum suffumigatum. *Albo cum uino dat ne digestio tardet. Pruritus, acoras, maculas,* elixatura eius delet. Si carice iuncta bibatur, sudorem eicit. *Luxatis uel contusis superaddita membris lana repleta prius oleo iunctis et aceto,* succis eius. Decoctio ipsius in uino frequenti potu *mortiferos morsus* fugat. Cum mulsa potatur aconita.[9] De succo eius et cepis et rossiriaco confectio talis ad solem in ere ponitur Phebo ente in Leone. Sic .xiiii. diebus feruere. Exinde subdita lecto non patitur nocuum accedere.[10]

Lauandula, herba odorifera unde et libris et uestibus imponi aptissima.[11]

Saluia saluberrima trita cum lilifago, uetonica, tanetico, feniculo, cerfolio, marrubio, absinthio, centaurea, plantagine, lappa. Hec omnia *amplo uase lo*{91va}*ca*, uino pleno. Hinc bibe cotidie ciffulum in mane. Hec medicina .X. herbarum dicitur contra quodlibet morbum.[12]

Sanicla dicitur quod uulnera sanet. Hec omnia penetrans per plagam exit qualiter bibitur. At <c>apite sauciato cauenda est ne uulnera querendo pelliculam cerebri perforet et cerebrum turbando sauciatum interficiat.[13]

Costus herba hortensis nomen habens a costo quod species est quia speciosa est et bene redolens, escis preelecta. Eius radix oleo uel aqua cocta stomacum et uentrem constipatum salubriter soluit.[14]

Est alia que dicitur costus Anglica que a Gallis despectiue Scottorum dicitur herba. Condimentis tamen et odoribus grata. Purpureo uino mixta *pectoris ardores, cordis dolores* sedat. Empicis et pleureticis cum melle prodest.[15]

---

9 A verb is missing from this sentence, most likely *premit* (*cf.* 1.7, line 37).

10 1.7, 9–17, 19–24, 20–34

11 1.8, 1–4

12 1.9, 28–35

13 1.15, 1–2, 10–14

14 1.16, 1–3, 5–9

15 1.17, 1–3, 5, 7–8, 10

Personatia est herba que a grecis persopes, a uulgo beta uocatur. *Cum uino ueteri morsus anguinos*, et colubrinos sanat. *Radix diu trita cum sale menstrua purgat*; radix eius cum spina siccis nata locis equali pondere commixta morsum canis rabidi curat. Preterea sumpto ciatho bete et duobus ciathis mellis, uetus ulcus sanatur.[16]

Est alia beta *minor foliis, effigie*, uiribus, si tamen *dolor aut uulnus capud turbauerit*, cito subuenit. Vnde et omnibus capitis medicaminibus simul et Theorodicon additur. Theodoricon est precisoum antidotum contra capitis passionem.[17]

Petroselinum greci triannem uocant. Hec *apio similis est foliis, uirtute, colore*, non tamen adeo fortis nec adeo uiridis. Sic dicitur quod petram pota repellat. Antidotis adhibetur. Hec est optima arietinis carnibus, sociata puleio, nasturcio, uel potius illi que ius danna {91vb} uulgo dicitur. Addito costo, modico pipere, hec arietino iure conficiantur et erit sapor optimus. Ad porcinam uero carnem aliter: petroselinum, lilifagum, satirea, nasturcium (si desit ius danna). Conterantur his succis; adde piper et cuminum. *Sic porcina tibi caro frigida* iocundissime *comedatur*.[18]

Solsequia grece elitropia dicitur, cui est flos aureus. Vix bruma superabilis sed qui et meridie aperitur nocte clauditur. Cacumen eius ad solem tam orientem quam occidentem uergitur. Hic quacumque die uidebitur uidentem febris acuta non inuadet et quicumque predictam febrem patitur folium dimidiumque folii suma[n]t, *bis genito sumptam macerent, potent maceratam. Hoc in principio* prodesse dicunt *si luxus cuiquam contingat* solesequii folia potata succurrent. Puluis eius uel herbe succus in uino bibitus omne uenenum destruit.[19]

Paruenca humilis et parua matrem tegit, ornat. Aerem fugiens terre incumbit, unde et pro mutuo habet quolibet tempore flores in mediis etiam niuibus, purpureis uiolis uix cedentes. Tactu dicitur puellas allicere. Victoriola etiam uocatur quia guttam uincit; *cesas in uulnere carnes uincire fertur*.[20]

---

16 1.18, 1–2, 5–12
17 1.19, 1–8
18 1.21, 2–3, 8, 10, 12–13, 18, 21–2, 24–6, 28–31
19 1.22, 2–8, 10–11, 14–21
20 1.23, 2–4, 10, 12–15, 17–18, 28–30

Mirtus in palude oritur calida tamen et uenerem mouens. Hec licet amara grata tamen, nam eius decoctio cum tisana et succo plantaginis ad terciam partem decocta dissentericos et ciliacos curat. Si poma quercus his apponantur, tormina omnia sedantur, si uicturus sit eger.[21]

Mandragora<m> humana[m] per omnia membra imitatur figuram. Vere nouo crines eius frondescent; fine estatis fatiscunt. Asserit quidam quod qui eam uelli audierit *moritur ut herba*, nisi eam *circumfodiunt nectuntque canem, fugientes*, {92ra} ad corpus mandragore; *canis esuriens petit escas longius positas*; *hec ru<m>pitur*, moritur ille. Succus huius fronti illinitur; capitis dolorem amputat. Nardino oleo iunctum et auri infusum dolorem curat. Preterea sume scripulum *de pede dextro*, de manu dextra tantumdem, puluis inde factus cum mero tritus et bibitus per septem dies podagram sanat, tumorem sedat. Contractos neruos reuocat uncia corporis trita et oleo perfusa; contractis membris succurrit. Item scripulum de corpore *in aqua calida prodest donare caduco. Eius sarticulum collo suspenditur egri, sicque filadericum*[22] *quidam fidunt superatum.*[23]

Acinum, quod uulgus cancrum dicit, que licet sit amara, stomaco tamen dulcis est, licet *aspera tactu*, matrici tamen lenis, licet *non splendida uisu*, splendida tamen uesano, quia dementiam pellit. Ex hac et ruta simul maceratis cum uino pocio hec amentem sanum reddit. Menstrua purgat, partum accelerat.[24]

Carui *uirtute, colore, figura* cerefoliis consimilis est, enim utrique *uis acris et ignea ualde*, color ceruleus. *Foliorum summa* his cesa uides. *Mouet uenerem, locium deducit habundans* carui, menstrua solum. *Sapor est gratissimus illi, perdit enim pretium* carui presente cuminum.[25]

Saxifraga saxa frangit ut petroselinum. His *iunctis et nodellis cerasorum, hec in aqua calida tribues petram patienti.* Nichil ad hoc utilius dum petra tenera est; febrem eciam pellit.[26]

---

21 1.25, 8–11, 13–16, 18

22 An attempt at *filacterium*.

23 2.1, 10–17, 19–33, 35–6

24 2.4, 1–11

25 2.6, 2–7

26 2.8, 1–5, 9

Pigmentum herba uulgo dicitur eo quod potibus mixta gratum saporem tribuit, adeo quod melle addito altera pigmenta habeantur. Nec mirum cum apes ita oblectet ut si *lac foliis iungas et uasa perungas*, examen retineatur.[27]

{92rb} Fraga nil adeo locium prouocat uel menstrua.[28]

Pipera et dumis effetis plurimum <subditur> ramorum multitudine. Flore **** ****ur, flore exiguo, et denso. Vis eius est: uulnera mundat, sanat, colorat.[29]

Benedicta que et auricula leporina uulnera purgat, carne replet, colorat, guttam expugnat.[30]

Conferba cum frustis carnis in aeno decocta, conglutinat illa. Membris luxatis, contusis prodest. Oxigaro iuncta stomacum curat. *Splen iuuat, os nodat, tussim fugat, intima curat.*[31]

Viole hiemales circa natale diuinum florent, predictis uiolis pares habet flores parem uirtutem, *sed foliis magis ista patet, magis illa uirescit.*[32]

Basilisca herba quodlibet uenenum pote[n]tur pota expugnat, cum eciam basilisci uenenum deuincat qui *solo flatu uirus effundit*, unde et nomen habet.[33]

Taneticum pectus et quelibet interiora purgat.[34]

---

27 2.13, 1–7

28 2.15, 4–5

29 2.18, 1–2, 5–6, 8. The upper right corner of this folio is badly worn, rendering some words illegible. The word *subditur* is conjectural, based on the use of that word in 2.18, line 1, and the *-ur* abbreviation visible before the *ra-* of *ramorum*. After the first *flore*, *niueo* would be expected, based on 2.18, line 6 (*flos niueus*), and the Excerptor's conversion to the ablative, but there are clearly two words after that first *flore*, neither of which seems to be *niueo*. The second word seems to be a verb ending with the *-ur* abbreviation.

30 2.19, 1–2, 6–9

31 2.20, 17, 21–4

32 2.21, 2, 4–6

33 2.22, 4–5, 7, 9

34 2.24, 3–4

Millemorbia species solet nimphee dici a uulgo fiola. Plagis preualet ut conferba, lumen acuit ut ruta, guttam extinguit ut leporina, uirus urget ut basilea.[35]

Macedonia, id est Alexandria, a plebe ut olus comeditur. Sola sanguinis fluxum restringit. Si ea iuncta puleio et papaueris frondibus uentrem foueas, omnem eius dolorem amputabis.[36]

Yreos et yris sunt consimiles ut thima et thime, nisi quod *rarior et carior est postrema priore, gratior et que latior est maiorque nitore*.[37]

Balsamum que et terralis et sisimbria dicitur, decore, sapore, odore grata. Hec pota febrem pellit. In aqua calida anhelis succurrit. In uino dolorem uesice et stranguiria curat.[38]

Radix herba raphano uirtute et gustu consimilis, sed paulo debilior. Vrinam mouet, pectus confortat et interiora, unde et tempore Martii salubriter comeditur.[39]

{92va} Sclarega dat dulci calide *uires et odorati fermenta saporis*. Vocem clarificat, pulmoni et uisceribus prodest.[40]

Est sclarega minor cuius succus cum lacte niuee capelle pectus optime curat.[41]

Piretrum terrestre sapore et uiribus omnino equatur piretro speciei, et eodem modo utendum est eo ut predicto.[42]

Febrefugia eo quod febrem fuget dicta est. Hanc quidam centauream maiorem uocant, quidam uero artemesiam, eptaphilos.[43]

---

35 3.5, 3, 5–10

36 3.7, 5–7, 9–12

37 3.9, 1–2, 5–6

38 3.12, 1–8

39 3.14, 1, 3–6

40 3.21, 1–5

41 3.22, 3–4

42 3.18. This one line summarizes the idea of Henry's entire poem, lines 1–27.

43 3.4, 1–2, 6–9

Iacinctus flos est ceruleus uulnera curans, contusa et luxata sanans.
Narcisus flos est roseus feruores reprimens. *Si capud inde laues, febres extinguit acutas.*[44]

Ameos alte crescit, semina habens parua per que resurgit, calore suo febrem cotidianam extinguit. Omnibus morbis ex frigiditate uenientibus obsistit. *Vrine, lateri, renibus apta.*[45]

Psillia frigida esse hinc probantur: sume in hieme modicum niuis trociscum et in seminibus psillii pone; nec poterit solis feruore resolui, tanta est herbe frigiditas. Constat *igitur quod morbos calidos enecat*, ut febrem tercianam, podagram calidam, cephalargiam.[46]

Lupinum amarum est. Qui huius legumen post gustauerit tutus erit ab ebrietate. Cum absinthio et prassio, uino confectum lumbricos pellit.[47]

Fenugrecum *duritias mollit collecturasque resoluit* melius cum altea et malua. *Item semen lini cum polline,* iunctum fenugreco, hoc agit. Item fenugrecum cum caule et aceto cataplasma arteri cos dolores mollit, podagram lenit.[48]

Git, .iiii. aduersis cornibus elatis, oritur in summo, grana miri saporis habens qui panem ualde meliorat.[49]

Gazara arbor et herba putatur, interiores dolores mire lenit. Radix uino iuncta *uomitus ingentes trahit morbumque repellit*. Difficilis est tamen medicina.[50]

Quatuor ut constans aquilis 'aquileia' uocatur; purior argento sic 'argentilla' uocatur. Non argentille color est argenteus, at purpura cedit [*cedit*] *ei. Mire gramen*, specie[i] *'herba puellaris'* eciam uocatur uel propter formam uel quia puellas fecundat uel <quia os redo>{92vb}lens facit.[51]

---

44 4.1–2, 22–3, 26–7, 29
45 4.8, 2, 4, 6–7, 10–12
46 4.9, 1–8, 10–12
47 4.11, 4–5, 8–10
48 4.12, 2–3, 5, 7–9
49 4.14, 2–5
50 4.15, 1, 4–8
51 4.17, 1–7. The bottom of this folio is badly rubbed and illegible. The supplied reading of 'quia os redo-' is based on the fact that there is space for only six to eight characters at the end of the final line in the rubbed space after the abbreviated 'uel,' and because the top of the next column clearly begins 'lens.' The sense is supplied from the final line of the poem (4.17, 8): 'uel quia mansum oris semen meliorat odores.'

Meu quoque diureticum est. Diuretica dicunt queque locium lacessent. Neufreticos calore suo curat.[52]

Valeriana ualidis *assurgit frondibus que strictum corpus obumbrans uerticibus latis crispata cacumine paruo* semina parua locat. Valeriana multa ualet. In uino trita et bibita febrem acutam soluit. Preterea guttam et magnos sanat liuores superaddita.[53]

Herba fera uel palma a uulgo Sancte Marie sigillum appellatur, merito precellit statura, magis effigie magisque colore, odore uero alios uincit odores. Hec pigmentis gratissima, gustu dulcissima. Venerem eciam cohercet.[54]

Lactea lacteridis qua nulla uirentior herba est uentrem soluit acute.[55]

---

52 4.19, 1–3
53 4.21, 1–10
54 4.24, 1–5, 7–8, 17
55 4 Epilogue 1, 10–11

Bibliography

Primary Sources

Abū Ma'shar. *Introductorium maius in astronomiam*. Venice 1506.

Adelard of Bath. *Conversations with His Nephew*. Ed. and trans. Charles Burnett. Cambridge: Cambridge University Press, 1998.

Agnus Castus. A Middle English Herbal Reconstructed from Various Manuscripts. Ed. Gösta Brodin. Uppsala: Lundequist, 1950.

Alan of Lille. *The Plaint of Nature*. Trans. with commentary by James J. Sheridan. Mediaeval Sources in Translation 26. Toronto: Pontifical Institute of Mediaeval Studies, 1980.

Aldhelm. *The Riddles of Aldhelm*. Ed. James Hall Pitman. New Haven: Yale University Press, 1925.

Alexander Neckham. *Alexandri Neckam De naturis rerum libri duo. With the Poem of the Same Author, De laudibus divinae sapientiae*. Ed. Thomas Wright. Rerum Britannicarum Medii Aevi Scriptores 34. London: Longman, Green, Longman, Roberts, and Green, 1863.

Alphita, a Medico-Botanical Glossary. Ed. J. L. G. Mowat. Anecdota Oxoniensia. Mediaeval and Modern Series, vol. 1, part 2. Oxford: Clarendon Press, 1887.

Anthimus. *Anthimi De observatione ciborum ad Theodoricum regem Francorum epistula*. Ed. and trans. Eduard Liechtenhan. Corpus medicorum Latinorum 8. 1. Berlin: In aedibus Academiae Scientiarum, 1963.

[*Antidotarium Nicolai*] *Eene Middelnederlandsche Vertaling van het Antidotarium Nicolaï (Ms. 15624–15641, Kon. Bibl. te Brussel)*. Ed. W. S. van den Berg. Leiden: Brill, 1917.

Augustine, Saint. *Sermones*. Ed. Miguel Fuertes Lanero. Obras Completas de San Agustín 7, 10, 23–6. Madrid: Editorial Católica, 1981–5.

Bartholomaeus Anglicus. *De genuinis rerum coelestium, terrestrium, et inferarum proprietatibus*. Frankfurt 1601; repr. under the title *De rerum proprietatibus*, Frankfurt am Main: Minerva, 1964.

Benedictus Crispus. *Poematium medicum*. PL 89. 369–374.

Bernard of Cluny. *Scorn for the World: Bernard of Cluny's* De Contemptu Mundi. Ed. and trans. Ronald Pepin. East Lansing, MI: Colleagues Press, 1991.

Bernardus Claravallensis. *Tractatus de gradibus humilitatis et superbiae*. PL 182. 939–72.

Bernardus Silvestris. *Cosmographia*. Ed. Peter Dronke. Leiden: Brill, 1978.

—. *The* Cosmographia *of Bernardus Silvestris*. Trans. Winthrop Wetherbee. New York: Columbia University Press, 1973.

Boethius. *De consolatione philosophiae*. In *The Theological Tractates; The Consolation of Philosophy*. Ed. and trans. H. F. Stewart and E. K. Rand. Loeb Classical Library. Cambridge, MA: Harvard University Press, 1962.

Calcidius. [*Commentarius in Timaeum Platonis*] *Timaeus a Calcidio translatus commentarioque instructus*. Ed. J. H. Waszink. Plato Latinus 4. London: Warburg Institute; Leiden: Brill, 1962.

'Capitulare de villis': see *Kapitularien*

[*Circa instans*] *Liber de simplici medicina dictus Circa instans*. In Johannes Serapion, *Practica Jo[hannis] Serapionis dicta Breviarium*, fols. 186r–211v. Venice 1497.

—. *Das Arzneidrogenbuch* Circa Instans *in einer Fassung des XIII. Jahrhunderts aus der Universitätsbibliothek Erlangen*. Ed. Hans Wölfel. Inaugural-Dissertation. Berlin: Preilipper, 1939.

Claudian. *Claudii Claudiani Carmina*. Ed. John Barrie Hall. Leipzig: Teubner, 1985.

Collectio Salernitana. Ossia documenti inediti, e trattati di medicina appartenenti alla scuola medica Salernitana. Ed. Salvatore de Renzi. 5 vols. Naples: Tip. del Filiatre-Sebezio, 1852–9; repr. Bologna: Forni, 1967.

Constantine the African. *Liber graduum*. In *Constantini Africani . . . Opera*, 2. 342–87. 2 vols. Basel 1536–9.

—. *Liber graduum*. In Isaac Israeli, *Opera omnia Ysaac*, 2. 78r–86r. Lyons 1515.

—. *Tratado médico de Constantino el Africano. Constantini Liber de Elephancia*. Ed. Ana Isabel Martín Ferreira. Serie Lingüística y filología 26. Valladolid: Universidad de Valladolid, 1996.

Culpeper, Nicholas. *Culpeper's Complete Herbal*. London: Foulsham, 1880.

[*Cyranides*] *Textes latins et vieux français relatifs aux Cyranides*. Ed. Louis Delatte. Liège: Faculté de philosophie et lettres, 1942.

Dioscorides. *Pedanii Dioscuridis Anazarbei, De materia medica libri quinque*. Ed. Max Wellmann. 3 vols. Berlin: Weidmann, 1906–14; repr. Berlin: Weidmann, 1958.

—. *De materia medica*. Trans. Lily Y. Beck. Altertumswissenschaftliche Texte und Studien 38. Hildesheim: Olms-Weidmann, 2005.

—. *Dioscoride latino. Materia medica libro primo*. Ed. H. Mihaescu. Iasi, Romania: Terek, 1938.

— [Latin Alphabetical Dioscorides]. *Index librorum in presenti volumine contentorum Dyoscoridis exactissimi indagatoris fidelissimique scriptoris virtutum simplicium medicinarum liber CCCCCCCXVII continens capitula: cum nonnullis additionibus Petri Paduanensis in margine libri notatis. Eiusdem Dyoscoridis de naturis et virtutibus aquarum tractatus unus*. Colle 1478; repr. Lyons 1512. [Unglossed version in Cambridge, Jesus College, MS Q. D. 2 (44), fols. 17–145.]

— [Latin Dioscorides]. 'Der Longobardische Dioskorides des Marcellus Virgilius.' Ed. Konrad Hofmann and T. M. Auracher. *Romanische Forschungen* 1 (1882), 49–105. Continued by Hermann Stadler, 'Dioscorides Longobardus,' *Romanische Forschungen* 10 (1897), 181–247, 369–446; 11 (1899), 1–121; 13 (1901), 161–243; with indices in 14 (1903), 601–636.

Du Cange, Charles du Fresne. *Glossarium latino-germanicum mediae et infimae aetatis*. Ed. Lorenz Diefenbach. Frankfurt: Baer, 1857.

Firmicus Maternus, Julius. *Mathesis*. Ed. and trans. Pierre Monat. 3 vols. Paris: Les Belles Lettres, 1992–7.

Galen. *Claudii Galeni Opera Omnia*. Ed. Karl Gottlob Kühn. 20 vols in 22. Leipzig: Cnobloch, 1821–33.

Gargilius Martialis. *Gargilii Martialis quae extant*. Vol. 1: *Fragmenta ad holera arboresque pomiferas pertinentia*. Ed. Sebastian Condorelli. Biblioteca di Helikon. Testi e studi 11. Rome: L'Erma di Bretschneider, 1977.

—. *Les remèdes tirés des légumes et des fruits* [*Medicinae ex holeribus et pomis*]. Ed. and trans. Brigitte Maire. Paris: Belles lettres, 2002.

Henry, Archdeacon of Huntingdon. *Historia Anglorum: The History of the English People*. Ed. and trans. Diana Greenway. Oxford: Clarendon Press, 1996.

Henry Daniel. *Aaron*. London, British Library, MS Additional 27329.

—. *Aaron*. London, British Library, MS Arundel 42.

Here men may se the vertues off herbes. A Middle English Herbal (MS. Bodley 483, ff. 57r–67v). Ed. Pol Grymonprez. Scripta 3. Brussels: Scripta, 1981.

Hermes Trismegistus. *Hermes Latinus* IV.2. *Textus Medici*. Ed. Paolo Lucentini. Corpus Christianorum Continuatio Mediaevalis 144A. Turnhout: Brepols, forthcoming.

Hildebert of Lavardin. *Carmina Minora*. Ed. A. B. Scott. Editio altera. Munich: Saur, 2001.

Hildegard of Bingen. *Physica*. Strasbourg 1533.

Horace. *Odes and Epodes*. Ed. and trans. Niall Rudd. Loeb Classical Library. Cambridge, MA: Harvard University Press, 2004.

—. *Satires, Epistles and Ars Poetica*. Trans. H. Rushton Fairclough. Loeb Classical Library. Cambridge, MA: Harvard University Press, 1929.

Ḥunayn ibn Isḥāq [Johannitius]. 'Johannicius. Isagoge ad Techne Galieni.' Ed. Gregor Maurach. *Sudhoffs Archiv* 62 (1978), 148–74.

[*Ilias Latina*] *Baebii Italici Ilias Latina. Introduzione, Edizione Critica, Traduzione Italiana e Commento*. Ed. and trans. Marco Scaffai. Bologna: Pàtron, 1982.

Isidore of Seville. *Etymologiarum sive originum libri XX*. Ed. W. M. Lindsay. Oxford: Clarendon Press, 1911.

—. *Isidori Hispalensis Versus*. Ed. José María Sánchez Martín. Corpus Christianorum Series Latina 113A. Turnhout: Brepols, 2000.

Jerome, Saint. *Sancti Eusebii Hieronymi Epistulae*. Editio altera. Ed. Isidorus Hilberg and Margit Kamptner. CSEL 54–6. Vienna: Verlag der Österreichischen Akademie der Wissenschaften, 1996.

Johannes de Hauvilla. *Architrenius*. Ed. and trans. Winthrop Wetherbee. Cambridge: Cambridge University Press, 1994.

Johannes Serapion [Yúhānnā Ibn Serapion]: see *Circa instans*

Johannitius: *see* Ḥunayn ibn Isḥāq

Juvenal. [*Satires*]. In *Juvenal and Persius*, ed. and trans. Susanna Morton Braund. Loeb Classical Library. Cambridge, MA: Harvard University Press, 2004.

Juvencus. *Gai Vetti Aquilini Iuuenci Evangeliorum libri quattuor*. Ed. J. Huemer. CSEL 24. Vienna: Tempsky; Leipzig: Freitag, 1891.

Kapitularien. Ed. Reinhard Schneider. Göttingen: Vandenhoeck u. Ruprecht, 1968.

Lateinische Hymnen des Mittelalters, grösstentheils aus Handschriften schweizerischer Klöster als Nachtrag zu den Hymnensammlungen von Mone, Daniel und Andern. Ed. Gall Morel. Einsiedeln: Benziger, 1868.

The Laud Herbal Glossary. Ed. J. Richard Stracke. Amsterdam: Rodopi, 1974.

Le Neve, John. *Fasti Ecclesiae Anglicanae, 1066–1300*. Vol. 3: *Lincoln*. Ed. Diana Greenway. London: Institute of Historical Research; Athlone Press, 1977.

Leechdoms, Wortcunning, and Starcraft of Early England. Ed. Thomas Oswald Cockayne. 3 vols. Rerum Britannicarum Medii Aevi Scriptores 35. London: Longman, Green, Longman, Roberts, and Green, 1864–6.

Lenz, F. W. 'Das pseudo-ovidische Gedicht *De medicamine aurium*'. In *Ovidiana: Recherches sur Ovide*, publiée à l'occasion du bimillénaire du poète par Niculae I. Herescu avec le concours de D. Adamesteanu, Vasile Cristea, E. Lozovan, 526–40. Paris: Belles lettres, 1958.

Liber Eliensis. Ed. E. O. Blake. Camden Third Series 92. London: Offices of the Royal Historical Society, 1962.

Lucan. [*De bello civili*] *The Civil War (Pharsalia)*. Ed. A. E. Housman. Trans. J. D. Duff. Loeb Classical Library. Cambridge, MA: Harvard University Press, 1962.

Lucretius. *De rerum natura*. Trans. W. H. D. Rouse. Loeb Classical Library. Cambridge, MA: Harvard University Press, 1947.

Macer Floridus. *Macer Floridus De viribus herbarum*. Ed. Ludwig Choulant. Leipzig: Voss, 1832. Repr. with German translation in *Höhepunkte der Klostermedizin. Der 'Macer Floridus' und das Herbarium des Vitus Auslasser*, trans. Johannes Gottfried Mayer and Konrad Goehl (Holzminden: Reprint-Verlag Leipzig, 2001); German translation only in *Kräuterbuch der Klostermedizin. Der 'Macer Floridus': Medizin des Mitteralters*, trans. Johannes Gottfried Mayer and Konrad Goehl (Holzminden: Reprint-Verlag Leipzig, 2003).

—. *A Middle English Translation of Macer Floridus De viribus herbarum*. Ed. Gösta Frisk. Uppsala: Almqvist & Wiksells boktryckeri, 1949.

—. *Der deutsche 'Macer'. Vulgatfassung mit einem Abdruck des lateinischen Macer Floridus 'De viribus herbarum'*. Ed. Bernhard Schnell with William Crossgrove. Tübingen: Niemeyer, 2003.

—. [*Spuria macri*] *Floridi Macri De viribus herbarum. Capita X, e codice MS. Guelferbitano chartaceo, ao. 1508 exarato*. In *Walafridi Strabi hortulus Carmen ad cod. ms veterumque editionum fidem recensitum, lectionis varietate notisque instructum. Accedunt analecta ad antiquitates florae germanicae et capita aliquot Macri nondum edita*, ed. F. A. Reuss. Würzburg: Stahel, 1834.

Marbode of Rennes. *Marbode of Rennes' (1035–1123) 'De lapidibus' Considered as a Medical Treatise with Text, Commentary, and C. W. King's Translation, Together with Text and Translation of Marbode's Minor Works on Stones*. Ed. John M. Riddle. Sudhoffs Archiv, Beiheft 20. Wiesbaden: Steiner, 1977.

—. *De lapidibus*. PL 171: 1738–70.

—. *De ornamentis verborum. Liber decem capitulorum. Retorica, mitologia et moralità di un vescovo poeta (secc. XI–XII)*. Ed. Rosario Leotta and Carmelo Crimi. Florence: SISMEL, edizioni del Galluzzo, 1998.

—. *Lapidario (Liber lapidum)*. Ed. and trans. María Esthera Herrera. Paris: Belles lettres, 2005.

Marcellus Empiricus. *Marcelli de medicamentis liber* [*Über Heilmittel*]. 2nd ed. Ed. Max Niedermann and Eduard Liechtenhan. Trans. Jutta Kollesch and Diethard Nickel. 2 vols. Corpus medicorum Latinorum 5. Berlin: Akademie-Verlag, 1968.

Marius. *On the Elements*. Ed. and trans. Richard C. Dales. Berkeley: University of California Press, 1976.

Martial. *Epigrams*. Ed. and trans. D. R. Shackleton Bailey. 3 vols. Loeb Classical Library. Cambridge, MA: Harvard University Press, 1993.

—. *Liber Spectaculorum*. Ed. and trans. Kathleen M. Coleman. Oxford: Oxford University Press, 2006.

Mesue the Elder: *see* Yūhannā ibn Māsawayh

Middle English Lyrics: Authoritative Texts, Critical and Historical Backgrounds, Perspectives on Six Poems. Ed. Maxwell S. Luria and Richard L. Hoffman. New York: W. W. Norton & Company, 1974.

Nemesius of Emesa. *Nemesii episcopi Premnon physicon sive, [Peri physeōs anthrōpoy], liber a N. Alfano archiepiscopo Salerni in Latinum translatus*. Ed. Karl Immanuel Burkhard. Leipzig: Teubner, 1917.

Oribasius. *Oeuvres d'Oribase*. Ed. U. C. Bussemaker and C. Daremberg. 6 vols. Paris: Imprimerie nationale, 1851–76.

—. *Oribasius Latinus (Erster Teil)*. Ed. Henning Mørland. Symbolae Osloenses, Supplement 10. Oslo: Brogger, 1940.

Orientius. *Carmina*. Ed. Robinson Ellis. In *Poetae christiani minores*. CSEL 16. Vienna: Tempsky, 1888.

Ovid. *Amores. Medicamina faciei femineae. Ars amatoria. Remedia amoris*. Ed. and trans. E. J. Kenney. Oxford: Clarendon Press, 1961.

—. *Metamorphoses*. Trans. Frank Justus Miller. 2 vols. Loeb Classical Library. Cambridge, MA: Harvard University Press, 1951.

Persius. *Satires*. In *Juvenal and Persius*, ed. and trans. Susanna Morton Braund. Loeb Classical Library. Cambridge, MA: Harvard University Press, 2004.

Peter of Blois. *The Later Letters of Peter of Blois*. Ed. Elizabeth Revell. Auctores Britannici Medii Aevi 13. Oxford: Published for the British Academy by Oxford University Press, 1993.

Platearius: see *Circa instans*

Pliny the Elder. *Natural History*. Ed. and trans. H. Rackham, W. H. S. Jones, and D. E. Eichholz. 10 vols. Loeb Classical Library. Cambridge, MA: Harvard University Press, 1938–63.

Porphyry. *Categoriarum supplementa: Porphyrii Isagoge translatio Boethii et anonymi fragmentum vulgo vocatum "Liber sex principiorum"*. Ed. L. Minio-Paluello. Bruges: Desclée de Brouwer, 1966.

The Prose Salernitan Questions, Edited from a Bodleian Manuscript (Auct. F.3.10). Ed. Brian Lawn. Auctores Britannici Medii Aevi 5. London: Published for The British Academy by the Oxford University Press, 1979.

Proverbs, Sentences, and Proverbial Phrases. Ed. Bartlett Jere Whiting and Helen Wescott Whiting. Cambridge, MA: Belknap Press of Harvard University Press, 1968.

[*Psalmi Turonenses*] 'Die Psalmenparaphrase eines Anonymus aus Marmoutier.' Ed. Peter Orth (26 November 2007). MGH Poetae Latini medii aevi 6, Nachträge zu den Poetae aevi Carolini, Ergänzende Texte. <http://www.mgh.de/~Poetae/Texte/Psalmi-Turonenses.pdf>. Accessed 10 January 2010.

Pseudo-Apuleius. *Antonii Musae De herba vettonica liber, Pseudoapulei Herbarius, Anonymi De taxone liber, Sexti Placiti Liber medicinae ex animalibus*. Ed. Ernst Howald and Henry E. Sigerist. Corpus medicorum Latinorum 4. Leipzig: Teubner, 1927.

Pseudo-Bartholomaeus Mini de Senis. *Tractatus de herbis (MS London, British Library, Egerton 747)*. Ed. Iolanda Ventura. Florence: SISMEL, edizioni del Galluzzo, 2009.

Pseudo-Dioscorides. 'Pseudo-Dioscoridis *De herbis femininis*.' Ed. Heinrich F. Kästner. *Hermes* 31 (1896), 578–636, with 'Addendum' in *Hermes* 32 (1897), 160.

Pseudo-Galen. *Alfabetum Galieni*. In *Galeni Opera Omnia. Galeno ascripti libri*, fols. 88–101. Venice: Valgrisi, 1562.

—. *Liber de anatomia parua*. In *Galeni opera ex sexta Iuntarum editione. Spurii Galeno ascripti libri*. Venice: Giunta, 1586.

Pseudo-Oribasius. *Oribasii Medici de Simplicibus Libri Quinque*, Book 4. In *Physica S. Hildegardis*, 122–233. Strasbourg 1533.

Pseudo-Ovid: *see* Lenz

Pseudo-Pliny. *Physica Plinii Bambergensis (Cod. Bamb. med. 2, fol. 93v–232r)*. Ed. Alf Önnerfors. Hildesheim: Olms, 1975.

—. *Plinii Secundi Iunioris Qui feruntur De medicina libri tres*. Ed. Alf Önnerfors. Corpus medicorum Latinorum 3. Berlin: In aedibus Academiae Scientiarum, 1964.

Pseudo-Theodori i.e. Anonymi ex libris Galeni epitomae De simplici medicina. Ed. Valentin Rose. In *Theodori Prisciani Euporiston libri III*, ed. V. Rose, 401–23. Leipzig: Teubner, 1894.

Pseudo-Virgil. *Culex*. In *Virgil*, vol. 2: *Aeneid Books 7–12, Appendix Vergiliana*. Ed. and trans. H. Rushton Fairclough. Rev. G. P. Goold. Loeb Classical Library. Cambridge, MA: Harvard University Press, 2000.

Quintus Serenus. *Liber Medicinalis*. Ed. and trans. R. Pépin. Paris: Presses universitaires de France, 1950.

Rabanus Maurus. *De rerum naturis*. PL 111: 9–614.

Regimen Sanitatis Salernitanum. Gesundheitsregeln der Schule von Salerno. L'École de Salerne. Texte zur Geschichte der Präventivmedizin 1. Basel: Braun, Gesellschaft für Präventivmedizin, 1981.

Robert Cricklade. *Roberti Crikeladensis Defloratio Naturalis historiae Plinii Secundi*. Ed. Bodo Näf. Berlin: Peter Lang, 2002.

Rufinus. *The Herbal of Rufinus*. Ed. Lynn Thorndike, assisted by Francis S. Benjamin, Jr. Chicago: University of Chicago Press, 1946.

Salvatore de Renzi: see *Collectio Salernitana*

Scribonii Largi Compositiones. Ed. Sergio Sconocchia. Leipzig: Teubner, 1983.

Sinonoma Bartholomei. Ed. J. L. G. Mowat. Anecdota Oxoniensia. Mediaeval and Modern Series, Vol. 1, Part 1. Oxford: Clarendon Press, 1882.

Statius. *Silvae*. Ed. and trans. D. R. Shackleton Bailey. Loeb Classical Library. Cambridge, MA: Harvard University Press, 2003.

—. *Thebaid. Achilleid*. Ed. and trans. D. R. Shackleton Bailey. 2 vols. Loeb Classical Library. Cambridge, MA: Harvard University Press, 2003.

The Trotula: *A Medieval Compendium of Women's Medicine*. Ed. and trans. Monica H. Green. Philadelphia: University of Pennsylvania Press, 2001.

Venantius Fortunatus. *Venanti Honori Clementiani Fortunati presbyteri italici Opera poetica*. Ed. Friedrich Leo. Berlin: Weidmann, 1881.

Virgil. *Aeneid*. In *Virgil*, rev. ed. with new introduction, ed. and trans. H. Rushton Fairclough, rev. G. P. Goold. Loeb Classical Library. 2 vols. Cambridge, MA: Harvard University Press, 1999–2000.

Walahfrid Strabo. *Hortulus*. Ed. Cataldo Roccaro. Palermo: Herbita, 1979.

—. *Hortulus: The Little Garden*. Trans. Raef Payne, with commentary by Wilfrid Blunt. Pittsburgh, PA: Hunt Botanical Library, 1966.

William of Conches. *De philosophia mundi*. PL 172: 39–102.

Yūhannā ibn Māsawayh, Abū Zakariyā. *Le Livre des axiomes médicaux (Aphorismi)*. Édition du texte arabe et des versions latines avec traduction française et lexique, Danielle Jacquart and Gérard Troupeau. Geneva: Droz; Paris: Champion, 1980.

Secondary Sources

Anderson, Frank J. 'New light on *Circa instans*.' *Pharmacy in History* 20 (1978), 65–69.

André, Jacques. *Les noms de plantes dans la Rome antique*. Paris: Belles lettres, 1985.

Baader, Gerhard. 'Early medieval Latin adaptations of Byzantine medicine in Western Europe.' *Dumbarton Oaks Papers* 38, Symposium on Byzantine Medicine (1984), 251–9.

Banham, Debby. 'Arestolobius, the Patriarch of Jerusalem and bark that comes from Paradise: What did the Orient mean to compilers of Old English medical collections?.' In *Proceedings of the Thirty-Eighth International Congress on the History of Medicine, 1–6 September* 2002, ed. Nil Sari *et al.*, 459–68. 3 vols. Ankara: International Society for the History of Medicine, 2005.

Beccaria, Augusto. *I codici di medicina del periodo presalernitano (secoli IX, X e XI)*. Rome: Edizioni di Storia e letteratura, 1956.

Bénédictins du Bouveret. *Colophons de manuscrits occidentaux des origines au XVIe siècle*. 6 vols. Spicilegii Friburgensis Subsidia 2–7. Fribourg: Éditions Universitaires, 1965–1982.

Bierbaumer, Peter. *Der botanische Wortschatz des Altenglischen*. 3 vols. Frankfurt: Peter Lang, 1975–9.

Black, Winston. 'Henry of Huntingdon's lapidary rediscovered and his *Anglicanus ortus* reassembled'. *Mediaeval Studies* 68 (2006), 43–87.

—. '"I will add what the Arab once taught": Constantine the African in Northern European medical verse.' In *Herbs and Healers from the Ancient Mediterranean through the Medieval West: Essays in Honor of John M. Riddle*, ed. Anne Van Arsdall and Timothy Graham. Aldershot: Ashgate, forthcoming.

The British Pharmaceutical Codex. Council of the Pharmaceutical Society of Great Britain. London: Pharmaceutical Press, 1907–1973.

Burnett, Charles and Danielle Jacquart, eds. *Constantine the African and 'Alī ibn al-'Abbās al-Maǧūsī. The* Pantegni *and Related Texts*. Studies in Ancient Medicine 10. Leiden: Brill, 1994.

Bylebyl, Jerome J. 'The medical meaning of *physica*.' *Osiris*, 2nd series, 6 (1990), 16–41.

Caiazzo, Irene. 'Un inedito commento sulla *Isagoge Iohannitii* conservato a Parigi.' In *La Scuola Medica Salernitana. Gli autori e i testi. Convegno internazionale, Università degli studi di Salerno, 3–5 novembre 2004*, ed. Danielle Jacquart and Agostino Paravicini Bagliani, 93–123. Florence: SISMEL, edizioni del Galluzzo, 2007.

Cameron, M. L. *Anglo-Saxon Medicine*. Cambridge Studies in Anglo-Saxon England 7. Cambridge: University of Cambridge Press, 1993.

—. 'The sources of medical knowledge in Anglo-Saxon England.' *Anglo-Saxon England* 11 (1983), 135–55.

Chenu, Marie-Dominique. 'Nature and man: The Renaissance of the twelfth century.' In M.-D. Chenu, *Nature, Man, and Society in the Twelfth Century. Essays on New Theological Perspectives in the Latin West*, ed. and trans. Jerome Taylor and Lester K. Little, 1–48. Medieval Academy Reprints for Teaching 37. Toronto: University of Toronto Press in association with the Medieval Academy of America, 1997.

Choulant, Ludwig. *Handbuch der Bücherkunde für die ältere Medizin*. Leipzig 1841; repr. Graz: Akademische Druck- u. Verlagsanstalt, 1956.

La Collectio Salernitana *di Salvatore De Renzi. Convegno internazionale, Università degli Studi di Salerno, 18–19 giugno 2007*. Ed. Danielle Jacquart and Agostino Paravicini Bagliani. Edizione Nazionale La Scuola Medica Salernitana 3. Florence: SISMEL, Edizioni del Galluzzo, 2008.

Collins, Minta. *Medieval Herbals: The Illustrative Traditions*. British Library Studies in Medieval Culture. London: British Library; Toronto: University of Toronto Press, 2000.

Cristofolini, Giovanni and Umberto Mossetti. 'Interpretation of plant names in a late medieval medical treatise.' *Taxon* 47 (1998), 305–19.

Crossgrove, William C. 'Textual criticism in a fourteenth-century scientific manuscript.' In *Studies on Medieval* Fachliteratur. *Proceedings of the Special Session on Medieval Fachliteratur of the Sixteenth International Congress on Medieval Studies, Kalamazoo, Michigan (U.S.A.), May 10, 1981*, ed. William Eamon, 45–58. Brussels: Omirel, UFSAL, 1982.

—. 'Zur Datierung des "Macer Floridus".' In *Licht der Natur. Medizin in Fachliteratur und Dichtung. Festschrift für Gundolf Keil zum 60. Geburtstag*, ed. Josef Domes, Bernhard D. Haage and Werner E. Gerabek, 55–63. Göppingen: Kümmerle, 1994.

Curtis, Robert I. *Garum and Salsamenta: Production and Commerce in Materia Medica*. Studies in Ancient Medicine 3. Leiden: Brill, 1991.

Curtius, Ernst Robert. *European Literature and the Latin Middle Ages*. Trans. Willard R. Trask. Bollingen Series 36. New York: Harper & Row, 1953.

Daems, Willem F. *Nomina simplicium medicinarum ex synonymariis medii aevi collecta. Semantische Untersuchungen zum Fachwortschatz hoch- und spätmittelalterlicher Drogenkunde*. Studies in Ancient Medicine 6. Leiden: Brill, 1993.

Demaitre, Luke. *Doctor Bernard de Gordon: Professor and Practitioner*. Studies and Texts 51. Toronto: Pontifical Institute of Mediaeval Studies, 1980.

Dictionary of Greek and Roman Biography and Mythology. Ed. William Smith. 3 vols. Boston: Little, Brown and Co., 1870.

Dictionary of Medieval Latin from British Sources. Ed. R. E. Latham, D. R. Howlett, *et al.* 13 fascicles. London: Published for the British Academy by Oxford University Press, 1975–.

Dronke, Peter. 'Bernard Silvestris, Natura, and personification.' *Journal of the Warburg and Courtauld Institutes* 43 (1980), 16–31. Repr. in Peter Dronke, *Intellectuals and Poets in Medieval Europe* (Rome: Edizioni di storia e letteratura, 1992), 41–61.

—. *Fabula: Explorations into the Uses of Myth in Medieval Platonism*. Leiden: Brill, 1974.

—. *Medieval Latin and the Rise of European Love-Lyric*. 2nd ed. 2 vols. Oxford: Clarendon Press, 1968.

—. 'New approaches to the School of Chartres.' *Anuario de estudios medievales* 6 (1969), 117–40.

—. *Poetic Individuality in the Middle Ages. New Departures in Poetry, 1000–1150*. 2nd ed. London: Westfield College, University of London Committee for Medieval Studies, 1986.

Economou, George D. *The Goddess Natura in Medieval Literature*. Cambridge, MA: Harvard University Press, 1972. Reprinted with new introduction and updated bibliography, Notre Dame, IN: University of Notre Dame Press, 2002. Page references are to the 2002 edition.

Effe, Bernd. *Dichtung und Lehre. Untersuchungen zur Typologie des antiken Lehrgedichts*. Munich: Beck, 1977.

Fassler, Margot. 'Mary's Nativity, Fulbert of Chartres, and the *Stirps Jesse*: Liturgical innovation circa 1000 and its afterlife.' *Speculum* 75 (2000), 389–434.

Fischer, Hermann. *Mittelalterliche Pflanzenkunde*. Munich: Verlag der Münchner Drucke, 1929.

Fischer, Klaus-Dietrich. 'A mirror for deaf ears? A medieval mystery.' *Electronic British Library Journal* (2008), Article 9, <http://www.bl.uk/eblj/2008articles/article9.html>. Accessed 25 June 2009.

Flood, Bruce P., Jr. 'Macer Floridus: A medieval herbalism.' PhD diss., University of Colorado, 1968.

—. 'The medieval herbal tradition of "Macer Floridus".' *Pharmacy in History* 18 (1976), 62–6.

—. 'Pliny and the medieval "Macer" medical text.' *Journal of the History of Medicine and Allied Sciences* 32 (1977), 395–402.

Friedman, John B. 'Alice of Bath's astral destiny: A re-appraisal.' *Chaucer Review* 35 (2000), 166–81.

García-Ballester, Luis. 'Introduction: Practical medicine from Salerno to the Black Death.' In *Practical Medicine from Salerno to the Black Death*, ed. Luis García-Ballester, Roger French, Jon Arrizabalaga, and Andrew Cunningham, 1–29. Cambridge: Cambridge University Press, 1994.

Glaze, Florence Eliza. 'Gariopontus and the Salernitans: Textual traditions in the eleventh and twelfth centuries.' In *La* Collectio Salernitana *di Salvatore De Renzi*, ed. Jacquart and Paravicini Bagliani, 149–90.

Green, Monica H. 'Flowers, poisons and men: Menstruation in Medieval Western Europe.' In *Menstruation: A Cultural History*, ed. Andrew Shail and Gillian Howie, 51–64. Basingstoke: Palgrave Macmillan, 2005.

—. 'Rethinking the manuscript basis of Salvatore de Renzi's *Collectio Salernitana*: The corpus of medical writings in the "long" twelfth century.' In *La* Collectio Salernitana *di Salvatore De Renzi*, ed. Jacquart and Paravicini Bagliani, 15–60.

—. 'Salerno on the Thames: The genesis of Anglo-Norman medical literature.' In *Language and Culture in Medieval Britain: The French of England, c.1100–c.1500*, ed. Jocelyn Wogan-Browne, with Carolyn Collette, Maryanne Kowaleski, Linne Mooney, Ad Putter, and David Trotter, 220–31. Woodbridge: York Medieval Press, 2009.

Greenway, Diana. 'Authority, convention, and observation in Henry of Huntingdon's *Historia Anglorum*.' *Anglo-Norman Studies* 18, Proceedings of the Battle Conference 1995 (1996), 105–22.

—. 'Henry of Huntingdon as poet: The *De herbis* rediscovered.' *Medium Ævum* 74 (2005), 329–32.

Grieve, Maud. *A Modern Herbal. The Medicinal, Culinary, Cosmetic and Economic Prop-*

erties, Cultivation and Folklore of Herbs, Grasses, Fungi, Shrubs and Trees with All Their Modern Scientific Uses. 2 vols. New York: Harcourt, Brace, 1931; repr. Middlesex: Penguin, 1980.

Harig, Georg. *Bestimmung der Intensität im medizinischen system Galens: ein Beitrag zur theoretischen Pharmakologie, Nosologie und Therapie in der galenischen Medizin*. Berlin: Akademie-Verlag, 1974.

Harvey, John H. 'The first English garden book: Mayster Jon Gardener's treatise and its background.' *Garden History* 13 (1985), 83–101.

—. 'Henry Daniel: A scientific gardener of the fourteenth century.' *Garden History* 15 (1987), 81–93.

—. 'The square garden of Henry the Poet.' *Garden History* 15 (1987), 1–11.

—. 'Vegetables in the Middle Ages.' *Garden History* 12 (1984), 89–99.

Haye, Thomas. *Das lateinische Lehrgedicht im Mittelalter. Analyse einer Gattung*. Mittellateinische Studien und Texte 22. Leiden: Brill, 1997.

Hunt, R. W. and A. G. Watson. *Bodleian Library Quarto Catalogues*, vol. 9: *Digby Manuscripts*, part 2: *Notes on Macray's Descriptions of the Manuscripts*. Oxford: Bodleian Library, 1999.

Hunt, Tony. *Anglo-Norman Medicine*. Vol. 1: *Roger Frugard's Chirurgia and the Practica brevis of Platearius*. Cambridge: Brewer, 1994.

—. *Plant Names of Medieval England*. Cambridge: Brewer, 1989. [= Hunt]

—. *Popular Medicine in Thirteenth-Century England*. Cambridge: Brewer, 1990.

—. *Teaching and Learning Latin in Thirteenth-Century England*. 3 vols. Cambridge: Brewer, 1991.

Jacquart, Danielle. 'À l'aube de la renaissance médicale des XIe–XIIe siècles: L'*Isagoge Johannitii* et son traducteur.' *Bibliothèque de l'École des Chartes* 144 (1986), 209–40.

Johnson, Lesley. 'Return to Albion.' *Arthurian Literature* 13 (1995), 19–40.

Jolly, Karen Louise. *Popular Religion in Late Saxon England: Elf Charms in Context*. Chapel Hill, NC: University of North Carolina Press, 1996.

Jordan, Mark D. 'The construction of a philosophical medicine: Exegesis and argument in Salernitan teaching on the soul.' *Osiris*, 2nd series, 6 (1990), 42–61.

Kealey, Edward J. *Medieval Medicus: A Social History of Anglo-Norman Medicine*. Baltimore: Johns Hopkins University Press, 1981.

—. *Roger of Salisbury, Viceroy of England*. Berkeley: University of California Press, 1972.

Keiser, George R. 'Reconstructing Robert Thornton's herbal.' *Medium Ævum* 65 (1996), 35–53.

—. 'Through a fourteenth-century gardener's eyes: Henry Daniel's herbal.' *Chaucer Review* 31 (1996), 58–75.

—. 'Verse introductions to Middle English medical treatises.' *English Studies* 84 (2003), 301–17.

Kristeller, Paul Oskar. 'The school of Salerno: Its development and its contribution to the history of learning.' *Bulletin of the History of Medicine* 17 (1945), 138–94. Translated by Antonio Cassesi, with additions, as *Studi sulla Scuola medica Salernitana* (Naples: Istituto Italiano per gli Studi Filosofici, 1986).

Langslow, D. R. 'The language of poetry and the language of science: the Latin poets and "Medical Latin".' In *Aspects of the Language of Latin Poetry*, ed. J. N. Adams and R. G. Mayer, 183–225. Proceedings of the British Academy 93. Oxford: Oxford University Press, 1999.

—. *The Latin Alexander Trallianus: The Text and Transmission of a Late Latin Medical Book*. Journal of Roman Studies Monographs 10. London: Society for the Promotion of Roman Studies, 2006.

—. *Medical Latin in the Roman Empire*. Oxford: Oxford University Press, 2000.

Lapidge, Michael. *Anglo-Latin Literature, 900–1066*. London: Hambledon Press, 1993.

—. 'Some Latin poems as evidence for the reign of Athelstan.' *Anglo-Saxon England* 9 (1981), 61–98.

Latham, R. E. *Revised Medieval Latin Word-List from British and Irish Sources*. 1965; repr. with supplement, London: Published for The British Academy by the Oxford University Press, 1980.

Lawn, Brian. *The Salernitan Questions. An Introduction to the History of Medieval and Renaissance Problem Literature*. Oxford: Clarendon Press, 1963.

Leland, John. *De uiris illustribus / On Famous Men*. Ed. and trans. James P. Carley, with the assistance of Caroline Brett. Studies and Texts 172; British Writers of the Middle Ages and the Early Modern Period 1. Toronto: Pontifical Institute of Mediaeval Studies; Oxford: Bodleian Library, 2010.

—. *Joannis Lelandi antiquarii De rebus Britannicis collectanea*. Ed. T. Hearne. 2nd ed. 6 vols. London 1770.

Lieberknecht, Sieglinde. *Die* Canones *des Pseudo-Mesue. Eine mittelalterliche Purgantien-Lehre*. Quellen und Studien zur Geschichte der Pharmazie 71. Stuttgart: Wissenschaftliche Verlagsgesellschaft, 1995.

Longnon, Auguste. *Pouillés de la Province de Sens*. Paris: Imprimerie Nationale, 1904.

Maaz, Wolfgang. *Lateinische Epigrammatik im hohen Mittelalter. Literarhistorische Untersuchungen zur Martial-Rezeption*. Spolia Berolinensia 2. Hildesheim: Weidmann, 1992.

MacKinney, Loren C. 'Medieval medical dictionaries and glossaries.' In *Medieval and Historiographical Essays in Honor of James Westfall Thompson*, ed. James Lea Cate and Eugene N. Anderson, 240–68. Chicago: University of Chicago Press, 1938.

Macray, William D. *Catalogi codicum manuscriptorum Bibliothecae Bodleianae, pars nona: codices a viro clarissimo Kenelm Digby, Eq. Aur., anno 1634 donatos, complectens: adiecto indice nominum et rerum*. Oxford: Clarendon Press, 1883.

Manitius, Max. *Geschichte der lateinischen Literatur des Mittelalters*. 3 vols. Munich: Beck, 1911–31.

Martin, Janet. 'Classicism and style in Latin literature.' In *Renaissance and Renewal in the Twelfth Century*, ed. Robert L. Benson and Giles Constable, with Carol D. Lanham, 537–68. Medieval Academy Reprints for Teaching 26. Cambridge, MA: Harvard University Press, 1982; repr. Toronto: Published by the University of Toronto Press in association with the Medieval Academy of America, 1991.

Marvin, Julia. 'Albine and Isabelle: Regicidal queens and the historical imagination of the Anglo-Norman prose *Brut* chronicles.' *Arthurian Literature* 18 (2001), 143–91.

Matheson, Lister M. '*Médecin sans frontières*? The European dissemination of John of Burgundy's plague treatise.' *ANQ* 18/3 (2005), 17–28.

Meyer, E. H. F. *Geschichte der Botanik*. 4 vols. Königsberg: Gebrüder Bornträger, 1854–7.

McKeon, Richard. 'Medicine and philosophy in the eleventh and twelfth centuries: The problem of elements.' *The Thomist* 24 (1961), 211–56.

McVaugh, Michael R. 'Surface meanings: The identification of apostemes in medieval surgery'. In *Medical Latin from the Late Middle Ages to the Eighteenth Century. Proceedings of the European Science Foundation Exploratory Workshop in the Humanities, Organized under the Supervision of Albert Derolez in Brussels on 3 and 4 September 1999*, ed. Wouter Bracke and Herwig Deumens, 13–29. Brussels: Koninklijke Academie voor Geneeskunde van België, 2000.

Moreno Olalla, David. '*The fautys to amende*: On the interpretation of the *explicit* of Sloane 5, ff. 13–57, and related matters'. *English Studies* 88 (2007), 119–42.

Mørland, Henning. *Die lateinischen Oribasiusübersetzungen*. Symbolae Osloenses, Supplement 5. Oslo: Brøgger, 1932.

O'Boyle, Cornelius. *The Art of Medicine. Medical Teaching at the University of Paris, 1250–1400*. Education and Society in the Middle Ages and Renaissance 9. Leiden: Brill, 1998.

—. *Thirteenth- and Fourteenth-Century Copies of the* Ars Medicine. *A Checklist and Contents Descriptions of the Manuscripts*. Articella Studies 2. Cambridge: Cambridge Wellcome Unit for the History of Medicine, 1998.

O'Neill, Ynez Violé. 'William of Conches and the cerebral membranes'. *Clio Medica* 2 (1967), 13–21.

Opsomer-Halleux, Carmélia. 'The medieval garden and its role in medicine'. In *Medieval Gardens*, ed. Elisabeth B. MacDougall, 93–114. Dumbarton Oaks Colloquium on the History of Landscape Architecture 9. Washington, DC: Dumbarton Oaks Research Library and Collection, 1986.

Otter, Monika. *Inventiones: Fiction and Referentiality in Twelfth-Century English Historical Writing*. Chapel Hill, NC: University of North Carolina Press, 1996.

—. '*Prolixitas temporum*: Futurity in medieval history narratives'. In *Reading Medieval Culture: Essays in Honor of Robert W. Hanning*, ed. Robert Stein and Sandra Prior, 45–67. Notre Dame, IN: University of Notre Dame Press, 2005.

Parker, Holt. 'Vergil's mysterious *siler*: A possible identification from a lousy clue'. *The Classical Quarterly* 56 (2006), 623–9.

Partner, Nancy. 'Henry of Huntingdon: Clerical celibacy and the writing of history'. *Church History* 42 (1973), 467–75.

—. *Serious Entertainments: The Writing of History in Twelfth-Century England*. Chicago: University of Chicago Press, 1977.

Patera, Adolf and Antonín Podlaha. *Soupis rukopisu Knihovny Metropolitní kapitoly pražské*. 2 vols. Prague: Nákl. Ceské akademie císare Frantiska Josefa pro vedy, slovesnost a umení, 1910–22.

Pollington, Stephen. *Leechcraft. Early English Charms, Plant Lore, and Healing*. Norfolk: Anglo-Saxon Books, 2000.

Raby, F. J. E. *A History of Secular Latin Poetry in the Middle Ages*. 2 vols. Oxford: Clarendon Press, 1934; repr. Oxford: Sandpiper Press, 1997.

Resak, Cyrill. *Odo Magdunensis, der Verfasser des 'Macer Floridus' und der deutsche Leipziger Macer Text*. Leipzig: Robert Noske, 1917.

Riddle, John M. 'Byzantine commentaries on Dioscorides'. *Dumbarton Oaks Papers* 38, Symposium on Byzantine Medicine (1984), 95–102. Repr. in Riddle, *Quid pro quo*, Article 13.

—. 'Dioscorides'. *Catalogus translationum et commentariorum: Mediaeval and Renaissance Latin Translations and Commentaries* 4 (1980), 1–143.

—. *Dioscorides on Pharmacy and Medicine*. History of Science Series 3. Austin: University of Texas Press, 1985.
—. *Eve's Herbs: A History of Contraception and Abortion in the West*. Cambridge, MA: Harvard University Press, 1997.
—. 'The Latin Alphabetical Dioscorides.' *Proceedings of the XIIIth International Congress of the History of Science, Moscow, Aug. 18–24, 1971*, Acts Section 4, 204–9. Moscow: Nauka, 1974. Repr. in Riddle, *Quid pro quo*, Article 4.
—. 'Lithotherapy in the Middle Ages. Lapidaries considered as medical texts.' *Pharmacy in History* 12 (1970), 39–50. Repr. in Riddle, *Quid pro quo*, Article 3.
—. 'Pseudo-Dioscorides' *Ex herbis femininis* and early medieval medical botany.' *Journal of the History of Biology* 14 (1981), 43–81. Repr. in Riddle, *Quid pro quo*, Article 9.
—. *Quid pro quo: Studies in the History of Drugs*. Aldershot: Ashgate, 1992.
—. 'Theory and practice in medieval medicine.' *Viator* 5 (1974), 157–84.
Rigg, A. G. 'Henry of Huntingdon's herbal.' *Mediaeval Studies* 65 (2003), 213–92.
—. 'Henry of Huntingdon's metrical experiments.' *Journal of Medieval Latin* 1 (1991), 60–72.
—. *A History of Anglo-Latin Literature, 1066–1422*. Cambridge: Cambridge University Press, 1992.
Rippinger, Léon. 'À propos de quelques noms de maladies chez Celse et Scribonius Largus.' In *Études de linguistique générale et de linguistique latine offertes en hommage à Guy Serbat*, 207–18. Bibliothèque de l'information grammaticale 6. Paris: Société pour l'information grammaticale, 1987.
Rohde, Eleanour Sinclair. *The Old English Herbals*. London: Longmans, Green, 1922.
Rose, Valentin. 'Ptolemaeus und die Schule von Toledo.' *Hermes* 8 (1874), 327–49.
Runia, David T. *Philo and the Church Fathers*. Leiden: Brill, 1995.
Ruppel, Bernd. 'Heinrichs von Huntingdon verschollenes Gedicht "De herbis".' *Mittellateinisches Jahrbuch* 32 (1997), 211.
—. 'Ein verschollenes Gedicht des 12. Jahrhunderts: Heinrichs von Huntingdon "De herbis".' *Frühmittelalterliche Studien* 31 (1997), 197–213.
Rusche, Philip G. 'The sources for plant names in Anglo-Saxon England and the Laud Herbal Glossary.' In *Health and Healing from the Medieval Garden*, ed. Peter Dendle and Alain Touwaide, 128–44. Woodbridge: Boydell, 2008.
Schnell, Bernhard. 'Übersetzungen in der Fachliteratur. Zum "Älteren Deutschen Macer".' *Wolfram-Studien* 14: Übersetzen im Mittelalter (1996), 185–207.
Schöner, Erich. *Das Viererschema in der antiken Humoralpathologie*. Sudhoffs Archiv, Beiheft 4. Wiesbaden: Steiner, 1964.
Sharpe, Richard. *A Handlist of the Latin Writers of Great Britain and Ireland before 1540*. Publications of the Journal of Medieval Latin 1. Turnhout: Brepols, 1997; repr. with additions and corrections, Turnhout: Brepols, 2001.
—. 'List of identifications.' British Medieval Library Catalogues. <http://www.history.ox.ac.uk/sharpe/index.htm>
Silverstein, Theodore. '*Elementatum*: Its appearance among the twelfth-century cosmogonists.' *Mediaeval Studies* 16 (1954), 156–62.
—. 'Guillaume de Conches and Nemesius of Emessa: On the sources of the "new science" of the twelfth century.' In *Harry Austryn Wolfson: Jubilee Volume on the Occasion of His Seventy-Fifth Birthday*, 2.719–34. 3 vols. Jerusalem: American Academy for Jewish Research, 1965.

Singer, Charles. 'The herbal in antiquity and its transmission to later ages.' *The Journal of Hellenic Studies* 47 (1927), 1–52.

Siraisi, Nancy G. *Medieval & Early Renaissance Medicine: An Introduction to Knowledge and Practice*. Chicago: University of Chicago Press, 1990.

Smallwood, T. M. 'The transmission of charms in English, Medieval and Modern.' In *Charms and Charming in Europe*, ed. Jonathan Roper, 11–31. Basingstoke: Palgrave Macmillan, 2004.

Stadler, H. 'Die Quellen des Macer Floridus.' *Archiv für die Geschichte der Naturwissenschaften und der Technik* 1 (1908), 52–65.

Stannard, Jerry. 'Alimentary and medicinal uses of plants.' In *Medieval Gardens*, ed. Elisabeth B. MacDougall, 69–91. Dumbarton Oaks Colloquium on the History of Landscape Architecture 9. Washington, DC: Dumbarton Oaks Research Library and Collection, 1986.

—. 'Benedictus Crispus, an eighth century medical poet.' *Journal of the History of Medicine and Allied Sciences* 21 (1966), 24–46. Repr. in Jerry Stannard, *Pristina Medicamenta: Ancient and Medieval Botany*, ed. Katherine E. Stannard and Richard Kay, Article 10. Aldershot: Ashgate, 1999.

—. 'A fifteenth-century botanical glossary.' *Isis* 55 (1964), 353–67.

—. *Herbs and Herbalism in the Middle Ages and Renaissance*. Ed. Katherine E. Stannard and Richard Kay. Aldershot: Ashgate, 1999.

—. 'Medieval herbals and their development.' *Clio Medica* 9 (1974), 23–33. Repr. in Stannard, *Herbs and Herbalism*, Article 3.

—. 'Medieval reception of classical plant names.' *Revue de Synthèse*, 3rd series, 89 (1968), 153–62. Repr. in Stannard, *Herbs and Herbalism*, Article 1.

—. 'Rezeptliteratur as *Fachliteratur*.' In *Studies on Medieval* Fachliteratur. *Proceedings of the Special Session on Medieval Fachliteratur of the Sixteenth International Congress on Medieval Studies, Kalamazoo, Michigan (U.S.A.), May 10, 1981*, ed. William Eamon, 59–73. Brussels: Omirel, UFSAL, 1982.

—. 'The theoretical bases of medieval herbalism.' *Medical Heritage* 1 (1985), 186–98. Repr. in Stannard, *Herbs and Herbalism*, Article 4.

— and Peter Dilg. 'Camerarius' contributions to medicine and pharmacy: Observations on his *De Theriacis et Mithridateis Commentariolus*.' In *Joachim Camerarius (1500–1574): Beiträge zur Geschichte des Humanismus im Zeitalter der Reformation*, ed. Frank Baron, 152–86. Munich: Fink, 1978. Repr. in Jerry Stannard, *Pristina Medicamenta: Ancient and Medieval Botany*, ed. Katherine E. Stannard and Richard Kay, Article 12. Aldershot: Ashgate, 1999.

Steadman, John M. 'Perseus upon Pegasus and *Ovid Moralized*.' *Review of English Studies*, New Series, 9 (1958), 407–10.

Sternberg, Kaspar. *Abhandlung über die Pflanzenkunde in Böhmen*. 2 vols. Prague: Haase, 1817–18.

Texts and Transmission: A Survey of the Latin Classics. Ed. L. D. Reynolds. Oxford: Clarendon Press, 1983.

Thomas, Alfred. *Anne's Bohemia: Czech Literature and Society, 1310–1420*. Foreword by David Wallace. Minneapolis, MN: University of Minnesota Press, 1998.

Thorndike, Lynn. *A History of Magic and Experimental Science*. 8 vols. New York: Macmillan, 1923–58.

— and Pearl Kibre. *A Catalogue of Incipits of Mediaeval Scientific Writings in Latin*. Rev. ed. Cambridge, MA: Mediaeval Academy of America, 1963.

Touwaide, Alain. 'Latin crusaders, Byzantine herbals.' In *Visualizing Medieval Medicine and Natural History, 1200–1550*, ed. Jean A. Givens, Karen M. Reeds and Alain Touwaide, 25–50. Aldershot: Ashgate, 2006.

—. 'Oreibasios.' In *Der neue Pauly: Enzyklopädie der Antike*, ed. Hubert Cancik and Helmuth Schneider, 9. 15–16. 16 vols. in 19. Stuttgart: Metzler, 1996–2003.

Usher, Jonathan. 'Simona and Pasquino: "Cur moriatur homo cui salvia crescit in horto?".' *MLN* 106 (1991), 1–14.

Van Arsdall, Anne. 'Exploring what was understood by "mandragora" in Anglo-Saxon England.' In *Old Names—New Growth. Proceedings of the 2nd ASPNS Conference, University of Graz, Austria, 6–10 June 2007, and Related Essays*, ed. Peter Bierbaumer and Helmut W. Klug, 57–74. Frankfurt am Main: Peter Lang, 2009.

—. *Medieval Herbal Remedies. The* Old English Herbarium *and Anglo-Saxon Medicine*. New York: Routledge, 2002.

—, Helmut W. Klug and Paul Blanz. 'The mandrake plant and its legend: A new perspective.' In *Old Names – New Growth. Proceedings of the 2nd ASPNS Conference, University of Graz, Austria, 6–10 June 2007, and Related Essays*, ed. Peter Bierbaumer and Helmut W. Klug, 285–346. Frankfurt am Main: Peter Lang, 2009.

Voigts, Linda E. 'Anglo-Saxon plant remedies and the Anglo-Saxons.' *Isis* 70 (1979), 250–68.

Wallis, Faith. 'The ghost in the *Articella*: A twelfth-century commentary on the Constantinian *Liber Graduum*.' In *Herbs and Healers from the Ancient Mediterranean through the Medieval West: Essays in Honor of John M. Riddle*, ed. Anne Van Arsdall and Timothy Graham. Aldershot: Ashgate, forthcoming.

Walther, Hans. *Initia carminum ac versuum Medii Aevi posterioris Latinorum. Alphabetisches Verzeichnis der Versanfänge mittellateinischer Dichtungen*. 2nd ed. Göttingen: Vandenhoeck & Ruprecht, 1969.

—. *Proverbia sententiaeque Latinitatis Medii Aevi. Lateinische Sprichwörter und Sentenzen des Mittelalters in alphabetischer Anordnung*. 6 vols. Göttingen: Vandenhoeck & Ruprecht, 1963–9.

Watson, Gilbert. *Theriac and Mithridatium: A Study in Therapeutics*. London: Wellcome Historical Medical Library, 1966.

Wellmann, M. 'Sextius Niger, eine Quellenuntersuchung zu Dioscorides.' *Hermes* 24 (1889), 530–69.

Wetherbee, Winthrop. 'Philosophy, cosmology, and the twelfth-century Renaissance.' In *A History of Twelfth-Century Western Philosophy*, ed. Peter Dronke, 21–53. Cambridge: Cambridge University Press, 1988.

—. *Platonism and Poetry in the Twelfth Century: The Literary Influence of the School of Chartres*. Princeton: Princeton University Press, 1972.

Wolska-Conus, Wanda. 'Stéphanos d'Athènes et Stéphanos d'Alexandrie: Essai d'identification et de biographie.' *Revue des études byzantines* 47 (1989), 5–89.

Ziolkowski, Jan M. '*Amaritudo mentis*: The Archpoet's interiorization and exteriorization of bitterness in its twelfth-century contexts.' In *Codierungen von Emotionen im Mittelalter*, ed. C. Stephen Jaeger and Ingrid Kasten, 98–111. Berlin: De Gruyter, 2003.

—. 'Classical influences on medieval Latin views of poetic inspiration.' In *Latin Poetry and the Classical Tradition: Essays in Medieval and Renaissance Literature*, ed. Peter Godman and Oswyn Murray, 15–38. Oxford: Clarendon Press, 1990.

Indices

Four indices (Index herbarum et medicinarum, Index membrorum et aegritudinum, Index personarum et locorum, Index uocabulorum usualium) have been compiled to help readers interested not only in plants, medicines, and diseases as they appear in the *Anglicanus ortus* but also in the vocabulary and frequency of word usage of Henry as an Anglo-Latin poet. Each index is keyed only to Latin words in the text (given in the infinitive for verbs or nominative singular for nouns and adjectives). A few important topics are listed in English in the indices in italic typeface; *e.g. amulets*; *self-reference*; *war imagery*.

Each citation in the index is given as a poem number followed by one or more line numbers. The citations themselves are separated by semicolons. Poem numbers consisting of two numbers are from Books 1–4 of the *Anglicanus ortus*; *e.g.*, 1.7, 28 refers to poem 1.7, line 28, and 2.9, 23 refers to poem 2.9, line 23. (Note that poem 4.1–2 is a single poem treating two flowers, and is always listed as such; *e.g.* 4.1–2, 4.) Poem numbers consisting of three numbers are from Books 5–6, since those books are separated into two sections each; *e.g.*, 5.2.6, 10 refers to poem 5.2.6, line 10, and 6.2.15, 8–9 refers to poem 6.2.15, lines 8–9.

In the first index, of herbs and medicines, citations given in bold typeface refer to the poem dedicated to the herb or spice in question.

The prose prologue is abbreviated as Pr.Prol. and the line numbers refer only to the Latin, not to the English translation. The various verse prologues and interludes are abbreviated as 1.Prol., 2.Prol., *etc.*; and 5.Int., 6.Int. The epilogues to Books 4 and 6 are abbreviated 4.Ep.1, 4.Ep.2 and 6.Ep.

Index herbarum et medicinarum

Numbers in bold type refer to the main entry for that herb or spice.

Index membrorum et aegritudinum

Index personarum et locorum

Index uocabulorum usualium